Handbook of Small Animal Radiology and Ultrasound

T0383264

Commissioning Editor: Robert Edwards
Development Editor: Louisa Welch
Project Manager: Vijayakumar Sekar
Designer: Kirsteen Wright
Illustration Manager: Gillian Richards

Handbook of Small Animal Radiology and Ultrasound

Techniques and Differential Diagnoses

Ruth Dennis MA, VetMB, DVR, DipECVDI, MRCVS
Animal Health Trust, Newmarket, UK

Robert M. Kirberger BVSc, MMedVet(Rad), DipECVDI
Onderstepoort Veterinary Academic Hospital, University of Pretoria, South Africa

Frances Barr MA, VetMB, PhD, DVR, DipECVDI, MRCVS
School of Veterinary Science, University of Bristol, Bristol, UK

Robert H. Wrigley BVSc, MS, DVR, DipACVR, DipECVDI, MRCVS
University Veterinary Teaching Hospital, University of Sydney, Australia

Foreword by Donald E. Thrall DVM, PhD

SECOND EDITION

Illustrations by Debbie Maizels and Jonathan Clayton-Jones

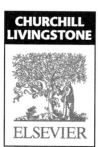

CHURCHILL LIVINGSTONE

ELSEVIER

Edinburgh   London   New York   Oxford   Philadelphia   St Louis   Sydney   Toronto   2010

CHURCHILL
LIVINGSTONE
ELSEVIER

First edition © Harcourt Publishers Limited 2001
Second edition © Elsevier Limited 2010.

ISBN 978-0-7020-2894-6

British Library Cataloguing in Publication Data
A catalogue record for this book is available from the British Library

Library of Congress Cataloging in Publication Data
A catalog record for this book is available from the Library of Congress

Notice
Neither the publisher nor the authors assume any responsibility for any loss or injury and/or damage to persons or property arising out of or related to any use of the material contained in this book. It is the responsibility of the treating practitioner, relying on independent expertise and knowledge of the patient, to determine the best treatment and method of application for the patient.

The Publisher

ELSEVIER your source for books, journals and multimedia in the health sciences

www.elsevierhealth.com

Working together to grow
libraries in developing countries

www.elsevier.com | www.bookaid.org | www.sabre.org

ELSEVIER BOOK AID International Sabre Foundation

Printed and bound by CPI Group (UK) Ltd, Croydon, CR0 4YY

Transferred to digital print 2013

The
Publisher's
policy is to use
**paper manufactured
from sustainable forests**

Contents

Foreword   vii
Preface   ix
Acknowledgements   xi

1. Skeletal system: general   1

2. Joints   39

3. Appendicular skeleton   51

4. Head and neck   85

5. Spine   115

6. Lower respiratory tract   145

7. Cardiovascular system   175

8. Other thoracic structures: pleural cavity, mediastinum, thoracic oesophagus, thoracic wall   199

9. Other abdominal structures: abdominal wall, peritoneal and retroperitoneal cavities, parenchymal organs   229

10. Gastrointestinal tract   267

11. Urogenital tract   297

12. Soft tissues   331

Appendix   341
    Radiographic faults   341
    Ultrasound terminology and artefacts   343
    Geographic distributions of diseases   347

Index   353

Foreword

I am honoured to introduce the second edition of the *Handbook of Small Animal Radiology and Ultrasound: Techniques and Differential Diagnoses*, written by Ruth Dennis, Robert Kirberger, Frances Barr and Robert Wrigley. Each of these highly qualified radiologists is a seasoned expert, having taught the principles of imaging to veterinary students and residents for many years. Their experience in transmitting knowledge about how to interpret diagnostic images, coupled with collective decades of clinical acumen, provides a level of credibility matched by few other textbooks focused on facilitating the image interpretation process.

Personally, for nearly 40 years, I have struggled with determining how to best instruct people efficiently in image interpretation. I have come to the conclusion that everyone learns a bit differently and at a different rate. The effectiveness of different instructional methodologies also varies between students. Most radiologic imaging instruction is based on actual patient material, i.e. images of sick animals that have been produced in the clinic. In this work the message is based on drawings where the pathologic alteration of tissue is demarcated clearly. Though not identical to the clinical images of patients, these drawings make it crystal clear exactly what is happening in the patient that leads to the appearance of various tissue alterations in real radiographic and sonographic images. Understanding tissue alterations at this basic level will be an asset to many who struggle with image interpretation in the clinic.

The main function of this book is unchanged; that being the intent to order one's thought process after the radiographic or sonographic abnormalities have been categorized. In other words, once imaging abnormalities have been identified, lists of considerations are provided for each sign. These considerations can then be compared to the history, signalment and physical and clinical findings allowing rational prioritization of real diseases. This prioritization can then be used to tailor further diagnostic tests or therapeutic interventions. One fact about imaging is that if one has never heard of a disease, it cannot be diagnosed. Consultation with this resource will increase ones familiarity with possibilities that need to be considered.

As before, this book is not an all-inclusive imaging text, nor will it be useful without some pre-existing experience in imaging interpretation. However, this does not detract from the value of this work – on the contrary, this resourceful publication fills a much-needed gap by enhancing the maturation of the image interpreter. The most competent radiologists are not just readers of roentgen signs. They are consultants to animal owners, practitioners and other specialists. Effective consultation requires making sense of the observed roentgen signs. Information contained herein facilitates taking imaging abnormalities from the descriptive to the interpretive and formulating that information into an effective consultation.

Donald E. Thrall, DVM, PhD
Diplomate ACVR (Radiology, Radiation Oncology), Professor, Department of Molecular Biomedical Sciences, College of Veterinary Medicine, North Carolina State University, Raleigh, NC, USA

Preface

Body systems can only respond to disease or injury in a limited number of ways and therefore it is often impossible to make a specific diagnosis based on a single test, such as radiography. Successful interpretation of radiographs and ultrasonograms depends on the recognition of abnormalities, the formulation of lists of possible causes for those abnormalities and a plan for further diagnostic tests, if appropriate. This handbook is intended as an *aide memoire* of differential diagnoses and other useful information in small animal radiology and ultrasound, in order to assist the radiologist to compile as complete a list of differential diagnoses as possible. Schematic line drawings of many of the conditions as well as normal anatomy and variants are included, to complement the text.

The authors hope that this book will prove useful to all users of small animal diagnostic imaging, from specialist radiologists through general practitioners to veterinary students. However it is intended to supplement, rather than replace, the many excellent standard textbooks available and a certain degree of experience in the interpretation of images is presupposed.

The book is divided into sections representing body systems, and for various radiographic and ultrasonographic abnormalities possible diagnoses are listed in approximate order of likelihood, including those due to normal anatomical variation and technical or iatrogenic causes. Conditions which principally or exclusively occur in cats are indicated as such, although many of the other diseases listed may occur in cats as well as in dogs. Infectious and parasitic diseases which are not ubiquitous but which are confined to certain parts of the world are indicated by an asterisk *, and the reader should consult the Table of Geographic Distribution of Diseases in the Appendix for further information. Details of radiographic technique (including contrast studies) are included and guidance on ultrasonographic technique and a description of the normal ultrasonographic appearance of organs is given. This second edition of our book has been expanded considerably with much extra information about techniques and normal anatomy, many new differential diagnoses, more detailed description of many of the diseases included, updating of the Table of Geographic Distribution of Diseases and expanded Further Reading sections. An addition to the Appendix is a section on digital radiographic film faults, which is reproduced with kind permission from the journal *Veterinary Radiology and Ultrasound*. New illustrations by our artist Debbie Maizels are included, to add to those from the first edition drawn by Jonathan Clayton-Jones, and we are indebted to them both for their excellent diagrammatic reproduction of the radiographs and ultrasonograms.

A book such as this can never hope to be complete, as new conditions are constantly being recognized and described. The authors apologise for any omissions there may be and would welcome comments from readers for possible future editions.

Acknowledgements

Our thanks go to Professor Don Thrall for kindly agreeing to write the foreword to this second edition. We also wish to acknowledge assistance and advice from Dr. Gerhard Steenkamp (dental radiology), Dr. Nerissa Stander (gastrointestinal ultrasonography) and Professor Banie Penzhorn (geographic distribution of diseases), all from the Faculty of Veterinary Science, University of Pretoria. Figures 9.6, 9.14, 9.15, 9.17, 9.18, and 9.19 have been reproduced, with permission, from Chapter 32 'Abdominal Masses' by Charles R. Root in *Textbook of Veterinary Diagnostic Radiology* 2nd edition, edited by Donald E. Thrall and published by Saunders. Finally, we would like to thank the many people at Elsevier who have supported us throughout this project.

Ruth Dennis
Newmarket, UK
November 2009

Chapter 1

Skeletal system: general

CHAPTER CONTENTS

General   1
1.1 Radiographic technique for the skeletal system   1
1.2 Anatomy of bone: general principles   2
1.3 Ossification and growth plate closures   3
1.4 Response of bone to disease or injury   3
1.5 Patterns of focal bone loss (osteolysis)   4
1.6 Patterns of osteogenesis: periosteal reactions   6
1.7 Principles of interpretation of skeletal radiographs   7
1.8 Features of aggressive versus non-aggressive bone lesions   8
1.9 Fractures: radiography, classification and assessment of healing   9

Bones   14
1.10 Altered shape of long bones   14
1.11 Dwarfism   15
1.12 Delayed ossification or growth plate closure   15
1.13 Increased radiopacity within bone   16
1.14 Periosteal reactions   18
1.15 Bony masses   19
1.16 Osteopenia   21
1.17 Coarse trabecular pattern   22
1.18 Osteolytic lesions   22
1.19 Expansile osteolytic lesions   24

1.20 Mixed osteolytic–osteogenic lesions   25
1.21 Multifocal diseases   28
1.22 Lesions affecting epiphyses   29
1.23 Lesions affecting physes   30
1.24 Lesions affecting metaphyses   31
1.25 Lesions affecting diaphyses   33

GENERAL

1.1 RADIOGRAPHIC TECHNIQUE FOR THE SKELETAL SYSTEM

The skeletal system lends itself well to radiography, but it must be remembered that only the mineralized components of bone are visible. The osteoid matrix of bone is of soft tissue radiopacity and cannot be assessed radiographically; this makes up 30–35% of adult bone. Articular cartilage is also of soft tissue opacity and is not seen on survey radiographs (see arthrography, 2.1). Lesions in the skeletal system may be radiographically subtle, and so attention to good radiographic technique is essential.

1. Highest definition film–screen combination consistent with the thickness of the area or appropriate digital radiography algorithm.
2. No grid is necessary except for the proximal limbs and spine in larger dogs; in smaller joints, insufficient scattered radiation is produced to warrant the use of a grid, and the presence of grid lines may obscure fine detail.

3. Accurate positioning and centring with a small object–film distance to minimize geometric distortion and blurring due to the penumbra effect.
4. Close collimation to enhance radiographic definition by minimizing scatter, and for radiation safety.
5. Correct exposure factors to allow examination of soft tissues as well as bone.
6. Beware of hair coat debris creating artefactual shadows.
7. Radiograph the opposite limb for comparison if necessary.
8. Use wedge filtration techniques if a whole limb view is required (e.g. for angular limb deformity); use a special wedge filter or intravenous fluid bags.
9. Optimum viewing conditions – dry films, darkened room, bright light and dimmer facility, glare around periphery of film masked off.
10. Use a magnifying glass for fine detail; use bone specimens, a film library and radiographic atlases.
11. For analogue film, ensure good processing technique to optimize contrast and definition.
12. With digital radiography, manipulation of image size and greyscale is readily performed.

1.2 ANATOMY OF BONE: GENERAL PRINCIPLES (Fig. 1.1A and B)

Apophysis – Non-articular bony protuberance for attachment of tendons and ligaments; a separate centre of ossification.

Articular cartilage – Soft tissue opacity, therefore appears radiolucent compared with bones (unless mineralizing through disease). Provides longitudinal growth of epiphyses.

Cancellous bone – Spongy bone consisting of a meshwork of bony trabeculae; found in epiphyses, metaphyses and small bones. A coarse trabecular pattern is seen where forces are constant and a fine trabecular pattern where they are variable. The greater surface area compared with cortical bone results in a 40 times greater rate of remodelling in response to disease or injury. The cancellous bone of skull is called *diploë*.

Cortex – Compact lamellar bone formed by intramembranous ossification from periosteum. Uniformly radiopaque. Thickest where the circumference of the bone is smallest, where attached soft tissues exert stress or on the concave side of a curved bone and taper to nothing in the metaphyseal region.

Diaphysis – The shaft of a long bone; a tube of cortical bone surrounding medullary cavity and cancellous bone.

Endosteum – Similar to periosteum but thinner, and lines large medullary cavities; it may produce bone in some circumstances (e.g. fractures).

Epiphysis – The end of a long bone bearing the articular surface, which forms from a separate centre of ossification; cancellous bone with a denser subchondral layer.

Medullary cavity – Fatty bone marrow space in the mid-diaphysis; radiolucent and homogeneous.

Metaphysis – Between the physis and diaphysis; cancellous bone. In the young animal, it remodels bone from the growth plate into the diaphyseal cortex, hence its external surface may be irregular, especially in large dogs; this is known as the *cut-back zone* and should not be mistaken for a periosteal reaction or pathological osteolysis (Fig. 1.1A).

Nutrient foramen – Seen as a radiolucent line running obliquely through the cortex and carrying major blood vessels; its consistent location in long bones reflects relative growth in length from the two ends of the bone (it originates centrally in the fetus). Occasionally it may be in an aberrant location.

Periosteum – Fibroelastic connective tissue surrounding bone except at articular surfaces and where muscle fibres and tendons insert; its inner layer produces bone by intramembranous ossification causing increase in bone diameter.

Physis – Cartilaginous growth plate present in young animals and seen radiographically as a radiolucent band. Endochondral ossification at the physis results in increased length of the bone. Its width reduces with progressing ossification; after skeletal maturity, it may be seen as a sclerotic line or physeal scar. It provides longitudinal growth of metaphyses and diaphyses.

Sesamoids – Small bony structures lacking periosteum that form in tendons near joints; thought to reduce friction at sites of direction changes.

Subchondral bone – Thin, dense layer of bone beneath articular cartilage; appears more radiopaque than adjacent bone.

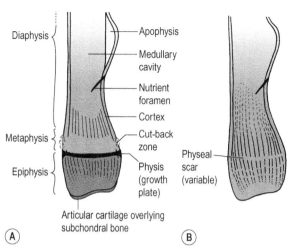

Figure 1.1 (A) Anatomical features of an immature long bone; (B) anatomical features of a mature long bone.

1.3 OSSIFICATION AND GROWTH PLATE CLOSURES

- Skeletal mineralization in dogs and cats begins about two-thirds of the way through pregnancy.
- This occurs in a preformed cartilage matrix for most of the skeleton by endochondral ossification; the skull forms within membranes by intramembranous ossification.
- At birth, ossification is seen radiographically only in diaphyses and skull bones; joints appear wide because epiphyses are still cartilaginous and therefore radiolucent.
- Subsequently, ossification centres appear in epiphyses, apophyses and small bones.
- These secondary ossification centres show ragged margination as ossification progresses.
- As skeletal maturity approaches, secondary ossification centres enlarge and become smoother in outline, and physes and the apparent joint spaces therefore become narrower.
- Some terminology: *achondroplasia*, absence of cartilage development; *chondrodysplasia*, disordered cartilage development; *skeletal dysplasia*, disordered skeletal development.

Growth plate closure times (dog)

Radiographic growth plate closure times are variable, and so a general range is given for each site. In an individual animal, closure times will normally be the same in right and left limbs (see Table 1.1).

1.4 RESPONSE OF BONE TO DISEASE OR INJURY

Regardless of cause, the pathology of bone response is essentially the same. There are only two mechanisms: bone loss (focal, osteolysis; diffuse, osteopenia) and bone production (osteogenesis). A combination of both processes may also occur. Bone is laid down and remodels according to Wolff's law – bone is deposited at sites where it is required and resorbed where it is not; this also explains the orientation of trabeculae.

1. Bone loss (see 1.5 and 1.16)

- Recognized radiographically after approximately 7–10 days.
- Only the mineralized component of bone is visible radiographically, and 30–60% of mineral content must be lost before being detected radiographically.
- Radiography is therefore not a sensitive tool for detecting minor bone loss.
- Focal bone loss is easier to see than diffuse bone loss, by comparison with adjacent normal bone.
- Bone loss is easier to see in cortical bone than in cancellous bone, as cortical bone is more radiopaque.
- *Osteopenia* is a radiological term describing a generalized reduction in bone radiopacity. It is due to two different pathological processes:
  - *osteomalacia* – insufficient or abnormal mineralization of organic osteoid
  - *osteoporosis* – normal proportions of osteoid and mineral component, but reduced amounts.

- Technical factors such as radiographic exposure and processing must be taken into account when diagnosing osteopenia – compare the radiopacity of bone with the radiopacity of the soft tissues.

Table 1.1 Growth plate closure times in dogs[a]	
	GROWTH PLATE CLOSURE TIME
Scapular tuberosity	4–7 months
Proximal humerus	
Greater tubercle to humeral head	4 months
Proximal epiphysis	10–13 months
Distal humerus	
Medial to lateral condyle	8–12 weeks
Medial epicondyle	6 months
Condyle to diaphysis	5–8 months
Proximal radius	5–11 months
Distal radius	6–12 months
Proximal ulna	
Olecranon	5–10 months
Anconeal process	3–5 months
Distal ulna	6–12 months
Accessory carpal bone physis	10 weeks–5 months
Proximal metacarpal I (dewclaw)	6 months
Distal metacarpal II–V	5–7 months
Phalanges (proximal P1, proximal P2 only)	4–6 months
Pelvis	
Acetabulum	4–6 months
Iliac crest	1–2 years (or may remain open permanently)
Tuber ischii	8–10 months
Proximal femur	
Femoral head	6–11 months
Greater trochanter	6–10 months
Lesser trochanter	8–13 months
Distal femur	6–11 months
Proximal tibia	
Medial to lateral condyle	6 weeks
Tibial tuberosity to condyles	6–8 months
Tuberosity and condyles to diaphysis	6–12 months
Distal tibia	
Main physis	5–11 months
Medial malleolus of distal tibia	5 months
Proximal fibula	6–12 months
Distal fibula	5–12 months
Tuber calcis	11 weeks–8 months
Vertebral endplates	6–9 months

[a]In the cat, growth plates fuse later, especially in neutered animals.
Sources: Sumner-Smith, G. (1966) Observations on epiphyseal fusion of the canine appendicular skeleton. *Journal of Small Animal Practice* 7, 303–312.
Ticer, J.W. (1975) *Radiographic Technique in Small Animal Practice*. Philadelphia: Saunders.

2. Bone production (see 1.6)

- *Sclerosis* or *osteosclerosis* used as a radiological term describes increased bone radiopacity. It can be due to two different pathological processes:
  - *increased density of bone* (e.g. sequestrum, subchondral compaction, enlargement of trabeculae)
  - *Superimposed* periosteal or endosteal reaction.
- Apparent sclerosis may also be caused by superimposition of bones (e.g. overlapping fracture fragments).
- *Sclerosis* is also a pathological term meaning literally 'hardening of tissue' and refers to organs becoming hard and useless due to an excess of connective tissue; it is often applied to the central nervous system. Caution should therefore be exercised when using this word in a radiological sense in order that the meaning is clear.

3. Mixed reactions

- Many lesions combine osteolysis and new bone production to variable degrees.
- New bone may predominate and obscure underlying minor osteolysis.
- Conversely, superimposition of irregular new bone may create areas of relative radiolucency that mimic osteolysis.
- Consider also the possibility of two pathological processes being present simultaneously (e.g. synovial cell sarcoma in a joint with pre-existing osteoarthrosis).

1.5 PATTERNS OF FOCAL BONE LOSS (OSTEOLYSIS)

Bone loss may be recognized 7–10 days after an insult. It is easier to recognize in cortical than in trabecular bone and is more obvious if focal. Categorizing the type of osteolysis helps in differential diagnosis by suggesting the aggressiveness or activity of the disease process (see 1.8).

1. Geographic osteolysis (Fig. 1.2)

- A single large area or confluence of several smaller areas, usually more than 10 mm in diameter.
- Clearly marginated, i.e. there is a narrow zone of transition to normal bone.

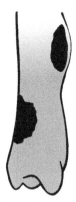

Figure 1.2 Geographic osteolysis.

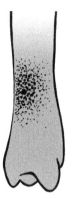

Figure 1.4 Permeative osteolysis.

- Sclerotic margins may be present if the body is attempting to wall off the lesion.
- Usually affects both the medullary cavity and the cortex.
- The overlying cortex may be thinned and displaced outwards due to a lesion that is expansile (see 1.19 and Figs 1.25 and 1.26).
- Usually due to a benign or non-aggressive, low-grade lesion such as a bone cyst, pressure atrophy or a benign dental tumour.

2. Moth–eaten osteolysis (Fig. 1.3)

- Multiple areas of osteolysis, often varying in size and usually 3–10 mm in diameter.
- May coalesce to form geographic osteolysis in the centre of the lesion.
- Less well defined, with a wider zone of transition to normal bone.
- The cortex is often irregularly eroded.
- Due to a more aggressive disease process such as a malignant tumour or osteomyelitis.

3. Permeative osteolysis (Fig. 1.4)

- Numerous small pinpoint areas of osteolysis, 1–2 mm in diameter.
- Poorly defined, with a wide zone of transition to normal bone – areas of osteolysis are more spread out at the periphery.
- Mainly recognized in the cortex (hard to see in the medulla because of its trabecular pattern).
- The cortex is irregularly eroded from the endosteal side.
- Due to a highly aggressive disease process such as a very active malignant tumour or fulminant (often fungal) osteomyelitis.

4. Mixed pattern of osteolysis (Fig. 1.5)

Often more than one type of osteolysis is recognized (e.g. central geographic osteolysis surrounded by moth-eaten and permeative zones); the nature of the lesion is denoted by the most aggressive type of osteolysis present.

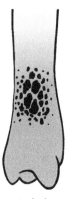

Figure 1.3 Moth-eaten osteolysis.

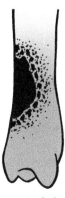

Figure 1.5 Mixed pattern osteolysis.

5. Osteopenia (diffuse reduction in bone radiopacity – see also 1.16)

- Due to osteomalacia or osteoporosis (see 1.4).
- Differential diagnoses are overexposure, overdevelopment, other causes of fogging.
- Reduced radiopacity of bone compared with soft tissues (ghostly bones).
- Thin, shell-like cortices.
- Coarse trabecular pattern, as smaller trabeculae are resorbed.
- Apparent sclerosis of subchondral bone, especially in vertebral endplates, as these are relatively spared and therefore show high contrast with the osteopenic bone.
- Double cortical line due to intracortical bone resorption is occasionally seen.
- If in a limb due to disuse, the epiphyses and small bones are affected predominantly.
- Pathological folding fractures may occur, seen as sclerotic lines.

1.6 PATTERNS OF OSTEOGENESIS: PERIOSTEAL REACTIONS

Periosteal new bone is also usually recognized 7–10 days after an insult (earlier in young animals). Identifying its nature helps in differential diagnosis by suggesting the aggressiveness of the disease process (see 1.8).

There are two main groups of periosteal reactions: continuous and interrupted (Figs 1.6 and 1.7). However, these represent arbitrary division of a spectrum of periosteal reactions.

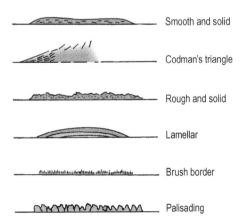

Figure 1.6 Continuous periosteal reactions.

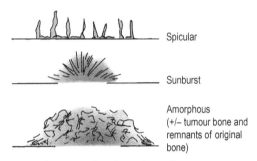

Figure 1.7 Interrupted periosteal reactions.

1. Continuous periosteal reactions

Often slow disease processes that allow new bone to form in an orderly fashion. Usually represent a benign or healed process but may also be seen early in a more aggressive disease or at the edge of an overtly aggressive lesion. Described below in order of increasing aggressiveness.

- Smooth and solid (e.g. chronic mild trauma, remodelled more active new bone, panosteitis, healed subperiosteal haematoma).
- Codman's triangle – solid triangle of new bone at the edge of a more active lesion, due to bony infilling beneath advancing periosteal elevation. Often at the diaphyseal edge of a primary malignant bone tumour.
- Rough and solid (e.g. trauma, adjacent soft tissue inflammation). May settle to become smooth.
- Lamellar – periosteum elevated by exudate or haemorrhage and produces a single line of new bone parallel to the cortex that fills in with time, becoming solid, for example early metaphyseal osteopathy (hypertrophic osteodystrophy).
- Lamellated ('onion skin') – late stage, after recurrent episodes of periosteal elevation due to sequential insults creating several layers of new bone, for example late metaphyseal osteopathy (hypertrophic osteodystrophy), fungal osteomyelitis.
- Palisading (thick brush-like) – solid chunks of new bone perpendicular to the cortex (e.g. hypertrophic osteopathy, craniomandibular osteopathy).
- Brush border (thin brush-like, 'hair on end') – periosteum lifted fairly rapidly over an extensive area of cortex with new bone laid down along the perpendicularly oriented Sharpey's fibres (e.g. adjacent soft tissue inflammation, acute osteomyelitis, early neoplasia).

2. Interrupted periosteal reactions

Represent an aggressive disease process (e.g. malignant neoplasia or osteomyelitis).

Rapidly changing lesions breaching the cortex and periosteum with no time for orderly repair. Variable in radiopacity and depth and may be in short, disconnected segments. Often associated with underlying cortical lysis.

- Spicular – wisps of new bone extending out into soft tissue, roughly perpendicular to the cortex.
- Sunburst – radiating spicular pattern, deepest centrally; indicates a focal lesion erupting through the cortex and extending into soft tissues.
- Amorphous – not a periosteal reaction as such, but fragments of new bone that are variable in size, shape and orientation; often cannot be differentiated from remnants of displaced original bone and tumour bone produced by osteosarcomas.

1.7 PRINCIPLES OF INTERPRETATION OF SKELETAL RADIOGRAPHS

Bone has a limited response to disease or insult, and so lesions with different aetiologies may look similar radiographically, for example neoplasia and osteomyelitis. A definitive diagnosis may not be possible without further tests or biopsy. The radiologist must examine radiographs methodically, identify changes, recognize patterns and then formulate lists of differential diagnoses. Patient type, history, clinical signs, blood parameters, geographic location (current or previous), change of the lesion with time and response to treatment must be considered. Radiographs should be oriented consistently on the viewer to promote familiarity with the normal appearance, and bone specimens and radiographic atlases used for reference.

A useful mnemonic for differential diagnosis of aetiology is VITAMIN D:

V vascular
I inflammatory or infectious
T trauma
A anomalous
M metabolic
I idiopathic
N neoplastic
D degenerative

Features to consider when interpreting skeletal radiographs include the following:

1. Distribution of lesions.
   a. Generalized or diffuse changes.
      - Metabolic or nutritional disease.
      - Neoplasia (e.g. widespread osteolysis – multiple myeloma; widespread sclerosis – lymphoma).
   b. Whole limb.
      - Disuse.
   c. Focal lesions.
      - Congenital or developmental.
      - Trauma.
      - Infection or inflammation.
      - Neoplasia.
   d. Symmetrical lesions.
      - Metabolic disease.
      - Haematogenous osteomyelitis.
      - Metaphyseal osteopathy (hypertrophic osteodystrophy).
      - Hypertrophic osteopathy.
      - Bilateral trauma.
      - Metastatic tumours.
2. Number of lesions.
   a. Monostotic.
      - Congenital or developmental.
      - Trauma.
      - Localized infection (trauma, iatrogenic).
      - Neoplasia (primary bone tumour, soft tissue tumour distant from joint, solitary metastasis).
   b. Polyostotic (see 1.21).
3. Location of lesions (see 1.22–1.25).
   a. Epiphysis (e.g. various arthritides, chondrodysplasias, osteochondrosis, soft tissue tumours affecting joints).
   b. Physis – mainly young animals (e.g. haematogenous osteomyelitis, trauma, premature closures, rickets).
   c. Metaphysis, e.g. haematogenous osteomyelitis, metaphyseal osteopathy (hypertrophic osteodystrophy), primary malignant bone tumours.
   d. diaphysis (e.g. trauma, panosteitis, hypertrophic osteopathy, metastatic tumours).
4. Presence and type of osteolysis (see 1.5 and Figs 1.2–1.5).

5. Presence and type of osteogenesis (see 1.6 and Figs 1.6 and 1.7).
   a. Periosteal.
   b. Endosteal.
   c. Trabecular.
   d. Neoplastic – in bone-producing tumours.
   e. Heterotopic – ossification in an abnormal location.
   f. Dystrophic – ossification in previously damaged soft tissue.
6. Zone of transition between lesion and normal bone.
   a. Short – well-demarcated lesion, abrupt transition to normal bone; usually benign or non-aggressive disease.
   b. Long – poorly demarcated lesions, gradual transition to normal bone; usually aggressive disease.
7. Soft tissue changes.
   a. Muscle atrophy.
   b. Soft tissue swelling.
   c. Joint effusions.
   d. Displacement or obliteration of fascial planes or fat pads.
   e. Soft tissue emphysema.
   f. Soft tissue mineralization.
   g. Radiopaque foreign bodies.
   h. Abnormalities in other body systems (e.g. lung metastases).
8. Rate of change on sequential radiographs and presence of response to treatment. The time interval between radiographic studies is arbitrary and determined by the apparent activity or aggression of the lesion and the age of the animal – active lesions may change within a few days, and both bone loss and new bone production occur more rapidly in young animals.

1.8 FEATURES OF AGGRESSIVE VERSUS NON-AGGRESSIVE BONE LESIONS

An aggressive lesion is one that extends rapidly into adjacent normal bone with no or minimal visible host response attempting to confine the lesion (Table 1.2 and Figs 1.8 and 1.9). Assessment of this activity is essential in order to compile a realistic list of differential diagnoses. Lesions may change their status with time or in response to treatment. Intermediate grades of aggression exist through a spectrum (e.g. chronic osteomyelitis, low-grade malignancy).

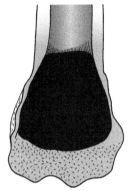

Figure 1.8 Non-aggressive osteolytic bone lesion, with geographic osteolysis, short zone of transition, intact overlying cortex and smooth periosteal reaction.

Table 1.2 Radiographic features of aggressive versus non-aggressive bone lesions[a]	
NON-AGGRESSIVE	**AGGRESSIVE**
For example uncomplicated trauma, degenerative or resolving lesion, benign neoplasia, bone cyst	For example malignant neoplasia, fulminant osteomyelitis
Well demarcated	Poorly demarcated
Narrow, distinct zone of transition	Wide, indistinct zone of transition
Absent or geographic osteolysis	Permeative osteolysis
Cortex may be displaced and thinned but rarely broken	Cortex interrupted
Continuous solid or smooth periosteal reaction	Interrupted, irregular periosteal reaction
± surrounding sclerosis	No surrounding sclerosis
Static or slow rate of change	Rapid rate of change

[a]If mixed signs are present, the lesion should be categorized according to its most aggressive feature.

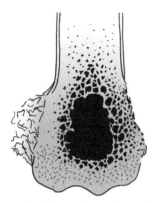

Figure 1.9 Aggressive bone lesion, with a mixed pattern of osteolysis, long zone of transition, cortical erosion and interrupted periosteal reaction.

1.9 FRACTURES: RADIOGRAPHY, CLASSIFICATION AND ASSESSMENT OF HEALING

Causes of fractures

1. Trauma (direct or indirect, e.g. avulsion).
2. Pathological; spontaneous or following minor trauma to weakened bone.
   a. Neoplasia.
   b. Bone cyst.
   c. Osteomyelitis.
   d. Diffuse osteopenia such as nutritional secondary hyperparathyroidism (usually folding fractures).
   e. Brittle or fragile bones, for example osteopetrosis (see 1.13.15), osteogenesis imperfecta (see 1.16.13).
   f. Incomplete ossification of the humeral condyle – Spaniels (see 3.4.5. and Fig. 3.4).
   g. Empty screw hole.
3. Stress protection – weakened bone at the end of an orthopaedic plate.
4. Fatigue fracture – due to repeated stress on a bone, especially metacarpals and metatarsals in racing greyhounds.
5. Defect in bone due to biopsy or surgery, or after plate removal.

Radiography

- Obtain at least two radiographs, including views at 90° to one another (orthogonal views).
- Include joints above and below to check for joint involvement and rotation of fragments.
- In young animals, examine growth plates for signs of injury; after trauma to the antebrachium, re-radiograph after 3 weeks to check for signs of premature closure of the distal ulnar physis.
- Radiograph the opposite leg for assessment of true bone length if surgery is planned.
- Use a horizontal beam if necessary (e.g. if pain, spinal instability or thoracic trauma prevent dorsal recumbency).
- Increase exposure factors if soft tissue swelling is present.
- Thoracic and abdominal studies are often required in cases of road accident or falls from high buildings (e.g. to detect pulmonary contusion, ruptured diaphragm, pneumothorax or bladder rupture).
- If hairline fractures are suspected but not seen, repeat the radiographs 7–10 days later (or use scintigraphy).
- Stressed views may be needed to detect fracture (sub)luxations or collateral ligament damage (see 2.1 and Fig. 2.2).
- Remember that radiographs give no information about damage to articular cartilage or surrounding soft tissues.

Radiographic signs of fractures

1. Disruption of the normal shape of bone or of the cortex or trabecular pattern.
2. Radiolucent fracture lines can be mimicked by:
   a. nutrient foramen
   b. overlying fascial plane fat
   c. skin defect or gas in fascial planes – open fracture
   d. normal growth plate or skull suture
   e. Mach line – dark lines along edge of two overlapping bones due to an optical illusion
   f. grid line artefact from damaged grid.
   NB: hairline or minimally displaced fractures radiating along the shaft from the main fracture site may be seen only if parallel to X-ray beam; this may require additional views.
3. Increased radiopacity of cortex and medulla if the fracture is folding or impacted or if fragments override.

4. Small, free fragments of variable size can be mimicked by:
   a. unusual centres of ossification
   b. inconsistently present sesamoids
   c. multipartite sesamoids
   d. dirt on the animal's hair coat
   e. debris within soft tissues.
      (a)–(c) are usually bilateral, so if in doubt radiograph the opposite limb for comparison.
5. Ballistics, foreign material and gas – compound fractures.
6. Evidence of fracture healing – see below.
7. Muscle atrophy and disuse osteopenia.

   Reasons for overlooking fractures include incorrect exposure or processing, non-displacement of fracture fragments, insufficient number of views, confusion with growth plates and fracture reduced by positioning.

Classification of fractures

1. Closed, or open or compound (therefore risk of infection, especially if the skin has broken outside to inside).
2. Simple (single fracture), comminuted (three or more fragments), multiple (fracture lines do not connect; same bone or different bones) or segmental (two or more separate fracture lines in a single bone).
3. Transverse, oblique, spiral, longitudinal or irregular.
4. Complete (entire bone width) or incomplete (one cortex only).
   a. Greenstick fracture – convex side cortex; alternatively defined as a fracture with minimal separation between fragment ends and periosteum remains intact.
   b. Torus fracture – concave side fracture.
5. Chip fracture (no or one articular surface involved) or slab fracture (two articular surfaces involved).
6. Articular – within the limits of the joint capsule, whether or not the fracture line crosses the articular surface. Young animals are over-represented due to the presence of relatively weak growth plates. Alternatively, non-articular.
7. Avulsion (traction by soft tissue attachment) – usually at an apophysis.

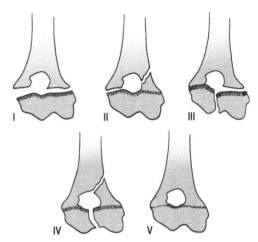

Figure 1.10 Salter–Harris classification of growth plate fractures. Type I: separation through the growth plate (e.g. proximal femur); also known as slipped epiphysis or epiphysiolysis. Type II: a metaphyseal fragment remains attached to the epiphysis (e.g. distal femur). Type III: fracture through the epiphysis into the growth plate (rare). Type IV: fracture through the epiphysis and metaphysis crossing the growth plate (e.g. distal humerus). Type V: crush injury to the growth plate (may not be radiographically visible initially but leads to growth disturbance) (e.g. distal ulna).

8. Fatigue or stress fracture – one cortex only, from repeated minor trauma.
9. Impaction or compression fracture – shortening of bone due to stress along its length, or one fragment driven into another; especially vertebrae.
10. Fracture (sub)luxation – fracture with associated soft tissue injury causing joint instability or displacement.
11. Salter–Harris fractures (Fig. 1.10) – fractures involving unfused growth plates; may lead to growth disturbances (e.g. shortening or angulation of bone). They can occur surprisingly late in neutered cats, as the growth plates remain open longer than in entire animals.

Assessment of fracture: at the time of injury

1. Location – which bone, which anatomical area of the bone?
2. Age of fracture (if not known) – assess sharpness of fracture margins and look for evidence of healing.
3. Type of fracture – see above.

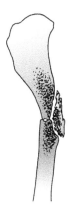

Figure 1.11 Pathological fracture: diffuse rarefaction of bone around a tibial fracture site due to metastatic neoplasia.

4. Displacement of fragments – distal relative to proximal fragment (e.g. distracted, impacted, overriding).
5. Underlying bone radiolucency or loss of normal architecture, for evidence of pathological fracture (Fig. 1.11).
6. Involvement of joints – subsequent osteoarthritis may occur.
7. Presence of foreign material.
8. Soft tissue changes.
9. Injuries elsewhere in body (e.g. with pelvic trauma, check for bladder or urethral rupture; thoracic pathology).

Assessment of fracture: immediate post-operative radiographs

1. Degree of reduction – at least 50% bone contact on orthogonal views is needed for healing.
2. Alignment.
   a. Medial–lateral and cranial–caudal.
   b. Rotational alignment – include joints above and below.
3. Adequacy of implant type, size and placement.
4. Joints – congruency, lack of entry by implants.
5. Presence of cancellous bone grafts.
6. Soft tissues.

(Useful mnemonic: ABCDS – alignment, bone, cartilage, device, soft tissues; alternatively, consider the four A's – apposition, alignment, angulation, apparatus).

Fracture healing

NB: need two orthogonal views to assess healing, as the fracture may appear bridged on one view and not on another. Healing occurs more rapidly in young animals.

1. *Primary bone healing* – direct bridging of the fracture by osseous tissue, re-establishing cortex and medulla without intermediate callus. Occurs with a high degree of reduction and stabilization of the fracture site. Stages 1, 2 and 5 (Fig. 1.12).
2. *Secondary bone healing* – unstructured bone laid down in soft tissue as a callus and subsequently remodelled. Stages 1–5 (Fig. 1.12).

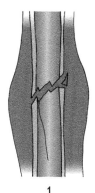 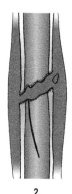 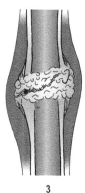 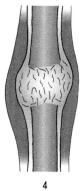 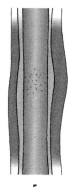

1   2   3   4   5

Figure 1.12 The five stages of fracture healing. Stage 1: sharp fragments, hairline fracture lines easily overlooked, marked soft tissue swelling. Stage 2: fracture margins becoming blurred; hairline fractures more obvious; reduced soft tissue swelling. Stage 3: unstructured bony callus with partial bridging of fracture line. Stage 4: callus becoming more solid; early remodelling. Stage 5: continued remodelling results in reduction in callus size.

- Stage 1 (recent injury): sharp fracture ends; well-defined fragments; soft tissue swelling; disruption to skin and soft tissue emphysema if the fracture is compound (open).
- Stage 2 (approximately 1–2 weeks): reducing soft tissue swelling; fracture line blurred due to hyperaemia and bone resorption; hairline fractures widened and more obvious; early, indistinct periosteal reaction, especially in young animals.
- Stage 3 (approximately 2–3 weeks): abundant, unstructured bony callus forming (size depends on the type of fracture, location, use of limb, stability at site, vascularization); partial bridging of fracture line; structurally strong.
- Stage 4 (approximately 3–8 weeks): continued filling in of the fracture line; early remodelling of the callus.
- Stage 5 (approximately 8 weeks on): continued remodelling and reduction in size of callus; restoration of cortices and trabecular pattern; the limb may straighten slightly if malunion occurred originally.

Assessment of fracture: subsequent examinations

1. The intervals at which follow-up radiographs are obtained depend on the age of the patient, the severity of the injury, the nature of the repair and the condition of the patient. Usually 2- to 3-week intervals for young animals and 4–6 weeks for mature animals are adequate.
2. Use the same radiographic technique as for the original radiographs, for comparison (may need to reduce exposure factors if soft tissue is less due to reduction of swelling or muscle atrophy).
3. Alignment of fragments.
4. Position and integrity of implants – migration, bending, cracking or fracture of implants may occur.
5. Stability of fracture site – evidence of instability following surgical repair includes migration of implants, radiolucent haloes around screws and pins (differential diagnoses are infection, bone necrosis from high-speed drill, artefactual radiolucent halo around metallic implants in some digital images).
6. Stage of fracture healing.
7. Amount of callus, for example active fractures may be hypertrophic (moderate to large

amount of callus) or oligotrophic (little callus), whereas inactive fractures show no callus or atrophy of bone ends.
8. Evidence of infection – osteolysis especially around implants, unexpected periosteal reactions (differential diagnosis is periosteal stripping), sequestrum formation, soft tissue swelling ± emphysema.
9. Evidence of secondary joint disease.
10. Evidence of disuse – muscle atrophy, osteopenia.
11. The six A's – apposition, alignment, angulation, apparatus, activity of bone healing and architecture of bone and surrounding soft tissue.

Complications of fracture healing

1. Delayed union – longer than expected time to heal for the type and location of fracture, but evidence of bone activity is present.
   a. Disuse.
   b. Instability.
   c. Poor reduction.
   d. Poor nutrition.
   e. Old age.
   f. Infection.
   g. Poor vascularity.
   h. Large intramedullary pin.
   i. Presence of a sequestrum.
   j. Undetected underlying pathology (e.g. neoplasia).
2. Non-union – fracture healing has apparently ceased without uniting the fragments, usually 10–12 weeks post fracture; bone ends smooth with sealed medullary cavity. Predisposed to by movement or infection at the fracture site.
   a. Non-viable or biologically inactive, for example atrophic (dying back) (Fig. 1.13) – no callus, pointed bone ends; especially the radius and ulna in toy breeds of dog that have been treated with external co-optation or intramedullary pinning; also dystrophic or necrotic non-union (devitalized intermediate fragment), defect non-union (significant bone defect).
   b. Viable or biologically active, for example hypertrophic ('elephant's foot') (Fig. 1.14) – new bone surrounds bone ends but does not cross the fracture line, giving a bell-shaped appearance; fragment ends parallel;

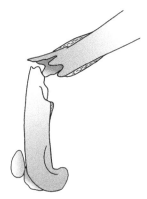

Figure 1.13 Atrophic non-union of a femoral fracture.

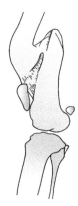

Figure 1.15 Malunion of a femoral fracture.

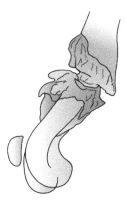

Figure 1.14 Hypertrophic non-union of a femoral fracture.

medullary cavity may appear sealed; also lesser degrees of callus or absent callus (oligotrophic).

Both types may form a false joint in which the fragment ends are contoured (e.g. one is concave and the other is convex or pointed).

3. Malunion (Fig. 1.15) – bones fuse but with incorrect alignment. Subsequent remodelling may correct the malunion to some extent. Joints proximal and distal to the site may become arthritic due to altered stresses.
4. Excessive callus formation.
   a. Movement at fracture site.
   b. Infection.
   c. Periosteal stripping.
   d. Incorporation of bone grafts.
5. Ossification of stripped periosteum, especially in young animals (e.g. rhino horn or bucket handle callus often seen on caudal aspect of femur); not usually a clinical problem.
6. Osteomyelitis – leads to delayed or non-union; differential diagnosis is exuberant callus due to instability at the fracture site.
7. Sequestrum formation – a devitalized piece of bone that will impede healing and/or lead to sinus formation. Seen radiographically as a sharply defined fragment of dense bone with a surrounding radiolucent space containing pus. May be surrounded by a sclerotic involucrum attempting to wall off the process.
8. Fracture disease – a clinical syndrome with joint stiffness and muscle wastage due to disease; radiographs show osteopenia.
9. Neoplastic transformation – may be years later, especially if metallic implants are present or healing was complex. The mechanism is not known but is possibly due to chronic inflammation. Usually in fractures sustained at 1–3 years of age.
10. Metallosis – a sterile, chronic, proliferative osteomyelitis that may result from reaction to metallic implants, especially if dissimilar metals have been combined; less common in domestic animals than in humans due to their shorter lifespan.

Ultrasonographic assessment of fracture healing

Ultrasonography can be used to assess soft tissues and bony surfaces of fractures and calluses, both at the time of injury and during the healing process. Ultrasonography permits detection of healing earlier than with radiography and therefore can prevent unnecessarily long limb immobilization. Vascularity of tissues can be assessed with power Doppler.

Stages of fracture healing detected ultrasonographically roughly correspond to those seen radiographically as follows.

- Stage 1 (recent injury): homogeneous, hypoechoic soft tissue in the gap between the fragment ends.
- Stage 2 (1–2 weeks): heterogeneous, hypoechoic soft tissue in the fracture gap.
- Stage 3 (2–3 weeks; callus formation): heterogeneous, irregular appearance with hyperechoic areas indicating the start of mineralization earlier than is seen radiographically.
- Stage 4 (3–8 weeks): heterogeneous callus becoming continuous and lamellar.
- Stage 5 (8 weeks on): a continuous, smooth, hyperechoic line represents the healed cortex, and intramedullary implants can no longer be identified.

BONES

1.10 ALTERED SHAPE OF LONG BONES

See also section 1.15, *Bony masses*.

1. Bowing of bone(s).
   a. 'Normal' in chondrodystrophic breeds (e.g. Basset Hound, Bulldog and Dachshund); especially radius and ulna. Long bones in affected breeds often have prominent apophyses as well (enthesiopathies – osteophytes at ligamentar insertions) (Fig. 1.16).
   b. Growth plate trauma resulting in uneven growth.
   c. Radius – passive bowing due to shortening of ulna and secondary bowstring effect (see 3.5.4 and Fig. 3.13).
   d. Chondrodysplasias (dyschondroplasias) are recognized in numerous breeds and in the Domestic Short-haired cat (see 1.22.7). Failure of normal endochondral ossification leads to bowing of long bones, especially the radius and ulna, and epiphyseal changes result in arthritis.
   e. Rickets; bowing of long bones, especially the radius and ulna.

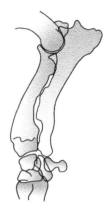

Figure 1.16 'Normal' radius and ulna of a chondrodystrophic dog, showing bowing of the long bones, prominence of apophyses, enthesiopathies and bony proliferation in the interosseus space.

   f. Congenital hypothyroidism; bowing of long bones, especially the radius and ulna; seen especially in Boxers (see 1.22.9). Disturbed epiphyseal ossification may also lead to a change in shape and subsequent osteoarthritis.
   g. Asymmetric bridging of a growth plate, resulting in uneven growth, for example severe periosteal reaction in metaphyseal osteopathy (hypertrophic osteodystrophy), surgical staple left in too long.
   h. Tension from shortened soft tissues (e.g. quadriceps contracture).
   i. Altered stresses due to bone or joint disease elsewhere in limb.
   j. Hemimelia (rare) – either radius or ulna absent (usually radial agenesis), putting abnormal stress on the remaining bone.

2. Angulation of bone.
   a. Traumatic folding (greenstick) fracture.
   b. Pathological fracture.
      - Primary, secondary or pseudohyperparathyroidism (see 1.16.4 and Fig. 1.20).
      - Neoplasia, especially if mainly osteolytic (primary, secondary, multiple myeloma) (see 1.18.2, 1.19.1, 1.20.1 and Figs 1.21–1.24 and 1.27).
      - Enchondromatosis (see 1.19.1).
      - Bone cyst (see 1.19.2 and Fig. 1.26).
      - Osteomyelitis (see 1.20.2 and Figs 1.28 and 1.29).

- Severe osteopenia (see 1.16).
- Osteogenesis imperfecta (see 1.16.13).
c. Malunion.
3. Abnormally straight bone (e.g. radius, due to premature closure of the distal radial growth plate). Long bones are normally very straight in some larger dog breeds.
4. Expansion or irregular margination of bone.
   a. Osteochondroma (single) or multiple cartilaginous exostoses (multiple) (see 1.15.2 and Fig. 1.19).
   b. Enchondromatosis (see 1.19.1).
   c. Other expansile tumour (see 1.19.1 and Fig. 1.25).
   d. Bone cyst (see 1.19.2 and Fig. 1.26).
   e. Late, remodelled metaphyseal osteopathy (hypertrophic osteodystrophy; see 1.24.4 and Fig. 1.31B).
   f. Disseminated (diffuse) idiopathic skeletal hyperostosis – mainly spine but also extremital periarticular new bone and enthesiopathies (see 5.4.5).
   g. Insertion tendonopathies.
      - 'Normal' in chondrodystrophic breeds (see 1.10.1 and Fig. 1.16).
      - Pathological (see Ch. 3).

1.11 DWARFISM

1. Proportionate dwarfism.
   a. Pituitary dwarfism; mainly German Shepherd dog, also reported in the Miniature Pinscher, Spitz and Covelian Bear dog. May be hypothyroid too (see below).
   b. GM_1-gangliosidosis – English Springer Spaniels.

2. Disproportionate dwarfism.
   a. Chondrodysplasias (see 1.22.7).
   b. Hypothyroidism; mainly Boxer (see 1.22.9).
   c. Rickets or hypovitaminosis D (see 1.23.8 and Fig. 1.30).
   d. Zinc-responsive chondrodysplasia in the Alaskan Malamute and possibly other northern breeds.
   e. Hypervitaminosis D – a massive intake in a young animal causes retarded growth, bone deformity and osteopenia, although death from renal failure is more likely; cats are more sensitive to toxicity.
   f. Cats – mucopolysaccharidosis – especially cats with Siamese ancestry; rarely occurs in dogs but mucopolysaccharidosis type VII is reported to cause disproportionate dwarfism in dogs (see 5.4.9).
   g. Cats – mucolipidosis type II (rare).
   h. Cats – hypervitaminosis A in young cats – reduced length of long bones due to abnormality of physeal cartilage.

1.12 DELAYED OSSIFICATION OR GROWTH PLATE CLOSURE

Delayed ossification is mainly recognized in epiphyses, carpal and tarsal bones. The various conditions listed here may be difficult to differentiate, and chondrodysplasias are often initially misdiagnosed as rickets. However, rickets does not manifest until after weaning, whereas other conditions begin to develop before weaning. Table 1.3 summarizes the radiographic changes that may be present in animals with growth disturbances, but the subject is complex.

Table 1.3 Radiographic changes that may be present in animals with growth disturbances					
	EPIPHYSEAL DYSPLASIA	WIDE PHYSES	LATE-CLOSING PHYSES	OSTEOPENIA	STUNTING
Chondrodysplasia	Yes	Yes	Some	No	Yes
Congenital hypothyroidism	Yes	Yes	Yes	No	Yes
Hypervitaminosis A in immature cats	No	No	No	Yes	Yes
Pituitary dwarfism	Yes	Yes	Yes	No	Yes
Mucopolysaccharidosis	Yes	Irregular	Not reported	Yes	Possible
Rickets	No	Yes	Yes	Yes	Yes

1. Chondrodysplasias – effect on growth plate closure time is variable (see 1.22.7).
2. Congenital hypothyroidism – especially Boxers (see 1.22.9).
3. Pituitary dwarfism – especially German Shepherd dogs.
4. Rickets.
5. Hypervitaminosis D – a massive intake in a young animal causes retarded growth, bone deformity and osteopenia, although death from renal failure is more likely; cats are more sensitive to toxicity.
6. Copper deficiency.
7. Cats – mucopolysaccharidosis, especially in cats with Siamese ancestry; rarely affects dogs (see 5.4.9).
8. Cats – neutering delays growth plate closure, especially in male cats.

1.13 INCREASED RADIOPACITY WITHIN BONE

It may be difficult to differentiate increased radio-pacity within a bone from increased radiopacity due to superimposition of surrounding new bone. Both will produce a radiographic increased opacity often referred to as *(osteo)sclerosis*.

1. Technical factors causing artefactual increased radiopacity.
   a. Underexposure (too low a kV or mAs).
   b. Underdevelopment.
   c. Intensifying screen marks.
2. Normal.
   a. Normal metaphyseal condensation in the metaphysis of skeletally immature animals; also incorrectly termed 'idiopathic osteodystrophy'.
   b. Subchondral bone.
   c. Physeal scar – a fine radiopaque line persisting for variable lengths of time after the growth plate has closed; however, its presence is not a reliable indicator of the animal's age.
3. Artefactual.
   a. Superimposition of periosteal new bone – examine the orthogonal view.
   b. Superimposition of soft tissues – look beyond the bone margins to see if soft tissue lines continue.

4. Neoplasia.
   a. Primary malignant bone tumour of blastic type, although usually there is some evidence of osteolysis as well (see 1.20.1).
   b. Bone metastases – may be sclerotic or osteolytic; often at atypical sites for primary tumours (e.g. diaphyses); often multiple in one bone or polyostotic (see 1.20.1 and Fig. 1.22).
   c. Certain myeloproliferative disorders (see 1.13.15).
   d. Cats – feline leukaemia-induced medullary osteosclerosis – rare; likely to be widespread in the skeleton.
   e. Cats – feline lymphoma may cause medullary osteosclerosis – rare; likely to be widespread in the skeleton.
5. Osteomyelitis – more likely to be a mixed lesion including osteolysis (see 1.20.2 and Figs 1.28 and 1.29). If due to haematogenous spread, there are likely to be multiple, possibly bilaterally symmetrical lesions.
   a. Bacterial.
   b. Fungal.
   c. Protozoal – leishmaniasis* – periosteal and intramedullary bone proliferation in diaphyses and flat bones, provoked by chronic osteomyelitis; mixed, aggressive bone lesions; also erosive and non-erosive joint lesions.
6. Panosteitis (Fig. 1.17) – usually immature or young adult (5–18 months old, occasionally older); especially German Shepherd dogs, although other breeds can be affected; male

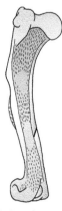

Figure 1.17 Panosteitis in a humerus: patches of increased medullary radiopacity, coarse trabeculation and smooth periosteal reaction.

preponderance. The aetiology is unknown. Clinical signs are of cyclical shifting leg lameness, which may be acute and severe with pain on bone palpation; also lethargy, anorexia and pyrexia. The condition is self-limiting but may have a protracted course. Lesions are seen in diaphyses and metaphyses of long bones, and several patterns of increased radiopacity may occur.

- Ill-defined medullary patches often near the nutrient foramen; main differential diagnosis is osteomyelitis.
- Coarse, sclerotic trabecular pattern.
- Increased radiopacity due to superimposed periosteal reaction, which occurs in a minority of cases.
- Narrow transverse sclerotic lines as recovery occurs; differential diagnosis is growth arrest lines.
   Radiographic signs may lag behind clinical signs and may be absent in early or mild cases; bone scintigraphy may be helpful in such cases.

7. Growth arrest lines – fine, transverse sclerotic lines due to periods of arrested and increased growth, of no clinical significance; differential diagnosis is panosteitis.

8. Metaphyseal osteopathy (hypertrophic osteodystrophy) – young dogs, especially the distal radius and ulna; initially radiolucent metaphyseal bands ± sclerotic borders; later superimposed periosteal new bone adds to increased radiopacity (see 1.24.4 and Fig. 1.31).

9. Fractures – if impaction of bone or overlapping of fragments occurs, a sclerotic band rather than a bone defect may be seen.
   a. Folding fractures.
      – Greenstick fractures (single cortex) in young animals.
      – Osteopenia, especially nutritional secondary hyperparathyroidism (see 1.16.4 and Fig. 1.20).
   b. Compression or impaction fractures – especially vertebrae; predisposed to by osteopenia.
   c. Superimposition of overridden fragments seen on one radiographic projection but shown to be displaced using orthogonal view.
   d. Healing fracture.

10. Osteopenia (see 1.16) – sparing of subchondral bone and bone along epiphyseal and metaphyseal margins of growth plates creates *apparent* sclerotic bands, which are probably artefactual and arise from increased contrast with the osteopenic bone.

11. Lead poisoning – in rare cases, thin sclerotic bands are seen in the metaphyses of long bones and vertebrae of young animals suffering lead poisoning; also causes osteopenia.

12. Canine distemper – bands of metaphyseal sclerosis paralleling the physis may been seen; differential diagnosis is metaphyseal osteopathy (hypertrophic osteodystrophy; possible link between this and canine distemper vaccination in Weimaraners).

13. Hypervitaminosis D – alternating areas of sclerosis and bone resorption in metaphyses and diaphysis together with periosteal and endosteal new bone; however, bone changes are rare, as the animal is more likely to show soft tissue mineralization and to die from renal failure (see 12.2).

14. Bone infarcts – rare; multiple irregular sclerotic patches in medullary cavities of limb bones and cranial diploë; may be associated with, or lead to, osteosarcoma. Mainly smaller breeds (e.g. Shetland Sheepdog, Miniature Schnauzer). Cause unknown, possibly vascular disease leading to hypoxia.

15. Osteopetrosis (osteosclerosis fragilis, marble bone disease, chalk bones) – rare disease in which primary and/or secondary spongiosa persists in marrow cavities due to a defect in osteoclastic resorption; produces a diffuse increase in bone radiopacity (osteosclerosis) with coarsening of trabeculae, thickening of cortices and progressive obliteration of the medullary cavity; the bones are brittle, and pathological fractures may occur. May cause anaemia if medullary cavities are severely compromised (myelophthistic anaemia).
   a. Congenital.
      – Autosomal recessive gene, usually lethal but some animals may survive into adulthood.
      – Hereditary anaemia in the Basenji.
      – Sclerosing bone dysplasia – an inherited subset of osteochondrodysplasia causing generalized osteosclerosis with obliteration of nasal turbinates and nasolacrimal duct obstruction.

b. Acquired (the disease is poorly understood, and it is not known whether all such cases are truly acquired or whether some represent a late manifestation of an inherited disease).
  - Chronic dietary excess of calcium.
  - Chronic vitamin D toxicity.
  - Myelofibrosis.
  - Idiopathic.
16. Osteoid osteoma has been described in the humerus of a dog and the mandible of a cat and is a benign lesion consisting of vascular osteoid tissue in the medullary cavity surrounded by an area of sclerotic bone. These are well described in humans, occurring usually in males under 25 years in the femur and tibia.
17. Cats – diffuse osteosclerosis of the skeleton may be seen as an incidental finding or associated with renal failure, leukaemia, myeloproliferative disease or systemic lupus erythematosus.

1.14 PERIOSTEAL REACTIONS

Periosteal reactions forming new bone may be localized or diffuse depending on the aetiology. Localized periosteal reactions appearing as bony masses are also described in Section 1.15. In some cases, periosteal elevation caused by underlying pathology may be visualized ultrasonographically, and fine needle aspiration may be performed using ultrasound guidance.

1. Trauma.
  a. Direct blow to the cortex, producing periosteal stimulation (a single episode or repetitive milder trauma).
  b. Periosteal tearing or elevation associated with fractures; especially young animals.
  c. Subperiosteal haematoma – often caudal skull in dogs with prominent nuchal crest; also sometimes in dogs with coagulopathies (e.g. Dobermann Pinschers with von Willebrand's disease).
  d. Reactive (e.g. beneath a lick granuloma).
2. Infection (more likely to produce a diffuse reaction in young animals in which the periosteum is loosely attached).
  a. Bacterial – often solitary and associated with an open wound (trauma, surgery); focal anaerobic osteomyelitis occurs following bite wounds, with a small central sequestrum surrounded by a raised, ring-like periosteal reaction. May be multifocal if haematogenous spread.
  b. Fungal – may be multifocal due to haematogenous spread; more often mixed osteolytic–proliferative lesion (see 1.20.2 and Figs 1.28 and 1.29).
  c. Protozoal.
    - Leishmaniasis* – a spectrum of periosteal reactions varying from smooth to irregular; also intramedullary sclerosis, mixed bone lesions and erosive or non-erosive joint disease.
    - Hepatozoonosis* – chronic myositis, debilitation and death, often with periosteal reactions varying from subtle to dramatic. Mainly *Hepatozoon americanum*, which produces periosteal new bone on long bones, ilium and vertebrae, probably via a humoral mechanism. The main differential diagnosis is hypertrophic osteopathy, but the distribution of lesions is different, usually affecting more proximal limb sites and/or the axial skeleton.
  d. Cats – feline tuberculosis – various *Mycobacterium* species (rare). Also mixed lesions, discospondylitis and arthritis.
3. Neoplasia – early malignancy (primary bone, metastatic or soft tissue tumours before osteolysis becomes apparent). Follow-up radiography may help to distinguish neoplasia from infection or trauma.
4. Panosteitis – severe cases may show a mild, smooth or lamellated periosteal reaction on the diaphyses (see 1.13.6 and Fig. 1.17). The diagnosis is usually obvious from the signalment and clinical signs and the presence of typical medullary lesions.
5. Metaphyseal osteopathy (hypertrophic osteodystrophy) – advanced cases show bilateral collars of periosteal new bone and paraperiosteal soft tissue mineralization around the metaphyses, which may obscure the characteristic mottled metaphyseal band (see 1.24.4 and Fig. 1.31). Subsequent remodelling causes thickening of metaphyses. In severe cases, the adjacent physis may become bridged, resulting in a subsequent angular limb deformity.
6. Hypertrophic (pulmonary) osteopathy (HPO, Marie's disease) (Fig. 1.18) – florid periosteal

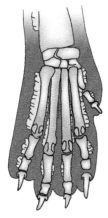

Figure 1.18 Hypertrophic pulmonary osteopathy: palisading periosteal new bone mainly on abaxial surfaces of bones, with overlying diffuse soft tissue swelling.

new bone on the diaphyses of long bones, usually beginning distally in the limb, although can extend proximally to scapula or pelvis; bilaterally symmetrical, with overlying soft tissue swelling due to oedema. In the digits, it is most severe on the abaxial margins of digits II and V. The new bone may appear in several patterns: palisading, irregular, brush border, lamellated or smooth and solid depending on the stage of the disease. The thorax and abdomen should be imaged to look for an underlying lesion. This is usually primary or secondary pulmonary neoplasia, but a variety of other causes have been implicated, including non-neoplastic pulmonary disease, other intrathoracic masses, oesophageal disease (especially neoplastic transformation of *Spirocerca lupi* granulomas), infective endocarditis and bladder neoplasia. Theories as to cause include pulmonary shunting, vagal nerve stimulation, humoral substances produced by neoplastic cells and megakaryocyte or platelet clumping. The diagnosis is usually obvious from the nature and distribution of the periosteal reaction and detection of a primary lesion. HPO is rare in cats. The main differential diagnosis is hepatozoonosis* (see 1.14.2).

7. Craniomandibular osteopathy (mainly Terriers, especially West Highland White Terrier, but seen sporadically in other breeds) – florid periosteal new bone on the skull, particularly the mandible and tympanic bullae (see 4.11.1 and Fig. 4.6). Masses of paraperiosteal new bone

adjacent to distal ulnar metaphyses, similar to metaphyseal osteopathy (hypertrophic osteodystrophy), are occasionally seen (see 3.5.16 and Fig. 3.14).

8. Cats – hypervitaminosis A – focal periosteal new bone around vertebrae (mainly cervical or thoracic), joints (especially elbow and stifle), sternum, ribs and occipital bone. May lead to joint ankylosis. Usually young adult cats on raw bovine liver diets; differential diagnosis is mucopolysaccharidosis.

9. Cats – mucopolysaccharidosis – mainly spinal changes similar to hypervitaminosis A (see 2.5.14 and 5.4.9). Differential diagnosis is hypervitaminosis A. Rare in dogs.

1.15 BONY MASSES

See also Sections 1.10, *Altered shape of long bones*, and 1.14, *Periosteal reactions*.

Differential diagnoses for bony masses include mixed osteoproductive–osteolytic lesions in which new bone predominates and obscures underlying lysis, and soft tissue mineralization that is close to or superimposed over bone, for example calcinosis circumscripta (see 12.2.2 and Fig. 12.1).

1. Trauma.
   a. Exuberant, localized periosteal reaction following direct injury.
   b. Large fracture callus – due to movement, infection, periosteal stripping.
   c. Hypertrophic non-union – bone defect at the fracture line should be evident.
   d. Rhino horn callus from periosteal stripping caudal to the femur, associated with femoral fracture.

2. Neoplasia.
   a. Osteochondroma (when single) or osteochondromatosis or multiple cartilaginous exostoses (when multiple) (Fig. 1.19). Rare: a skeletal dysplasia rather than a true neoplastic process. In dogs, seen when skeletally immature at osteochondral junctions, for example long bone metaphyses (often bilateral), ribs and costochondral junctions, pelvis and vertebrae. Hereditary tendency for multiple lesions; especially Terriers. Generally smooth, cauliflower-like or nodular projections with cortex and medulla continuous with underlying bone, but may appear more granular and

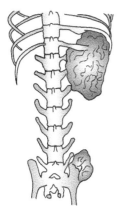

Figure 1.19 Multiple cartilaginous exostoses (dog): expansile masses arising from a rib and the wing of the ilium.

aggressive during the active growth phase. Lesions in long bones may be more irregular than those elsewhere, and those arising at growth plates may cause limb shortening or angular limb deformities. While still ossifying, they may appear not to be attached to underlying bone and may mimic calcinosis circumscripta (see 12.2.2 and Fig. 12.1). Osteochondromata in ribs may mimic healing rib fractures. Growth of osteochondromata ceases at skeletal maturity, but malignant transformation to osteosarcoma or chondrosarcoma has been reported. In cats, seen in young, mature animals, usually 2–4 years old at diagnosis; possibly with a viral aetiology (test for feline leukaemia virus). Lesions are similar to those in dogs. They arise from the perichondrium of flat or irregular bones such as the skull, ribs and pelvis and may continue to grow, becoming more aggressive; as in dogs, malignant transformation may occur. Also reported as amorphous and linear opacities in the surrounding soft tissues. In older cats, osteocartilaginous exostoses, often around the elbows, may represent the same condition.

b. Osteoma (benign) – rare, usually skull; often younger dogs; especially Mastiff types. Dense, bony mass without underlying osteolysis.

c. Ossifying fibroma – skull.

d. Multilobular tumour of bone (syn. osteochondrosarcoma, chondroma rodens) – skull (see 4.6.3 and Fig. 4.3); often have a characteristic stippled appearance.

e. Predominantly osteoblastic primary malignant bone tumour – mainly metaphyses of long bones; also skull.

f. Parosteal or juxtacortical osteosarcoma (see 3.11.12 and Fig. 3.29) – rare; radiographically and pathologically distinct from other osteosarcomata. Slow-growing, sclerotic, smooth or lobulated, non-aggressive or low-grade malignant bony mass arising from periosteal connective tissue with little or no underlying osteolysis; seen especially around the stifle on the caudal aspect of the distal femur but also reported affecting other long bones, skull, vertebrae and ribs. Periosteal and high-grade surface osteosarcomas also occur on the outside of bones but are more aggressive in appearance and behaviour.

3. Enthesiopathies (osteophytes forming within ligamentar insertions).
   a. Normal prominence of apophyses in chondrodystrophic breeds; bilaterally symmetrical (see 1.10.1 and Fig. 1.16).
   b. Enthesiopathies in individuals of other breeds suffering from chondrodysplasias; bilaterally symmetrical.
   c. Enthesiopathies in specific tendon and ligament attachments (see Ch. 3).
   d. Disseminated or diffuse idiopathic skeletal hyperostosis (DISH) – spurs of new bone mainly on the spine but also periarticular new bone and enthesiopathies in the limbs (see 5.4.5).

4. Proliferative joint diseases may result in bony masses associated with joints (see also 2.5).
   a. Severe osteoarthritis.
   b. Disseminated idiopathic skeletal hyperostosis.
   c. Synovial osteochondromatosis (see 2.8.18 and Fig. 2.7).
   d. Cats – osteochondromata or osteocartilaginous exostoses – especially the elbows.
   e. Cats – hypervitaminosis A; especially the elbow and stifle, although spinal changes predominate (see 5.4.8).
   f. Cats – mucopolysaccharidosis (see 2.5.14 and 5.4.9).

5. Craniomandibular osteopathy – masses of periosteal new bone on the skull, mainly mandibles and tympanic bullae; occasionally see limb changes (see 3.5.16, 4.10.1 and Figs 3.14 and 4.6).

6. Calvarial hyperostosis in Bullmastiffs (see 4.6.2).

1.16 OSTEOPENIA

Osteopenia is a radiographic term meaning reduction in radiographic bone radiopacity. This may be due to *osteoporosis* (reduced bone mass but normal ratio of organic matrix and inorganic salts) or *osteomalacia* (organic matrix present in excess due to failure of mineralization), and these cannot be differentiated radiographically. This section lists differential diagnoses for diffuse osteopenia usually affecting the whole skeleton, or in the case of disuse, a whole limb. More localized areas of osteopenia are described in Section 1.18, *Osteolytic lesions*. Focal osteopenia is more easily recognized than diffuse osteopenia, due to contrast with surrounding normal bone. However, radiography is relatively insensitive for bone loss, because approximately 30–60% of the mineral content of bone must be lost before being radiographically evident.

Osteopenia is most readily apparent in parts of the skeleton with high bone turnover, such as trabeculated bone in the metaphyses and epiphyses of long bones, vertebrae and the skull. The radiographic signs of osteopenia are:

- a reduction in bone radiopacity compared with soft tissues
- thinning of cortices, sometimes with a double cortical line
- relative sparing of subchondral bone leading to apparent sclerosis, especially in the endplates of the vertebrae and adjacent to physes
- coarse trabeculation due to resorption of smaller trabeculae
- pathological folding or compression fractures, which are seen as distortion of the contour of the bone and bands of increased opacity.

Most causes of osteopenia are metabolic diseases, and the aetiology may be complex. The condition is reversible if the cause is corrected. Osteopenia may also be mimicked by incorrect technical factors during radiography.

1. Technical factors causing artefactual osteopenia (see Appendix).
   a. Overexposure.
   b. Overdevelopment.
   c. Fogging of the film (numerous causes).
2. Artefactual due to changes in the thickness of overlying soft tissue.
   a. Reduction in overlying soft tissue, leading to relative overexposure of the bone (e.g. in a limb with chronic disuse) – compare with the opposite limb if possible.
   b. Increase in surrounding soft tissue in obese dogs, especially affecting spinal radiographs; the increased kV required produces more Compton scatter, resulting in loss of visualization of trabeculae and apparent osteopenia.
3. Disuse (limb) – paralysis, fracture or severe lameness; often most severe distal to a fracture and affecting particularly epiphyses and the cuboidal bones of the carpus and tarsus.
4. Hyperparathyroidism (osteitis fibrosa cystica, fibrous osteodystrophy). Metastatic calcification may occur secondarily in soft tissues such as the kidneys, gastric rugae and major blood vessels (see 12.2).
   a. Nutritional secondary hyperparathyroidism (juvenile osteoporosis, butcher's dog disease) (Fig. 1.20) – especially seen in young animals due to high skeletal activity. Seen after weaning when on a high-meat diet that is low in calcium and high in phosphorus. Clinical signs of lameness, lordosis and para- or tetraplegia due to folding fractures occur. More common in cats than in dogs.
   b. Renal secondary hyperparathyroidism (renal rickets, renal osteodystrophy) – chronic renal failure in young animals with renal dysplasia or in older animals with chronic renal disease; mainly affects the skull, causing rubber jaw (see 4.9.5 and Fig. 4.5), but other skeletal changes may also be seen as above.
   c. Primary hyperparathyroidism – rare; parathyroid gland hyperplasia or neoplasia.
   d. Pseudohyperparathyroidism; hypercalcaemia of malignancy – various neoplastic causes, especially lymphoma and

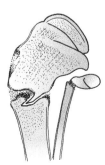

Figure 1.20 Nutritional secondary hyperparathyroidism: folding fractures in an osteopenic tibia and fibula.

anal sac adenocarcinoma; also mammary adenocarcinoma, myeloma, gastric squamous cell carcinoma, thyroid adenocarcinoma, testicular interstitial cell tumours.

   e. Other causes of secondary hyperparathyroidism (e.g. pregnancy and lactation, vitamin D deficiency, acidosis, osteomalacic anticonvulsant therapy).

5. Corticosteroid excess.
   a. Hyperadrenocorticism – Cushing's disease.
   b. Iatrogenic – long-term corticosteroid administration.
6. Senility – especially aged cats.
7. Chronic protein deprivation or loss.
   a. Starvation.
   b. Liver disease.
   c. Malabsorption.
8. Hyperthyroidism.
9. Diabetes mellitus.
10. Panosteitis – not a true osteopenia but residual changes include paucity of trabeculae in long bones, giving a hollow appearance, although the cortices are of normal thickness and radiopacity.
11. Rickets – probably via associated nutritional secondary hyperparathyroidism (see 1.23.8 and Fig. 1.30).
12. Multiple myeloma (plasma cell myeloma) – genuine osteopenia; also apparent osteopenia due to confluence of areas of osteolysis (see 1.18.2 and Fig. 1.24).
13. Osteogenesis imperfecta – a rare inherited type I collagen defect characterized by osteopenia and excessive bone fragility and resulting in multiple pathological fractures; it may occur with dentinogenesis imperfecta, in which teeth also fracture. Seen in young animals, so the main differential diagnosis is nutritional secondary hyperparathyroidism.
14. Lead poisoning in immature animals; sclerotic metaphyseal lines may also be seen.
15. Hypervitaminosis D – a massive intake in a young animal can produce osteopenia with bone deformity and retarded growth, but the main changes are soft tissue calcification (see 12.2).
16. Copper deficiency.
17. Prolonged high-dose anticonvulsant therapy – primidone, phenytoin and phenobarbitone in humans, although effects in animals are not proven; due to liver damage and effect on vitamin D production.
18. Cats – hypervitaminosis A – osteopenia due to reduced periosteal activity, disuse and concomitant nutritional secondary hyperparathyroidism; however, the proliferative spine and joint changes predominate.
19. Cats – mucopolysaccharidosis and mucolipidosis – as hypervitaminosis A; may occur rarely in dogs (see 5.4.9).

1.17 COARSE TRABECULAR PATTERN

1. Osteopenia – osteopenia is most apparent in areas of trabecular bone, because here bone turnover is highest. Small trabeculae are resorbed first, leaving a coarse trabecular pattern due to the remaining larger trabeculae. For causes, see Section 1.16.
2. Panosteitis – coarse, sclerotic trabeculae may be seen in large or small patches or arising from the endosteal surface of the cortices (see 1.13.6 and Fig. 1.17). In a dog of suggestive age and breed, this finding is usually considered pathognomonic for the disease.
3. Distal ulnar and/or radial metaphyseal changes consisting primarily of thickened trabeculae have been described as an incidental finding in young Newfoundland dogs in Norway (see 3.4.11).
4. Multiple myeloma (plasma cell myeloma) – the disease may produce multiple confluent osteolytic lesions and osteopenia, which together can create an apparent coarse trabecular pattern (see 1.18.2 and Fig. 1.24).
5. Osteopetrosis (see 1.13.15).

1.18 OSTEOLYTIC LESIONS

Ultrasonography is increasingly being used for various areas of the skeletal system. Although the ultrasound beam cannot penetrate normal bone, it can show areas of superficial osteolysis such as cortical defects, allowing the needle to be guided into the bone for fine needle aspiration biopsy, which will sometimes give a cytological diagnosis. Adjacent soft tissue masses may also be aspirated under ultrasound guidance. The procedure does not always require general anaesthesia and is therefore rapid and cost-effective as well as being less invasive than a bone biopsy. However, a negative ultrasound-guided fine needle aspiration biopsy does not rule out neoplasia and should be followed by a tissue core biopsy and histological analysis.

1. Artefactual.
   a. Superimposition of skin defect or gas in an open wound.
   b. Superimposition of anal sac gas on the ischium on ventrodorsal pelvic radiographs.
2. Neoplasia (see 1.19.1 and 1.20.1).
   a. Primary malignant bone tumour of osteolytic type (especially in cats) (Fig. 1.21), although usually there is some evidence of new bone production as well.
   b. Bone metastases (Fig. 1.22) – may be osteolytic or sclerotic; usually in atypical sites for primary tumours (e.g. diaphyses); often multiple in one bone or polyostotic. Metastatic carcinoma is predominantly osteolytic without accompanying new bone. Any primary tumour may metastasize, but mammary tumours are over-represented.
   c. Malignant soft tissue tumour invading bone (Fig. 1.23) – usually soft tissue swelling and cortical destruction starting subperiosteally are obvious. If near a joint, more than one bone may be affected (see 2.4.7 and Fig. 2.4). Haemangiosarcoma, synovial sarcoma, histiocytic sarcoma (malignant histiocytosis), plasmacytoma and liposarcoma are predominantly osteolytic with an aggressive

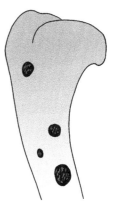

Figure 1.22 Bone metastases: multiple osteolytic lesions in atypical sites for primary neoplasia.

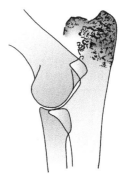

Figure 1.23 Malignant soft tissue tumour invading bone: osteolysis predominates, and more than one bone may be involved.

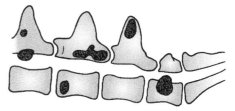

Figure 1.24 Multiple myeloma in a dog, producing several discrete punched-out areas of osteolysis in lumbar vertebrae.

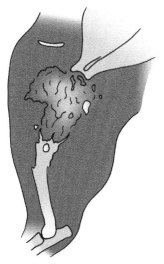

Figure 1.21 Osteolytic osteosarcoma of the proximal humerus in a cat: severe bone destruction with pathological fracture.

appearance. Infiltrative lipoma or liposarcoma will have a characteristic fat opacity.
   d. Lymphoma – usually predominantly osteolytic lesions, which may be multifocal; tendency for pathological fracture.
   e. Multiple myeloma (plasma cell myeloma) (Fig. 1.24) – discrete, punched-out osteolytic areas of variable size and lacking any sclerotic margin; usually multiple, confluent

or polyostotic, less often solitary. Where lesions are confluent, the affected bone has a polycystic or marbled appearance or may appear osteopenic with coarse trabeculation. Mainly affects pelvis, spine, ribs, and long bones. Pathological fractures are common.

3. Infection, osteomyelitis (see 1.20.2 and Figs 1.28 and 1.29).
   a. Bacterial.
      – Osteolytic halo around infected teeth due to periapical granuloma; differential diagnosis is renal secondary hyperparathyroidism (see 4.9.5 and Fig. 4.5).
      – Around sequestra.
      – Around metallic implants; differential diagnoses are movement, bone necrosis due to heat from high-speed drill, artefact around metallic implant on some digital radiographs.
      – At fracture sites, especially following an open wound.
      – Haematogenous osteomyelitis, especially in metaphyses; differential diagnosis is metaphyseal osteopathy (hypertrophic osteodystrophy) (see 1.24.4 and 1.24.5 and Figs 1.31 and 1.32).
   b. Fungal* – usually spread by the haematogenous route and therefore likely to be multiple lesions.
   c. Protozoal – leishmaniasis* – may cause severe osteolytic arthritis.
4. Trauma.
   a. Superimposition of skin defect or gas in open wound.
   b. Fracture line before full bridging.
   c. Osteolytic halo around surgical implants caused by infection, movement or bone necrosis due to the use of a high-speed drill; also artefactual on some digital radiographs.
   d. Stress protection – a localized area of osteopenia and bone weakness at the end of a bone plate.
5. Pressure atrophy – a smoothly bordered area of superficial bone loss due to pressure from an adjacent mass (e.g. rib tumour, mass between digits, elastic band around limb).
6. Fibrous dysplasia – rare fibro-osseous defect of bone thought to be developmental in origin as mainly seen in young animals; mono- or polyostotic osteolytic lesions that may undergo pathological fracture. Often the adjacent mid-radial and mid-ulnar diaphyses.

7. Idiopathic multifocal osteopathy – one report of four adult Scottish Terriers in which there was multifocal absence of bone, mainly affecting the spine. However, it was unclear whether this was true osteolysis or failure of the bone to form.

8. Osteolytic lesions at specific locations.
   a. Metaphyseal osteopathy (hypertrophic osteodystrophy; see 1.24.4 and Fig. 1.31).
   b. Metaphyseal osteomyelitis (see 1.24.5 and Fig. 1.32).
   c. Retained cartilaginous cores (see 1.24.3, 3.5.3 and Fig. 3.12) – not truly osteolytic but areas of non-ossification of cartilage.
   d. Large osteochondrosis lesions – not truly osteolytic but areas of non-ossification of cartilage.
   e. Avascular necrosis of the femoral head (Legg–Calvé–Perthes disease) – young dogs of Terrier breeds – may affect both hips (see 3.9.4 and Fig. 3.24).
   f. Intraosseous epidermoid cysts – rare in bone; usually osteolytic; distal phalanges and vertebrae.
   g. Physeal dysplasia, slipped capital femoral epiphysis and feline femoral neck metaphyseal osteopathy with subsequent bone resorption of the femoral neck (see 3.9.6 and 3.9.10 and Fig. 3.25).

1.19 EXPANSILE OSTEOLYTIC LESIONS

The following lesions are likely to be *expansile*, that is, they are osteolytic lesions arising within bones, which displace the cortex progressively outwards and cause predominantly thinning rather than frank lysis of the cortex. Pathological fracture may occur. They are usually benign or of low-grade malignancy.

1. Neoplasia.
   a. Giant cell tumour (osteoclastoma) (Fig. 1.25) – a rare tumour usually seen in the epiphyses and metaphyses of long bones, especially the distal ulna. Expansile, osteolytic lesion with multiloculated, septate appearance and variable transition to normal bone. May look identical to a bone cyst, but the patients are usually older.

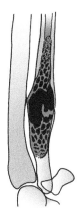

Figure 1.25 Expansile bone lesion: giant cell tumour of the distal ulna. Although malignant, the lesion does not appear particularly aggressive.

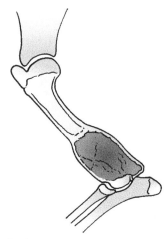

Figure 1.26 Benign bone cyst in the distal humerus of a skeletally immature dog, producing an expansile bone lesion with non-aggressive characteristics.

    b. Rarely, other non-osteogenic malignancies may appear expansile.

    c. Enchondroma (single) or enchondromatosis (multiple) – syn. osseous chondromatosis, dyschondroplasia, Ollier's disease. Rare; larger breeds. A benign but debilitating condition in which foci of physeal cartilage are displaced through the metaphyses into the diaphyses, causing weakening of the bone due to expansile, non-ossified lesions; animals usually present while immature due to pathological fractures.

    d. Osteochondroma or multiple cartilaginous exostoses – may appear expansile because the cortex is continuous with underlying bone (see 1.15.2 and Fig. 1.19).

2. Benign bone cysts (Fig. 1.26) – rare, mainly young dogs of large breeds; male predominance; often distal radius or ulna. Expansile, often septated, osteolytic lesions that may appear identical to giant cell tumours, although affected dogs are generally younger. The lesion is likely to be confined to the metaphysis, not crossing the growth plate, although it may migrate along the diaphysis with skeletal maturity. Usually single (unicameral, monostotic), occasionally multiple (polyostotic).

3. Aneurysmal bone cysts appear similar but are due to vascular anomalies such as arteriovenous fistulae or vascular defects resulting from trauma or neoplasia; an enlarged nutrient foramen may be seen. Usually older animals. Doppler ultrasound through the thin cortices may demonstrate blood flow.

4. Fibrous dysplasia (see 1.18.6) – may be expansile.

5. Bone abscess – rare.

1.20 MIXED OSTEOLYTIC–OSTEOGENIC LESIONS

Because bone can respond to disease or injury only by loss of bone or by production of new bone, diseases of different aetiology can appear very similar radiographically. One of the main challenges for the radiologist is to distinguish between neoplasia and infection, although it may be impossible to do this with certainty, and a biopsy, follow-up radiographs or other tests may be required. There may be an equal combination of bone destruction and new bone production, and the mixed nature of the lesion may be obvious; in other cases, one or other process may predominate.

    Ultrasound-guided fine needle aspiration of bone lesions that involve osteolysis is possible and may give a cytological diagnosis (see 1.18).

1. Neoplasia.

    a. Primary malignant bone tumour (Fig. 1.27) – primary malignant bone tumours are usually confined to single bones and rarely cross joints. Eighty per cent are osteosarcoma; also chondrosarcoma, fibrosarcoma and tumours arising from soft tissue elements such as haemangiosarcoma, histiocytic sarcoma and liposarcoma. It is impossible to differentiate

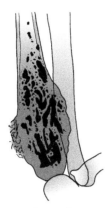

Figure 1.27 Primary malignant bone tumour: osteosarcoma of the distal radius. A mixed osteolytic–proliferative lesion of aggressive appearance.

histological types radiographically. In dogs, osteosarcoma usually arises in long bone metaphyses in larger breeds (especially the proximal humerus and distal radius, the thoracic limb being affected twice as often as the pelvic limb), although any bone including the axial skeleton may be affected by malignancy. Most are endosteal in origin, but periosteal and parosteal osteosarcomas may occur. Affected dogs are usually middle- to old-aged, although a smaller population is affected at 1–2 years of age. Primary malignant bone tumours are usually mixed osteolytic–proliferative and aggressive with a wide transition zone to normal bone, although some lesions may appear almost entirely osteolytic (osteoclastic type) or proliferative (osteoblastic type). New bone production varies from minimal to florid, and in the case of osteosarcoma includes tumour bone as well as reactive bone. High-grade tumours tend to show more cortical destruction and surrounding soft tissue swelling than low-grade tumours. Pathological fracture may occur. Lung metastases are common in most dog breeds, although in small dogs the tumours may be less aggressive and less likely to metastasize. In cats, osteosarcomas tend to be mainly osteolytic and are more often seen in the pelvis and pelvic limb. They are less aggressive in their behaviour than in larger dogs, with a relatively low metastatic rate. Osteosarcomas may occasionally arise at the site of previous

fractures, chronic infection, infarcts or radiation therapy, sometimes years later.

b. Bone metastases – mixed, fairly aggressive lesions, although lysis or sclerosis may predominate strongly and periosteal reaction may be minimal; usually in atypical sites for primary tumours, such as diaphyses; often multiple in one bone or polyostotic. Rarer than in humans; usually from primary tumours of epithelial type such as mammary or prostate. The main differential diagnosis is osteomyelitis, especially where fungal diseases are endemic; sclerotic lesions may mimic panosteitis, although patients with metastases are likely to be older. Scintigraphy using technetium-99m methylene diphosphonate is more sensitive for bone metastases than is radiographic screening.

c. Malignant soft tissue tumour invading bone – osteolysis usually predominates, although there may be some bony reaction or pre-existing osteoarthritis. If arising near a joint, more than one bone may be affected (see 1.18.2, 2.4.7 and Figs 1.23 and 2.4).

d. Neoplastic transformation at the site of a previous fracture – rare but well recognized in humans and animals. Usually several years after internal fixation – postulated causes include the presence of a metallic implant or chronic low-grade infection. Radiographic signs are of an active and aggressive lesion superimposed over obvious previous fracture; differential diagnosis is chronic infection.

e. Benign bone tumours may occasionally show lysis as well as a bony mass (osteoma, osteochondroma) or bone reaction as well as lysis (enchondroma).

2. Infection – bone inflammation and infection (osteomyelitis) generally produces a mixed osteolytic–proliferative bone lesion, although the proportions of bone loss and new bone production vary. The lesions are often hard to differentiate from neoplasia, but soft tissue swelling is often more marked with infection. Small pockets of gas may be seen if gas-producing organisms are present.

a. Bacterial.
    – Solitary lesions in older animals are usually associated with a known wound, surgery, extension from soft tissue

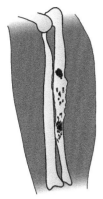

Figure 1.28 Acute osteomyelitis in the ulna of a cat, following a dog bite: a mixed, aggressive lesion with marked surrounding soft tissue swelling. The two focal radiolucent areas are the result of injury caused by the canine teeth of the attacking animal.

infection or a migrating foreign body. In the acute stage, osteomyelitis is a mixed, fairly aggressive lesion but is more likely to show a surrounding sclerotic zone (due to walling off) than is neoplasia (Fig. 1.28). Chronic or resolving osteomyelitis appears less aggressive, and new bone formation may predominate. Sequestrum or involucrum formation is an occasional finding (Fig. 1.29). Pathological fractures are less common than with neoplasia. Osteomyelitis predisposes to delayed or non-union of fractures and causes

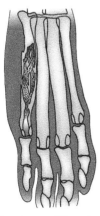

Figure 1.29 Chronic osteomyelitis and sequestrum formation in the metatarsus of a cat, following a cat bite. This lesion is less aggressive in nature and appears partly walled off.

osteolysis around surgical implants. Differential diagnoses are movement of implant, necrosis from high-speed drill, artefact around metallic implants on some digital radiographs.

- Multiple lesions, often bilaterally symmetrical, are seen with haematogenous osteomyelitis, which is more common in young animals. Especially in metaphyses due to sluggish blood flow. Aggressive osteolytic lesions result, with surrounding sclerosis and/or periosteal reaction; pathological fracture may occur. Differential diagnosis is metaphyseal osteopathy (hypertrophic osteodystrophy) in young dogs (see 1.24.4 and 1.24.5 and Figs 1.31 and 1.32).
- A mycetoma is a localized, suppurative, granulomatous, inflammatory lesion with sinus formation, which shows a predilection for skin, subcutis, fascia and bone. Lesions usually develop following traumatic implantation of soil organisms into the tissues. The cause may be bacterial (actinomycotic mycetoma) or fungal (eumycotic mycetoma).

b. Fungal – usually spread haematogenously, producing single or multiple lesions, again often metaphyseal. Usually aggressive, mixed osteolytic–proliferative bone lesions. Main differential diagnosis is metastatic neoplasia, but with fungal infection the patient is more likely to be systemically ill; also consider bacterial osteomyelitis.
  - Coccidioidomycosis* – pyrexia and depression with respiratory, skin, ocular and skeletal lesions; 90% of the bone lesions are in the appendicular skeleton, mainly in the distal ends of long bones.
  - Blastomycosis* – affects mainly large-breed, young male dogs, causing a spectrum of syndromes as above; 30% of dogs have bone involvement, with lesions usually solitary and distal to the elbow or stifle.
  - Aspergillosis* – as well as destructive rhinitis, other aggressive bone lesions (e.g. discospondylitis) and pneumonia have been reported in the German Shepherd dog and immunocompromised patients in areas where other fungal diseases are not endemic (e.g. the UK).

- Histoplasmosis* – various systemic illnesses (mainly gastrointestinal in the dog); rarely causes osteolytic or mixed bone lesions.
  - Cryptococcosis* – usually part of a more generalized disease process, especially in immunosuppressed patients.
  - Mycetoma – see above.
  c. Protozoal – leishmaniasis* – may cause multifocal, often bilateral bone lesions that are mainly diaphyseal periosteal reactions and increased intramedullary radiopacity, especially near the nutrient foramen; another common presentation is erosive or non-erosive joint disease (see 2.4.12).
  d. Cats – feline tuberculosis – various *Mycobacterium* species (rare). Skin and lung lesions predominate but occasionally aggressive mixed bone lesions are seen; also periosteal reactions, discospondylitis and osteoarthritis.
3. Trauma.
  a. Healing fracture – partial bridging of the fracture line with resorption of damaged bone.
  b. Osteomyelitis at a fracture site.
  c. Late neoplastic transformation at a fracture site.
4. Metaphyseal osteopathy (hypertrophic osteodystrophy) – lesions in metaphyses only; differential diagnosis is metaphyseal osteomyelitis (see 1.24.4 and 1.24.5 and Figs 1.31 and 1.32).
5. Multifocal idiopathic pyogranulomatous bone disease – sterile, polyostotic bone disease thought to be part of the group of histiocytic diseases.
6. Canine leucocyte adhesion deficiency (CLAD) (see 1.24.9).

Differentiating malignant bone neoplasia from osteomyelitis

- The degree and extent of osteolysis is usually greater in malignancy, and the cortex is more likely to be breached.
- Pathological fracture is therefore more likely with neoplasia.
- Periosteal new bone formation is much more irregular in neoplasia, with a tendency to form spicules, often radiating out from the centre of the lesion, whereas with osteomyelitis the new bone tends to be more solid and extensive.

- A Codman's triangle of new bone at one end of the lesion is more likely to be associated with neoplasia.
- Sequestrum formation may occur with osteomyelitis but not neoplasia.
- Most primary malignant bone tumours affect only a single bone and rarely cross joints.
- Soft tissue swelling is often more extensive with acute osteomyelitis, and gas bubbles may be seen due to gas-producing organisms.
- The thorax should be radiographed to check for lung metastases if there is a suspicion of neoplasia.
- Ultrasonography may be used to look for abdominal metastases.

1.21 MULTIFOCAL DISEASES

Multifocal diseases may produce more than one lesion in the same bone (monostotic) or may affect multiple bones (polyostotic). For multifocal joint diseases, see 2.7.

Multiple lesions of increased radiopacity (see 1.13)

1. Panosteitis (see 1.13.6 and Fig. 1.17).
2. Sclerotic bone metastases.
3. Haematogenous osteomyelitis, especially fungal.
4. Bone infarcts – rare.
5. Osteopetrosis – rare (see 1.13.15).

Multiple lesions of reduced radiopacity (see 1.18 and 1.19)

6. Osteolytic bone metastases.
7. Disseminated histiocytic sarcoma – especially Rottweilers.
8. Multiple myeloma (plasma cell myeloma) (see 1.18.2 and Fig. 1.24).
9. Enchondromatosis (see 1.19.1).
10. Lymphoma – may occasionally produce multiple or polyostotic osteolytic bone lesions; prone to pathological fracture.
11. Multiple bone cysts (more often single) (see 1.19.2 and Fig. 1.26).
12. Metaphyseal osteopathy (hypertrophic osteodystrophy) – early cases show a

radiolucent metaphyseal band (see 1.24.4 and Fig. 1.31).

13. Metaphyseal osteomyelitis (see 1.24.5 and Fig. 1.32).

14. Disuse osteopenia – seen especially in epiphyses and small bones.

Multiple lesions of mixed radiopacity (see 1.20)

15. Bone metastases.

16. Haematogenous osteomyelitis.

   a. Fungal*.

   b. Bacterial, especially in young animals.

   c. Protozoal – leishmaniasis*.

17. Multifocal idiopathic pyogranulomatous bone disease.

Multiple mineralized or bony masses

18. Multiple cartilaginous exostoses (multiple osteochondromata) (see 1.15.2 and Fig. 1.19).

19. Calcinosis circumscripta – usually single, occasionally multiple; in soft tissues close to but not attached to bone (see 12.2.2 and Fig. 12.1).

20. Synovial osteochondromatosis – masses around joints (see 2.8.18 and Fig. 2.7).

21. Cats – hypervitaminosis A (cats over 2 years old on raw bovine liver diet) – leads to masses around joints; mainly spinal new bone but may also see exostoses near the limb joints, especially the elbow, and on the occipital bone.

1.22 LESIONS AFFECTING EPIPHYSES

See also Chapter 2 for joint diseases in general, Chapter 3 for specific joints and Chapter 5 for vertebral epiphyseal lesions.

Lesions usually affecting single or few epiphyses

1. Fractures (see 1.9 and Fig. 1.10) – usually Salter–Harris growth plate fractures in skeletally immature animals; types III and IV cross the epiphysis, causing disruption to the articular surface with variable displacement of the fragment. In skeletally mature animals, the commonest epiphyseal fracture is the lateral humeral condylar fracture seen especially in Spaniel breeds (see 3.4.17 and Fig. 3.10).

2. Remodelling of epiphyses due to altered stresses following angular limb deformities and traumatic subluxations (e.g. of the distal radial epiphysis following radiocarpal subluxation as a result of premature closure of the distal ulnar growth plate); may be bilateral in giant breeds.

3. Disuse osteopenia (see 1.16.3) – due to fracture or paralysis of a limb; the osteopenia usually affects the distal limb most severely, with loss of bone radiopacity especially in epiphyses and cuboidal bones (e.g. non-union of radial or ulnar fractures in toy breeds of dog, with severe osteopenia in the carpus and distal limb epiphyses). Disuse osteopenia is reversible if the cause is corrected.

4. Giant cell tumour (osteoclastoma) (see 1.19.1 and Fig. 1.25).

5. Irregularity or osteolysis of the articular surface of an epiphysis (see 2.4–2.6).

   a. Osteochondrosis – may be bilateral or in other joints.

   b. Septic arthritis – in multiple joints if of haematogenous origin.

   c. Chronic osteoarthritis – may affect more than one joint depending on the underlying cause.

   d. Soft tissue tumour near a joint.

   e. Avascular necrosis of the femoral head (Legg–Calvé–Perthes disease) – young dogs of Terrier breeds, especially West Highland White Terrier – may affect both hips (see 3.9.4 and Fig. 3.24).

   f. Dysplasia epiphysealis hemimelica – seen in humans as a growth disorder involving preferentially the medial compartment of the lower limbs; epiphyseal hypertrophy and lack of ossification. One case has been described in a Boxer, affecting a medial femoral condyle.

Lesions usually affecting numerous epiphyses

These include diseases that result in epiphyseal dysplasia or dysgenesis, often together with other widespread skeletal defects such as delayed growth plate closure, long bone curvature and dwarfism.

6. Normal skeletal immaturity – endochondral ossification occurs from the centre of epiphyses and apophyses, and in the young animal the

bone surface may appear ragged and irregular due to normal, incomplete ossification (particularly the humeral greater tubercle and femoral condyles); compare with other animals of similar age.

7. Chondrodysplasias (dyschondroplasias) recognized in numerous breeds (e.g. Alaskan Malamute, Australian Shepherd dog**, Beagle, Bedlington Terrier**, Cocker Spaniel, Dachshund, Dobermann**, English Pointer, English Springer Spaniel**, French Bulldog, German Short-haired Pointer, Irish Setter, Japanese Akita, Labrador**, Miniature Poodle, Newfoundland, Norwegian Elkhound, Pyrenean Mountain dog, Saint Bernard, Samoyed**, Scottish Deerhound, Scottish Terrier, Shetland Sheepdog, Swedish Lapphund**; **may be with ocular defects as well. Cats – Domestic Short-hair.

8. Chondrodysplasias are inherited abnormalities of endochondral ossification that produce generalized stippling and fragmentation of epiphyses on radiographs and that lead to secondary osteoarthritis. Clinically, they may mimic rickets but may be seen prior to weaning and in related animals on different diets; radiographically, rickets does not show epiphyseal changes, just physeal widening and long bone bowing. Multiple epiphyseal dysplasia (stippled epiphyses, dysplasia epiphysealis punctata) – inherited deficiency of ossification of epiphyses, apophyses and cuboidal bones; especially Beagle and Miniature Poodle.

9. Congenital hypothyroidism – especially the Boxer. A congenital disease resulting in disproportionate dwarfism; differential diagnosis is chondrodysplasia. Affected dogs suffer from epiphyseal dysgenesis leading to secondary osteoarthritis, delayed growth plate closure and shortened, bowed limbs. Facial and spinal changes are also seen (see 5.3.11).

10. Pituitary dwarfism – some cases show epiphyseal dysplasia, although this may be due to concurrent hypothyroidism.

11. Mucopolysaccharidosis types I, VI and VII – especially cats with Siamese ancestry; facial and spinal lesions with varying degrees of epiphyseal dysplasia and secondary osteoarthritis, especially in the shoulders and hips (see 5.4.9). Rarely occurs in dogs, but

mucopolysaccharidosis type I (Plott Hound) and II (Pointers) are reported to cause epiphyseal dysplasia and periarticular bony proliferations and type VII to affect vertebral epiphyses.

12. Cats – mucolipidosis type II – rare; less severe epiphyseal lesions reported.

1.23 LESIONS AFFECTING PHYSES

Loss of physeal line

1. Poor positioning, so the growth plate is not parallel to the X-ray beam.
2. Premature closure of the growth plate due to trauma.
   a. Salter–Harris type V crushing injury – probably responsible for 'idiopathic' premature closure of the distal ulnar growth plate in giant breeds; may be bilateral (see 3.5.4 and Fig. 3.13).
   b. Bridging of the margin of a growth plate due to superimposed periosteal new bone; may be seen with metaphyseal osteopathy (hypertrophic osteodystrophy; see 1.24.4 and Fig. 1.31).

Widening of physeal lines: single

3. Salter–Harris type I fracture with displacement (see 1.9.11 and Fig. 1.10).
4. Infection (physitis) – although haematogenous osteomyelitis more often occurs in metaphyses due to sluggish blood flow in these areas. May be associated with a portosystemic shunt. Vertebral physitis is recognized in younger dogs, affecting caudal lumbar physes.

Widening of physeal lines: generalized

Affected animals are often stunted and may also have epiphyseal dysplasia leading to secondary osteoarthritis. Physeal lesions are often most severe in the distal radius and ulna due to the normally rapid growth rate at these sites.

5. Chondrodysplasias – variable effects on growth plates, with widening, ragged margination and delayed closure in some affected animals. Often initially misdiagnosed as rickets.
6. Congenital hypothyroidism – wide and irregular growth plates with delayed closure, particularly in the spine (see 5.3.11); especially the Boxer.

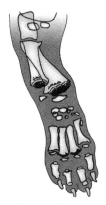

Figure 1.30 Rickets: thoracic limb of a young puppy, showing changes especially in the distal radial and ulnar growth plates.

7. Pituitary dwarfism – some cases may show wide and irregular growth plates with delayed closure, perhaps due to concomitant hypothyroidism.
8. Rickets (juvenile osteomalacia) (Fig. 1.30).
   a. Now rare, due to a dietary deficiency of phosphorus or vitamin D and seen after weaning.
   b. Hypovitaminosis D due to failure to absorb vitamin D (e.g. extrahepatic biliary atresia or common bile duct obstruction in young animals).
   c. Hypovitaminosis D due to failure to metabolize vitamin D – vitamin D-dependent rickets types I and II are due to gene mutations leading to errors of vitamin D metabolism.
   d. Renal dysplasia preventing final hydroxylation pathway to create active metabolite.
   Physes are wide transversely and longitudinally due to failure of ossification and accumulation of unmineralized osteoid; metaphyses flare laterally and show beaked margins due to continued periosteal bone growth. Long bones are shortened and may be bowed, leading to stunting; osteopenia may be present due to concomitant nutritional secondary hyperparathyroidism. Unlike hereditary chondrodysplasias, the epiphyses are normal.
9. Infection – haematogenous physitis may affect more than one growth plate.
10. Copper deficiency.

Masses arising at physes

11. Osteochondroma (single) or multiple cartilaginous exostoses (multiple) – arise at osteochondral junctions in young dogs, so are often seen protruding from the site of previous growth plates (see 1.15.2 and Fig. 1.19).

1.24 LESIONS AFFECTING METAPHYSES

1. Normal cut-back zone – area of cortical remodelling adjacent to the physis in young dogs, which results in an irregular bone surface (see 1.3 and Fig. 1.1A).
2. Neoplasia.
   a. Primary malignant bone tumours (e.g. osteosarcoma) – the long bone metaphyses are a strong predilection site, especially the proximal humerus and distal radius in giant dog breeds (see 1.20.1 and Fig. 1.27).
   b. Osteochondroma (single) or multiple cartilaginous exostoses (multiple) – in young dogs, arising at osteochondral junctions and therefore often protruding from the metaphyses (see 1.15.2 and Fig. 1.19).
   c. Enchondromatosis – persistent segments of physeal cartilage are displaced through metaphyses into diaphyses, producing multiple, expansile, osteolytic lesions that may undergo pathological fracture (see 1.19.1).
3. Retained cartilaginous cores – retention of physeal cartilage in metaphyses due to incomplete endochondral ossification, producing conical or candle flame-shaped radiolucent areas with fine, sclerotic margins in the distal ulnar metaphyses (occasionally the distal radius or femur). Giant breeds, often bilateral; may coexist with retarded growth or premature closure of the distal ulnar growth plate, but a causal relationship is not certain (see 3.5.3 and Fig. 3.12).
4. Metaphyseal osteopathy (syn. hypertrophic osteodystrophy (MOD), skeletal scurvy, Möller–Barlow's disease) (Fig. 1.31A and B) – skeletally immature (usually 2–8 months old) dogs of larger breeds, with a higher incidence in the German Shepherd dog, Irish Setter, Weimaraner, Great Dane and Chesapeake Bay Retriever; male preponderance in some

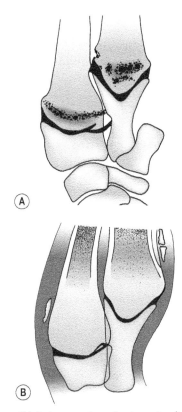

(A)

(B)

Figure 1.31 (A) Early metaphyseal osteopathy (hypertrophic osteodystrophy): a mottled band of radiolucency in the metaphysis parallel to the growth plate. (B) Late metaphyseal osteopathy (hypertrophic osteodystrophy): the metaphyses are surrounded by successive layers of periosteal and paraperiosteal new bone, the deeper layers becoming remodelled into the cortex. Superimposition of new bone creates a sclerotic appearance.

reports. The aetiology is unknown, but the disease can be associated with a high plane of nutrition. Pain, heat and swelling are found at metaphyses; the patient is depressed, febrile and anorexic, but the condition is usually self-limiting. Radiography shows a radiolucent band ± narrow sclerotic margins, or a mottled band, crossing metaphyses parallel to but not involving the growth plate (note: the normal periphery of the conical distal ulnar growth plate should not be mistaken for a transverse radiolucent band). Later, subperiosteal haemorrhages provoke collars of mineralization and paraperiosteal new bone that may become large and deforming. The distal radius and ulna are most severely

affected. Differential diagnoses are metaphyseal osteomyelitis, normal cut-back zone in large dogs (areas of ill-defined cortical irregularity due to remodelling of bone), unusual manifestation of craniomandibular osteopathy, canine leucocyte adhesion disorder; lead poisoning if the band appears mainly sclerotic.

5. Infection – usually produces metaphyseal lesions if the infection is spread haematogenously, especially in young animals due to sluggish blood flow at these sites; likely to be multifocal and often bilaterally symmetrical.
   a. Bacterial – metaphyseal osteomyelitis (Fig. 1.32) is an unusual condition in young dogs with aggressive, osteolytic metaphyseal lesions that may undergo pathological fracture; definitive diagnosis requires blood culture; differential diagnosis is metaphyseal osteopathy (hypertrophic osteodystrophy).
   b. Fungal* – aggressive, usually mixed lesions.
6. Bone cysts – often metaphyseal (see 1.19.2 and Fig. 1.26).
7. Chondrodysplasias, rickets and other growth abnormalities (see 1.12) – often metaphyses are widened due to abnormal endochondral ossification at the growth plate.
8. Distal ulnar and/or radial metaphyseal changes have been described as an incidental finding in young Newfoundland dogs in Norway (see 3.5.11).

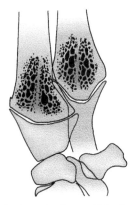

Figure 1.32 Metaphyseal osteomyelitis: the osteolysis is more diffuse and aggressive than with metaphyseal osteopathy.

9. Canine leucocyte adhesion deficiency – an inherited disease in the Irish Setter causing osteolytic or mixed osteolytic–proliferative lesions in metaphyses, especially the distal radius and ulna, and skull changes similar to craniomandibular osteopathy; clinical signs include gingivitis, lameness, mandibular swelling and lymphadenopathy.
10. Craniomandibular osteopathy – rarely see additional masses of paraperiosteal new bone adjacent to distal ulnar metaphyses; may mimic metaphyseal osteopathy (hypertrophic osteodystrophy) (see 3.5.14, 4.10.1 and Figs 3.14 and 4.6).
11. Lead poisoning – rarely see radiographic lesions; thin, transverse sclerotic bands in metaphyses.

1.25 LESIONS AFFECTING DIAPHYSES

Conditions that are mainly seen in diaphyses are listed in this section, although some of these lesions may also produce changes in other parts of the skeleton.

Thinning of cortices

1. Osteopenia – various causes (see 1.16). Also results in reduced bone radiopacity, coarse trabecular pattern and folding fractures.
2. Expansile lesion within medullary cavity, for example bone cyst, giant cell tumour, enchondroma (see 1.19 and Figs 1.25 and 1.26). The cortex is displaced outwards and is smoothly thinned but may not be interrupted.
3. Osteolytic lesions (e.g. neoplasia, osteomyelitis). The cortex is irregularly thinned and often interrupted.
4. Pressure atrophy – a smoothly bordered area of superficial bone loss due to pressure from an adjacent mass (e.g. rib tumour, mass between digits).
5. Convex side of a bowed long bone.
6. Atrophic non-union of a fracture.

Thickening of cortices

7. Remodelling periosteal reaction – numerous causes (see 1.14).

8. Hypertrophic osteopathy (Marie's disease; see 1.14.6 and Fig. 1.18) – a specific cause of periosteal reaction.
9. Healing fracture.
10. Chronic osteomyelitis and involucrum formation.
11. Leishmaniasis* – periosteal and intramedullary bone proliferation in diaphyses and flat bones provoked by chronic osteomyelitis; increased medullary radiopacity often near the nutrient foramina. Erosive and non-erosive polyarthritis are also seen.
12. Concave side of bowed long bone in response to increased load.
13. Congenital hypothyroidism – especially Boxers; shortened, bowed radius and ulna with thickened cortices and increased medullary radiopacity (see 5.3.11).
14. Osteopetrosis and certain myeloproliferative disorders – rare (see 1.13.15).

Interruption of cortices

15. Fracture.
16. Neoplasia.
17. Osteomyelitis.
18. Large expansile lesion.
19. Biopsy site.
20. Site of drill hole or implant removal.

Radiolucent lines in diaphyses

21. Artefacts
    a. Overlying skin defect.
    b. Overlying fat or gas in fascial planes.
    c. Mach effect from other superimposed bones.
22. Nutrient foramen – location usually known anatomically; compare with the opposite limb if in doubt.
23. Fissure fractures.

Sclerotic lines in diaphyses (see 1.13)

24. Growth arrest lines.
25. Panosteitis.
26. Fractures – if impaction of bone or overlapping of fragments occurs, a sclerotic band rather than a bone defect may be seen.
    a. Folding fractures.

- Greenstick fractures (single cortex) in young animals.
- Osteopenia, especially due to nutritional secondary hyperparathyroidism.

b. Compression or impaction fractures – especially vertebrae.

c. Superimposition of overridden fragments seen on one radiographic projection but shown to be displaced using the orthogonal view.

d. Healing fracture.

Osteolytic areas in diaphyses (see 1.18 and 1.19)

27. Neoplasia.

a. Bone metastases – may be predominantly osteolytic; often multiple in one bone or polyostotic.

b. Multiple myeloma (plasma cell myeloma) – usually multiple, discrete osteolytic lesions affecting more than one bone.

c. Malignant soft tissue tumour invading bone – osteolysis usually predominates.

d. Osteolytic primary bone tumour extending into the diaphysis or in an atypical location (usually they are metaphyseal).

e. Lymphoma.

28. Infection – mixed lesions are more common than purely osteolytic lesions, although a bone abscess (rare) may appear as a well-defined radiolucent area with a sclerotic margin.

29. Bone cysts – discrete, expansile lesions; rare.

30. Enchondromatosis – discrete, expansile lesions; rare.

Sclerotic areas in diaphyses (see 1.13)

31. Neoplasia.

a. Bone metastases – may be predominantly sclerotic; often multiple in one bone or polyostotic.

b. Osteoproductive primary bone tumour extending into the diaphysis or in an atypical location (usually they are metaphyseal).

c. Certain myeloproliferative disorders.

d. Lymphoma – may rarely cause medullary osteosclerosis.

e. Cats – feline leukaemia-induced medullary osteosclerosis – rare; likely to be widespread in the skeleton.

32. Osteomyelitis – haematogenous osteomyelitis may produce ill-defined patches of sclerosis.

33. Panosteitis.

34. Healing fractures.

35. Bone infarcts.

36. Osteopetrosis – rare; affects the whole skeleton but is most obvious radiographically in the diaphyses.

Mixed osteolytic–osteogenic lesions in diaphyses (see 1.20)

37. Neoplasia.

a. Bone metastases – may be mixed lesions, although they are often predominantly osteolytic or sclerotic; often multiple in one bone or polyostotic.

b. Malignant soft tissue tumour invading bone.

c. Neoplastic transformation at the site of a previous fracture.

d. Mixed primary bone tumour in an atypical location (usually they are metaphyseal).

38. Infection.

39. Trauma.

a. Healing fracture.

b. Infected fracture.

c. Neoplastic transformation at the site of a previous fracture.

Altered shape of diaphyses (see 1.10)

Further reading

General

Papageorges, M., 1991. How the Mach phenomenon and shape affect the radiographic appearance of skeletal structures. Vet. Radiol. 32, 191–195.

Papageorges, M., Sande, R.D., 1990. The Mach phenomenon. Vet. Radiol. 32, 191–195.

Thompson, K., 2007. Bones and joints. In: Maxie, M.G. (Ed.), Jubb, Kennedy and Palmer's Pathology of Domestic Animals, fifth ed, vol. 1. Saunders, New York.

Weinstein, J.M., Mongil, C.M., Rhodes, W.H., Smith, G.K., 1995. Orthopedic conditions of the Rottweiler – Part II. Compend. Contin. Educ. Pract. Veterinarian (Small Animal) 17, 925–938.

Weinstein, J.M., Mongil, C.M., Smith, G.K., 1995. Orthopedic conditions of the Rottweiler – Part I. Compend. Contin. Educ. Pract. Veterinarian (Small Animal) 17, 813–830.

Skeletal ultrasonography

Britt, T., Clifford, C., Barger, A., Moroff, K., Drobatz, K., Thacher, G., Davis, G., 2007. Diagnosing appendicular osteosarcoma with ultrasound-guided fine-needle aspiration: 36 cases. J. Small Anim. Pract. 48, 145–150.

Kramer, M., Gerwing, M., Hach, V., Schimke, E., 1997. Sonography of the musculoskeletal system in dogs and cats. Vet. Radiol. Ultrasound 38, 139–149.

Risselada, M., Karmer, M., de Rooster, O., Taeymans, O., Verleyen, H., van Bree, H., 2005. Ultrasonographic and radiographic assessment of uncomplicated secondary fracture healing of long bones in dogs and cats. Vet. Surg. 34, 9–107.

Samii, V.F., Nyland, T.G., Werner, L. L., Baker, T.W., 1999. Ultrasound-guided fine-needle aspiration biopsy of bone lesion: a preliminary report. Vet. Radiol. Ultrasound 40, 82–86.

Normal anatomy, normal variants and artefacts

Fagin, B.D., Aronson, E., Gutzmer, M.A., 1992. Closure of the iliac crest ossification centre of dogs. J. Am. Vet. Med. Assoc. 200, 1709.

Root, M.V., Johnston, S.D., Olson, P. N., 1997. The effect of prepubertal and postpubertal gonadectomy on radial physeal closure in male and female domestic cats. Vet. Radiol. Ultrasound 38, 42–47.

Congenital and developmental diseases; diseases of young animals

Campbell, B.G., Wootton, J.A.M., Krook, J., DeMarco, J., Minor, R. R., 1997. Clinical signs and diagnosis of osteogenesis imperfecta in three dogs. J. Am. Vet. Med. Assoc. 211, 183–187.

Demko, J., McLaughlin, R., 2005. Developmental orthopedic disease. Vet. Clin. North Am. Small Anim. Pract. 35, 1111–1135.

Konde, L.J., Thrall, M.A., Gasper, P., Dial, S.M., McBiles, K., Colgan, S., Haskins, M., 1987. Radiographically visualized skeletal changes associated with mucopolysaccharidosis VI in cats. Vet. Radiol. 28, 223–228.

Muir, P., Dubielzig, R.R., Johnson, K.A., 1996. Panosteitis. Compend. Contin. Educ. Pract. Veterinarian (Small Animal) 18, 29–33.

Muir, P., Dubielzig, R.R., Johnson, D.G., Shelton, D.G., 1996. Hypertrophic osteodystrophy and calvarial hyperostosis. Compend. Contin. Educ. Pract. Veterinarian (Small Animal) 18, 143–151.

Rørvik, A.M., Tiege, J., Ottesen, N., Lingaas, F., 2008. Clinical, radiographic, and pathologic abnormalities in dogs with multiple epiphyseal dysplasia: 19 cases (1991–2005). J. Am. Vet. Med. Assoc. 233, 600–606.

Scott, H., 1998. Non-traumatic causes of lameness in the forelimb of the growing dog. In Pract. 20, 539–554.

Scott, H., 1999. Non-traumatic causes of lameness in the hindlimb of the growing dog. In Pract. 21, 176–188.

Trowald-Wigh, G., Ekman, S., Hansson, A., Hedhammar, A., Hard af Segerstad, C., 2000. Clinical, radiological and pathological features of 12 Irish Setters with canine leucocyte adhesion deficiency. J. Small Anim. Pract. 41, 211–217.

Metabolic bone disease (some overlap with above)

Allan, G.S., Huxtable, C.R.R., Howlett, C.R., Baxter, R.C., Duff, B.R.H., Farrow, B.R.H., 1978. Pituitary dwarfism in German Shepherd dogs. J. Small Anim. Pract. 19, 711–729.

Buckley, J.C., 1984. Pathophysiologic considerations of osteopenia. Compend. Contin. Educ. Pract. Veterinarian (Small Animal) 6, 552–562.

Dennis, R., 1989. Radiology of metabolic bone disease. Vet. Ann. 29, 195–206.

Dunn, M.E., Blond, L., Letard, D., DiFruscia, R., 2007. Hypertrophic osteopathy associated with infective endocarditis in an adult boxer dog. J. Small Anim. Pract. 48, 99–103.

Godfrey, D.R., Anderson, R.M., Barber, P.J., Hewison, M., 2005. Vitamin D-dependent rickets type II in a cat. J. Small Anim. Pract. 46, 440–444.

Johnson, K.A., Church, D.B., Barton, R.J., Wood, A.K.W., 1988. Vitamin D-dependent rickets in a Saint Bernard dog. J. Small Anim. Pract. 29, 657–666.

Konde, L.J., Thrall, M.A., Gasper, P., Dial, S.M., McBiles, K., Colgan, S., Haskins, M., 1987. Radiographically visualized skeletal changes associated with mucopolysaccharidosis VI in cats. Vet. Radiol. 28, 223–228.

Lamb, C.R., 1990. The double cortical line: a sign of osteopenia. J. Small Anim. Pract. 31, 189–192.

Saunders, H.M., Jezyk, P.K., 1991. The radiographic appearance of canine congenital hypothyroidism: skeletal changes with delayed treatment. Vet. Radiol. 32, 171–177.

Tanner, E., Langley-Hobbs, S.J., 2005. Vitamin D-dependent rickets type 2 with characteristic radiographic changes in a 4-month-old kitten. J. Feline Med. Surg. 7, 307–311.

Tomsa, K., Glaus, T., Hauser, B., Flueckiger, M., Arnold, P., Wess, C., Reusch, C., 1999. Nutritional secondary hyperparathyroidism in six cats. J. Small Anim. Pract. 40, 533–539.

Infective and inflammatory conditions

Agut, A., Corzo, N., Murciano, J., Laredo, F.G., Soler, M., 2003. Clinical and radiographic study of bone and joint lesions in 26 dogs with leishmaniasis. Vet. Rec. 153, 648–652.

Canfield, P.J., Malik, R., Davis, P.E., Martin, P., 1994. Multifocal idiopathic pyogranulomatous bone disease in a dog. J. Small Anim. Pract. 35, 370–373.

Dunn, J.K., Dennis, R., Houlton, J.E.F., 1992. Successful treatment of two cases of metaphyseal osteomyelitis in the dog. J. Small Anim. Pract. 33, 85–89.

Macintire, D.K., Vincent-Johnson, N., Dillon, A.R., Blagburn, B., Lindsay, E.M., Whitley, E.M., Banfield, C., 1997. Hepatozoonosis in dogs: 22 cases (1989–1994). J. Am. Vet. Med. Assoc. 210, 916–922.

Stead, A.C., 1984. Osteomyelitis in the dog and cat. J. Small Anim. Pract. 25, 1–13.

Turrel, J.M., Pool, R.R., 1982. Bone lesions in four dogs with visceral leishmaniasis. Vet. Radiol. 23, 243–249.

Neoplasia

Blackwood, L., 1999. Bone tumours in small animals. In Pract. 21, 31–37.

Dubielzig, R.R., Biery, D.N., Brodey, R.S., 1981. Bone sarcomas associated with multifocal medullary bone infarction in dogs. J. Am. Vet. Med. Assoc. 179, 64–68.

Gibbs, C., Denny, H.R., Kelly, D.F., 1984. The radiological features of osteosarcoma of the appendicular skeleton of dogs: a review of 74 cases. J. Small Anim. Pract. 25, 177–192.

Gibbs, C., Denny, H.R., Lucke, V.M., 1985. The radiological features of non-osteogenic malignant tumours of bone in the appendicular skeleton of the dog: a review of 34 cases. J. Small Anim. Pract. 26, 537–553.

Gorra, M., Burk, R.L., Greenlee, P., Weeren, F.R., 2002. Osteoid osteoma in a dog. Vet. Radiol. Ultrasound 43, 28–30.

Jacobson, L.S., Kirberger, R.M., 1996. Canine multiple cartilaginous exostoses: unusual manifestations and a review of the literature. J. Am. Anim. Hosp. Assoc. 32, 45–51.

Lamb, C.R., Berg, J., Schelling, S.H., 1993. Radiographic diagnosis of an expansile bone lesion in a dog. J. Small Anim. Pract. 34, 239–241.

Matis, U., Krauser, K., Schwartz-Porsche, A.V., Putzer-Brenig, A. V., 1989. Multiple enchondromatosis in the dog. Vet. Com. Orthop. Traumatol. 4, 144–151.

Russel, R.G., Walker, M., 1983. Metastatic and invasive tumors of bone in dogs and cats. Vet. Clin. North Am. 13, 163–180.

Schrader, S.C., Burk, R.L., Lin, S., 1983. Bone cysts in two dogs and a review of similar cystic bone lesions in the dog. J Am Vet Med Assoc 182, 490–495.

Schultz, R.M., Puchalski, S.M., Kent, P.F., Moore, P.F., 2007. Skeletal lesions of histiocytic sarcoma in nineteen dogs. Vet. Radiol. Ultrasound 48, 539–543.

Turrel, J.M., Pool, R.R., 1982. Primary bone tumors in the cat: a retrospective study of 15 cats and a literature review. Vet. Radiol. 23, 152–166.

Wrigley, R.H., 2000. Malignant versus nonmalignant bone disease. Vet. Clin. North Am. Small Anim. Pract. 30, 315–348.

Trauma

Anderson, M.A., Dee, L.G., Dee, J.F., 1995. Fractures and dislocations of the racing greyhound – Part I. Compend. Contin. Educ. Pract. Veterinarian (Small Animal) 17, 779–786.

Anderson, M.A., Dee, L.G., Dee, J.F., 1995. Fractures and dislocations of the racing greyhound – Part II. Compend. Contin. Educ. Pract. Veterinarian (Small Animal) 17, 899–909.

Langley-Hobbs, S., 2003. Biology and radiological assessment of fracture healing. In Pract. 25, 26–35.

Sande, R., 1999. Radiography of orthopaedic trauma and fracture repair. Vet. Clin. North Am. Small Anim. Pract. 29, 1247–1260.

Miscellaneous

Baines, E., 2006. Clinically significant developmental radiological changes in the skeletally immature dog: 1. Long bones. In Pract. 28, 188–199.

Canfield, P.J., Malik, R., Davis, P.E., Martin, P., 1994. Multifocal idiopathic pyogranulomatous bone disease in a dog. J. Small Anim. Pract. 35, 370–373.

Hanel, R.M., Graham, J.P., Levy, J.K., Buergelt, C.D., Creamer, J., 2004. Generalized osteosclerosis in a cat. Vet. Radiol. Ultrasound 45, 318–324.

Hay, C.W., Dueland, R.T., Dubielzig, R.R., Bjorenson, J.E., 1999. Idiopathic multifocal osteopathy in four Scottish terriers (1991–1996). J. Am. Anim. Hosp. Assoc. 35, 62–67.

Kramers, P., Flueckiger, M.A., Rahn, B.A., Cordey, J., 1988. Osteopetrosis in cats. J. Small Anim. Pract. 29, 153–164.

Morgan, J.P., Stavenborn, M., 1991. Disseminated idiopathic skeletal hyperostosis (DISH) in a dog. Vet. Radiol. 32, 65–70.

O'Brien, S.E., Riedesel, E.A., Miller, L.D., 1987. Osteopetrosis in an adult dog. J. Am. Anim. Hosp. Assoc. 23, 213–216.

Wright, M.W., Hudson, J.S.A., Hathcock, J.T., 2003. Osteopetrosis in cats: clarification of a misnomer. Vet. Radiol. Ultrasound 44, 106 (abstract).

Chapter 2

Joints

CHAPTER CONTENTS

2.1 Radiography of joints: technique and interpretation 39
2.2 Soft tissue changes associated with joints 41
2.3 Altered width of joint space 42
2.4 Osteolytic (erosive) joint disease 42
2.5 Proliferative joint disease 44
2.6 Mixed osteolytic–proliferative joint disease 45
2.7 Conditions that may affect more than one joint 45
2.8 Mineralization in or near joints 46

2.1 RADIOGRAPHY OF JOINTS: TECHNIQUE AND INTERPRETATION

Technique

Lesions in joints may be radiographically subtle, and so attention to good radiographic technique is essential.

1. Highest definition film–screen combination consistent with the thickness of the area or appropriate digital radiography algorithm.
2. No grid is necessary except for the shoulder and hip joints in large dogs.
3. Accurate positioning and centring, with a small object–film distance to minimize geometric distortion and blurring due to the penumbra effect.
4. Straight radiographs in two planes are usually required (i.e. orthogonal views), with oblique views as necessary.
5. Close collimation to enhance radiographic definition by minimizing scatter, and for radiation safety.
6. Correct exposure factors to allow examination of soft tissues as well as bone.
7. Beware of hair coat debris creating artefactual shadows.
8. Radiograph the opposite joint for comparison if necessary.
9. Use of stressed views (traction, rotation, sheer, hyperextension/flexion and fulcrum-assisted) and weight-bearing or simulated weight-bearing views for the detection of subluxation and altered joint width – great care with radiation safety is needed if the

patient is manually restrained. The vacuum phenomenon may occur with traction views of the shoulder, hip and spine (see 2.2.13).

10. For analogue film, ensure good processing technique to optimize contrast and definition.

Arthrography (negative, positive, double contrast)

Indications
Detection of the extent of the joint capsule or of rupture of the joint capsule; examination of the bicipital tendon sheath (shoulder joint); assessment of cartilage thickness and flap formation; detection of synovial masses and intra-articular filling defects such as radiolucent joint 'mice'; to see if a mineralized body is intra-articular. Most often performed in the shoulder joint.

Preparation
General anaesthesia; survey radiographs; sterile preparation of the injection site.

Technique (shoulder)
Insert a 20- to 22-gauge short-bevel needle 1 cm distal to the acromion and direct it caudally, distally and medially into the joint space. Joint fluid may flow freely or require aspiration; obtain a sample for laboratory analysis.

- Positive contrast arthrogram – inject 2–7 mL of 100–150 mg I/mL isotonic iodinated contrast medium (e.g. a non-ionic medium such as iohexol) depending on the patient size, withdraw the needle and apply pressure to the injection site; manipulate the joint gently to ensure even contrast medium distribution; take mediolateral, caudocranial and cranioproximal–craniodistal (skyline) radiographs. Use lower volumes for assessment of the joint space only and higher volumes for the biceps tendon sheath.
- Negative contrast arthrogram – use air.
- Double-contrast arthrogram – use a small volume of positive contrast medium followed by air.

Technical errors on arthrography
Contrast medium not entering the joint space but injected into surrounding soft tissues; insufficient or too much contrast medium used; gas bubbles mimicking radiolucent joint mice.

Interpretation of joint radiographs
1. Use optimum viewing conditions – for analogue films a darkened room, bright light and dimmer facility, magnifying glass, glare around periphery of film masked off.
2. With digital images, manipulation of greyscale and size is readily performed but beware of digital artefacts.
3. Compare with the contralateral joint and use radiographic atlases and bone specimens.
4. Consider patient signalment and associated clinical and laboratory findings.

Assess the following.
5. Number of joints affected (e.g. single – trauma, sepsis or neoplasia; bilateral – osteochondrosis, bilateral trauma; multiple – systemic or immune-mediated disease).
6. Alignment of bones forming the joint; examine bones and joints proximally and distally.
7. Epiphyseal shape and joint space congruity.
8. Joint space width (changes reliable only if severe or if weight-bearing views obtained).
9. Articular surface contour – remodelling, erosion.
10. Subchondral bone opacity – sclerosis, erosion, cyst formation, osteopenia.
11. Joint space opacity – gas, fat, mineralization, foreign material.
12. Presence of osteoarthrosis (see 2.5 and Fig. 2.6).
13. Soft tissue changes (may be more obvious radiographically than clinically).
    a. Increased soft tissue – concept of 'synovial mass', as synovial tissue and synovial fluid cannot be differentiated on survey radiographs.
    b. Reduced soft tissue – muscle wastage due to disuse (especially in the thighs).
14. Other articular and periarticular changes.
    a. Intra- and periarticular mineralization (see 2.8).
    b. Joint mice (apparently loose, mineralized articular bodies, although they may in fact be attached to soft tissue).
    c. Intra-articular fat pads reduced by synovial effusion.
    d. Fascial planes and sesamoids displaced by effusions and soft tissue swelling.
    e. Periarticular chip and avulsion fractures.
    f. Periarticular osteolysis.
    g. Periarticular new bone other than due to osteoarthrosis.

2.2 SOFT TISSUE CHANGES ASSOCIATED WITH JOINTS

Soft tissue swelling

Differentiation between joint effusion and surrounding soft tissue swelling may not be possible except in the stifle joint, but both are often present. A joint effusion will compress or displace any intra-articular fat and adjacent fascial planes and is limited in extent by the joint capsule; the effusion may be visible only when the radiograph is examined using a bright light. Periarticular swelling may be more extensive and will obliterate fascial planes. Occasionally, arthrography may reveal soft tissue pathology even when survey radiographs are normal, for example in synovial sarcoma or villonodular synovitis.

1. Joint effusion or soft tissue swelling (Fig. 2.1).
   a. External trauma.
   b. Damage to an intra-articular structure such as a cruciate ligament or meniscus.
   c. Early osteochondrosis confined to cartilage; medial coronoid disease.
   d. Early septic arthritis.
   e. Systemic lupus erythematosus (SLE) – usually multiple joints, symmetrical.
   f. Early rheumatoid arthritis (canine idiopathic erosive polyarthritis – see 2.4.8 and Fig. 2.5).
   g. Ehrlichiosis*.
   h. Lyme disease* (*Borrelia burgdorferi* infection).
   i. Polyarthritis–polymyositis syndrome, especially Spaniel breeds.
   j. Polyarthritis–meningitis syndrome – Weimaraner, German Short-haired Pointer, Boxer, Bernese Mountain dog, Japanese Akita, also cats.
   k. Heritable polyarthritis of the adolescent Japanese Akita.
   l. Polyarteritis nodosa – stiff Beagle disease.
   m. Drug-induced polyarthritis, especially certain antibiotics (e.g. fluoroquinolones such as enrofloxacin).
   n. Immune-mediated vaccine reactions.
   o. Other idiopathic polyarthritides.
   p. Chinese Shar Pei fever syndrome – short-lived episodes of acute pyrexia and lameness with mono- or pauciarticular joint pain and swelling of the tarsi and carpi; occasionally enthesiopathies.
2. Recent haemarthrosis.
   a. Trauma.
   b. Coagulopathy.
3. Joint capsule thickening.
4. Periarticular oedema, haematoma, cellulitis, abscess, fibrosis.
5. Soft tissue tumour.
6. Synovial cysts – herniation of joint capsule, bursa or tendon sheath. Infrequent, and usually associated with degenerative joint changes. In cats, described only at the elbow.
7. Soft tissue callus – large dogs, especially elbows.
8. Villonodular synovitis – often bone erosion at the chondrosynovial junction too.
9. Cats – various erosive and non-erosive feline polyarthritides; the latter showing soft tissue swelling only.

Gas in joints

10. Fat mistaken for gas.
11. Superimposed skin defect.
12. Post arthrocentesis.
13. Vacuum phenomenon – seen in humans in joints under traction, when gas (mainly nitrogen) diffuses out from extracellular fluid. In dogs, reported only in the shoulder, hip, intervertebral disc spaces and intersternebral or sternocostal spaces and only in the presence of joint disease (e.g. shoulder osteochondrosis, degenerative joint disease and chronic disc disease).
14. Open wound communicating with the joint.
15. Infection with gas-producing bacteria.

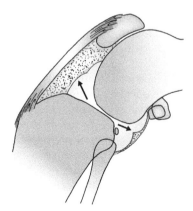

Figure 2.1 Joint effusion: stifle. The effusion is seen as a soft tissue radiopacity compressing the patellar fat pad and displacing fascial planes caudal to the joint (arrows).

2.3 ALTERED WIDTH OF JOINT SPACE

Decreased joint space width

1. Artefactual – X-ray beam not centred over the joint space, or joint space not parallel to X-ray beam.
2. Artefactual – flexed joint in craniocaudal or caudocranial view.
3. Articular cartilage erosion due to severe, chronic degenerative joint disease.
4. Articular cartilage erosion due to rheumatoid disease; usually multiple joints (see 2.4.8 and Fig. 2.5).
5. Periarticular fibrosis.
6. Advanced septic arthritis with erosion of articular cartilage and collapse of subchondral bone (see 2.4.6 and Fig. 2.3).
7. Cats – arthropathy is seen in some cases of acromegaly (growth hormone-secreting pituitary tumour). Cartilage hypertrophy and hyperplasia lead to osteoarthrosis. In early cases, the joint space may be widened due to cartilage thickening, but in later stages the joint space collapses.

Increased joint space width

8. Traction during radiography.
9. Skeletal immaturity and incomplete epiphyseal ossification.
10. Severe joint effusion.
11. Recent haemarthrosis.
12. Subluxation.
13. Intra-articular soft tissue mass.
14. Intra-articular pathology causing subchondral osteolysis (e.g. osteochondrosis, septic arthritis, soft tissue tumour, rheumatoid arthritis).
15. Various epiphyseal dysplasias (see 1.22.7–12).
16. Cats – early acromegalic arthropathy (see above).

Asymmetric joint space width

17. Normal variant in some joints, dependent on positioning (e.g. caudocranial views of the shoulder and stifle).
18. Congenital subluxation or dysplasia.
19. Collateral ligament rupture (Fig. 2.2) – stressed views may be required to demonstrate subluxation.

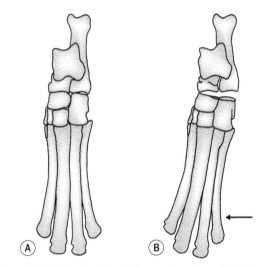

Figure 2.2 Lateral collateral ligament rupture of the tarsus: (A) the unstressed dorsoplantar view appears normal; (B) subluxation of the intertarsal joint space caused by laterally applied stress.

20. Asymmetric narrowing or widening of the joint space due to other pathology – see above.

2.4 OSTEOLYTIC (EROSIVE) JOINT DISEASE

1. Apparent osteolysis due to incomplete epiphyseal ossification in the young animal.
2. Apparent osteolysis due to abnormalities of ossification (see epiphyseal dysplasias, 1.22.7–12).
3. Artefactual in cases of severe osteoarthrosis, when superimposition of irregular amounts of new bone creates areas of relative lucency, mimicking osteolysis. Diagnosis of neoplasia or sepsis superimposed over osteoarthrosis may be very difficult radiographically.
4. Osteochondrosis – focal subchondral lucencies at specific locations, mainly the shoulder, elbow, stifle and tarsus in young, larger breed dogs; often bilateral. There is a male preponderance, and affected dogs are often rapidly growing and on a high plane of nutrition. Also see joint effusion ± mineralized cartilage flap, fragmentation of subchondral bone, joint mice, subchondral sclerosis, secondary osteoarthrosis (see 3.2.4, 3.4.6–9, 3.11.4 and 3.13.1). Note: this is not true osteolysis but rather failure of primary ossification of subchondral bone.

5. Legg–Calvé–Perthes disease (avascular necrosis of the femoral head) – patchy osteolysis and collapse of femoral head in young, small-breed dogs; often bilateral (see 3.9.4).
6. Septic arthritis (bacterial or fungal) (Fig. 2.3) – usually involves the articular surfaces of both or all bones of a joint and is associated with joint effusion ± limb cellulitis. Multiple joints may be affected if the infection has been spread haematogenously, which is more common in younger animals. Animals with multifocal pathology are more likely to be systemically ill. Pre-existing joint disease may predispose a joint to sepsis, for example after dentistry. In such cases, radiographs may be hard to interpret but the animal is usually very lame, with clinical signs more severe than with degenerative or neoplastic joint disease. Radiographic signs in established cases include joint effusion and periarticular swelling, changes in joint space width, subchondral erosions and sclerosis, peri-articular new bone and soft tissue mineralization. Arthrocentesis is important for diagnosis.
7. Soft tissue tumour (Fig. 2.4) – if at or near a joint will usually affect more than one bone, causing multiple areas of discrete osteolysis; the articular surfaces may be spared, as cartilage is protective, with osteolysis predominantly at sites of soft tissue attachment – this is an important sign to help distinguish from sepsis.
   a. Synovial sarcoma; uncommon in dogs and rare in cats. Mainly middle-aged and older large breeds of dog, and most often affects

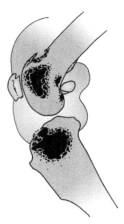

Figure 2.4 Soft tissue tumour around the stifle joint: osteolysis in several bones, joint effusion and surrounding soft tissue swelling. The articular surfaces are relatively spared (cf. Fig. 2.3).

the elbow and stifle; may be a large soft tissue component.
   b. Other periarticular soft tissue tumours; if liposarcoma then a characteristic fat opacity will be recognized.
8. Rheumatoid arthritis (canine idiopathic erosive polyarthritis) (Fig. 2.5) – immune-mediated, erosive, symmetrical polyarthritis; progressive and deforming; usually small to medium middle-aged dogs and rare in cats; many joints may be affected, but there is a predilection for the carpus and tarsus. Radiographic changes are progressive and include joint effusion and soft tissue swelling, changes in joint space width, subchondral osteolysis and cyst formation, osteolysis at sites of soft tissue attachment, worsening osteoarthrosis, periarticular calcification, juxta-articular osteopenia and eventual (sub)luxation, malalignment, collapse or ankylosis of the joint.
9. Osteopenia (e.g. disuse, metabolic) – epiphyses and carpal or tarsal bones are especially affected (see 1.16).
10. Chronic haemarthrosis – usually also with secondary osteoarthrosis.
11. Villonodular synovitis – intracapsular, nodular synovial hyperplasia thought to be due to trauma. Smooth, cup-shaped areas of osteolysis at the chondrosynovial junction; intra-articular mass can be shown by arthrography or ultrasonography.

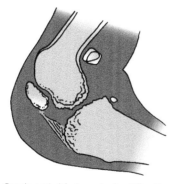

Figure 2.3 Septic arthritis in a dog's stifle: there is ragged osteolysis of articular surfaces, severe joint effusion and surrounding soft tissue swelling.

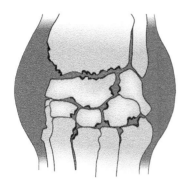

Figure 2.5 Rheumatoid arthritis affecting the carpus: widening of joint spaces (they may also be narrowed), subchondral osteolysis and surrounding soft tissue swelling.

12. Leishmaniasis* – 30% of affected dogs develop locomotor problems including severe osteolytic joint disease, which may affect multiple joints. Main differential diagnoses are septic arthritis, rheumatoid arthritis.
13. *Mycoplasma* polyarthritis – immunosuppressed or debilitated animals; also *M. spumans* polyarthritis in young greyhounds.
14. Subchondral cysts associated with osteoarthrosis – an occasional finding.
15. Severe drug-induced polyarthritis progressing from cartilage to subchondral bone (e.g. fluoroquinolones such as enrofloxacin).
16. Cats – feline metastatic digital carcinoma – multiple digits or feet, primary lesion in lung. Differential diagnosis is paronychia (see 3.7.11 and 3.7.13, and Fig. 3.18).
17. Cats – feline tuberculosis – various *Mycobacterium* species; occasionally affects the skeletal system – osteolytic joint disease and osteoarthrosis; also periostitis and mixed bone lesions.

2.5 PROLIFERATIVE JOINT DISEASE

The term *osteoarthritis* implies the presence of an inflammatory component to the disease process, whereas *osteoarthrosis* is generally used to imply a non-inflammatory condition. However, the two conditions may exist together and cannot be differentiated radiographically, and so the terms are often used synonymously. In some cases, new bone proliferation may be accompanied by marked remodelling of underlying bone. Severe proliferative joint disease may lead to ankylosis.

1. Osteoarthrosis secondary to elbow and hip dysplasia (see 3.4.6–9 and 3.4.19, 3.9.3, and Figs 3.11 and 3.21).
2. Osteoarthrosis secondary to damaged articular soft tissues (e.g. strained or ruptured cranial cruciate ligament; Fig. 2.6).
3. Osteoarthrosis secondary to osteochondrosis – typical breeds and joints, may be bilateral (3.2.4, 3.4.6–9, 3.11.4 and 3.13.1).
4. Primary (idiopathic) osteoarthrosis – an ageing change, but less common in small animals than in humans; mainly the shoulder and elbow.
5. Osteoarthrosis secondary to growth abnormalities (see 1.22.7–12).
6. Osteoarthrosis secondary to trauma or other abnormal stresses (e.g. angular limb deformities).
7. Osteoarthrosis secondary to repeated haemarthroses (may also see osteolysis).
8. Enthesiopathies at specific locations, although these may not be clinically significant (e.g. enthesiopathy of the short radial collateral ligament in the greyhound; see 3.6.11 and Fig. 3.16).
9. Neoplasia – single joints, large bony masses adjacent to joint.
   a. Osteoma – rare in small animals.
   b. Parosteal osteosarcoma – mainly proliferative, unlike other osteosarcomas (see 1.15.2 and 3.11.12 and Fig. 3.29).
10. Disseminated idiopathic skeletal hyperostosis – large dogs, mainly spondylotic lesions in the spine but may also affect appendicular joints, causing osteoarthrosis, enthesiopathies and

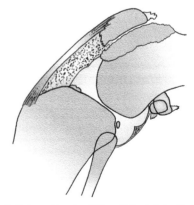

Figure 2.6 Osteoarthrosis of the stifle: joint effusion and periarticular osteophytes.

prominence of tuberosities and trochanters (see 5.4.5).

11. Synovial osteochondromatosis – mineralized intra- and periarticular bodies ± osteoarthrosis (see 2.8.18 and Fig. 2.7).

12. Systemic lupus erythematosus – very mild osteoarthrosis may occur in chronic cases.

13. Cats – hypervitaminosis A – raw liver diet; mainly spinal new bone (see 5.4.8) but may also see exostoses near the limb joints at insertions of tendons and ligaments, especially the elbow.

14. Cats – mucopolysaccharidoses (see 5.4.9) – mainly spinal changes similar to hypervitaminosis A but also osteoarthrosis secondary to epiphyseal dysplasia. Epiphyses become broad and irregular, and the osteoarthrosis may appear rather aggressive. Rare in dogs.

15. Cats – osteochondromata or osteocartilaginous exostoses – especially the elbows.

16. Cats – acromegalic arthropathy (see 2.3.7).

17. Cats – *Cryptococcus neoformans* has been reported to cause bilateral proliferative tarsal lesions.

18. Cats – osteochondrodysplasia of the Scottish Fold cat (see 3.7.8).

2.6 MIXED OSTEOLYTIC–PROLIFERATIVE JOINT DISEASE

1. Soft tissue neoplasia – osteolysis usually predominates, but there may be some periosteal reaction or the tumour may be superimposed over pre-existing osteoarthrosis, as patients are usually older (see 2.4.7 and Fig. 2.4). Osteolysis is mainly at sites of soft tissue attachment.

2. Rheumatoid arthritis (canine idiopathic erosive polyarthritis) – osteolytic or mixed joint lesions affecting mainly small joints such as carpus and tarsus (see 2.4.8 and Fig. 2.5).

3. Legg–Calvé–Perthes disease (avascular necrosis of the femoral head) with secondary osteoarthrosis – hip only (see 3.9.4 and Fig. 3.24).

4. Septic arthritis (see 2.4.6 and Fig. 2.3) – especially if chronic or if superimposed over pre-existing osteoarthrosis.

5. Chronic or repeated haemarthroses – animals with bleeding disorders, often multiple joints.

6. Leishmaniasis* – mainly osteolytic.

7. Villonodular synovitis (see 2.4.11).

8. Cats – feline non-infectious erosive polyarthritis.

9. Cats – feline tuberculosis.

10. Cats – periosteal proliferative polyarthritis (Reiter's disease); especially carpi and tarsi. Rare in dogs.

2.7 CONDITIONS THAT MAY AFFECT MORE THAN ONE JOINT

For further details of conditions that affect specific joints, see Chapter 3.

1. Elbow and hip dysplasia – often bilateral (see 3.4.6–9 and 3.9.2 and Figs 3.5–3.8, 3.11 and 3.21).

2. Osteochondrosis – primary lesions and secondary osteoarthrosis; mainly shoulder, elbow, stifle and tarsus in larger breed dogs. Often bilateral and may affect more than one pair of joints (see 3.2.4, 3.4.6–9, 3.11.4 and 3.13.1).

3. Primary osteoarthrosis – an ageing change, but less common in small animals than in humans; mainly the shoulder and elbow; often bilateral or multiple joints affected.

4. Stifle osteoarthrosis secondary to cruciate ligament disease or patellar subluxation; often bilateral (see 2.5.2 and Fig. 2.6, and 3.11.17).

5. Rheumatoid arthritis – erosive or mixed joint lesions affecting small joints especially (see 2.4.8 and Fig. 2.5).

6. Systemic lupus erythematosus – usually mild soft tissue swelling only; multiple joints, symmetrical.

7. Haematogenous bacterial or fungal septic arthritis – mixed osteolytic–proliferative changes.

8. Leishmaniasis* – erosive joint disease.

9. Chronic or repeated haemarthroses – animals with bleeding disorders.

10. Disseminated idiopathic skeletal hyperostosis – large dogs, mainly spondylotic lesions in the spine but may also affect appendicular joints,

causing osteoarthrosis, enthesiopathies and prominence of tuberosities and trochanters (see 5.4.5).

11. Skeletal dysplasias (e.g. chondrodysplasias, pituitary dwarfism and congenital hypothyroidism); multiple joints affected (see 1.22.7–12).

12. Multiple epiphyseal dysplasia (stippled epiphyses, dysplasia epiphysealis punctata) – inherited deficiency of ossification of epiphyses, apophyses and cuboidal bones; especially Beagle and Miniature Poodle.

13. Rocky Mountain spotted fever* (*Rickettsia rickettsii* infection).

14. Ehrlichiosis*.

15. Lyme disease* (*Borrelia burgdorferi* infection) – usually a shifting monoarticular or pauciarticular condition rather than a true polyarthritis.

16. Polyarthritis–polymyositis syndrome, especially Spaniel breeds.

17. Polyarthritis–meningitis syndrome – Weimaraner, German Short-haired Pointer, Boxer, Bernese Mountain dog, Japanese Akita, also cats.

18. Heritable polyarthritis of the adolescent Japanese Akita.

19. *Mycoplasma* polyarthritis – immunosuppressed or debilitated animals; also *M. spumans* polyarthritis in young greyhounds.

20. Chinese Shar Pei fever syndrome – short-lived episodes of acute pyrexia and lameness with mono- or pauciarticular joint pain and swelling of tarsi and carpi; occasionally enthesiopathies.

21. Polyarteritis nodosa – stiff Beagle disease.

22. Drug-induced polyarthritis, especially certain antibiotics.

23. Immune-mediated vaccine reactions.

24. Cats – feline non-infectious erosive and non-erosive polyarthritides.

25. Cats – feline calicivirus.

26. Cats – periosteal proliferative polyarthritis (Reiter's disease); especially carpi and tarsi. Rare in dogs.

27. Cats – hypervitaminosis A – raw liver diet; mainly spinal new bone but may also see exostoses near the limb joints, especially the elbow (see 5.4.8).

28. Cats – mucopolysaccharidoses (see 2.5.14 and 5.4.9).

29. Cats – feline tuberculosis.

30. Cats – osteochondromata or osteocartilaginous exostoses – especially the elbows.

2.8 MINERALIZATION IN OR NEAR JOINTS

Normal anatomical structures

1. Small sesamoid in tendon of *abductor pollicis longus et indicus proprius* muscle, medial aspect of carpus.

2. Sesamoids of metacarpo- or metatarsophalangeal joints (one dorsal, two palmar and plantar).

3. Patella.

4. Fabellae in heads of gastrocnemius muscle – caudal aspect of distal femur; medial much larger than lateral in cats and some small dogs.

5. Popliteal sesamoid – caudolateral aspect of stifle or proximal tibia; may be absent in small dogs.

6. Epiphyseal, apophyseal and small bone centres of ossification in young animals.

7. Cats – clavicles.

Normal variants: occasional findings of no clinical significance

These are likely to be bilateral, so if there is doubt as to their significance, radiograph the other leg.

8. Accessory centres of ossification – usually larger dogs, for example caudal glenoid rim, anconeus, dorsal aspect of wing of ilium (often remains unfused), craniodorsal margin of acetabulum.

9. Occasional sesamoids – for example sesamoid craniolateral to elbow (in humeroradial ligament, lateral collateral ligament, *supinator* or *ulnaris lateralis* muscles).

10. Bipartite or multipartite sesamoids – for example palmar metacarpophalangeal sesamoids 2 and 7 commonly seen in Rottweilers; medial fabella of stifle (see 3.7.4 and Fig. 3.17 and 3.11.2); differential diagnosis is traumatic fragmentation.

11. Rudimentary clavicles in some larger breed dogs.

12. Stifle meniscal calcification or ossification –
especially old cats (may also be associated with
lameness in some animals).

Mineralization likely to be clinically significant

See also Chapter 3 for details of specific joints.

13. Osteochondrosis – mineralized cartilage
flaps and osteochondral fragments
(joint mice).
14. Fractures.
    a. Avulsion fractures.
    b. Chip fractures.
    c. Fractured osteophytes from pre-existing
       osteoarthrosis.
15. Calcifying tendinopathy.
16. Meniscal calcification or ossification (stifle; see
3.11.19).
17. Synovial osteochondromatosis
(chondrometaplasia) (Fig. 2.7) – primary,
or secondary to joint disease; osteochondral
nodules form in synovial connective
tissue of a joint, bursa or tendon sheath.
Uncommon, but reported in both the dog
(shoulder, hip, stifle and tarsus) and cat.
May be rather dramatic and suggest
malignancy.
18. Calcinosis circumscripta – usually young
German Shepherd dogs; masses of stippled
calcified material in soft tissues over limb
prominences; also in the neck and tongue (see
12.2.2 and Fig. 12.1).
19. Severe osteoarthrosis or osteoarthritis –
dystrophic calcification of soft tissues around
joint; other arthritic changes seen too.
    a. Severe degenerative joint disease.
    b. Rheumatoid arthritis.
    c. Septic arthritis.
    d. Steroid arthropathy following intra-articular
       steroid injection.
20. Myositis ossificans – heterotopic bone
formation in muscle (see 12.2.3).

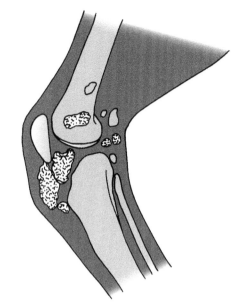

Figure 2.7 Synovial osteochondromatosis in the stifle of a cat. Extensive, nodular mineralization in the soft tissues of the stifle joint. The patella is slightly displaced.

    a. Primary idiopathic.
    b. Secondary to trauma.
21. Chondrocalcinosis or pseudogout
(calcium pyrophosphate deposition
disease) – uncommon, unknown
aetiology; older dogs. May affect single or
multiple joints, causing marked, acute-onset
lameness. Radiographs may be normal or
may show punctate areas of mineralization.
Diagnosed by the presence of crystals on
arthrocentesis.
22. Von Willebrand heterotopic
osteochondrofibrosis in Dobermann Pinschers
(hip see 3.9.12).
23. Extraskeletal osteosarcoma has been
reported as arising from the synovium of
the elbow in one dog, and produced
multiple periarticular and articular
mineralized bodies without evidence of
osteolysis.

Further reading

General

Carrig, C.B., 1997. Diagnostic imaging of osteoarthritis. Vet. Clin. North Am. Small Anim. Pract. 27, 777–814.

Farrow, C.S., 1982. Stress radiography: applications in small animal practice. J. Am. Vet. Med. Assoc. 181, 777–784.

Hoskinson, J.J., Tucker, R.L., 2001. Diagnostic imaging of lameness in small animals. Vet. Clin. North Am. Small Anim. Pract. 31, 165–180.

Various sections in: Ettinger, S.J., Feldman, E.C., 2005. Textbook of Veterinary Internal Medicine, sixth ed. Saunders, Philadelphia.

Techniques and normal anatomy

Muhumuza, L., Morgan, J.P., Miyabayashi, A.O., Atilola, A.O., 1988. Positive-contrast arthrography – a study of the humeral joints in normal beagle dogs. Vet. Radiol. 29, 157–161.

Congenital and developmental disease; diseases of young animals

Baines, E., 2006. Clinically significant developmental radiological changes in the skeletally immature dog: 2. Joints. In Pract. 28, 247–254.

Demko, J., McLaughlin, R., 2005. Developmental orthopedic disease. Vet. Clin. North Am. Small Anim. Pract. 35, 1111–1135.

Morgan, J.P., Wind, A., Davidson, A.P., 1999. Bone dysplasias in the Labrador retriever: a radiographic study. J. Am. Anim. Hosp. Assoc. 35, 332–340.

Rørvik, A.M., Tiege, J., Ottesen, N., Lingaas, F., 2008. Clinical, radiographic, and pathologic abnormalities in dogs with multiple epiphyseal dysplasia: 19 cases (1991–2005). J. Am. Vet. Med. Assoc. 233, 600–606.

Various authors, 1998. Osteochondrosis. Vet. Clin. North Am. Small Anim. Pract. 28 (1).

Infective and inflammatory conditions

Bennett, D., 1988. Immune-based erosive inflammatory joint disease of the dog: canine rheumatoid arthritis. 1. Clinical, radiological and laboratory investigations. J. Small Anim. Pract. 28, 779–797.

Bennett, D., Nash, A.S., 1988. Feline immune-based polyarthritis: a study of thirty-one cases. J. Small Anim. Pract. 29, 501–523.

Bennett, D., Taylor, D.J., 1988. Bacterial infective arthritis in the dog. J. Small Anim. Pract. 29, 207–230.

Gunn-Moore, D.A., Jenkins, P.A., Lucke, V.M., 1996. Feline tuberculosis: a literature review and discussion of 19 cases caused by an unusual mycobacterial variant. Vet. Rec. 138, 53–58.

Hanson, J.A., 1998. Radiographic diagnosis – Canine carpal villonodular synovitis. Vet. Radiol. Ultrasound 39, 15–17.

Marti, J.M., 1997. Bilateral pigmented villonodular synovitis in a dog. J. Small Anim. Pract. 38, 256–260.

May, C., 2005. Diagnosis and management of bacterial infective arthritis in dogs and cats. In Pract. 27, 316–321.

May, C., Hammill, J., Bennett, D., 1992. Chinese Shar Pei fever syndrome: a preliminary report. Vet. Rec. 131, 586–587.

Owens, J.M., Ackerman, N., Nyland, T., 1978. Roentgenology of arthritis. Vet. Clin. North Am. Small Anim. Pract. 8, 453–464.

Ralphs, S.C., Beale, B., 2000. Canine idiopathic erosive polyarthritis. Compend. Contin. Educ. Pract. Veterinarian (Small Animal) 22, 671–677.

Tisdall, P.L.C., Martin, P., Malik, R., 2007. Cryptic disease in a cat with painful and swollen hocks. J. Feline Med. Surg. 9, 418–423.

Neoplasia

Clements, D.N., Kelly, D.F., Philbey, A.W., Bennett, D., 2005. Arthrographic diagnosis of shoulder joint masses in two dogs. Vet. Rec. 156, 254–255.

McGlennon, N.J., Houlton, J.E.F., Gorman, N.T., 1988. Synovial sarcoma in the dog – a review. J. Small Anim. Pract. 29, 139–152.

Thamm, D.H., Mauldin, E.A., Edinger, D.T., Lustgarten, C., 2000. Primary osteosarcoma of the synovium in a dog. J. Am. Anim. Hosp. Assoc. 36, 326–331.

Whitelock, R.G., Dyce, J., Houlton, J.E.F., Jeffries, A.R., 1997. A review of 30 tumours affecting joints. Vet. Com. Orthop. Traumatol. 10, 146–152.

Trauma

Macias, C., McKee, M., 2003. Articular and periarticular fractures in the dog and cat. In Pract. 25, 446–465.

Owens, J.M., Ackerman, N., Nyland, T., 1978. Roentgenology of joint trauma. Vet. Clin. North Am. Small Anim. Pract. 8, 419–451.

Miscellaneous conditions

Agut, A., Corzo, N., Murciano, J., Laredo, F.G., Soler, M., 2003. Clinical and radiographic study of bone and joint lesions in 26 dogs with leishmaniasis. Vet. Rec. 153, 648–652.

Akselen, B., Hol, J., 2007. Quinolone-related arthropathy in a 12 week old Pyrenean Mountain dog – clinical and radiographic findings. Eur. J. Companion Anim. Pract. 17, 149–151.

Allan, G.S., 2000. Radiographic features of feline joint diseases. Vet. Clin. North Am. Small Anim. Pract. 30, 281–302.

De Haan, J.J., Andreasen, C.B., 1992. Calcium crystal-associated arthropathy (pseudogout) in a dog. J. Am. Vet. Med. Assoc. 200, 943–946.

Forsyth, S.F., Thompson, K.G., Donald, J.J., 2007. Possible pseudogout in two dogs. J. Small Anim. Pract. 48, 174–176.

Gregory, S.P., Pearson, G.P., 1990. Synovial osteochondromatosis in a Labrador retriever bitch. J. Small Anim. Pract. 31, 580–583.

Kramer, M., Gerwing, M., Hach, V., Schimke, E., 1997. Sonography of the musculoskeletal system in dogs and cats. Vet. Radiol. Ultrasound 38, 139–149.

Mahoney, P.N., Lamb, C.R., 1996. Articular, periarticular and juxtaarticular calcified bodies in the dog and cat: a radiological review. Vet. Radiol. Ultrasound 37, 3–19.

Morgan, J.P., Stavenborn, M., 1991. Disseminated idiopathic skeletal hyperostosis (DISH) in a dog. Vet. Radiol. 32, 65–70.

Prymak, C., Goldschmidt, M.H., 1991. Synovial cysts in five dogs and one cat. J. Am. Anim. Hosp. Assoc. 27, 151–154.

Short, R.P., Jardine, J.E., 1993. Calcium pyrophosphate deposition disease in a Fox Terrier. J. Am. Anim. Hosp. Assoc. 29, 363–366.

Stead, A.C., Else, R.W., Stead, M.C.P., 1995. Synovial cysts in cats. J. Small Anim. Pract. 36, 450–454.

Weber, W.J., Berry, C.R., Karmer, R. W., 1995. Vacuum phenomenon in twelve dogs. Vet. Radiol. Ultrasound 36, 493–498.

White, J.D., Martin, P., Hudson, D., Clark, R., Malik, R., 2004. What is your diagnosis? (synovial cyst). J. Feline Med. Surg. 6, 339–344.

Chapter 3

Appendicular skeleton

CHAPTER CONTENTS

3.1 Scapula   52
3.2 Shoulder   53
3.3 Humerus   55
3.4 Elbow   55
3.5 Radius and ulna (antebrachium, forearm)   60
3.6 Carpus   63
3.7 Metacarpus, metatarsus and phalanges   65
3.8 Pelvis and sacroiliac joint   67
3.9 Hip (coxofemoral joint)   68
3.10 Femur   71
3.11 Stifle   71
3.12 Tibia and fibula   77
3.13 Tarsus (hock)   77

This chapter describes conditions that are most commonly associated with specific bones or joints. Lack of inclusion of a condition under an anatomical area may not mean that it cannot occur there, simply that this area is not a predilection site; for example synovial sarcomas most often arise around the elbow and stifle, although they may arise near any synovial joint. Conditions that may occur in any joint (e.g. infectious arthritis) are described in Chapter 2, *Joints*.

For each anatomical area, the conditions are listed in the following order:

● artefacts and normal anatomical variants
● congenital or developmental
● metabolic
● infective
● inflammatory
● neoplastic
● traumatic
● degenerative
● miscellaneous conditions.

Conditions that most closely resemble each other radiographically are indicated by 'differential diagnosis'. Conditions involving joints are listed under the relevant bone but described more fully under the appropriate joint.

Joint trauma tends to affect the weakest area, hence physeal fractures occur in skeletally immature animals and ligamentous damage in older animals; young dogs rarely suffer from ligament trauma.

In many cases in which there is doubt as to the presence of genuine pathology, always consider radiographing the opposite limb for comparison.

Useful terminology

Amelia – absence of a limb.

Brachymyelia – abnormally short limb.

Dimelia – duplication of a limb.

Dysmelia – congenital deformity of a limb.

Ectromelia – absence of part of a limb.

Hemimelia – absence of the distal part of a limb; also used to denote absence of radius or ulna or tibia or fibula.

Meromelia – incomplete limb development.

Micromelia – abnormally small limb.

Notomelia – accessory limb attached to the back.

Peromelia – as dysmelia.

Phocomelia – absence of the proximal portion of a limb.

Adactyly – absence of a digit.

Brachydactyly – reduced size of outer digits.

Dactomegaly – abnormally large digit.

Ectrodactyly – absence of part or all of a digit; also used to describe split hand (lobster claw) deformity.

Polydactyly – supernumerary digit(s).

Polymyelia – supernumerary limb.

Polypodia – supernumerary feet.

Syndactyly – fusion of digits.

Valgus – lateral deviation of a limb distal to an abnormal growth plate or fracture malunion.

Varus – medial deviation of a limb distal to an abnormal growth plate or fracture malunion.

Ultrasonography of the musculoskeletal system

The use of ultrasonography is now well documented for investigation of musculotendinous lesions, although it requires considerable experience. High-frequency transducers of 7.5 MHz or more are required, and linear transducers give contact over a larger area.

The appearance of a normal tendon in longitudinal section is a band of medium echogenicity with parallel hyperechoic lines representing the fibrillar texture of the tendon, and in transverse section is of a round to ovoid structure with central inhomogeneities. The peritenon appears as a hyperechoic, continuous line. Acute and chronic tendinitis, tenosynovitis, mineralization, partial or complete tendon ruptures and tendon dislocations can be detected, and tendon healing after injury can be monitored.

Normal muscle is hypoechoic to anechoic with fine, oblique echogenic striations. Muscle injuries can be detected, their appearance varying with age of the injury; as with tendons, healing can be monitored.

Joints may be assessed ultrasonographically provided that an acoustic window can be found, although often only small areas can be seen. The bone surface, articular cartilage, synovium and synovial fluid may be recognized, but ligaments are usually too small to see. Joint effusion, chronic synovitis, articular cartilage defects, joint mice, chronic synovitis and osteophytes may be identified.

Ultrasonography may be used to examine the surface of bones and soft tissue lesions such as abscesses, haematomas, foreign bodies and soft tissue tumours, allowing ultrasound-guided aspiration in many cases.

See the further reading list for more information.

3.1 SCAPULA

Views

Mediolateral (ML); ML with dorsal displacement of the limb; caudocranial (CdCr); distoproximal – dorsal recumbency with the affected limb pulled caudally so the scapula is vertical and the shoulder joint is flexed to 90°.

Development

The ossification centre of the scapular body is present at birth, and the scapular tuberosity appears at 7 weeks; fusion occurs at 4–7 months.

1. Ossification centre of the scapular tuberosity (supraglenoid tubercle) fuses to the body of the scapula by 4–7 months; differential diagnosis is fracture.
2. Chondrosarcoma – flat bones are predisposed (scapula, pelvis, cranium, ribs).
3. Scapular fractures. Usually young, medium to large breeds of dog and after major trauma; often concurrent thoracic injuries.
   a. Scapular body – non-articular.
   b. Scapular spine – non-articular.
   c. Scapular neck – non-articular.
   d. Scapular tuberosity (supraglenoid tubercle) – usually avulsed by biceps brachii tendon in skeletally immature animals, articular; differential diagnosis is separate centre of ossification.
   e. Other glenoid fractures; articular.

3.2 SHOULDER

Views

ML; ML with pronation and/or supination; CdCr; flexed cranioproximal–craniodistal oblique (CrPr–CrDiO) for the intertubercular groove through which biceps tendon runs; arthrography (see 2.1). On the CdCr view, the joint space is often wider medially.

Ultrasonography

The use of ultrasonography for shoulder disease has been described (see *Further reading*).

1. Clavicles – clearly seen in cats; smaller and less mineralized in dogs, but rudimentary structures are sometimes visible, especially on the CdCr view of the shoulder; bilaterally symmetrical.
2. Caudal circumflex humeral artery seen end on caudoventral to the joint, surrounded by fat; differential diagnosis is poorly mineralized joint mouse.
3. Separate ossification centre of glenoid – small, crescentic mineralized opacity adjacent to the caudal rim of the glenoid; may fuse to the scapula or persist throughout life; may be an incidental finding but differential diagnosis is osteochondrosis (OC) of glenoid (see 3.2.5 below). However, incomplete ossification of the caudal glenoid has recently been reported as causing lameness in a number of larger breed dogs of varying ages, especially the Rottweiler. Possibly associated with minor trauma, abnormal growth and OC (or osteochondritis dissecans, OCD). Damage to the medial glenohumeral ligament may also be present. Radiographs show a bony fragment adjacent to the caudal glenoid margin ± secondary osteoarthrosis.
4. Osteochondrosis of the humeral head; also called OCD if there is evidence of cartilage flap formation (Fig. 3.1) – young dogs mainly 5–7 months old of larger breeds; Border Collies, Labradors and Great Danes over-represented; male preponderance; often bilateral. Reported only twice in cats. Radiographic signs include flattening or concavity of the caudal third of the humeral articular surface ± subchondral lucency or sclerosis, overlying mineralized cartilage flap. In chronic cases joint mice may be seen, usually in the caudal joint pouch but

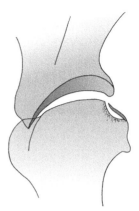

Figure 3.1 Shoulder osteochondritis dissecans with secondary osteoarthrosis: subchondral bone erosion affecting the caudal part of the humeral head, an overlying mineralized cartilage flap and an osteophyte on the caudal articular margin of the humerus.

also in the biceps tendon sheath or the subscapular joint pouch (CdCr view), as well as mild secondary osteoarthrosis. The presence of the vacuum phenomenon (see 2.2.13) is highly suggestive of an OC lesion. Arthrography is helpful in demonstrating thickening and irregularity of the articular cartilage layer, non-mineralized cartilage flap formation and non-mineralized joint mice. Ultrasonography can also be used to show OCD lesions, joint mice, joint effusions and new bone.

5. Osteochondrosis of the glenoid rim – unusual – separate mineralized fragment adjacent to articular rim; differential diagnosis is separate centre of ossification, but usually larger.
6. Congenital shoulder luxation or subluxation (Fig. 3.2) – rare, mainly miniature and toy breeds of dog, especially the Toy Poodle; may be bilateral. Usually present at 3–10 months of age, but older animals may show luxation after minor trauma. The humerus is normally displaced medially due to underdevelopment of the medial labrum of the scapular glenoid, but spontaneous reduction may occur on positioning for radiography. Radiographic signs include a flattened, underdeveloped glenoid with progressive remodelling of articular surfaces leading to osteoarthrosis; differential diagnosis is trauma at an early age.
7. Traumatic shoulder luxation – uncommon, unilateral. The humerus is usually displaced medially or laterally, occasionally cranially or

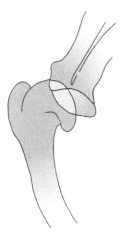

Figure 3.2 Congenital shoulder luxation or remodelling following trauma at a very early age: the glenoid of the scapula and the humeral head are both deformed, with loss of congruity of the joint space; superimposition of the two bones on the mediolateral view implies luxation in the sagittal plane.

caudally. With sagittal displacement, ML radiographs show a slight overlap of the scapula and humerus with loss of the joint space; on CdCr radiographs, the luxation is obvious unless spontaneous reduction has occurred; differential diagnosis is normal medial widening of the shoulder joint space on a CdCr view, especially if poorly positioned and particularly in smaller dog breeds. Check also for associated chip fractures.

8. Fractures involving the shoulder joint.
   a. Scapular tuberosity (supraglenoid tubercle) – Salter–Harris type I growth plate fracture in a skeletally immature animal, or bone fracture in a mature animal. May be avulsed by biceps brachii tendon. Differential diagnosis is separate centre of ossification.
   b. Other articular glenoid fractures.
   c. Salter–Harris type I fracture of the proximal humeral epiphysis in young animals – rare.
   d. Articular fracture of the proximal humeral epiphysis – rare.
9. Biceps brachii tendon rupture – acute or gradual onset; partial or complete; Bernese Mountain Dog and Rottweiler predisposed. Diagnosed by positive contrast arthrography or ultrasonography. With ultrasonography of complete tendon rupture, there is an area that is hypo- to anechoic due to bleeding between the tendon ends, which are swollen,

hyperechoic and heterogeneous. With partial rupture, the tendon is swollen and of irregular echotexture with tendon sheath effusion.

10. Biceps brachii tendon sheath rupture – reported in two Labradors. Rupture of the tendon sheath distally, diagnosed by positive contrast arthrography that showed leakage of contrast medium distally, outlining the proximal part of the muscle belly.
11. Shoulder osteoarthrosis – usually osteophytes on the caudal glenoid rim and caudal articular margin of the humeral head. The amount of new bone formation is often relatively mild. Joint mice may be visible in the caudal joint pouch and may become very large in old dogs. Some may develop into synovial osteochondromas.
    a. Primary – ageing change; often clinically insignificant.
    b. Secondary – for example following OC (OCD).
12. Calcifying tendinopathy – usually supraspinatus and biceps brachii tendons (Fig. 3.3); changes in the infraspinatus tendon and bursa and coracobrachialis tendon are also reported. Mainly medium to large, middle-aged dogs, especially Rottweilers and Labradors; aetiology unknown. Mild, chronic or intermittent lameness or clinically silent. May be bilateral. Radiographic signs include areas of mineralization in the region of the affected tendon or bursa; differential diagnosis is rudimentary clavicles or joint mice

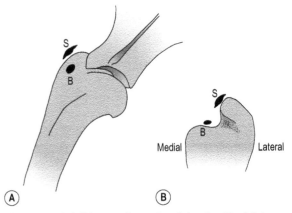

Figure 3.3 Calcifying tendinopathy of the shoulder joint: (A) mediolateral view and (B) cranioproximal–craniodistal oblique view (right shoulder). Calcification is seen as a radiopaque area radiographically, although shown here in black. B, in biceps brachii tendon; and S, in supraspinatus tendon or its bursa slightly more cranial, lateral and proximal.

in the biceps tendon sheath. Orthogonal radiographs (ML and CdCr) are essential to differentiate lesions within the bicipital groove from those medial or lateral to the shoulder, and the CrPr–CrDiO view and arthrography are also helpful in identifying the tendon of origin. Radiographs of the opposite shoulder should be obtained for comparison. Bicipital calcifying tendinopathy may be associated with tenosynovitis (see 3.2.13). Ultrasonography of the tendons may be helpful in showing fibre disruption, areas of mineralization (hyperechoic foci with distal acoustic shadowing) and joint capsule or tendon sheath effusion.

13. Bicipital tenosynovitis and bursitis – signalment as above. Radiographs may be normal or may show ill-defined sclerosis and new bone in the intertubercular groove, enthesiophytes on the supraglenoid tubercle and mild osteoarthrosis. Arthrography may show reduced or irregular filling of the biceps tendon sheath due to synovial villous hypertrophy. Ultrasonography may be used to demonstrate fluid distension of the bursa and tendon sheath and changes within the tendon itself.

3.3 HUMERUS

Views

ML; CdCr or craniocaudal (CrCd).

Development

The ossification centre of the humeral diaphysis is present at birth, and the proximal epiphysis appears at 1–2 weeks. Fusion of the greater tubercle to the humeral head occurs at 4 months and of the proximal epiphysis to the diaphysis at 10–13 months. At the distal end of the bone, the ossification centres of the medial and lateral parts of the humeral condyle appear at 2–3 weeks and of the medial epicondyle at 6–8 weeks; the two halves of the condyle fuse at 8–12 weeks, the medial epicondyle at 6 months and the condyle to the diaphysis at 5–8 months.

1. Compensatory overgrowth of the humerus – increase in humeral length compared with the contralateral limb has been described in dogs in which there is significant antebrachial shortening due to premature closure of radial and/or ulnar growth plates. The mechanism is thought to be secondary to either reduced physeal compression as a result of decreased weight bearing, or alteration in blood flow.

2. Panosteitis – the humerus is a predilection site (see 1.13.6 and Fig. 1.17).

3. Metaphyseal osteopathy (hypertrophic osteodystrophy) – proximal and distal humeral metaphyses are a minor site; the most obvious lesions are usually in the distal radius and ulna (see 1.24.4 and Fig. 1.31).

4. Primary malignant bone tumours (most commonly osteosarcoma) – the proximal humeral metaphysis is a predilection site (see 1.20.1 and Fig. 1.27); the distal humerus is very rarely affected.

5. Humeral fractures.
   a. Distal two-thirds of diaphysis – commonest area; usually spiral or oblique and may be comminuted, following the musculospiral groove; commonly associated with transient radial paralysis.
   b. Proximal third of diaphysis – usually a transverse fracture near the deltoid tuberosity.
   c. Salter–Harris type I fracture of the proximal humeral growth plate in skeletally immature animals.
   d. Distal epiphysis (see 3.4.17 and Fig. 3.10); may be secondary to incomplete ossification of the condyle, especially in Spaniels (see 3.4.5. and Fig. 3.4).
      – Lateral humeral condylar fracture.
      – Y fracture affecting both medial and lateral parts of the condyle.
      – Medial humeral condylar fracture.

3.4 ELBOW

Views

Flexed, extended and neutral ML; CrCd; CdCr, although results in magnification and blurring; craniolateral–caudomedial oblique (CrL–CdMO); craniomedial–caudolateral oblique (CrM–CdLO); arthrography. Oblique views may be obtained by pronating or supinating the limb.

Ultrasonography

Normal ultrasonographic anatomy of the canine elbow has been described (see *Further reading*).

1. Ossification centres visible in the elbow: medial and lateral parts of the distal humeral condyle, medial humeral epicondyle, anconeus, olecranon, proximal radial epiphysis; occasional small separate centre of ossification in the lateral humeral epicondyle seen on the CrCd view.
2. Elbow sesamoids – mineralized elbow sesamoids are commonly seen in both dogs (mainly larger breeds) and cats; small, smooth, round bodies craniolateral to the radial head; usually bilateral. Mainly in the supinator muscle but also reported in the annular ligament and lateral collateral ligament. Differential diagnoses are joint mice, chip fractures; should not be confused with a fragmented medial coronoid process.
3. Absence of the supratrochlear foramen of the distal humerus – occasionally noted in small, chondrodystrophic breeds of dog.
4. Cats – the supracondyloid foramen is present on the medial aspect of the distal humerus and is visible on a CrCd or CrL–CdMO radiograph; the brachial artery and median nerve pass through this foramen.
5. Incomplete ossification of the humeral condyle (Fig. 3.4) – especially English Springer Spaniels and American Cocker Spaniels but also seen in other Spaniel breeds and crosses and in some other pure breeds; male preponderance; often bilateral. Failure of fusion of the medial and lateral centres of ossification in the condyle

results in a residual sagittal cartilaginous plate that may be clinically silent or cause lameness in its own right as well as predisposing to condylar fractures (see 3.4.17 and Fig. 3.10). The fissure may be seen on CrCd or Cr 15° M–CdLO radiographs when the X-ray beam is parallel to the fissure, extending proximally from the articular surface to the physis and sometimes beyond into the supratrochlear foramen. Differential diagnosis is Mach effect along the edge of the superimposed olecranon (see 1.9).

6. Coronoid disease: fragmentation of the medial coronoid process of the ulna (FMCP) (Fig. 3.5) – part of the elbow dysplasia complex seen in young dogs of medium and large breeds, especially the Labrador, Golden Retriever, Bernese Mountain Dog, Rottweiler, Newfoundland; male preponderance; often bilateral. Lameness is first seen from 4–12 months of age. In some cases, initial lameness is not detected, particularly if bilateral disease is present, and the dog presents at an older age with osteoarthrosis. Predisposed to by elbow incongruity with widening of the humeroradial joint space, which puts increased pressure on the medial coronoid process. The diagnosis of FMCP and of humeral condylar OC is often made by identification of secondary osteoarthrosis in an appropriate patient rather than by visualization of a primary lesion (see 3.4.19 and Fig. 3.11); a specific diagnosis may not be possible without arthrotomy, arthroscopy or high-resolution CT

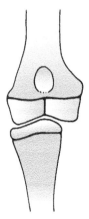

Figure 3.4 Incomplete condylar ossification of the right elbow on a craniocaudal view. A sagittal radiolucent line extends from the articular surface to the distal humeral growth plate. The ulna has been omitted for clarity.

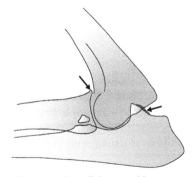

Figure 3.5 Fragmented medial coronoid process with early secondary osteoarthrosis: a small bone fragment is seen lying adjacent to the medial coronoid region of the ulna, which is flattened. Small osteophytes are present on the radial head and anconeal process (arrowed).

or magnetic resonance imaging. The primary radiographic findings are flattening, rounding or fragmentation of the process on the ML and Cr 15° L–CdMO views; the CrCd view shows not the process itself but a more medial projection of bone, which may be remodelled. 'Kissing' subchondral lesions may also be seen on the opposing articular surface of the humeral condyle; differential diagnosis is humeral OC (OCD).

7. Osteochondrosis (OCD) of the medial part of the distal humeral condyle (Fig. 3.6) – also part of the elbow dysplasia complex affecting the same breeds as above but with no gender predilection; often bilateral. The primary lesion is best seen on the CrCd view as subchondral bone flattening or irregularity, subchondral sclerosis, ± overlying mineralized cartilage flap; severe lesions may also be visible on the ML view; differential diagnosis is kissing lesion created by a fragmented medial coronoid process. Osteoarthrosis develops as with FMCP.

8. Ununited anconeal process (Fig. 3.7) – also part of the elbow dysplasia complex, although mainly in the German Shepherd Dog, Irish Wolfhound, Great Dane, Gordon Setter and Basset Hound; no gender predilection; often bilateral. Predisposed to by elbow incongruity with a slightly shorter ulna or longer radius putting pressure on the anconeus, but may also be due to trauma; some cases are bilateral. The

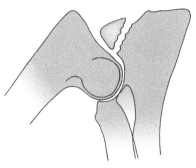

Figure 3.7 Ununited anconeal process: a large, triangular bone fragment is clearly seen, separated from the adjacent ulna.

separate centre of ossification for the anconeus usually fuses to the ulna between 3 and 5 months, and persistence of a radiolucent cleavage line beyond this time indicates separation. The flexed ML view is diagnostic, showing a substantial triangular bone fragment either adjacent to ulna or displaced proximally; chronic cases showing remodelling of the fragment and/or osteoarthrosis.

9. Elbow incongruity – seen in the various breeds predisposed to elbow dysplasia but especially in the Bernese Mountain Dog. Poor congruity between the humerus, radius and ulna puts increased pressure on the medial coronoid process or the anconeus and may lead to fragmentation or separation of these processes, respectively. Usually the humeroradial joint space is widened, best assessed on a CrCd view, as it is quite position-sensitive. May be seen alone or with FMCP, OC, ununited anconeal process ± osteoarthrosis. The clinical significance of incongruity alone is uncertain.

10. Medial epicondylar spurs (flexor tendon enthesiopathy) (Fig. 3.8) – usually larger breed dogs; may be bilateral; aetiology and significance not known and in some dogs is an incidental radiographic finding. The ML radiograph shows a distally projecting bony spur on the caudal aspect of the medial humeral epicondyle, or less commonly linear mineralization in adjacent soft tissues.

11. 'Ununited medial epicondyle' – unusual; aetiology not known but may be part of the elbow dysplasia complex, as similar breeds are affected, mainly young Labradors; may be bilateral. Single or multiple mineralized fragments of varying size and shape are seen

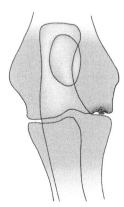

Figure 3.6 Humeral condylar osteochondritis dissecans (craniocaudal view of the right elbow): a shallow subchondral defect with adjacent sclerosis is seen in the medial part of the humeral condyle, with an overlying small mineralized cartilage flap.

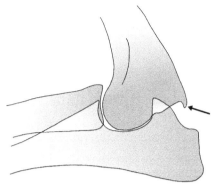

Figure 3.8 Medial epicondylar spur: a small, distally projecting enthesiophyte arises from the caudal aspect of the medial humeral epicondyle (arrowed).

at several locations near the medial epicondyle, sometimes with an adjacent bone defect. Secondary osteoarthrosis may be very minor. Some cases are radiographically similar to flexor enthesiopathies, and these may be different manifestations of the same condition. Box 3.1 describes the grading system recommended by the International Elbow Working Group for elbow dysplasia screening.

12. Elbow subluxation.
    a. Severe elbow incongruity (see 3.4.9).
    b. Secondary to relative shortening ± curvature of the ulna or radius, usually due to traumatic lesions at the distal growth plates or chondrodysplasia, and therefore recognized in young animals (see 3.5.4–7). Shortening of the ulna causes widening of the humeroulnar space distally and increased pressure on the anconeal process; shortening of the radius causes widening of the humeroradial space and of the humeroulnar space proximally, resulting in increased pressure on the medial coronoid process of the ulna.
    c. Distractio cubiti or dysostosis enchondralis in chondrodystrophic breeds (see 3.5.5).
    d. Congenital humeroulnar (sub)luxation – mainly small breeds of dogs (e.g. Pekinese) but also cats; male preponderance; often bilateral. Deformity is severe, with obvious limb dysfunction, and is therefore recognized at an early age (3–6 weeks). There is lateral displacement and 90° medial rotation of the ulna with a normal humeroradial articulation; the elbow is held

in flexion and the distal limb is pronated. Radiographically, the ulna is displaced laterally so its trochlear notch faces medially and is seen in profile on a CrCd view of the elbow; affected areas of bone are remodelled, and in chronic cases, osteoarthrosis develops.
    e. Congenital or developmental displacement of the radial head (Fig. 3.9) – mainly larger breeds of dog with no gender predilection; may be bilateral. May also be secondary to growth disturbances of the distal radius and ulna. Deformity is milder than with humeroulnar subluxation, although progressive degenerative joint changes develop. The radial head is (sub)luxated laterally or caudolaterally and is remodelled; the radius may appear longer than normal.
    f. Congenital complex elbow (sub)luxation – may be seen with other deformities such as ectrodactyly and split hand deformity (see 3.7.7).

13. Patella cubiti – a rare fusion defect through the trochlear notch of the ulna such that the olecranon and proximal ulnar metaphysis are separated from the rest of the ulna and

---

BOX 3.1   International Elbow Working Group grading system for elbow dysplasia

The International Elbow Working Group recommends the following grading system for elbow dysplasia screening based on the degree of secondary osteoarthrosis, from 12 months of age onwards:
- grade 0 – normal elbow, no osteoarthrosis or primary lesion
- grade 1 – mild osteoarthrosis with osteophytes < 2 mm
- grade 2 – moderate osteoarthrosis with osteophytes 2–5 mm
- grade 3 – severe osteoarthrosis with osteophytes > 5 mm.

Primary lesions described include malformed or fragmented medial coronoid process, ununited anconeal process, osteochondrosis (osteochondritis dissecans) of the humeral condyle and incongruity of the articular surfaces. Grading schemes in different countries vary in the number of radiographic views required and in their grading of primary lesions; the minimum requirement is a flexed mediolateral view of each elbow.

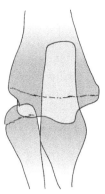

Figure 3.9 Congenital lateral luxation of the radial head (craniocaudal view of the right elbow): the radial head is markedly remodelled and no longer contoured to the humeral condyle.

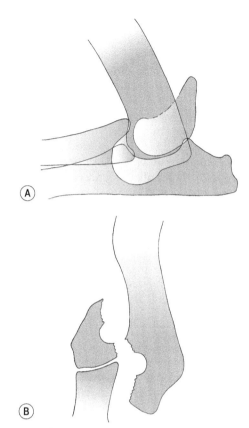

Figure 3.10 Lateral humeral condylar fracture: (A) on the mediolateral view, the medial and lateral parts of the humeral condyle are no longer superimposed; and (B) on the craniocaudal view (right elbow), the displaced fracture is clearly seen (the ulna has been omitted on this view for clarity). The radius remains articulating with the lateral condylar fragment, and these bones override the humeral shaft.

distracted by the triceps muscle; so-called because the fragment of bone is patella-shaped. May be bilateral. Differential diagnosis is avulsion fracture through the proximal ulnar growth plate or trochlear notch.

14. Cats – hypervitaminosis A; usually due to excessive ingestion of raw liver, leading to bony exostoses mainly on the spine, but the elbow is also a predilection site (see 5.4.8 and Fig. 5.8).

15. Synovial sarcoma (occasionally other soft tissue tumours, such as histiocytic sarcoma; see 2.4.7 and Fig. 2.4) – the elbow is a predilection site; mainly larger breeds of dog; differential diagnoses are severe osteoarthrosis, in which superimposition of new bone may mimic osteolysis; septic arthritis. The diagnosis may be difficult in cases in which tumour is superimposed over pre-existing osteoarthrosis. In the case of a tumour, a soft tissue mass may be palpable or radiographically visible adjacent to the joint.

16. Cats – osteocartilaginous exostoses are often seen around the elbow and may be bilateral. Possibly a type of osteochondroma (see 1.15.2 and Fig. 1.19).

17. Fractures involving the elbow joint.
    a. Lateral humeral condylar fracture (Fig. 3.10) – usually Spaniels and Spaniel crosses; often minor trauma only; may be bilateral. Young dogs or adults; in the latter, thought to be predisposed to by incomplete ossification between the medial and lateral parts of the humeral condyle (see 3.4.5 and Fig. 3.4), together with the increased loading of the lateral part of the condyle by its articulation with the radius and its weak attachment to the humeral shaft. Best seen on the CrCd view, but overriding of the fragments is also seen on the ML view. The most common elbow fracture, because the lateral condyle articulates with the radius and takes most of the load, and also because its epicondyle is relatively insubstantial.
    b. Y fractures of the humeral condyle – also Spaniels and predisposed to by incomplete ossification of the humeral condyle; the fracture line runs proximally between the medial and lateral parts of the condyle into the supratrochlear foramen, and then separate fracture lines emerge through the medial and lateral humeral cortices. Best seen on the CrCd view.

c. Medial humeral condylar fractures –
uncommon; also predisposed to by incomplete
ossification of the humeral condyle.

d. Salter–Harris type I fracture of the distal
humeral epiphysis in skeletally immature
animals – uncommon.

e. Olecranon fractures – through the proximal
ulnar physis in skeletally immature animals
(non-articular) or into the trochlear notch
(articular), both with distraction by triceps
muscle; differential diagnosis is patella
cubiti (see 3.4.13).

f. Proximal radial fracture – uncommon;
occasionally Salter–Harris type I fracture
through the physis in young animals.

g. Monteggia fracture – uncommon; a
proximal ulnar fracture (articular or non-
articular) with cranial luxation of the radius
and distal ulnar fragment.

18. Traumatic elbow luxation – usually due to a road
traffic accident or suspension by the limb from a
fence. ML radiographs may be almost normal,
but the CrCd view shows dislocation of radius or
ulna from humerus clearly; small avulsion or chip
fractures may also be seen. Usually the radius and
ulna luxate laterally as the large medial humeral
epicondylar ridge prevents medial luxation.
Ulnar luxation alone also reported.

19. Elbow osteoarthrosis (Fig. 3.11) – new bone
mainly on the anconeus and radial head (seen
on the ML view) and medial and lateral
humeral epicondyles (seen on the CrCd view).
Sclerosis of the ulnar trochlear notch is due to a
combination of increased bone density and
superimposition of osteophytes, and is seen
especially in dogs with fragmented coronoid

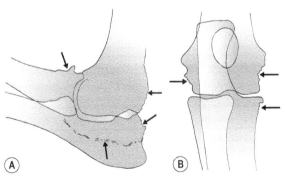

Figure 3.11 Elbow osteoarthrosis: (A) mediolateral and
(B) craniocaudal view (right elbow), showing periarticular
new bone (arrowed).

process. The lameness may be quite severe
with mild radiographic changes.

a. Primary – ageing change; radiographic
findings are usually minor.

b. Secondary – usually due to elbow dysplasia;
radiographic findings may be severe.

3.5 RADIUS AND ULNA (ANTEBRACHIUM, FOREARM)

Views

ML; CrCd.

Development

Radius – the ossification centre of the diaphysis is
present at birth; the proximal epiphysis appears
at 3–5 weeks and fuses to the diaphysis at 5–11
months; the distal epiphysis appears at 2–4 weeks
and fuses to the diaphysis at 6–12 months. Ulna –
the ossification centre of the diaphysis is present
at birth; the ossification centre of the anconeus
appears at about 11–12 weeks and fuses to the olecranon at 3–5 months in large dogs; the olecranon
appears at 8 weeks and fuses to the diaphysis at
5–10 months; the distal epiphysis appears at 2–4
weeks and fuses to the diaphysis at 6–12 months.
The distal ulnar physis is conical in the dog,
appearing V-shaped radiographically, and is flat
and horizontal in the cat.

1. Late closure of the radial growth plates in
neutered cats (males – distal only; females –
both proximal and distal); leads to an overall
longer radius than in entire cats.

2. Hemimelia (radial or ulnar agenesis) – one of
the paired bones is congenitally absent, usually
the radius; rare; usually unilateral. Medial
carpal bones and the first digit may also be
absent in the case of radial hemimelia; the
remaining bone shows variable shape changes.
Severe limb deformity and disability are
evident from birth. Possibly heritable, as
reported in several sibling cats.

3. Retained cartilaginous core, distal ulnar
metaphysis (Fig. 3.12) – common, often
bilateral, ossification defect in giant dog
breeds, in which a central core of distal growth
plate cartilage is slow to ossify, forming a
candle flame-shaped lucency with faintly
sclerotic borders. Implicated in growth
disturbances but may be a coincidental
finding, as often seen in normal dogs too.

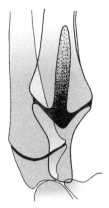

Figure 3.12 Retained cartilaginous core in the distal ulnar metaphysis: seen as a conical radiolucent area extending proximally from the growth plate.

4. Premature closure of the distal ulnar growth plate (radius curvus syndrome) (Fig. 3.13) – a common growth disturbance in young dogs of giant breeds, leading to angular limb deformity, often bilateral. The cause is usually not identified, so deemed idiopathic, but proposed mechanisms include:
   a. Salter–Harris type V crush injury of the distal ulnar growth plate – susceptible to such injury due to its deep conical shape,

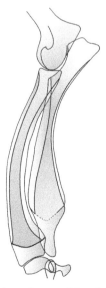

Figure 3.13 Premature closure of the distal ulnar growth plate: relative shortening of the ulna leading to cranial bowing of the antebrachium and often elbow and carpal subluxation. There is thickening of the adjacent radial and ulnar cortices.

which prevents lateral movement. May also occur unilaterally in other breeds.
   b. Metaphyseal OC or retained cartilaginous core.

Radiographs should include the whole antebrachium including the elbow and carpus, and show shortening of the ulna and distraction of the lateral styloid process from the carpus, craniomedial bowing of the radius and ulna with thickening of the adjacent radial and ulnar cortices, carpal subluxation and remodelling of the distal radius, carpal valgus and external rotation of the foot, and secondary elbow subluxation, usually of the distal aspect of the humeroulnar articulation. Carpal valgus may also be due to distal radius or ulna fracture or to developmental laxity of the short radial collateral ligament, and radiography permits differentiation of these conditions.

5. Distractio cubiti or dysostosis enchondralis – asynchronous growth of the radius and ulna in chondrodystrophic breeds (e.g. Bassett Hound), leading to elbow incongruity and pain; widening of the distal aspect of the humeroulnar articulation. Usually present with elbow lameness at about 12 months of age; may be bilateral.
6. Premature closure of the distal radial growth plate – trauma at or near the growth plate causes reduction in growth of the radius with shortening of the bone and subluxation of the elbow; widening of the humeroradial articulation ± increased width of the humeroulnar space proximally. Angular limb deformity is usually minor, and the main clinical problem is elbow pain.
   a. Symmetric closure – radius short and unusually straight, ulna may be slightly short too, elbow subluxation.
   b. Asymmetric closure – distal radius remodelled.
      – Lateral aspect (more common) – mimics premature closure of the distal ulnar growth plate with bowing of the radius and ulna and carpal valgus.
      – Medial aspect – carpal varus.
7. Premature closure of the proximal radial growth plate – rare; presumed to be due to trauma; radiographic signs as for 6a, but the

proximal radius may be obviously remodelled. Only 30% of the radial growth occurs proximally, therefore radial shortening is less severe than that following distal growth plate trauma.

8. Osteochondrodysplasias – various types of hereditary dwarfism are recognized in a number of dog breeds and in cats (see 1.22.7). Pathological and radiographic lesions are often most severe in the distal ulna and radius due to the high rate of growth at this site. The main abnormality is delayed growth at the distal ulnar growth plate, leading to shortening and bowing of the antebrachium. Some conditions may also resemble rickets radiographically (see 1.23.8 and Fig. 1.30). The pelvic limbs are less severely affected and may be normal.

9. Congenital hypothyroidism – causes dwarfism with radiographic changes similar to hereditary osteochondrodysplasias (see 1.22.9).

10. Radioulnar synostosis (fusion of the bones) leading to secondary radial head subluxation and external rotation of the foot has been described in a cat and is recognized in children. The radius and ulna are fused proximally at the interosseous space, preventing pronation–supination, and secondary elbow malformation results. May also occur following antebrachial fractures.

11. Bone remodelling in the distal ulnar and/or radial metaphyses has been described in Newfoundland dogs in Norway: 45% of dogs examined radiographically over a period of time showed islands of reduced opacity outlined by thickened trabeculae in the distal metaphyses at 6 months of age; the changes progressed up the diaphyses and persisted for up to 24 months of age. Aetiopathogenesis unclear. No clinical signs, but should not be mistaken for other conditions.

12. Metaphyseal osteopathy (syn. hypertrophic osteodystrophy) – young, rapidly growing dogs of larger breeds; lesions are usually most severe in the distal ulnar and radial metaphyses (see 1.24.4 and Fig. 1.31). Extensive periosteal and paracortical new bone may occasionally bridge growth plates, leading to angular limb deformities.

13. Panosteitis – the radius and ulna are predilection sites (see 1.13.6 and Fig. 1.17).

14. Rickets (syn. juvenile osteomalacia) – young animals after weaning; lesions usually most severe in the distal ulnar and radial growth plates (see 1.23.8 and Fig. 1.30).

15. Hypertrophic (pulmonary) osteopathy (syn. Marie's disease) – the radius and ulna may be affected by palisading periosteal new bone, although the distal limb is likely to be affected first (see 1.14.6 and Fig. 1.18).

16. Craniomandibular osteopathy – rarely, paracortical new bone may be seen surrounding the distal ulna and radius, mimicking metaphyseal osteopathy (Fig. 3.14), sometimes in the absence of the typical skull lesions, although in dogs of appropriate breed and age (see 4.10.1 and Fig. 4.6).

17. Canine leucocyte adhesion deficiency – a hereditary, fatal disease in Irish Setters, causing lesions similar to metaphyseal osteopathy and craniomandibular osteopathy.

18. Primary malignant bone tumours (most commonly osteosarcoma) – the distal radial metaphysis is the main predilection site, especially in large and giant dog breeds,

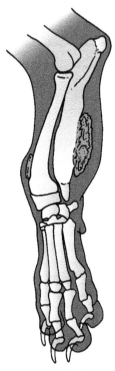

Figure 3.14 Lesions associated with craniomandibular osteopathy on the ulna and radius.

for example Great Dane, Irish Wolfhound (see 1.20.1 and Fig. 1.27).

19. Giant cell tumour (syn. osteoclastoma) – the distal ulnar metaphysis is a predilection site; differential diagnosis is solitary bone cyst (see 1.19.1 and Fig. 1.25).

20. Solitary bone cyst – the distal ulnar metaphysis is a predilection site; differential diagnosis is giant cell tumour (see 1.19.2 and Fig. 1.26).

21. Fractures of the antebrachium.
    a. Transverse fracture of the radius and ulna is very common; usually distal one-third.
    b. Fracture of one bone only occurs occasionally due to direct trauma.
    c. Fissure fracture of the cranial cortex of the radius mid-shaft after jumping from a height has been reported.
    d. Distal radial (medial styloid process) fractures usually occur as avulsion fractures of the short radial collateral ligaments and result in medial joint instability, detected on stressed radiographs.
    e. Distal ulnar (lateral styloid process) fractures may be associated with damage to the origins of the short ulnar collateral ligaments and result in lateral joint instability, detected on stressed radiographs.
    f. Avulsion of the origin of the dorsal radiocarpal ligament – racing Greyhounds; avulsion fragment from dorsomedial aspect of the distal radius.

22. Radial or ulnar fracture delayed union or non-union – common in toy dog breeds due to failure to use the injured limb; radiographs show atrophic non-union and disuse osteopenia (see 1.9 and 1.16).

3.6 CARPUS

Views

ML; flexed ML; dorsopalmar (DPa); dorsolateral–palmaromedial oblique; dorsomedial–palmarolateral oblique; stressed and weight-bearing views. Stressed views allow more accurate diagnosis of ligamentous injuries and should be obtained by using soft ties around the distal antebrachium and metacarpus and not by manual restraint. Oblique views of the carpus are helpful in interpretation, and similar radiographs of the normal leg for comparison are invaluable. On flexed ML radiographs, the antebrachiocarpal joint accounts for the majority of joint flexion, the middle carpal joint for some and the carpometacarpal joint for relatively little. The antebrachiocarpal joint normally also allows slight hyperextension.

Development

The ossification centres of the radial, ulnar and numbered carpal bones appear at 3–4 weeks; the body of the accessory carpal bone appears at 2 weeks and its epiphysis at 7 weeks, with fusion occurring at 10 weeks to 5 months.

1. Normal sesamoid in the insertion of abductor pollicis longus muscle on proximal metacarpal 1, seen on a DPa radiograph medial to the radial carpal bone; differential diagnosis is old chip fracture.

2. Developmental antebrachiocarpal subluxations – secondary to growth disturbances in the antebrachium and angular limb deformities; most commonly premature closure of the distal ulnar growth plate with cranial bowing of the radius, leading to articulation of the distal radius with the dorsoproximal margin of the radial carpal bone and remodelling of the distal radial epiphysis (see 3.5.4. and Fig. 3.13).

3. Carpal flexural deformity – skeletally immature dogs at about 6–12 weeks of age, especially the Dobermann. Thought to be due to relative shortening of flexor carpi ulnaris muscle. Radiographs are normal and are used to exclude bony pathology.

4. Cats – osteodystrophy of the Scottish Fold cat; changes are more severe in the pelvic limbs (see 3.7.8).

5. Rheumatoid arthritis – the carpus and tarsus are predilection sites; often bilateral (see 2.4.8 and Fig. 2.5).

6. Cats – various feline polyarthritides; the carpus and tarsus are predilection sites.

7. Chinese Shar Pei fever syndrome, also known as familial renal amyloidosis of Chinese Shar Pei dogs – mainly the tarsus, but the carpus is occasionally affected (see 3.13.6).

8. Carpal fractures – often associated with avulsions of tendons or ligaments, so what appear to be minor fractures may cause serious effects.
    a. Accessory carpal bone fractures (Fig. 3.15) – especially racing Greyhounds and other

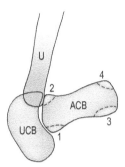

Figure 3.15 Diagrammatic representation of types 1–4 accessory carpal bone fractures (mediolateral view). ACB, accessory carpal bone; U, ulna; UCB, ulnar carpal bone.

athletic dogs; mainly the right carpus due to loading when running anticlockwise; best seen on extended and flexed ML radiographs. Five types are described:
- type 1 – accessoroulnar ligament avulsion from the base of the bone
- type 2 – avulsion of ligaments attaching to the radius and ulna, on the proximal border of the bone
- type 3 – avulsion of the origin of the accessorometacarpal ligaments
- type 4 – avulsion of the tendon of insertion of flexor carpi ulnaris muscle
- type 5 – comminuted.

Types 1, 2 and 5 are articular and may lead to osteoarthrosis of the accessoroulnar joint.
  b. Radial carpal bone fractures – may occur without known trauma, and Boxers are over-represented; may be bilateral; possibly due to a fusion defect of the three embryological centres of ossification in the bone (radial, intermediate and central, which normally fuse before birth). Usually sagittal or oblique sagittal fractures that are best seen on DPa views.
  c. Ulnar carpal bone fractures – rare; usually associated with ligamentous injury.
  d. Other carpal bones – small chip fractures on the dorsal aspect of the small, numbered carpal bones may result from hyperextension injuries, although may be hard to identify radiographically due to their small size and the complexity of the joint.
9. Carpal luxations and subluxations – carpal ligamentous injuries are more common than fractures and are usually the result

of a jump or fall, particularly high rise syndrome. Hyperextension and medial or lateral collateral instabilities are the most common injuries.
  a. Carpal overextension injuries or palmar ligament rupture – due to jumping from a height; also arise insidiously in older Shetland Sheepdogs and Collies; may be bilateral. Unstressed ML radiographs may appear normal, but with pressure from the palmar aspect or weight-bearing radiographs, overextension may be seen at any of the three carpal joints. Small chip fractures may be seen on the dorsal aspect of the radial carpal bone in cases of injury. Associated injuries such as proximal metacarpal 2 or 5 fractures or collateral ligament injuries may be seen as well. Chronic cases show secondary osteoarthrosis.
  b. Carpal overextension due to poor tone in the flexor tendons may be seen in skeletally immature dogs of larger breeds, especially the German Shepherd dog, but is not associated with bony radiographic changes.
  c. Antebrachiocarpal joint (sub)luxation – the carpus is usually displaced in a palmar direction; ± ligament damage and avulsion fractures; a serious injury.
  d. Radial carpal bone luxation – an uncommon injury that appears to be due to antebrachial joint hyperextension and rotation combined with rupture of the short radial collateral ligament and dorsal joint capsule; the radial carpal bone is displaced palmarly or palmaroproximally.
10. Collateral ligament trauma.
  a. Rupture of the collateral ligaments (short radial medially and short ulnar laterally) – medially and laterally stressed DPa radiographs are needed to confirm the injury. Radial (medial) collateral ligamentous injuries are more common, because the normal joint has up to 15° valgus deviation during weight bearing. Radiographs of chronic cases may show local soft tissue swelling and enthesiophyte formation at the origins and insertions of the ligaments.
  b. Avulsion fractures of the origins of the oblique and straight short radial collateral ligaments – especially racing Greyhounds; best seen on a DPa view. Chronic cases may

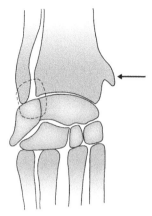

Figure 3.16 Enthesiopathy of the short radial collateral ligament (arrow): small spurs may be seen in racing Greyhounds; larger masses of new bone may be associated with carpal osteoarthrosis in other large breeds of dog.

show dystrophic mineralization and enthesiopathy (see below).

11. Enthesiopathy of the short radial collateral ligament (Fig. 3.16) – racing Greyhounds and sometimes other breeds, although not necessarily causing lameness. Remodelling and osteophyte production may be seen on the small bony tubercle that forms the proximal margin of the medial radial sulcus.

12. Abductor pollicis longus tenosynovitis – large dogs of varying ages in which chronic tendon sheath synovitis occurs, sometimes with bony stenosis caused by osteophytes on either side of the medial sulcus of the distal radius through which it passes; radiographic signs are of varying degrees of soft tissue swelling and bony proliferation along the course of the tendon sheath but do not correlate well with the degree of lameness. This muscle originates on the lateral margins of the radial and ulnar diaphyses and crosses the dorsal aspect of the distal radius obliquely, passing through the medial radial sulcus and between the two parts of the short radial collateral ligament to insert on the first digit.

13. Carpal osteoarthrosis and enthesiopathy – common in older dogs, especially of larger breeds, and also develops following trauma; radiographic changes may be much less severe than the clinical signs suggest. Often a focal, firm soft tissue swelling medial to the carpus, with underlying enthesiophytes on the medial

aspect of the distal radius and proximal second metacarpal bone. In severe cases, joint spaces may be irregular.

3.7 METACARPUS, METATARSUS AND PHALANGES

Views

ML; DPa or dorsoplantar (DPl); dorsolateral–palmaro- or plantaromedial oblique; dorsomedial–palmaro- or plantarolateral oblique; ML with digits separated using ties (splayed toe view).

Development

The ossification centres of the metapodial and phalangeal diaphyses are present at birth, and associated epiphyses are seen from 4–6 weeks, with fusion at 4–7 months. The proximal metapodial and distal phalangeal physes are closed at birth. Palmar or plantar sesamoids appear at 2 months and dorsal sesamoids at 4–5 months.

1. Artefacts created by radiopaque dirt on the foot, especially between the pads.
2. Radiopaque foreign bodies embedded in the pads (e.g. wire, glass).
3. Variation in the appearance of digit 1 (dew claw), especially in dogs that have undergone removal of this digit as puppies.
4. Sesamoid disease (Fig. 3.17) – especially young Rottweilers; fragmentation of the palmar metacarpal sesamoids (metatarsal less commonly), mainly sesamoids 2 and 7 (axial sesamoids of digits 2 and 5); unknown cause,

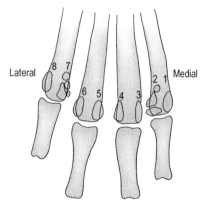

Figure 3.17 Fragmentation of the palmar metacarpophalangeal sesamoids: typically sesamoids 2 and 7.

but possibly abnormal endochondral ossification; lameness variable or absent, as these may be incidental findings, so check for other causes too. Scintigraphy has been reported to be useful in demonstrating significance. Differential diagnoses are congenital bipartite or multipartite sesamoids; fractures.

5. Polydactyly (e.g. six-toed cats); may be hereditary.

6. Syndactyly – lack of differentiation between two or more toes on single or multiple feet due to incomplete separation between soft tissues ± bone in utero; may be hereditary. May be complicated by other anomalies too. Radiographic signs may be dramatic, with complete or incomplete fusion of phalanges and metapodial bones, but lameness is unusual.

7. Ectrodactyly (split hand or lobster claw deformity) – seen sporadically in a number of dog breeds and in cats usually affecting one thoracic limb; very variable bony changes but appear grossly as a longitudinal cleft in the paw; hereditary in cats and unknown cause in dogs.

8. Cats – osteochondrodysplasia of the Scottish Fold cat – an inherited condition arising as a spontaneous mutation in a female British Short-hair in 1996, from which a new breed with folded ears was established. Both homozygotes and to a lesser extent heterozygotes are affected, developing deformities of the distal limbs and a short, thick and inflexible tail early in life. The pelvic limbs are usually more severely affected. Affected cats show inconsistently shortened and thickened metapodial bones, splayed phalanges; exostoses, ankylosing polyarthropathy and degenerative joint disease affect the tarsus, carpus, digits and tail; occasionally, there is osteolysis and a more aggressive radiographic appearance.

9. Hypertrophic (pulmonary) osteopathy (syn. Marie's disease) – affects the distal limbs initially, with periosteal new bone most obvious on the abaxial margins of metapodial bones and phalanges (see 1.14.6 and Fig. 1.18).

10. Calcinosis circumscripta – may affect the lower limbs, including the pads (see 12.2.2 and Fig. 12.1).

11. Paronychia (nail bed infection) and osteomyelitis of phalanx 3 – an osteolytic or mixed osteolytic–proliferative lesion affecting

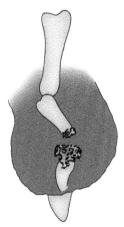

Figure 3.18 Paronychia or digital neoplasia: osteolysis of adjacent articular surfaces of phalanges 2 and 3, with surrounding soft tissue swelling.

P2–3 joint or P3; paronychia may affect multiple toes and often shows more extensive periosteal reaction; differential diagnoses are malignant neoplasia, intraosseous epidermoid cysts (see 3.7.13 and 3.7.14 and Fig. 3.18).

12. Malignant neoplasia of the metacarpal and metatarsal bones (e.g. osteosarcoma or soft tissue tumour) – an occasional occurrence.

13. Malignant neoplasia of the digits (Fig. 3.18) – osteolytic or mixed osteolytic–proliferative lesions with soft tissue swelling affecting phalanx 3 ± phalanx 2. Differential diagnoses are paronychia, osteomyelitis, intraosseous epidermoid cysts.
    a. Squamous cell carcinoma of nail bed – mostly large-breed dogs and unpigmented areas; primarily osteolytic and usually destroying bone from distal to proximal.
    b. Malignant melanoma – mainly pigmented areas.
    c. Cats – polyostotic digital metastases from pulmonary carcinoma; often multiple feet affected, predominantly weight-bearing digits.

14. Intraosseous epidermoid cysts – reported to affect phalanx 3 in dogs, although more common in the skin; unknown cause, but secondary to trauma in humans when arising in phalanges. Differential diagnoses are paronychia, osteomyelitis, malignant neoplasia.

15. Metacarpal and metatarsal fractures.
    a. Common traumatic injury, especially in the thoracic limb; often multiple, displaced and with minimal callus formation. Fractures of proximal metacarpal (metatarsal) 2 and 5 are associated with collateral ligament injury to the carpus (tarsus).
    b. Fractures of the first digit may cause lameness even though this digit is not weight bearing.
    c. Metatarsal 3 stress fracture of right pelvic limb occasionally seen in racing Greyhounds; minimally displaced, as supported by adjacent metatarsal bones.
16. Interphalangeal subluxations – racing Greyhounds, especially digit 5 of the left forefoot. May reduce spontaneously, leaving only soft tissue swelling.
    a. Distal interphalangeal joint – 'knocked-up' or 'sprung' toe; dorsal elastic ligament remains intact.
    b. Proximal interphalangeal joint.
17. Sesamoid fractures – usually palmar metacarpal sesamoids 2 and 7; especially the right forefoot in racing Greyhounds. Recent injuries show sharp fracture lines; fragments remodel with time. Differential diagnoses are congenital bipartite or multipartite bones; sesamoid disease in Rottweilers.
18. Osteoarthrosis of the digits – single, few or numerous joints affected, with varying amounts of new bone; usually older, active, large-breed dogs and may sometimes be severe, splaying the toes apart. Variable clinical signs.

3.8 PELVIS AND SACROILIAC JOINT

Views

Ventrodorsal (VD); laterolateral; oblique lateral to reduce superimposition of the two hemipelves. A tangential VD view angling the X-ray beam 20° cranially (ventro 20° cranial–dorsocaudal oblique) may give extra information in trauma cases.

Development

Ossification centres of the ilium, ischium and pubis are present at birth, and the acetabular bone appears at 7 weeks; fusion of these four bones at the acetabulum occurs at 4–6 months (Fig. 3.19).

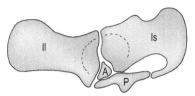

Figure 3.19 Main ossification centres of the pelvis (laterolateral view). A, acetabular bone; Il, ilium; Is, ischium; P, pubis.

The tuber ischii appear at 3 months and fuse to the ischia at 8–10 months; the caudal margin of the ischium often appears roughened, especially in larger dogs. The iliac crest appears at 4 months and may fuse at 1–2 years or may remain open longer (its appearance is highly variable). Occasionally, a triangular centre of ossification is seen from 7 months in the caudal part of the pelvic symphysis.

Sacroiliac joints

Sacroiliac disease is recognized as a cause of back pain in humans but is poorly documented in dogs. The sacroiliac joints consist of synovial joints ventrally and caudally, and rough, interdigitating fibrocartilaginous synchondroses dorsally. VD radiographs with the pelvic limbs extended only slightly caudally result in a horizontal orientation of the sacrum and are best for demonstrating dorsal, middle and ventral parts of the joints, while VD views with full pelvic limb extension angle the sacrum relative to the film and demonstrate the cranial part of the joints better. Changes that may be recognized radiographically include arthrosis, sclerosis, various degrees of mineralization leading to ankylosis, neoplasia and osteomyelitis.

1. Artefact – apparent osteolysis of the ischium on a VD view, due to superimposed gas in an anal sac.
2. Pelvic bone shape changes in Golden Retrievers with muscular dystrophy.
3. Neoplasia.
    a. Osteochondroma – especially the wing of the ilium, young dogs (see 1.15.2 and Fig. 1.19).
    b. Chondrosarcoma – flat bones are predisposed to chondrosarcoma, although other primary malignant tumours (e.g. osteosarcoma, fibrosarcoma) may also occur in the pelvis.
    c. Multiple myeloma (plasma cell myeloma) – the pelvis is a predilection site (see 1.18.2 and Fig. 1.24).

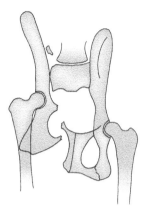

Figure 3.20 Pelvic fractures and unilateral sacroiliac separation in a cat.

4. Pelvic fractures (Fig. 3.20) – common traumatic injuries; usually multiple and displaced. Complications include concurrent lower urinary tract injury, sacrocaudal luxations and subsequent pelvic malunion leading to obstipation and dystocia. May also be accompanied by thoracic pathology, so abdominal and thoracic radiographs are advised.
5. Sacroiliac separation (Fig. 3.20) – a common injury, especially in cats; alone or associated with pelvic fractures. If bilateral, or if associated with ipsilateral pelvic fractures, cranial displacement of part of the pelvis may occur. Differential diagnosis is the normal radiolucency of the sacroiliac joint seen on a slightly oblique VD radiograph.
6. Cats – prepubic tendon avulsion following blunt trauma such as a road traffic accident; in some cases, an avulsed bone fragment may be seen cranial to the pubic brim.
7. Von Willebrand heterotopic osteochondrofibrosis in Dobermanns (see 3.9.12).

3.9 HIP (COXOFEMORAL JOINT)

Views

Extended VD; flexed (frog-legged) VD; ML with opposite leg abducted; laterolateral pelvis but hips superimposed; dorsal acetabular rim view; distraction VD view (PennHIP); stress applied craniodorsally to femora on a VD view.

1. Fovea capitis – focal area of irregularity on the femoral head for insertion of the teres ligament; variable in size and may be seen as flattening of the centre of the femoral head on a VD extended hip radiograph; should not be mistaken for evidence of hip dysplasia.
2. Accessory ossification centre of the craniodorsal margin of the acetabular rim – an occasional finding and may remain unfused; differential diagnosis is OC of the dorsal acetabular edge (see 3.9.5).
3. Hip dysplasia (Fig. 3.21) – a developmental and partly inherited condition of hip joint laxity, leading to subluxation, bony deformity and secondary degenerative changes; clinical signs are usually limited to larger breeds of dog (especially prevalent in the German Shepherd dog and Labrador), but radiographic changes may also be observed in small breeds and in cats (especially the Maine Coon). Radiographic screening programmes exist in a number of countries. The main radiographic signs include femoral head subluxation, shallow conformation of acetabulum, flattening of the cranial acetabular edge, new bone around the acetabular margins and femoral neck, recontouring of the femoral head and muscle wastage in severe cases. In cats, the changes predominantly affect the acetabulum rather than the femoral head and

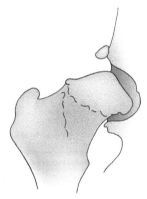

Figure 3.21 Severe hip dysplasia and secondary osteoarthrosis. The femoral head is subluxated and remodelled, and the acetabulum is shallow and irregular. New bone is present in the acetabular fossa, around the margins of the acetabulum, encircling the femoral neck and running vertically along the metaphyseal area as a caudolateral curvilinear osteophyte (a Morgan line).

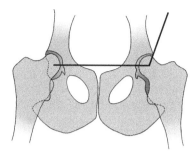

Figure 3.22 Method for measuring the Norberg angle. The base line joins the centres of the femoral heads, and then for each hip joint, a second line is taken from the femoral head centre to the junction between the cranial and dorsal acetabular edges. In normal hips, the angle between the lines is 105° or greater. Reduction in the Norberg angle denotes femoral head subluxation and/or a shallow acetabulum, in proportion to the degree of dysplasia present.

neck. Symmetrical VD radiographs are required, because lateral tilting of the pelvis may result in apparent subluxation of the hip joint closer to the table. The extended VD view is standard; some screening programmes also require a flexed VD radiograph. The degree of subluxation and the depth of the acetabulum together are evaluated by measuring the Norberg angle (Fig. 3.22). Normal values in the dog are > 105°, and in the cat, > 95°.

PennHIP scheme

Distraction index (DI) (Fig. 3.23) is a quantitative measurement of hip laxity calculated by comparing the position of the femoral head centre without and with traction applied to the hip joints using a fulcrum between the femora. DI of 0 means a fully congruent and non-lax joint; DI of 1, luxation. DI is a good predictor of subsequent hip osteoarthrosis, as hips with a DI of < 0.3 rarely develop secondary change.

Dorsal acetabular rim view

To assess dogs for suitability for triple pelvic osteotomy. The dog is positioned in sternal recumbency with the pelvic limbs pulled cranially, the femora parallel to the body and the tarsi elevated slightly from the table top. This causes flexion of the lumbosacral and hip joints, resulting in steep angulation of pelvis – the roof of the acetabulum is projected tangentially and its slope can be measured.

4. Legg–Calvé–Perthes disease (Perthes disease; avascular necrosis of the femoral head) (Fig. 3.24) – adolescent dogs of small breeds, especially terriers; no gender predisposition; usually unilateral but occasionally bilateral. Ischaemic necrosis of the femoral head with repair by fibrovascular tissue; probable autosomal recessive inheritance in some breeds (e.g. West Highland White Terrier). Radiographic signs include uneven radiopacity of the femoral head, leading to femoral head collapse, widening and irregularity of the joint space, varus deformity of the femoral neck, secondary osteoarthrosis and muscle wastage.

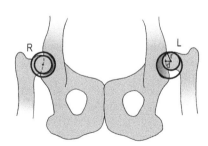

Figure 3.23 Calculation of the distraction index (DI). The right hip remains fully congruent with traction and the centre of the femoral head does not move; DI = 0. The left hip becomes subluxated with traction and the femoral head centre moves outwards; DI = distance moved *d*/radius of femoral head *r*. *(From the* Journal of the American Veterinary Medical Association, *with permission.)*

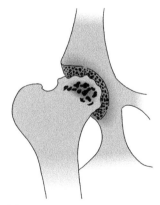

Figure 3.24 Advanced Perthes disease: the femoral head shows a moth-eaten radiopacity due to osteolysis and has collapsed, resulting in a wide and irregular joint space.

Differential diagnosis is intracapsular hip trauma, severe hip dysplasia (but atypical breeds), femoral head OC (OCD).

5. Osteochondrosis (OCD) – the hip joint is a highly unusual location.
   a. Femoral head – reported in Pekinese, Labrador and Border Collie; focal subchondral osteolysis ± mineralized flap formation. Differential diagnosis is Perthe's disease, although appears more focal.
   b. Dorsal acetabular rim – differential diagnosis is accessory ossification centre (see 3.9.2).
6. Physeal dysplasia with slipped capital femoral epiphysis, SCFE (also known as spontaneous femoral capital epiphyseal fracture) (Fig. 3.25) – mainly cats but occasionally in dogs. Uncommon condition of unknown aetiology, probably a cartilaginous physeal defect in which the femoral head displaces without significant trauma. Lameness may be insidious onset and progressive. Affected cats are usually less than 2 years old and predominantly overweight neutered males with an indoor lifestyle; dogs are usually about 1 year of age, also overweight neutered males, and Labradors and Shetland Sheepdogs are possibly over-represented. Unilateral or bilateral, or unilateral with the other hip affected at a later date. Radiographs show varying degrees of displacement or 'slippage' of the femoral head, with an open physis, changes in bone opacity of the femoral neck and in more chronic cases narrowing of the femoral neck due to bone resorption (apple core appearance). SCFE is well recognized in humans, mainly in obese adolescent boys, and in pigs (in this species known as epiphysiolysis and thought to be due to physeal OC).

7. Cats – feline femoral neck metaphyseal osteopathy; very similar to SCFE described above and may be a late stage of the same condition.
8. Mucopolysaccharidoses or mucolipidoses – may produce hip dysplasia, especially in cats.
9. Luxation of the hip – a common traumatic injury in skeletally mature dogs and cats; the femoral head usually displaces craniodorsally. Both lateral and VD radiographs are required to confirm the direction of displacement. Small avulsion fractures from the insertion of the teres ligament on to the femoral head may be seen in the acetabulum. Check for other pelvic or femoral fractures, sacroiliac separation and lower urinary tract damage. Chronic, unreduced hip luxation results in new bone on the ilial shaft and false joint formation.
10. Fractures involving the hip joint.
    a. Proximal femoral growth plate fractures – Salter–Harris type I or II (slipped epiphysis): this is the most common injury of the femoral head in immature dogs and cats and may require both extended and flexed VD radiographs for diagnosis, because the fracture may be reduced on one view. In skeletally immature animals, the only femoral head blood supply is via the joint capsule, so untreated intracapsular neck fractures or growth plate fractures will probably result in avascular necrosis of the femoral head and non-union. This leads to femoral neck resorption, producing an apple core appearance.
    b. Femoral neck fractures – intracapsular or extracapsular. In skeletally mature animals, blood supply via the medullary cavity exists and bone resorption is less likely.
    c Acetabular fractures – the femoral head displaces medially; secondary hip osteoarthrosis is likely.
    d. Femoral head avulsion fractures – small fragment of bone remaining attached to the teres ligament when the hip luxates.
    e. Physeal dysplasia and SCFE (epiphysiolysis – see 3.9.6 and Fig. 3.25).

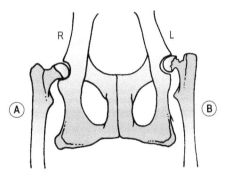

Figure 3.25 Slipped capital femoral epiphysis in a cat: (A) early and (B) late. (A) In the right hip, there is a radiolucent line in the region of the physis; (B) in the left hip, there is osteolysis of the femoral neck, producing an apple core appearance, with displacement between the femoral head and the rest of the femur.

11. Calcifying tendinopathy.
    a. Middle gluteal muscle (less commonly deep and superficial gluteal muscles) – one or more rounded, mineralized bodies near the greater trochanter of the femur, commonly seen on VD hip radiographs of larger dogs; clinically insignificant.
    b. Iliopsoas – a similar finding near the lesser trochanter.
    c. Biceps femoris – near the ischiatic tuberosity.
12. Von Willebrand heterotopic osteochondrofibrosis of Dobermann Pinschers – variably sized masses of mineralized tissue and/or periosteal reactions in the region of the hip joint, causing severely reduced range of motion. Thought to be due to microvascular bleeding in dogs with low levels of von Willebrand factor. Differential diagnosis is skeletal neoplasia.

3.10 FEMUR

Views

ML; CrCd.

Development

The ossification centre of the diaphysis is present at birth. Proximally, the femoral head appears at 2 weeks and the greater and lesser trochanters at 8 weeks, with fusion to the diaphysis at 6–11 months, 6–10 months and 8–13 months, respectively. Distally, the medial and lateral femoral condyles appear at 3 weeks and fuse to the diaphysis at 6–11 months.

1. Growth arrest lines – fine, transverse, sclerotic lines in the medullary cavity of larger dogs; no clinical significance. Differential diagnosis is previous panosteitis.
2. Compensatory overgrowth of the femur – increase in femoral length compared with the contralateral limb has been described in dogs in which there is significant tibial shortening due to premature closure of tibial growth plates. The mechanism is thought to be secondary to either reduced physeal compression as a result of decreased weight bearing, or alteration in blood flow.
3. Panosteitis – the femur is a predilection site (see 1.13.6 and Fig. 1.17).
4. Metaphyseal osteopathy (hypertrophic osteodystrophy) – the proximal and distal femoral metaphyses are a minor site; the most obvious lesions are usually in the distal radius and ulna (see 1.24.4 and Fig. 1.31).
5. Hypertrophic (pulmonary) osteopathy (Marie's disease) – the femur is a minor site (see 1.14.6 and Fig. 1.18).
6. Neoplasia.
    a. Primary malignant bone tumours (most commonly osteosarcoma) – the proximal femoral metaphysis is an occasional site, the distal metaphysis is affected more commonly, although the incidence is less than in the thoracic limb.
    b. Parosteal osteosarcoma – the distal femur is a predilection site (see 3.11.12 and Fig. 3.29).
    c. Infiltrative lipoma of thigh – swelling of thigh and displacement of muscle bellies by fat radiopacity; rarely see femoral osteolysis or new bone formation.
7. Femoral fractures.
    a. Diaphysis – common, often comminuted.
    b. Proximal femur (see 3.9.10).
    c. Greater trochanter avulsion; uncommon as a solitary lesion and more often associated with hip luxation.
    d. Distal femur (see 3.11.13).

3.11 STIFLE

Views

ML in various degrees of flexion; CrCd or CdCr; stressed views; flexed CrPr–CrDiO to skyline the trochlear groove.

Development

The patella ossification centre appears at 9 weeks and the fabellae and popliteal sesamoid at 3 months.

Ultrasonography

The use of ultrasonography for stifle joint disease has been described (see *Further reading*).

1. Popliteal sesamoid not mineralized – an occasional finding, especially in small dogs.
2. Fabella variants.
    a. Cats – the medial fabella is normally smaller than the lateral fabella and may be absent (also occasionally in toy dogs).

b. Non-ossification of the medial fabella – an occasional finding.

c. Bipartite or multipartite fabellae – two or more smooth, rounded fragments; differential diagnosis is old fabella fracture (no change over time if a developmental variant).

d. Distal displacement of one (usually medial) fabella, particularly in West Highland White and other small Terrier breeds.

3. Patella variants.

a. Congenital patella aplasia – reported in cats.

b. Cats – normal tapering, pointed distal pole of patella, not to be confused with new bone.

c. Bipartite or multipartite patella – two or more smooth, rounded fragments probably with some distraction; differential diagnosis is old patella fracture (no soft tissue swelling or change with time if developmental).

d. Patella alta – in some large, straight-legged dogs, the patella may lie very high or even proximal to the trochlear groove; also associated with medial patellar luxation.

e. Patella baja – opposite to above, and associated with lateral patellar luxation in similar breeds.

4. Osteochondrosis (OC or OCD) of the distal femur (Fig. 3.26) – similar breed, age and sex predisposition as other manifestations of OCD (OCD) and has been reported once in a domestic short-haired cat; may be bilateral; less common than thoracic limb OC (OCD).

a. Lateral femoral condyle (medial aspect) most common.

b. Medial femoral condyle.

c. Lateral trochlear ridge – rare; differential diagnosis is normal rough appearance of immature bone until about 4 months of age.

Radiographic signs of stifle OC (OCD) are similar to those of shoulder OC (OCD) and include stifle joint effusion (see 2.2.1 and Fig. 2.1), roughening or flattening of subchondral bone and underlying radiolucency, overlying mineralized cartilage flap, joint mice in various locations including the supratrochlear pouch, and minor osteoarthrosis.

5. Medial patellar luxation.

a. Congenital or developmental (Fig. 3.27) – usually toy dog breeds; in cats, it is unusual and may be incidental, although there is a genetic predisposition in the Devon Rex and Abyssinian. Much more common than later patellar luxation; may be unilateral or bilateral. Usually secondary to underlying developmental malalignment of the quadriceps mechanism, with decreased

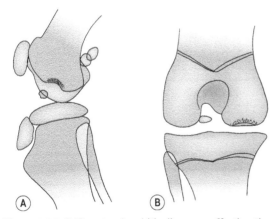

Figure 3.26 Stifle osteochondritis dissecans affecting the medial femoral condyle: (A) mediolateral and (B) craniocaudal views (right stifle). A subchondral erosion with adjacent sclerosis is seen on the medial femoral condyle, and a free mineralized body is present in the joint space. A joint effusion would also be present.

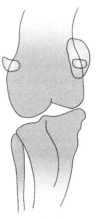

Figure 3.27 Congenital or developmental medial patellar luxation (craniocaudal view of the right stifle). The patella is displaced medially and rotated about its long axis; the distal femur and proximal tibia are bowed and the femorotibial joint space lies obliquely.

femoral head and neck anteversion and coxa vara, leading to outward rotation of the stifle (genu varum or bow-legged conformation). Diagnosis is based on palpation, with four grades of severity recognized. Radiographs may be useful to show the degree of limb deformity and secondary osteoarthrosis and may be normal in mild cases, although it is not clear which bony deformities are the cause and which the effect of patellar luxation. Radiographic signs include medial displacement of the patella (although this may reduce on positioning for a CrCd view), lateral bowing and external rotation of the distal third of the femur, mediolateral tilting of the femorotibial joint, medial displacement and remodelling of the tibial tuberosity, medial bowing of the proximal tibia and internal rotation of the tibial tuberosity, shallow trochlear groove with hypoplastic medial ridge and hypoplastic medial femoral condyle (seen on a CrPr–CrDiO view) and secondary osteoarthrosis.

b. Acquired – usually due to trauma and soft tissue damage; patella displaced (may reduce during positioning for radiography), but bones otherwise of normal appearance.

6. Lateral patellar luxation – much less common; usually larger breeds of dog.
   a. Due to trauma causing reduction in growth of the lateral aspect of the distal femur or proximal tibia.
   b. Secondary to hip deformity (increased anteversion and coxa valga) leading to inward rotation of the stifle (genu valgum or knock-kneed conformation). Radiographic signs are the opposite of those seen with medial patellar luxation.

7. Premature closure of the distal femoral growth plate – usually the lateral aspect, leading to genu valgum and lateral patellar luxation; may be associated with hip dysplasia.

8. Premature closure of the proximal tibial growth plate (tibial plateau deformans) (Fig. 3.28) – usually young adult dogs; various breeds including the Rough Collie and West Highland White Terrier; thought to be due to Salter–Harris type I or V injury to the growth plate. In severe cases, leads to inability to extend the stifle (resulting in a crouching pelvic limb stance) ± bow-legged

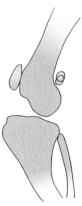

Figure 3.28 Premature closure of the proximal tibial growth plate (tibial plateau deformans): the proximal tibial articular surface slopes caudodistally and the fibula is bowed.

conformation; affected dogs usually present due to secondary rupture of the cranial cruciate ligament. Radiographic signs include remodelling of the tibial plateau, a caudodistal slope to the femorotibial joint space, caudal bowing of the fibula, secondary joint effusion and osteoarthrosis due to cruciate ligament damage.

9. Cats – hypervitaminosis A; the stifle may be a predilection site after the spine and elbow; differential diagnosis is synovial osteochondromatosis (see 3.11.18).

10. Idiopathic effusive arthritis or juvenile gonitis – especially the Boxer and Rottweiler, 1–3 years old; may be bilateral; idiopathic arthropathy may lead to rupture of the cranial cruciate ligament (see 3.11.14).

11. Synovial sarcoma (occasionally other soft tissue tumours) – the stifle is a predilection site (see 2.4.7 and Fig. 2.4); mainly larger breeds of dog. Differential diagnosis is severe osteoarthrosis, in which superimposition of new bone may mimic osteolysis; septic arthritis. The most significant radiographic sign may be displacement of the patella by a soft tissue mass.

12. Parosteal osteosarcoma (Fig. 3.29; see also 1.15.2) – rare: radiographically and pathologically distinct from other osteosarcomata. Slow-growing, smooth or lobulated, non-aggressive bony mass arising from the periosteum or parosteal connective tissue with little or no underlying osteolysis;

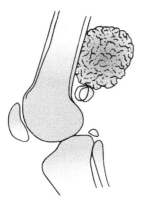

Figure 3.29 Parosteal osteosarcoma: a large, dense mass of unstructured bone lies caudal to the distal femur. Apparent absence of underlying osteolysis misleadingly suggests that this could be a benign lesion.

seen especially around the stifle on the caudal aspect of the distal femur.

13. Fractures involving the stifle joint.
    a. Distal femoral supracondylar fractures – Salter–Harris type I or II fractures of the distal femoral growth plate in skeletally immature animals; the femoral condyles usually rotate caudally; may heal as a malunion.
    b. Avulsion of the tibial tuberosity (Fig. 3.30) – Salter–Harris type I fracture of the tibial tuberosity growth plate.
       – Extrinsic; due to external trauma.
       – Intrinsic; with no or minor trauma; especially the Greyhound and English or Staffordshire Bull Terrier, may be

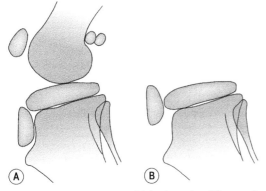

Figure 3.30 Avulsion of the tibial tuberosity: (A) normal unfused tibial tuberosity, (B) separation and proximal displacement.

bilateral; OC of the growth plate was found in one litter.
Radiographic signs include proximal displacement or rotation of the tibial tuberosity ± multiple small mineralized fragments, soft tissue swelling. Differential diagnosis is normal wide growth plate (compare with the opposite leg unless there are bilateral clinical signs).
    c. Proximal tibial growth plate fractures – Salter–Harris type I or II; the tibial tuberosity may remain attached or may separate, and the tibial shaft is usually displaced cranially; may heal as a malunion (see 3.11.8). Terrier breeds appear to be predisposed to combined tibial crest avulsion and Salter–Harris type II fracture of the proximal tibial epiphysis, the metaphyseal fragment being caudolateral or caudomedial.
    d. Fractured patella – due to a direct blow but may be spontaneous and bilateral in cats with preceding patellar sclerosis; if transverse, the fragments will distract. With a chronic lesion with fragment remodelling, the differential diagnosis is bipartite or multipartite patella.
    e. Fractured fabellae – spontaneous fracture of the lateral fabella is reported in dogs, especially in the Labrador, Golden Retriever and Border Collie. With a chronic lesion with fragment remodelling, the differential diagnosis is bipartite or multipartite fabella.
14. Cruciate ligament disease.
    a. Strained or ruptured cranial cruciate ligament – acute trauma or chronic strain, especially in large dogs with upright pelvic limb conformation; often bilateral. Radiographic signs include joint effusion, secondary osteoarthrosis (see 2.5.2, 3.11.17 and Figs 2.1 and 2.6), joint mice and dystrophic mineralization in the region of the ligament, remodelling of the tibial plateau at the site of attachment of the ligament, and cranial displacement of the tibia on the femur in severe cases. Tibial compression radiography has been described as being a highly sensitive test – with the stifle flexed at 90°, the hock is maximally flexed, causing cranial displacement of the tibia and distal displacement of the popliteal sesamoid in cases of cranial cruciate ligament damage. Tibial plateau angle (TPA) can be measured

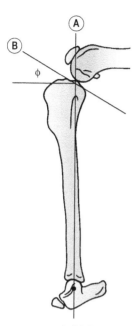

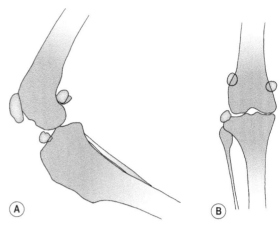

Figure 3.32 Avulsion of the tendon of origin of the long digital extensor muscle from its origin in the extensor fossa; a mineralized fragment is seen in the craniolateral aspect of the femorotibial joint space: (A) mediolateral view and (B) craniocaudal view (right stifle).

Figure 3.31 Measurement of tibial plateau angle (TPA). The vertical line 'A' is drawn through the centre of the tibial intercondylar eminences and the centre of the talus; it represents the functional axis of the tibia. The tibial plateau line 'B' joins the cranial and caudal margins of the medial tibial plateau. The TPA (Φ) is the angle between a line perpendicular to line A, and line B, at their intersection.

(Fig. 3.31); the literature is inconsistent as to whether dogs with cruciate disease have steeper angles, but measurement of TPA is used for planning tibial plateau levelling osteotomy (TPLO), which creates a more horizontal tibial plateau, thus reducing stress on the cranial cruciate ligament.

b. Avulsion of the insertion of the cranial cruciate ligament on to the tibial plateau – dogs < 2 years old, in which the ligament is stronger than the bone. Radiographic signs include joint effusion and a small mineralized fragment in the centre of the joint. Differential diagnoses are OC (OCD), secondary osteoarthrosis.

c. Partial avulsion of the origin of the cranial cruciate ligament – rare; small mineralized fragment in the intercondylar region of the distal femur and swelling of intracapsular soft tissues caudal to the patellar fat pad.

d. Avulsion of the origin or insertion of the caudal cruciate ligament – often associated with multiple stifle injuries, and isolated

injury is uncommon. Radiographic signs include joint effusion, caudal displacement of the tibia, mineralized fragment(s) in the caudal part of the femoral intercondylar fossa or caudal to the tibial plateau and secondary osteoarthrosis.

15. Tendon avulsions.

a. Avulsion of the origin of the long digital extensor muscle (Fig. 3.32) – usually skeletally immature dogs of larger breeds; may be no known trauma. Radiographic signs include a mineralized fragment adjacent or near to the extensor fossa of the distal femur, in the centre of the joint on the ML radiograph but shown to be lateral on the CrCd view; also a radiolucent bone defect in the extensor fossa; in some dogs, the defect is confined to soft tissue and there are no radiographic changes.

b. Avulsion of one or both heads of the gastrocnemius muscle (Fig. 3.33) – less common than distal injury to the Achilles tendon; may be bilateral; may be no known trauma; results in a plantigrade stance and hock hyperflexion if both the medial and lateral heads are affected. Radiographic signs include distal displacement of the associated fabella accentuated by hock flexion or in some cases only detected on hock flexion; in chronic cases, new bone on the distal femoral supracondylar tuberosities where the

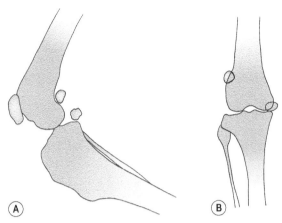

Figure 3.33 Avulsion of the medial head of gastrocnemius muscle, resulting in distal displacement of the medial fabella: (A) mediolateral view and (B) craniocaudal view (right stifle).

tendons arise, new bone around the associated fabella and dystrophic mineralization in surrounding soft tissues.

   c. Avulsion of the origin of the popliteal muscle – due to trauma, and may be associated with rupture of the cranial cruciate ligament; the CrCd radiograph may show an avulsed bone fragment and radiolucent bone defect on the lateral aspect of the lateral femoral condyle, with distal displacement of the popliteal sesamoid. Differential diagnosis is rupture of popliteal tendon itself or during tibial compression radiography in cases of damaged cranial cruciate ligament.

16. Other stifle ligamentous and soft tissue trauma.
   a. Collateral ligament rupture – medial or lateral stressed CrCd radiographs needed.
   b. Avulsion or rupture of the patellar ligament – proximal displacement of the patella exacerbated by stifle flexion, soft tissue swelling cranial to the infrapatellar fat pad. Tendon changes may also be visible using ultrasonography.
   c. Luxation of the stifle – rupture of cruciate and collateral ligaments; more common in cats; the tibia is usually displaced cranially.
   d. Quadriceps contracture – due to trauma or myositis and leads to stifle hyperextension and proximal displacement of the patella.

17. Stifle osteoarthrosis – a very common degenerative condition, especially in larger dogs; often bilateral; usually secondary to cranial cruciate ligament disease but also associated with OC (OCD), patellar luxation, trauma, etc. Radiographic signs include joint effusion that effaces the infrapatellar fat pad and displaces fascial planes caudal to the femorotibial joint, periarticular new bone at various sites (both poles of the patella, along the trochlear ridges of the distal femur, on the femoral epicondyles, at the extensor fossa of the lateral femoral condyle, around the fabellae and popliteal sesamoid and around the articular margins of the tibial plateau), intra-articular mineralization or 'loose bodies', subchondral sclerosis, subchondral cysts in the intercondyloid fossa and femorotibial joint space narrowing on weight-bearing radiographs (see 2.2.1 and 2.5.2 and Figs 2.1 and 2.6).

18. Synovial osteochondromatosis or synovial chondrometaplasia – an uncommon condition; the stifle is a predilection site, especially in cats and larger dogs (see 2.8.18 and Fig. 2.7). Differential diagnosis in cats is, hypervitaminosis A.

19. Meniscal calcification or ossification – uncommon, dogs or cats; idiopathic or secondary to trauma (often associated with ruptured cranial cruciate ligament); mineralized body of variable size in the cranial horn of the medial (commoner) or lateral meniscus.

20. Calcifying tendinopathy.
   a. Quadriceps.
   b. Gastrocnemius.

21. Mineralized bodies in or near the stifle joint (see 2.8).
   a. Normal sesamoids.
   b. Fragmented sesamoids.
   c. Osteochondrosis (OCD).
   d. Cruciate ligament damage.
     – Dystrophic mineralization of damaged tendon.
     – Avulsion fragments.
   e. Osteoarthrosis – fractured osteophytes or enthesiophytes.
   f. Fracture fragments.
   g. Avulsion of the long digital extensor, gastrocnemius or popliteal muscles.
   h. Meniscal calcification or ossification.
   i. Synovial osteochondromatosis.
   j. Pseudogout.
   k. Cats – hypervitaminosis A.

3.12 TIBIA AND FIBULA

Views

ML; CrCd.

Development

The ossification centres of both diaphyses are present at birth. Proximally, the medial and lateral tibial condyles appear at 3 weeks and the tibial tuberosity at 8 weeks; the condyles fuse together at 6 weeks, the tuberosity to the condyles at 6–8 months and the tuberosity and condyles to the diaphysis at 6–12 months. The proximal fibular epiphysis appears at 9 weeks and fuses to the diaphysis at 6–12 months. Distally, the tibial epiphysis appears at 3 weeks and the medial malleolus at 5 months, with fusion at 5–11 months; the fibular epiphysis appears at 2–7 weeks and fuses at 5–12 months.

1. Osteochondrodysplasias – various types of hereditary dwarfism in dogs and cats (see 1.22.7). The distal tibia is the second commonest site for lesions after the distal radius and ulna, although often the pelvic limbs are less severely affected than the thoracic limbs.
2. Pes varus – medial bowing of the distal tibia, resulting in deviation of the tarsus and phalanges towards the midline (varus deformity); unilateral or bilateral; thought to be genetic in the Dachshund but may also be due to trauma.
3. Metaphyseal osteopathy (hypertrophic osteodystrophy) – lesions may be seen in the proximal and distal tibial metaphyses, although less severe than in the distal radius and ulna (see 1.24.4 and Fig. 1.31).
4. Panosteitis – the tibia may be affected (see 1.13.6 and Fig. 1.17).
5. Rickets (juvenile osteomalacia) – the distal tibial growth plate is the second most severely affected site after the distal radius and ulna (see 1.23.8 and Fig. 1.30).
6. Hypertrophic (pulmonary) osteopathy (Marie's disease) – the tibia ± fibula may be affected by palisading periosteal new bone, although the distal portion of the limb is likely to be affected first (see 1.14.6 and Fig. 1.18).
7. Primary malignant bone tumours (most commonly osteosarcoma) – the proximal and distal tibial metaphyses are predilection sites, although less commonly affected than the humerus and radius.
8. Tibial and fibular fractures.
   a. Proximal tibia (see 3.11.13).
   b. Diaphyseal – in the tibia may spiral or create incomplete fissure fractures.
   c. Distal tibia (see 3.13.7).

3.13 TARSUS (HOCK)

Views

ML; flexed ML; DPl; flexed DPl to skyline trochlear ridges; dorsolateral–plantaromedial oblique; dorsomedial–plantarolateral oblique; stressed and weight-bearing views. Like the carpus, the tarsus is a complex joint and bone specimens or comparable views of the normal limb may be helpful in interpretation.

Development

The ossification centres of the talus and calcaneus are present at birth or appear within the first week of life; the remaining tarsal bones appear at 2–4 weeks; the tuber calcis appears at 6 weeks and fuses to the calcaneus between 11 weeks and 8 months.

Ultrasonography

The use of ultrasonography for disease of the common calcaneal (Achilles) tendon has been described (see *Further reading*).

1. Osteochondrosis (OCD) of the tibiotarsal joint – similar breed and age predisposition as other manifestations of OC but apparently no sex predisposition; Rottweiler, Labrador, English and Staffordshire Bull Terriers over-represented; may be bilateral; less common than thoracic limb OC.
   a. Medial trochlear ridge of talus (tibial tarsal bone) (Fig. 3.34), usually the proximal or plantar aspect – by far the commonest site. Radiographic signs include joint effusion and periarticular soft tissue swelling, flattening and fragmentation of the ridge with widening of tibiotarsal joint space medially, joint mice and marked secondary osteoarthrosis; variably visible on the DPl, extended and flexed ML views (may be better seen on ML views if the plantar aspect of the ridge is affected; the medial ridge is the smaller of the two).

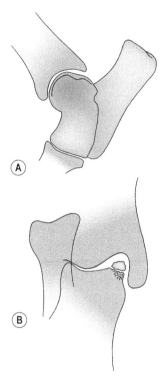

Figure 3.34 Osteochondritis dissecans of the medial trochlear ridge of the talus: (A) mediolateral (ML) and (B) dorsoplantar (DPl) view (right hock). The ML view shows flattening of one of the bony ridges; the DPl view identifies this as the medial ridge and shows subchondral radiolucency and overlying fragmentation with widening of the joint space.

    b. Lateral trochlear ridge of talus, usually the dorsal aspect – uncommon and harder to diagnose; Rottweiler and Golden Retriever predisposed. Oblique views and flexed DPl are helpful views, as this lesion is frequently missed on ML and DPl views. Differential diagnosis is avulsion of the fibular talar ligament.

    c. Fragmentation of the medial malleolus of the tibia – uncommon; possibly part of the OC complex and may be associated with medial trochlear ridge OC; Rottweiler predisposed.

2. Premature closure of the distal tibial growth plate – Rough Collie predisposed; usually the lateral aspect of the growth plate is more severely affected, leading to tarsal valgus (cow hocked conformation).

3. Cats – osteodystrophy of the Scottish Fold cat; the tarsi and hind paws are most severely affected (see 3.7.8).

4. Rheumatoid arthritis – the carpus and tarsus are predilection sites; often bilateral (see 2.4.8 and Fig. 2.5).

5. Cats – various feline polyarthritides; the carpus and tarsus are predilection sites.

6. Chinese Shar Pei fever syndrome, also known as familial renal amyloidosis of Chinese Shar Pei dogs – usually young dogs; unknown aetiology; fever often accompanied by acute synovitis of tarsal (less commonly carpal) joints; some dogs develop renal amyloidosis.

7. Tarsal fractures.

    a. Distal tibia – Salter–Harris type I fractures of the distal tibial growth plate.

    b. Medial or lateral malleolar fractures of the distal tibia and fibula – often with subluxation of the tibiotarsal joint space; stressed views may be required to demonstrate subluxation.

    c. Central tarsal bone fractures (Fig. 3.35) – especially racing Greyhounds, mainly right tarsus due to medial joint compression as running anticlockwise. May coexist with other tarsal fractures. Five types are described:

      – type 1 – non-displaced dorsal slab fracture; best seen on a ML view

      – type 2 – displaced dorsal slab fracture

      – type 3 – sagittal fracture; rare; best seen on a DPl view

      – type 4 – combined dorsal plane and sagittal fractures; the most common type

      – type 5 – severe comminution and displacement.

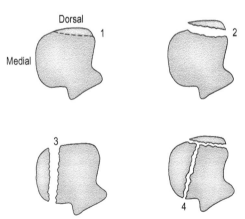

Figure 3.35 Classification of central tarsal bone fractures: cross-section of the right central tarsal bone.

d. Fibular tarsal bone (calcaneal) fractures – especially racing Greyhounds, right tarsus; often seen with central tarsal bone fractures or with proximal intertarsal joint subluxation; various locations of fracture, both simple and comminuted. Fractures through the tuber calcis may be distracted by the Achilles tendon.

e. Other tarsal bone fractures, for example of tibial tarsal bone (talus) or tarsal bone 4; rare except in racing Greyhounds, although cats may be predisposed to talar neck fractures.

f. Lateral talar ridge avulsion fractures at the insertion of the fibulotalar ligament.

8. Tarsal luxations and subluxations.

a. Tibiotarsal joint luxation – often with fracture of the medial or lateral malleolus of the tibia; stressed views may be needed (see 2.3.19 and Fig. 2.2).

b. Intertarsal and tarsometatarsal joint subluxation (Fig. 3.36) – traumatic; also arise insidiously in the Rough Collie, Shetland Sheepdog and Border Collie and may be bilateral in these dogs; may also be associated with rheumatoid arthritis (see 2.4.8 and Fig. 2.5) or systemic lupus erythematosus. Radiographic signs are best seen on a ML view and include soft tissue swelling, subluxation (stressed views may exacerbate), new bone especially on the plantar aspect of the tarsus, enthesiophyte formation and dystrophic soft tissue mineralization.

c. Central tarsal bone luxation has been reported; fracture of the plantar process of the bone may also be present; Border Collies possibly predisposed.

d. Dorsal tarsal instability due to rupture of the dorsal tarsal ligaments has been described as a racing injury in Greyhounds.

9. Lesions of the Achilles or common calcaneal tendon (common tendon of gastrocnemius and superficial digital flexor, with minor contributions from semitendinosus, gracilis and biceps femoris) (Fig. 3.37) – strain, rupture or avulsion of one or more components at or near the insertion on to the tuber calcis; mature, large-breed dogs, often overweight, may be bilateral. Radiographic signs include soft tissue swelling around the tendon and tuber calcis, a cap of proliferative new bone on the tuber calcis, avulsed fragments of bone and dystrophic mineralization in the tendon. Ultrasonography of the tendon may be helpful in showing fibre disruption and areas of mineralization, which produce bright echoes with acoustic shadowing (see 12.7.4 and Fig. 12.6).

10. Lateral luxation of the superficial digital flexor tendon – lateral displacement of the tendon from the tip of the tuber calcis due to tearing of its medial attachment, predisposed to by flattening of the bone at this site, as seen on the DPl view. Radiographs usually show soft tissue swelling only and no bony changes.

11. Tarsal osteoarthrosis – usually secondary to OC (OCD) or other underlying disease;

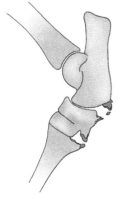

Figure 3.36 Chronic intertarsal subluxation with plantar new bone and soft tissue mineralization.

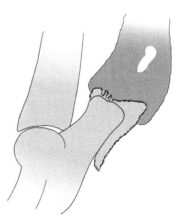

Figure 3.37 Chronic strain of the Achilles tendon: thickening of the tendon, dystrophic mineralization and calcaneal new bone.

radiographic changes may be milder than the clinical signs suggest. Smooth spurs of new bone on the dorsal aspect of the central and third tarsal bones and loss of clarity of the intervening joint space similar to bone spavin in horses are often an incidental finding in dogs but can sometimes be associated with lameness.

Further reading

Techniques and normal anatomy

Kramer, M., Gerwing, M., Hach, V., Schimke, E., 1997. Sonography of the musculoskeletal system in dogs and cats. Vet. Radiol. Ultrasound 38, 139–149.

Meier, H.T., Biller, D.S., Lora-Michiels, M., Hoskinson, J.J., 2001. Additional radiographic views of the thoracic limb in dogs. Compend. Contin. Educ. Pract. Veterinarian (Small Animal/Exotics) 23, 818–824.

Meier, H.T., Biller, D.S., Lora-Michiels, M., Hoskinson, J.J., 2001. Additional radiographic views of the pelvis and pelvic limb in dogs. Compend. Contin. Educ. Pract. Veterinarian (Small Animal/Exotics) 23, 871–878.

Muhumuza, L., Morgan, J.P., Miyabayashi, T., Atilola, A.O., 1988. Positive-contrast arthrography – a study of the humeral joints in normal beagle dogs. Vet. Radiol. 29, 157–161.

Slocum, B., Devine, T.M., 1990. Dorsal acetabular rim view for evaluation of the canine hip. J. Am. Anim. Hosp. Assoc. 26, 289–296.

Congenital and developmental diseases; diseases of young animals

Baines, E., 2006. Clinically significant developmental radiological changes in the skeletally immature dog: 1. Long bones. In Pract. 28, 188–199.

Demko, J., McLaughlin, R., 2005. Developmental orthopedic disease. Vet. Clin. North Am. Small Anim. Pract. 35, 1111–1135.

Hubler, M., Volkert, M., Kaser-Hotz, S., Arnold, S., 2004. Palliative irradiation of Scottish fold osteochondrodysplasia. Vet. Radiol. Ultrasound 45, 582–585.

Rochat, M.C., 2005. Emerging causes of canine lameness. Vet. Clin. North Am. Small Anim. Pract. 35, 1233–1239.

Various authors, 1998. Osteochondrosis. Vet. Clin. North Am. Small Anim. Pract. 28 (1).

Scapula

Jerram, R.M., Herron, M.R., 1998. Scapular fractures in dogs. Compend. Contin. Educ. Pract. Veterinarian (Small Animal) 20, 1254–1260.

Shoulder

Anderson, A., Stead, A.C., Coughlan, A.R., 1993. Unusual muscle and tendon disorders of the forelimb in the dog. J. Small Anim. Pract. 34, 313–318.

Barthez, P.Y., Morgan, J.P., 1993. Bicipital tenosynovitis in the dog – evaluation with positive contrast arthrography. Vet. Radiol. Ultrasound 34, 325–330.

Flo, G.L., Middleton, D., 1990. Mineralization of the supraspinatus tendon in dogs. J. Am. Vet. Med. Assoc. 197, 95–97.

Houlton, J.E.F., 1984. Osteochondrosis of the shoulder and elbow joints in dogs. J. Small Anim. Pract. 25, 399–413.

Krieglieder, H., 1995. Mineralization of the supraspinatus tendon: clinical observations in 7 dogs. Vet. Comp. Orthop. Traumatol. 8, 91–97.

Long, C.D., Nyland, T.G., 1999. Ultrasonographic evaluation of the canine shoulder. Vet. Radiol. Ultrasound 40, 372–379.

McKee, M., Macias, C., 2004. Orthopaedic conditions of the shoulder in the dog. In Pract. 26, 118–129.

McKee, M., Macias, C., May, C., Scurrell, E.J., 2007. Ossification of the infraspinatus tendon-bursa in 13 dogs. Vet. Rec. 161, 846–852.

Muir, P., Johnson, K.A., 1994. Supraspinatus and biceps brachii tendinopathy in dogs. J. Small Anim. Pract. 35, 239–243.

Siems, J.J., Breur, G.J., Blevins, W.E., Cornell, K.K., 1998. Use of two-dimensional real-time ultrasonography for diagnosing contracture and strain of the infraspinatus muscle in a dog. J. Am. Anim. Hosp. Assoc. 212, 77–80.

Stobie, D., Wallace, L.J., Lipowitz, A.J., King, V., Lund, E.M., 1995. Chronic bicipital tenosynovitis in dogs: 29 cases (1985–1992). J. Am. Vet. Med. Assoc. 207, 201–207.

van Bree, H., 1992. Vacuum phenomenon associated with osteochondrosis of the scapulohumeral joint in dogs: 100 cases (1985–1991). J. Am. Vet. Med. Assoc. 201, 1916–1917.

Vandevelde, B., van Ryssen, B., Saunders, J.H., Kramer, M., van Bree, H., 2006. Comparison of the ultrasonographic appearance of osteochondrosis lesions in the canine shoulder with radiography, arthrography and arthroscopy. Vet. Radiol. Ultrasound 47, 174–184.

Wernham, B.G.J., Jerram, R.M., Warman, C.G.A., 2008. Bicipital tenosynovitis in dogs. Compend. Contin. Educ. Veterinarians 30, 537–552.

Elbow

Anderson, A., Stead, A.C., Coughlan, A.R., 1993. Unusual muscle and tendon disorders of the forelimb in the dog. J. Small Anim. Pract. 34, 313–318.

Berry, C.R., 1992. Radiology corner: Evaluation of the canine elbow for fragmented medial coronoid process. Vet. Radiol. Ultrasound 33, 273–276.

Houlton, J.E.F., 1984. Osteochondrosis of the shoulder and elbow joints in dogs. J. Small Anim. Pract. 25, 399–413.

Kirberger, R.M., Fourie, S., 1998. Elbow dysplasia in the dog: pathophysiology, diagnosis and control. J S Afr. Vet. Assoc. 69, 43–54.

Lamb, C.R., Wong, K., 2005. Ultrasonographic anatomy of the canine elbow. Vet. Radiol. Ultrasound 46, 319–325.

Lowry, J.E., Carpenter, L.G., Park, R. D., Steyn, P.F., Schwarz, P.D., 1993. Radiographic anatomy and technique for arthrography of the cubital joint in clinically normal dogs. J. Am. Vet. Med. Assoc. 203, 72–77.

Mason, T.A., Lavelle, R.B., Skipper, S.C., Wrigley, W.R., 1980. Osteochondrosis of the elbow joint in young dogs. J. Small Anim. Pract. 21, 641–656.

May, C., Bennett, D., 1988. Medial epicondylar spur associated with lameness in dogs. J. Small Anim. Pract. 29, 797–803.

Milton, J.L., Montgomery, R.D., 1987. Congenital elbow dislocations. Vet. Clin. North Am. Small Anim. Pract. 17, 873–888.

Miyabayashi, T., Takiguchi, M., Schrader, S.C., Biller, D.S., 1995. Radiographic anatomy of the medial coronoid process of dogs.

J. Am. Anim. Hosp. Assoc. 31, 125–132.

Moores, A., 2006. Humeral condylar fractures and incomplete ossification of the humeral condyle in dogs. In Pract. 28, 391–397.

Murphy, S.T., Lewis, D.D., Shiroma, J.T., Neuwirth, L.A., Parker, R.B., Kubilis, P.S., 1998. Effect of radiographic positioning on interpretation of cubital joint congruity in dogs. Am. J. Vet. Res. 59, 1351–1357.

Robins, G.M., 1980. Some aspects of the radiographical examination of the canine elbow joint. J. Small Anim. Pract. 21, 417–428.

Radius and ulna

Clayton-Jones, D.G., Vaughan, L.C., 1970. Disturbance in the growth of the radius in dogs. J. Small Anim. Pract. 11, 453–468.

Ramadan, R.O., Vaughan, L.C., 1978. Premature closure of the distal ulnar growth plate in dogs – a review of 58 cases. J. Small Anim. Pract. 19, 647–667.

Rossi, F., Vignoli, M., Terragni, R., Pozzi, L., Impallomeni, C., Magnani, M., 2003. Bilateral elbow malformation in a cat caused by radio-ulnar synostosis. Vet. Radiol. Ultrasound 44, 283–286.

Trangerud, C., Sande, R.D., Rorvik, A.M., Indrebo, A., Grondalen, J., 2005. A new type of radiographic bone remodeling in the distal radial and ulnar metaphysis in 54 Newfoundland dogs. Vet. Radiol. Ultrasound 46, 108–113.

Carpus

Anderson, A., Stead, A.C., Coughlan, A.R., 1993. Unusual muscle and tendon disorders of the forelimb in the dog. J. Small Anim. Pract. 34, 313–318.

Grundmann, S., Montavon, P.M., 2001. Stenosing tenosynovitis of

the abductor pollicis longus muscle in dogs. Vet. Comp. Orthop. Traumatol. 14, 95–100.

Guilliard, M.J., 1998. Enthesiopathy of the short radial collateral ligaments in racing greyhounds. J. Small Anim. Pract. 39, 227–230.

Johnson, K.A., 1987. Accessory carpal bone fractures in the racing greyhound: classification and pathology. Vet. Surg. 16, 60–64.

Li, A., Bennett, D., Gibbs, C., Carmichael, N., Gibson, N., Owen, M., et al., 2000. Radial carpal bone fractures in 15 dogs. J. Small Anim. Pract. 41, 74–79.

Whitelock, R., 2001. Conditions of the carpus in the dog. In Pract. 23, 2–13.

Metacarpus, metatarsus and phalanges

Cake, M.A., Read, R.A., 1995. Canine and human sesamoid disease: a review of conditions affecting the palmar metacarpal/metatarsal sesamoid bones. Vet. Comp. Orthop. Traumatol. 8, 70–75.

Gottfried, S.D., Popovitch, C.A., Goldschmidt, M.H., Schelling, C., 2000. Metastatic digital carcinoma in the cat: a retrospective study of 36 cats (1992–1998). J. Am. Anim. Hosp. Assoc. 36, 501–509.

Homer, B.L., Ackerman, N., Woody, B.J., Green, R.W., 1992. Intraosseous epidermoid cysts in the distal phalanx of two dogs. Vet. Radiol. Ultrasound 33, 133–137.

Muir, P., Norris, J.L., 1997. Metacarpal and metatarsal fractures in dogs. J. Small Anim. Pract. 38, 344–348.

Read, R.A., Black, A.P., Armstrong, S.J., MacPherson, G.C., Peek, J., 1992. Incidence and clinical significance of sesamoid disease in Rottweilers. Vet. Rec. 130, 533–535.

Towle, H.A., Blevins, W.E., Tuer, L.R., Breur, G.J., 2007. Syndactyly in a litter of cats. J. Small Anim. Pract. 48, 292–296.

Voges, A.K., Neuwirth, L., Thompson, J.P., Ackerman, N., 1996. Radiographic changes associated with digital, metacarpal and metatarsal tumors, and pododermatitis in the dog. Vet. Radiol. Ultrasound 37, 327–335.

Pelvis

Brumitt, J.W., Essman, S.C., Kornegay, J.N., Graham, J.P., Weber, W.J., Berry, C.R., 2006. Radiographic features of golden retriever muscular dystrophy. Vet. Radiol. Ultrasound 47, 574–580.

Crawford, J.T., Manley, P.A., Adams, W.M., 2003. Comparison of computed tomography, tangential view radiography, and conventional radiography in evaluation of canine pelvic trauma. Vet. Radiol. Ultrasound 44, 619–628.

Dennis, R., Penderis, J., 2002. Radiology corner – Anal sac gas. Vet. Radiol. Ultrasound 43, 552–553.

Knaus, I., Briet, S., Kunzel, W., 2003. Appearance of the sacroiliac joint in ventrodorsal radiographs of the normal canine pelvis. Vet. Radiol. Ultrasound 44, 148–154.

Knaus, I., Briet, S., Kunzel, W., Mayrhofer, E., 2004. Appearance and incidence of sacroiliac joint disease in ventrodorsal radiographs of the canine pelvis. Vet. Radiol. Ultrasound 45, 1–9.

Hip

Adams, W.M., Dueland, R.T., Meinen, J., O'Brien, R.T., Guiliano, E.K., Nordheim, E.K., 1998. Early detection of canine hip dysplasia: comparison of two palpation and five radiographic methods. J. Am. Anim. Hosp. Assoc. 34, 339–347.

Breur, G.J., Blevins, W.E., 1997. Traumatic injury of the iliopsoas muscle in 3 dogs. J. Am. Vet. Med. Assoc. 210, 1631–1634.

Craig, L.E., 2001. Physeal dysplasia with slipped capital femoral epiphysis in 13 cats. Vet. Pathol. 38, 92–97.

Dueland, R.T., Wagner, S.D., Parker, R.B., 1990. von Willebrand heterotopic osteochondrofibrosis in Doberman Pinschers: five cases (1980–1987). J. Am. Vet. Med. Assoc. 197, 383–388.

Flückiger, M.A., Freidrich, G.A., Binder, H., 1999. A radiographic stress technique for evaluation of of coxofemoral joint laxity in dogs. Vet. Surg. 28, 1–9.

Gibbs, C., 1997. The BVA/KC scoring scheme for control of hip dysplasia: interpretation of criteria. Vet. Rec. 141, 275–284.

Hauptman, J., Prieur, W.D., Butler, H.C., Guffy, M.M., 1979. The angle of inclination of the canine femoral head and neck. Vet. Surg. 8, 74–77.

Johnson, A.L., 1985. Osteochondrosis dissecans of the femoral head of a Pekinese. J. Am. Vet. Med. Assoc. 187, 623–625.

Keller, G.G., Reed, A.L., Lattimer, J.C., Corley, E.A., 1999. Hip dysplasia: a feline population study. Vet. Radiol. Ultrasound 40, 460–464.

McDonald, M., 1988. Osteochondritis dissecans of the femoral head: a case report. J. Small Anim. Pract. 29, 49–53.

McNicholas, W.T., Wilkens, B.E., Blevins, W.E., Snyder, P.W., McCabe, G.P., Applewhite, A.A., et al., 2002. Spontaneous femoral capital physeal fractures in adult cats: 26 cases (1996–2001). J. Am. Anim. Hosp. Assoc. 221, 1731–1736.

Moores, A.P., Owen, M.R., Fews, D., Coe, R.J., Brown, P.J., Butterworth, S.J., 2004. Slipped capital femoral epiphysis in

dogs. J. Small Anim. Pract. 45, 602–608.

Nunamaker, D.M., Biery, D.N., Newton, C.D., 1973. Femoral neck anteversion in the dog: its radiographic appearance. J. Am. Vet. Radiol. Soc. 14, 45–48.

Perez-Aparicio, F.J., Fjeld, T.O., 1993. Femoral neck fractures and capital epiphyseal separations in cats. J. Small Anim. Pract. 34, 445–449.

Queen, J., Bennett, D., Carmichael, S., Gibson, N., Li, N., Payne-Johnson, C.E., et al., 1998. Femoral neck metaphyseal osteopathy in the cat. Vet. Rec. 142, 159–162.

Slocum, B., Devine, T.M., 1990. Dorsal acetabular rim radiographic view for evaluation of the canine hip. J. Am. Anim. Hosp. Assoc. 26, 289–296.

Smith, G.K., Biery, D.N., Gregor, T.P., 1990. New concepts of coxofemoral joint stability and the development of a clinical stress-radiographic method for quantitating hip joint laxity in the dog. J. Am. Vet. Med. Assoc. 196, 59–70.

Stifle

de Rooster, H., van Bree, H., 1999. Popliteal sesamoid displacement associated with cruciate rupture in the dog. J. Small Anim. Pract. 40, 316–318.

de Rooster, H., van Bree, H., 1999. Use of compression stress radiography for the detection of partial tears of the canine cranial cruciate ligament. J. Small Anim. Pract. 40, 573–576.

de Rooster, H., Van Ryssen, B., van Bree, H., 1998. Diagnosis of cranial cruciate ligament injury in dogs by tibial compression radiography. Vet. Rec. 142, 366–368.

Ferguson, J., 1997. Patellar luxation in the dog and cat. In Pract. 19, 174–184.

Gnudi, G., Bertoni, G., 2001. Echographic examination of the stifle joint affected by cranial cruciate ligament rupture in the dog. Vet. Radiol. Ultrasound 42, 266–270.

Kramer, M., Stengel, H., Gerwing, M., Schimke, E., Sheppard, C., 1999. Sonography of the canine stifle joint. Vet. Radiol. Ultrasound 40, 282–293.

Kramer, M., Gerwing, M., Michele, S., Schimke, E., Kindler, S., 2001. Ultrasonographic examination of injuries to the Achilles tendon in dogs and cats. J. Small Anim. Pract. 42, 531–535.

Lamb, C.R., Duvernois, A., 2005. Ultrasonographic anatomy of the normal canine calcaneal tendon. Vet. Radiol. Ultrasound 46, 326–330.

L'Eplattenier, H., Montavon, P., 2002. Patellar luxation in dogs and cats: pathogenesis and diagnosis. Compend. Contin. Educ. Pract. Veterinarian (Small Animal) 24, 234–239.

Macpherson, G.C., Allan, G.S., 1993. Osteochondral lesion and cranial cruciate ligament rupture in an immature dog stifle. J. Small Anim. Pract. 34, 350–353.

Montgomery, R.D., Fitch, R.B., Hathcock, J.T., LaPrade, R.F., Wilson, M.E., Garrett, P.D., 1995. Radiographic imaging of the canine intercondylar fossa. Vet. Radiol. Ultrasound 36, 276–282.

Muir, P., Dueland, R.T., 1994. Avulsion of the origin of the medial head of the gastrocnemius muscle in a dog. Vet. Rec. 135, 359–360.

Park, R.D., 1979. Radiographic evaluation of the canine stifle joint. Compend. Contin. Educ. Pract. Veterinarian (Small Animal) 1, 833–841.

Prior, J.E., 1994. Avulsion of the lateral head of the gastrocnemius muscle in a working dog. Vet. Rec. 134, 382–383.

Read, R.A., Robins, G.M., 1982. Deformity of the proximal tibia in dogs. Vet. Rec. 111, 295–298.

Reinke, J., Mughannam, A., 1994. Meniscal calcification and ossification in six cats and two dogs. J. Am. Anim. Hosp. Assoc. 30, 145–152.

Robinson, A., 1999. Atraumatic bilateral avulsion of the origins of the gastrocnemius muscle. J. Small Anim. Pract. 40, 498–500.

Skelly, C.M., McAllister, H., Donnelly, W., 1997. Avulsion of the tibial tuberosity in a litter of greyhound puppies. J. Small Anim. Pract. 38, 445–449.

Soderstrom, M.J., Rochat, M.C., Drost, W.T., 1998. Radiographic diagnosis: Avulsion fracture of the caudal cruciate ligament. Vet. Radiol. Ultrasound 39, 536–538.

Störk, C.K., Petite, A.F., Norrie, R.A., Polton, G.A., Rayward, R.M., 2009. Variation in position of the medial fabella in West Highland white terriers and other dogs. J. Small Anim. Pract. 50, 236–240.

Tanno, F., Weber, U., Lang, J., Simpson, D., 1996. Avulsion of the popliteus muscle in a Malinois dog. J. Small Anim. Pract. 37, 448–451.

Williams, J., Fitch, R.B., Lemarie, R.J., 1997. Partial avulsion of the origin of the cranial cruciate ligament in a four-year-old dog. Vet. Radiol. Ultrasound 38, 380–383.

Tarsus

Carlisle, C.H., Reynolds, K.M., 1990. Radiographic anatomy of the tarsocrural joint of the dog. J. Small Anim. Pract. 31, 273–279.

Carlisle, C.H., Robins, G.M., Reynolds, K.M., 1990. Radiographic signs of

osteochondritis dissecans of the lateral ridge of the trochlea tali in the dog. J. Small Anim. Pract. 31, 280–286.

Dee, J.F., Dee, J., Piermattei, D.L., 1976. Classification, management and repair of central tarsal fractures in the racing greyhound. J. Am. Anim. Hosp. Assoc. 12, 398–405.

Montgomery, R.D., Hathcock, J.T., Milton, J.L., Fitch, R.B., 1994. Osteochondritis dissecans of the canine tarsal joint. Compend. Contin. Educ. Pract. Veterinarian (Small Animal) 16, 835–845.

Mughannam, A.J., Reinke, J., 1994. Avulsion of the gastrocnemius tendon in three cats. J. Am. Anim. Hosp. Assoc. 30, 550–556.

Newell, S.M., Mahaffey, M.B., Aron, D.N., 1994. Fragmentation of the medial malleolus of dogs with and without tarsal osteochondrosis. Vet. Radiol. Ultrasound 35, 5–9.

Ost, P.C., Dee, J.F., Dee, L.G., Hohn, R.B., 1987. Fractures of the calcaneus in racing greyhounds. Vet. Surg. 16, 53–59.

Reinke, J.D., Mughannam, A.J., 1993. Lateral luxation of the superficial digital flexor tendon in 12 dogs. J. Am. Anim. Hosp. Assoc. 29, 303–309.

Reinke, J.D., Mughannam, A.J., Owens, J.M., 1993. Avulsion of the gastrocnemius tendon in 11 dogs. J. Am. Anim. Hosp. Assoc. 29, 410–418.

Rivers, B.J., Walter, P.A., Kramek, B., Wallace, L., 1997. Sonographic findings in canine common calcaneal tendon injury. Vet. Comp. Orthop. Traumatol. 10, 45–53.

Sjöström, L., Hakanson, N., 1994. Traumatic injuries associated with the short lateral collateral ligaments of the talocrural joint of the dog. J. Small Anim. Pract. 35, 163–168.

Chapter 4

Head and neck

CHAPTER CONTENTS

4.1 Radiographic technique for the skull   86
4.2 Breed and conformational variations of the skull and pharynx   87

Cranial cavity   88
4.3 Variations in shape of the cranial cavity   88
4.4 Variations in shape of the foramen magnum   88
4.5 Variations in radiopacity of the cranium   88
4.6 Variations in thickness of the calvarial bones; calvarial masses   89
4.7 Ultrasonography of the brain   90

Maxilla and premaxilla   90
4.8 Maxillary and premaxillary bony proliferation or sclerosis   90
4.9 Maxillary and premaxillary bony destruction or rarefaction   91
4.10 Mixed proliferative–osteolytic maxillary and premaxillary lesions   92

Mandible   92
4.11 Mandibular bony proliferation or sclerosis   92
4.12 Mandibular bony destruction or rarefaction   92
4.13 Mandibular fracture   93
4.14 Mixed proliferative–osteolytic mandibular lesions   93

Temporomandibular joint   93
4.15 Temporomandibular joint not clearly seen   94

4.16 Abnormalities of the temporomandibular joint   94

Ear   95
4.17 Abnormalities of the external ear canal   95
4.18 Variations in the wall of the tympanic bulla   96
4.19 Increased radiopacity of the tympanic bulla   96
4.20 Ultrasonography of the tympanic bulla   97

Nasal cavity   97
4.21 Variations in shape of the nasal cavity   97
4.22 Increased radiopacity of the nasal cavity   97
4.23 Decreased radiopacity of the nasal cavity   99

Frontal sinuses   99
4.24 Variations in shape of the frontal sinuses   100
4.25 Increased radiopacity of the frontal sinuses   100
4.26 Variations in thickness of the frontal bones   100

Teeth   101
4.27 Variations in the number of teeth   101
4.28 Variations in the shape of teeth   102
4.29 Variations in structure or radiopacity of the teeth   102
4.30 Periodontal radiolucency   102

4.31 Displacement or abnormal location
of teeth   102

Pharynx and larynx   103
4.32 Variations in the pharynx   103
4.33 Variations in the larynx   104
4.34 Ultrasonography of the larynx   104
4.35 Changes in the hyoid apparatus   105

Soft tissues of the head and neck   105
4.36 Thickening of the soft tissues of the head
and neck   105
4.37 Variations in radiopacity of the soft tissues
of the head and neck   105
4.38 Contrast studies of the nasolacrimal duct
(dacryocystorhinography)   106
4.39 Ultrasonography of the eye and orbit   106
4.40 Contrast studies of the salivary ducts
and glands (sialography)   109
4.41 Ultrasonography of the salivary glands   109
4.42 Ultrasonography of the thyroid and parathyroid
glands   110
4.43 Ultrasonography of the carotid artery
and jugular vein   110
4.44 Ultrasonography of lymph nodes of the
head and neck   110
4.45 Cervical oesophagus   111
4.46 Nasal dermoid sinus cyst   111

4.1 RADIOGRAPHIC TECHNIQUE FOR THE SKULL

A basic radiographic examination of the head and neck should include laterolateral and dorsoventral (DV) and/or ventrodorsal (VD) views. The DV is usually easier to position than the VD, as facial landmarks can be seen. Great care should be taken to achieve accurate positioning, and to facilitate this, general anaesthesia is usually required. A high-definition film–screen system or digital algorithm should be used, and a grid is not necessary. Positioning for views (c), (e) and (h) may be achieved using soft ties or a perspex positioning frame.

Additional specialized views are used to highlight specific areas of the head.

a. *Lateral oblique view*, with rotation of the skull about its long axis; for a left 30° dorsal–right ventral oblique or a right 30° dorsal–left ventral oblique, the skull is rotated about its long axis towards the DV position, and for a left 30° ventral–right dorsal oblique or a right 30° ventral–left dorsal oblique, it is rotated towards the VD position. Used to separate symmetrical head structures such as the jaws, dental arcades, tympanic bullae and frontal sinuses but requires two identically positioned radiographs, one for each side. For the teeth, the mouth may be open to reduce superimposition.

b. *Sagittal oblique* (left 20° rostral–right caudal oblique or a right 20° rostral–left caudal oblique), in which the nose is tilted up from a true lateral position, each demonstrating the dependent temporomandibular joint (TMJ) (Fig. 4.8).

c. *Rostrocaudal (RCd) closed mouth*, to skyline the frontal sinuses or cranium or to demonstrate the nasal cavities end on. The animal lies in dorsal recumbency with the head flexed, and using a vertical X-ray beam, the area of interest being profiled correctly using the light beam diaphragm.

d. *Caudorostral (CdR) horizontal beam view* for frontal sinuses. The animal is in sternal recumbency with the head raised to profile the frontal sinuses. This view may be used to demonstrate fluid lines within the sinuses.

e. *Rostro 30° ventral–dorsocaudal oblique* with open mouth and vertical head and X-ray beam, to demonstrate the tympanic bullae (also known as RCd open mouth; see Fig. 4.9).

f. *Special view for the feline tympanic bullae* (Fig. 4.10).

g. *Intraoral DV (occlusal)* for the nasal cavity, maxilla and premaxilla. Requires non-screen film or a thin, flexible cassette.

h. *Open mouth VD (ventro 20° rostral–caudodorsal oblique)* with open mouth, horizontal hard palate and X-ray beam angled dorsocaudally for demonstration of the nasal cavity; an alternative to (g) but allowing more caudal structures such as the cribriform plate to be included; especially useful in cats. Placing a sandbag under the neck may help in positioning (Fig. 4.12).

i. *Intraoral VD (occlusal)* for the mandible. Requires non-screen film or a thin, flexible cassette.

j. *Special views for teeth* (see p. 01).

k. *Lesion-oriented oblique view* – to skyline areas of deformity such as swellings.

4.2 BREED AND CONFORMATIONAL VARIATIONS OF THE SKULL AND PHARYNX

Breeds of dog can be divided into three groups:

1. *dolichocephalic breeds*, in which the nasal cavity is longer than the cranium (e.g. Irish Setter).
2. *mesaticephalic breeds*, in which the nasal cavity and cranium are of approximately equal length (e.g. Labrador).
3. *brachycephalic*, breeds in which the nasal cavity length is greatly reduced (e.g. Bulldog).

There are marked conformational variations in the skull, particularly between different breeds of dog but also to a lesser extent between different breeds of cat (Fig. 4.1). Brachycephalic breeds have a short maxilla, although the mandible may remain relatively long. The nasal cavity is correspondingly reduced in size, and the teeth may be crowded and displaced. The cranium is more domed, and the occipital protuberance and frontal sinuses are less prominent than in the longer-nosed breeds. The fontanelle and suture lines may remain open. On CT or MRI, many of these dogs are seen to have ventriculomegaly, i.e. subclinical hydrocephalus. Brachycephalic breeds of dog also show soft palate thickening, increased submandibular soft tissue mass and caudal displacement of the hyoid apparatus. Skull, facial and cranial indices have been described that express skull (facial or cranial) width as a percentage of length; brachycephalic dogs have higher indices than mesaticephalic and dolichocephalic dogs, especially for the facial area.

In cats, the cranium is relatively large and the tentorium osseum between the cerebral hemispheres and cerebellum is prominent on the lateral view. The tympanic bullae are large and contain a characteristic inner bony shell that divides the bulla into two portions, ventromedial and dorsolateral.

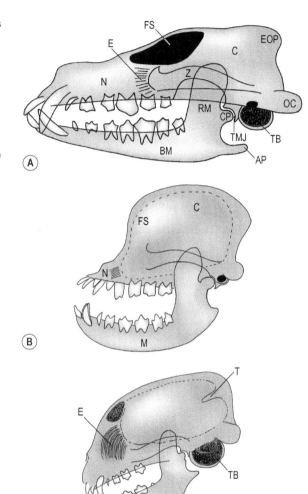

Figure 4.1 Normal lateral skulls. (A) Dolichocephalic dog (AP, angular process of mandible; BM, body of mandible; C, cranium or calvarium; CP, condyloid or articular process of mandible; E, ethmoturbinates; EOP, external occipital protuberance; FS, frontal sinus; N, nasal cavity; OC, occipital condyle; RM, ramus of mandible – its dorsal part is the coronoid process; TB, tympanic bulla; TMJ, temporomandibular joint; Z, zygomatic arch). (B) Brachycephalic dog (C, domed cranium; FS, absent or reduced frontal sinus; M, curved body of mandible; N, reduced nasal cavity with crowding of teeth). (C) Cat (E, ethmoturbinates; T, tentorium osseum; TB, large tympanic bulla with inner bony shell).

CRANIAL CAVITY

The cranial cavity is composed of the frontal, parietal, temporal and occipital bones; the cribriform plate of the ethmoid bone; and the bones forming the base of the skull (the sphenoid and basioccipital bones). The roof of the cranial cavity, formed by the frontal and parietal bones and part of the occipital bone, is known as the calvarium.

Views

a. Laterolateral.
b. Dorsoventral or ventrodorsal.
c. Lateral oblique.
d. Rostrocaudal.
e. Lesion-oriented oblique.

Normal appearance

The normal calvarium has slightly variable opacity, giving a copper-beaten appearance, due to variations in its thickness as it conforms to cerebral sulci and gyri. In small, dome-headed breeds such as the Chihuahua, the fontanelle and suture lines may remain open throughout life.

4.3 VARIATIONS IN SHAPE OF THE CRANIAL CAVITY

1. Breed-associated – brachycephalic breeds of dog and cat tend to have a domed calvarium; many have ventriculomegaly (subclinical hydrocephalus).
2. Congenital hydrocephalus (Fig. 4.2) – exaggeration of the domed shape, with thinning of the bones of the calvarium. The calvarial

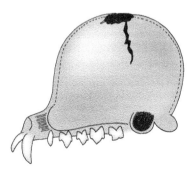

Figure 4.2 Congenital hydrocephalus: domed cranium with open fontanelle and suture lines.

bones may have a more uniform radiopacity than normal, lacking the usual copper-beaten appearance, and the fontanelle and suture lines are likely to remain open.
3. Bony masses (see 4.6.3 and Fig. 4.3).
4. Trauma – usually flattening or concavity of the calvarium seen on a lesion-oriented oblique view; fracture lines may be visible.
5. Thinning and caudal bulging of the occipital bone is seen in Cavalier King Charles Spaniels with caudal occipital malformation (Chiari syndrome), which is usually associated with syringohydromyelia, diagnosed using MRI.
6. Thickening and irregularity of the calvarium is seen in idiopathic calvarial hyperostosis of Bullmastiffs (see 4.6.2).

4.4 VARIATIONS IN SHAPE OF THE FORAMEN MAGNUM

1. Abnormal dorsal extension (keyhole shape) seen in occipital dysplasias; usually toy and miniature breeds of dog; may be associated with hydrocephalus and/or atlantoaxial malformations. Seen on a well-penetrated RCd view.

4.5 VARIATIONS IN RADIOPACITY OF THE CRANIUM

1. Decreased radiopacity of the cranium.
   a. Generalized.
      – Hyperparathyroidism – most commonly secondary to chronic renal disease but also secondary to nutritional imbalance or primary parathyroid disease (see 1.16.4 and 4.9.5 and Fig. 4.5).
   b. Localized.
      – Superimposed gas shadows in external ear canals.
      – Normal suture lines or vascular channels.
      – Fracture lines.
      – Neoplasia.
      – Pneumocephalus – usually ventricular.
2. Increased radiopacity of the cranium.
   a. Localized.
      – Trauma leading to periosteal new bone formation; subperiosteal haematoma in the nuchal crest area, which then mineralizes.
      – Neoplasia – osteoma or multilobular tumour of bone (MLTB – see 4.6.3 and

Fig. 4.3; well-defined, dense bony masses); osteochondroma or multiple cartilaginous exostoses (in cats, often involve the skull; rounded, well-mineralized juxtacortical masses); osteosarcoma (often predominantly proliferative in the skull).
  - Overlapping fracture fragments.
  - Foreign body reaction.
  - Calcification of a meningioma or hyperostosis of overlying cranial bone (especially in cats).
  - Myelographic contrast in the ventricular system and subarachnoid space – characteristic pattern following brain sulci.
  b. Generalized.
  - Increased radiopacity due to cranial bone thickening (see 4.6.2).
  - Craniomandibular osteopathy may cause calvarial thickening (see 4.11.1 and Fig. 4.6).
  - Osteopetrosis (see 1.13.15).
  - Idiopathic calvarial hyperostosis of Bullmastiffs (see 4.6.2).
3. Mixed or mottled radiopacity of the cranial bones – usually due to a mixture of bone production or soft tissue mineralization and osteolysis.
  a. Neoplasia – primary bone and soft tissue tumours tend to have varying proportions of bone destruction and bone proliferation or soft tissue mineralization. Examples are osteosarcoma, which tends to be predominantly proliferative at this site but with some destruction, and MLTB (osteochondrosarcoma), which is a dense mass with speckled mineralization and little osteolysis of underlying bone, most often involving the temporo-occipital region (see 4.6.3 and Fig. 4.3).
  b. Osteomyelitis – especially following trauma, and may be associated with meningitis.
  - Bacterial.
  - Fungal (e.g. cryptococcosis*) – predominantly osteolytic.

4.6 VARIATIONS IN THICKNESS OF THE CALVARIAL BONES; CALVARIAL MASSES

1. Thinning of the bones of the calvarium.
  a. Normal variant in small, brachycephalic breeds of dog, possibly due to subclinical hydrocephalus.
  b. Hydrocephalus (congenital or arising at a young age) – usually with a domed calvarium, open suture lines and fontanelle and a homogeneous 'ground glass' radiopacity. If there are open sutures, it may be possible to examine the brain ultrasonographically (see 4.7). Acquired hydrocephalus is unlikely to produce bony changes.
  c. Erosion by an adjacent mass.
2. Increased thickness of the bones of the calvarium.
  a. Normal variant in some breeds (e.g. Pit Bull Terrier).
  b. Healed fracture.
  c. Craniomandibular osteopathy (may affect parietal, frontal, occipital and temporal bones as well as the mandible – see 4.11.1 and Fig. 4.6).
  d. Hyperostosis (thickening and sclerosis) of the calvarium in young Bullmastiffs approximately 6–9 months of age – usually self-limiting and regresses at skeletal maturity; unknown aetiology, although it has some similarities to craniomandibular osteopathy and human infantile cortical hyperostosis. Affects mostly males but also reported in females and there may be a familial component. Femoral periostitis was also described in one dog.
  e. Meningioma in cats – may cause localized hyperostosis adjacent to the tumour; often best seen on a RCd view.
  f. Acromegaly in cats.
  g. Hypervitaminosis A in cats may give rise to occipital new bone (see 5.4.8).
3. Bony masses on the calvarium.
  a. Malignant neoplasia, for example osteosarcoma, chondrosarcoma, MLTB (also known as multilobular osteochondrosarcoma, chondroma rodens). Varying degrees of associated osteolysis. MLTB is an uncommon canine tumour that arises almost exclusively on the skull, mainly on the calvarium, maxilla and mandible. It is slow-growing and locally invasive, often recurring after excision. Metastasis may occur. Radiographically, it appears as a dense, mineralized mass with a nodular or stippled pattern and a variable degree of underlying osteolysis (Fig. 4.3).
  b. Benign neoplasia (e.g. osteoma) – rare in small animals.

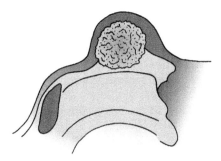

Figure 4.3 Multilobular tumour of bone (multilobular osteochondrosarcoma): a dense, mineralized mass with a stippled, broccoli-like appearance arises from the calvarium.

c. Osteochondroma (cartilaginous exostoses) – especially cats – (see 1.15.2).
d. Healing or healed trauma (e.g. fracture, subperiosteal haematoma).
e. Severe, localized osteomyelitis.

4.7 ULTRASONOGRAPHY OF THE BRAIN

Ultrasonographic examination of the brain is possible if there is an open fontanelle, and so can often be performed in young dogs and sometimes in adults of brachycephalic breeds. The brain itself appears hypoechoic and loosely granular in texture, while the interior of the cranial cavity is outlined by a well-defined echogenic line. It may be possible to identify the lateral ventricles as small anechoic foci, usually bilaterally symmetrical in size, shape and position. MRI and CT are, however, superior imaging techniques for imaging of intracranial structures.

Blood flow in the basilar artery (located by colour Doppler) can be evaluated via the cisterna magna. Flow in the ventrally located rostral or middle cerebral arteries can also be measured if there is an open fontanelle. Because absolute flows can be influenced by the angle between the incident sound and the artery, it is more usual to measure the resistive index (RI), which is the ratio of the difference between peak systolic and end diastolic velocities (V_s and V_d, respectively) and the peak systolic velocity:

$$RI = \frac{V_s - V_d}{V_s.}$$

The normal RI in the basilar artery in dogs is 0.56–0.75. RI correlates strongly with intracranial pressure, hence increased RI reflects raised intracranial pressure. Care should be taken in interpreting RI in animals under general anaesthesia or with cardiovascular disease.

1. Increased size of the lateral ventricles.
   a. Breed-associated; most brachycephalic breeds of dog have larger lateral ventricles than non-brachycephalic breeds.
   b. Hydrocephalus.
      – Congenital.
      – Acquired due to obstructive lesions such as tumours causing increased production of cerebrospinal fluid or preventing its caudal flow.
2. Increased RI.
   a. Hydrocephalus.
   b. Intracranial mass lesions.
   c. Intracranial bleeding.
   d. Brain oedema.
   e. Inflammatory brain disease.
   f. Raised systolic blood pressure.

MAXILLA AND PREMAXILLA

Views

a. Laterolateral (right and left sides are superimposed).
b. Lateral oblique.
c. Intraoral DV.
d. Intraoral DV with beam angled laterally for maxillary teeth.
e. Open mouth VD (ventro 10° rostral–dorsocaudal oblique) (Fig. 4.12).

4.8 MAXILLARY AND PREMAXILLARY BONY PROLIFERATION OR SCLEROSIS

1. Osteomyelitis – usually a mixture of bone proliferation and destruction.
   a. Secondary to dental disease.
   b. Secondary to chronic dacryocystitis and may be associated with cystic dilation of the nasolacrimal duct; dacryocystorhinography is indicated (see 4.38).
   c. Bacterial.
   d. Fungal.
2. Neoplasia – more often predominantly osteolytic (see below) but can be proliferative; some are exclusively proliferative, for example

MLTB (see 4.6.3 and Fig. 4.3). Nasal cavity neoplasia may produce apparent increase in radiopacity of the maxilla on the lateral radiograph.
3. Healing or healed maxillary or premaxillary fracture.

4.9 MAXILLARY AND PREMAXILLARY BONY DESTRUCTION OR RAREFACTION

1. Malignant neoplasia – all types may show some degree of bone proliferation but some are predominantly osteolytic. The osteolysis varies from localized and sharply marginated in appearance to diffuse; teeth in the area may be displaced, eroded or lost. The histological nature of the mass cannot be predicted from the radiographs.
   a. Squamous cell carcinoma (Fig. 4.4); commonest oral tumour in cats.
   b. Malignant melanoma; commonest oral tumour in dogs.
   c. Fibrosarcoma.
   d. Primary bone tumours, primarily osteosarcoma.
   e. Other oral sarcomas (e.g. leiomyosarcoma).
   f. Nasal cavity neoplasia eroding the surrounding bony case.
2. Non-malignant, odontogenic tumours – these do not metastasize but are locally invasive and therefore often radiographically indistinguishable from malignant tumours.

a. Acanthomatous ameloblastoma (acanthomatous epulis, basal cell carcinoma, adamantinoma) – dogs only.
   b. Ameloblastoma.
   c. Amyloid-producing odontogenic tumour.
   d. Complex and compound odontoma – include organized or disorganized dental tissue (see 4.12.2. and Fig. 4.7).
   e. Other rare odontogenic tumours.
3. Dentigerous or non-eruption cyst – expansile, radiolucent lesion containing tooth elements.
4. Periodontal disease and dental abscessation – radiolucent halo of osteolysis around the affected tooth root(s) (see 4.30.1 and 4.30.2 and Fig. 4.17).
5. Renal secondary hyperparathyroidism (rubber jaw, osteodystrophia fibrosa) (Fig. 4.5) – osteopenia secondary to chronic renal disease, especially renal dysplasia in young animals. The skull is affected primarily, and bones become osteopenic with a lace-like trabecular pattern and prominence of the nasal turbinates and soft tissue structures such as the soft palate. Bone mineral loss is especially marked around the teeth, with ill-defined haloes of rarefaction giving the impression of floating teeth. Rarely, primary or nutritional secondary hyperparathyroidism in adult animals may cause the same signs.
6. Nasolacrimal duct cysts – discrete radiolucency with a fine, sclerotic margin, communicating with the nasolacrimal duct on dacryocystorhinography (see 4.38).

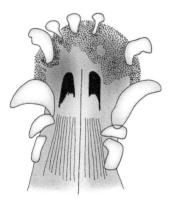

Figure 4.4 Squamous cell carcinoma of the premaxilla: mainly osteolytic with displacement, loss and erosion of teeth.

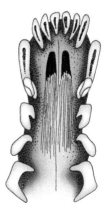

Figure 4.5 Renal secondary hyperparathyroidism: rarefaction of bone produces ill-defined radiolucent haloes around the teeth, giving the impression of floating teeth.

7. Maxillary cholesterol granuloma – identical in appearance to nasolacrimal duct cyst but no communication with the nasolacrimal duct.
8. Maxillary bone epithelial cyst – discrete osteolytic lesion, seen mainly in young dogs and not communicating with the nasolacrimal duct.
9. Maxillary giant cell granuloma – discrete osteolytic lesion, seen mainly in young dogs and not communicating with the nasolacrimal duct.
10. Fractures – check involvement of teeth, especially permanent tooth germs in young animals.

4.10 MIXED PROLIFERATIVE–OSTEOLYTIC MAXILLARY AND PREMAXILLARY LESIONS

1. Periodontal disease and dental abscessation – radiolucent halo of osteolysis around tooth root(s) and surrounding sclerosis.
2. Neoplasia – mixed osteolysis and new bone production; tumours of dental origin also contain highly opaque dental tissue.

MANDIBLE

Views

a. Laterolateral (mandibles are superimposed over each other).
b. Dorsoventral or ventrodorsal (partly obscured by maxillae).
c. Lateral oblique.
d. Intraoral VD.
e. Intraoral DV with beam angled laterally for mandibular teeth.

Normal appearance

The mandibles of brachycephalic breeds are markedly curved when seen on the lateral view, suggesting an attempt at shortening in order for the incisor teeth to approach those of the pre-maxilla (Fig. 4.1b). In elderly cats, the mandibular symphysis appears irregular on the intraoral view.

4.11 MANDIBULAR BONY PROLIFERATION OR SCLEROSIS

1. Craniomandibular osteopathy (Fig. 4.6) – florid periosteal new bone that remodels with time; immature dogs, primarily small breeds such as the West Highland White Terrier, Cairn Terrier and Scottish Terrier but occasionally large breeds; usually involves the mandible and/or the tympanic bullae but also sometimes the calvarium and frontal bones. The new bone is mainly palisading in appearance (see 1.6.1), and osteolysis is absent. Clinical signs often wax and wane, with bouts of pyrexia as well as swelling of the affected mandible(s); difficulty eating if the new bone encroaches on the TMJs.
2. Osteomyelitis – usually a mixture of bone proliferation and destruction.
   a. Secondary to dental disease or fracture.
   b. Bacterial.
   c. Fungal.
3. Neoplasia – more often predominantly osteolytic (see below) but can be proliferative; some are exclusively proliferative (e.g. osteoma). For MLTB, see 4.6.3 and Figure 4.3.
4. Healing or healed mandibular fracture.
5. Canine leucocyte adhesion deficiency – young Irish Setters (see 1.24.9).
6. Acromegaly (cats).

4.12 MANDIBULAR BONY DESTRUCTION OR RAREFACTION

1. Malignant neoplasia – as in maxilla (see 4.9.1 and Fig. 4.4).
2. Non-malignant, odontogenic tumours (see 4.9.2) (Fig. 4.7).
3. Dentigerous or non-eruption cyst; especially affecting PM1, with focal areas of mandibular osteolysis seen unilaterally or bilaterally; Boxers may be predisposed.

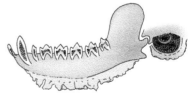

Figure 4.6 Craniomandibular osteopathy: florid periosteal new bone affecting the mandible and tympanic bulla.

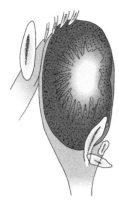

Figure 4.7 Tumour of dental origin: a complex odontoma in a young dog, seen as an expansile osteolytic bone lesion containing material of dental radiopacity.

4. Periodontal disease and dental abscessation – radiolucent halo of osteolysis around the affected root(s) (see 4.30.1 and Fig. 4.17). In severe cases may lead to pathological mandibular fracture.
5. Renal secondary hyperparathyroidism (rubber jaw) – osteopenia secondary to chronic renal disease (see 4.9.5 and Fig. 4.5).
6. Mandibular giant cell granuloma – discrete osteolytic lesion seen mainly in young dogs.

4.13 MANDIBULAR FRACTURE

1. Trauma.
   a. Symphyseal injury – most common in the cat; high rise syndrome (falling from a height) typically results in symphyseal separation and splitting of the hard palate, in conjunction with limb and soft tissue injuries.
   b. Fractures of the body of the mandible – check involvement of teeth, especially permanent tooth germs in young animals.
   c. Fractures of the ramus (also, depressed factures of the zygomatic arch may impinge on the ramus, causing problems opening the mouth).
   d. Fractures involving the TMJ; may cause subsequent TMJ ankylosis, especially in cats.
2. Pathological fracture.
   a. Through an area of severe periodontal disease or a dental abscess, especially in toy breeds of dog.

   b. Osteolytic tumour, for example squamous cell carcinoma, melanoma, lymphoma (especially cats).
   c. Renal secondary hyperparathyroidism.

4.14 MIXED PROLIFERATIVE–OSTEOLYTIC MANDIBULAR LESIONS

See 4.10. In cats especially, it is difficult to differentiate mandibular osteomyelitis from neoplasia, as both may produce osteolysis (sometimes with pathological fracture), sclerosis, periosteal new bone and erosion of teeth.

TEMPOROMANDIBULAR JOINT

The TMJ is a transversely elongated condylar synovial joint formed between the condylar process of the mandible and the mandibular fossa of the temporal bone. The fossa has a caudoventral extension, the retroarticular process, which prevents caudal luxation of the joint. The TMJ does not lie truly transversely but is angled slightly in a caudolateral to rostromedial direction. There is considerable variation in the precise orientation of the TMJ between breeds and individuals, with the joint lying more obliquely in brachycephalic animals. Accurate radiographic demonstration of the joint can be challenging due to these anatomical variations and to superimposition by other structures.

Views

a. Sagittal oblique (with mouth open and closed, Fig. 4.8). An angle of 10–30° in mesaticephalic and dolichocephalic breeds and an angle of 20–30° in brachycephalic breeds have been found to be optimal. Slight lateral rotation of about 10° may also help to prevent superimposition over the base of the skull.
b. Ventrodorsal or DV.

Normal appearance

On the sagittal oblique views, the mandibular condyle should be smoothly rounded, fitting closely into the glenoid (the smooth concavity in the petrous temporal bone), immediately rostral to the tympanic bulla.

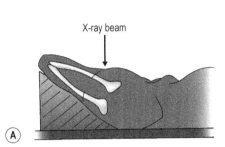
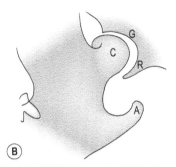

Figure 4.8 (A) Positioning for the sagittal oblique view of temporomandibular joint (TMJ): from a true lateral position, the nose is tilted upwards 10–30° depending on conformation (more tilt in brachycephalic breeds). (B) Normal appearance of the TMJ on a sagittal oblique view (A, angular process of mandible; C, condyle; G, glenoid or mandibular fossa of temporal bone; R, retroarticular process).

4.15 TEMPOROMANDIBULAR JOINT NOT CLEARLY SEEN

1. Incorrect positioning, especially use of the lateral oblique view (as for tympanic bullae) rather than the sagittal oblique view, as the X-ray beam does not pass through the joint space.
2. Technical factors.
   a. Underexposure.
   b. Underdevelopment.
3. Trauma.
   a. Fracture.
   b. Luxation or subluxation.
4. Periarticular new bone.
   a. Healing or healed fracture.
   b. Osteoarthritis.
   c. Ankylosis following trauma – especially cats after mandibular trauma; may be bilateral. Pseudoankylosis without radiographic changes can occur due to fibrosis as a result of haemarthrosis.
   d. Craniomandibular osteopathy (see 4.11.1 and Fig. 4.6); changes usually most marked along the mandibular ramus and on the tympanic bullae, but the TMJs may be involved secondarily.
   e. Canine leucocyte adhesion deficiency (young Irish Setters – see 1.23.7).
5. Destruction of articular surfaces.
   a. Infection – may extend from infection of the external or middle ear or from a para-aural abscess or wound.
   b. Neoplasia – primary bone tumour or invading soft tissue tumour; variable amounts of new bone too.

4.16 ABNORMALITIES OF THE TEMPOROMANDIBULAR JOINT

1. Irregular articular surfaces.
   a. Trauma.
      – Fracture; may lead to ankylosis secondary to haemarthrosis or callus, especially in cats.
      – Luxation or subluxation; usually unilateral, with condyle displaced rostrally and deviation of the mandible to the contralateral side; rarely, fracture of the retroarticular process allows caudal luxation.
   b. Osteoarthritis – narrowing of joint space and periarticular osteophytes may also be seen.
   c. Infection – may extend from infection of the external or middle ear or from a para-aural abscess or wound.
   d. Neoplasia – primary bone tumour or invading soft tissue tumour; variable amounts of new bone too.
2. Temporomandibular joint dysplasia – flattening ± abnormal angulation of the articular surfaces and absence of the retroarticular process are seen in some cases; especially the Basset Hound and Irish Setter. May be clinically silent in some dogs, especially the Cavalier King Charles Spaniel. On an open mouth VD view, the coronoid process of the mandible may be seen to impinge on the zygomatic arch, resulting in open mouth jaw locking. If the condition is unilateral, the impinging coronoid process is on the side contralateral to the TMJ dysplasia. Subluxation of the mandibular condyle may sometimes be seen by comparing open and closed mouth sagittal oblique radiographs.

EAR

Views

a. Dorsoventral or VD, for external ear canals and tympanic bullae (the DV is usually easier to position symmetrically, as facial landmarks can be seen). The petrous temporal bones and cranium are superimposed over the bullae, but comparison between right and left sides is possible.

b. Lateral oblique, skylining the dependent tympanic bulla.

c. Open mouth RCd for tympanic bullae (Fig. 4.9).

d. In the cat, a special view, the rostro 10° ventral– dorsocaudal oblique, has been described for the tympanic bullae (Fig. 4.10) and is technically easier than the RCd open mouth view used in dogs.

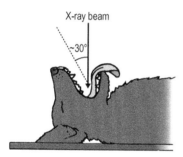

Figure 4.9 Positioning for the open mouth rostrocaudal view for the tympanic bullae. The hard palate lies about 30° beyond the vertical, but the precise position depends on the skull conformation. The endotracheal tube is usually removed for the exposure. Positioning aids are not shown.

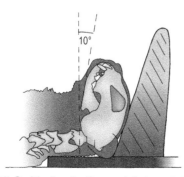

Figure 4.10 Positioning for the special view of the feline tympanic bullae.

Normal appearance

The normal external ear canals are seen as bands of gas lucency lateral to the tympanic bullae. The external ear canals and the pinnae may create confusing shadows on lateral and oblique radiographs. The walls of the tympanic bullae are seen as thin and regular bony structures, the cat also having an inner bony septum that divides the bulla incompletely into ventromedial and dorsolateral compartments.

Positive contrast canalography

The use of positive contrast medium has been described for assessment of the integrity of the tympanic membrane and for evaluation of stenotic ear canals. A small amount of non-ionic contrast medium such as iohexol is instilled into the ear canal and massaged. Presence of contrast medium in the bulla indicates rupture of the tympanic membrane, although false negative results may arise due to plugging of the ear canal with inflammatory debris.

Fistulography

If a para-aural abscess with discharging tracts is present, fistulography may be used to look for connection with the ear.

4.17 ABNORMALITIES OF THE EXTERNAL EAR CANAL

1. External ear canal not visible.
   a. Overexposure, overdevelopment or severe fogging of the film.
   b. Congenital absence of the ear canal (atresia).
   c. Occlusion of the canal by wax, debris or purulent material.
   d. Traumatic separation of the ear canal, usually between the annular and auricular cartilages; may give rise to otitis media and para-aural abscessation ± discharging sinuses.
   e. Previous surgical ablation of the canal.
   f. Occlusion of the canal by a soft tissue mass within or outside the canal.
      - Neoplasm.
      - Inflammatory polyp.
      - Para-aural abscess.
2. Narrowing of the external ear canal.

a. Hypertrophy and/or inflammation of the lining of the canal – due to acute or chronic otitis externa.

b. Compression of the canal by a para-aural mass or swelling.

3. Calcification of the external ear canal.

a. Normal – a small amount of orderly calcification of the cartilages encircling the canal may be normal in older dogs.

b. Sequel to chronic otitis externa.

c. Sequel to auditory canal atresia; may be associated with para-aural abscessation and draining sinuses.

d. Sequel to traumatic separation of the ear canal; may be associated with para-aural abscessation and draining sinuses.

4.18 VARIATIONS IN THE WALL OF THE TYMPANIC BULLA

1. Thickening of the wall of the tympanic bulla.

a. Normal variant in some brachycephalic breeds, for example Cavalier King Charles Spaniel, which has small bullae with relatively thickened walls.

b. Otitis media (middle ear disease; Fig. 4.11).

c. Inflammatory polyp – check for nasopharyngeal polyp too, especially in cats.

d. Craniomandibular osteopathy (see 4.11.1 and Fig. 4.6).

e. Neoplasia (usually with osteolysis too).
   - Squamous cell carcinoma.
   - Adenocarcinoma.

f. Canine leucocyte adhesion deficiency (young Irish Setters – see 1.24.9).

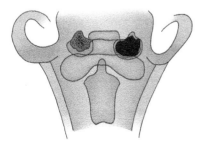

Figure 4.11 Otitis media: thickening of the bulla wall and increased radiopacity of the bulla lumen, seen here on an open mouth rostrocaudal radiograph.

2. Thinning or destruction of the wall of the tympanic bulla.

a. Neoplasia.
   - Squamous cell carcinoma.
   - Adenocarcinoma.
   - Lymphoma.

b. Severe otitis media with osteomyelitis.

c. Trapped ceruminous debris secondary to external auditory canal atresia.

d. Previous bulla osteotomy.

4.19 INCREASED RADIOPACITY OF THE TYMPANIC BULLA

1. Artefactual due to poor positioning on the open mouth RCd view, or superimposition of the tongue.

2. Increased radiopacity of the bulla – may be due to obliteration of air within the bulla and/or thickening of the bulla wall.

a. Accumulation of fluid in the bulla is a common finding in brachycephalic dogs on MRI, although radiographic findings in such cases have not been described.

b. Accumulation of fluid in the bulla may also be the result of auditory tube dysfunction (e.g. with trigeminal neuropathy or palatine defects).

c. Otitis media, usually with thickening of the bulla wall.

d. Inflammatory polyp, often with thickening of the bulla wall; may extend into the external ear canal or nasopharynx.

e. Neoplasia (see above).

f. Trapped ceruminous debris secondary to auditory canal atresia.

g. Cholesterol granuloma.

h. Cholesteatoma.

i. Otolithiasis – discrete, mineralized opacities within the bulla lumen probably due to mineralization of necrotic material due to current or previous otitis media; may be an incidental finding.

3. Increased radiopacity due to thickening of the bony bulla wall (see 4.18.1 and Fig. 4.11).

Note that radiography is relatively insensitive for detection of middle ear disease, and normal radiographs do not rule out the diagnosis. MRI (gold standard) and CT are preferred techniques.

4.20 ULTRASONOGRAPHY OF THE TYMPANIC BULLA

Ultrasonography can be used to detect fluid within the bulla and is more sensitive and specific than radiography in this respect. When fluid is present, the bulla lumen appears anechoic and the deep wall of the bulla is visible, but when the bulla contains air, sound is reflected from the bone–air interface at the superficial bulla wall and the lumen is not visible due to reverberation artefact. Saline may be infused into the ear canal to act as an acoustic window for visualization of the tympanic membrane.

NASAL CAVITY

Views

a. Intraoral DV (occlusal).
b. Open mouth ventro 20° rostral–dorsocaudal oblique (open mouth VD) (Fig. 4.12).
c. Dorsoventral or ventrodorsal (the mandibles are superimposed over the lateral parts of the nasal cavity).
d. Laterolateral (the right and left sides are superimposed over each other, but this view is useful for seeing changes in the overlying nasal bones and frontal sinuses).
e. Lateral oblique.
f. Rostrocaudal centred on nares.

Positive contrast rhinography using barium sulphate or iodinated contrast medium has been described

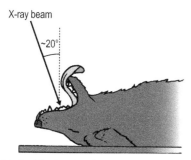

X-ray beam

~20°

Figure 4.12 Positioning for the open mouth ventrodorsal view for the nasal cavity. The X-ray beam is angled about 20° from the vertical. It is not usually necessary to remove the endotracheal tube. Positioning aids are not shown.

but not widely used. MRI and CT are far superior techniques, if available.

Normal appearance

The turbinate (conchal) pattern should be clearly delineated, and broadly symmetrical when comparing the right and left nasal cavities. In the rostral third of the nasal cavity, the turbinate pattern should consist of a fine linear pattern. In the middle third, the pattern becomes woven into an irregular honeycomb and the ovoid maxillary recesses can be seen laterally. In the caudal third, the pattern returns to a linear form. The bony part of the nasal septum (the vomer) divides the right and left nasal cavities. It is not unusual for the vomer and nasal septum to be curved or deviated in brachycephalic breeds and in cats. Rostrally, the paired palatine fissures are seen. On radiographs taken using a low exposure, the soft tissues of the nostrils can also be assessed.

Nasal radiographs may be highly suggestive of a specific disease in dogs but tend to be non-specific in cats, and biopsy is usually required. Nasal disease, especially nasal neoplasia, may be accompanied by changes in one or both frontal sinuses, and therefore the radiographic protocol should include appropriate frontal sinus views.

4.21 VARIATIONS IN SHAPE OF THE NASAL CAVITY

1. Breed variation.
2. Congenital deformity.
3. Trauma.
4. Mucopolysaccharidosis – inherited condition of the Domestic Short-haired cat, Siamese and Siamese crosses; broad, short maxilla, reduced or absent frontal sinuses, abnormal nasal conchae, hypoplasia of the hyoid apparatus (see also 1.22.11 and 5.4.9).

4.22 INCREASED RADIOPACITY OF THE NASAL CAVITY

1. Increased radiopacity with retention of the underlying turbinate pattern – usually bilateral, occasionally unilateral (Fig. 4.13).
   a. Underexposure.
   b. Underdevelopment.
   c. Recent nasal flushing.

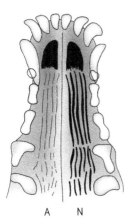

A   N

Figure 4.13 Unilateral rhinitis: the turbinate pattern is blurred compared with the normal side, and there is an overall increase in radiopacity. Confident diagnosis is harder if the changes are bilateral. A, affected side; N, normal nasal cavity.

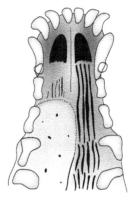

Figure 4.14 Nasal neoplasia: destruction of turbinate bones by a soft tissue radiopacity, with deviation and interruption of the nasal septum or vomer shadow; osteolysis of surrounding bones (maxilla, nasal bones and palate) may also occur.

d. Inflammatory rhinitis (e.g. lymphoplasmacytic, eosinophilic, neutrophilic, foreign body), although normal radiographs do not rule out rhinitis.
e. Hyperplastic rhinitis.
f. Rhinitis–bronchopneumonia syndrome in Irish Wolfhounds – aetiology unknown; may be immune-mediated or a primary ciliary defect and appears to be heritable. Most affected dogs show transient to persistent mucoid to mucopurulent nasal discharge of varying severity from birth, with bouts of bronchopneumonia.
g. Rhinitis associated with dental disease (see 4.28–4.30).
h. Nasal haemorrhage (coagulopathy, trauma, immune-mediated disease).
i. Small or recent nasal foreign body (unilateral).
j. Kartagener's syndrome (or immotile cilia syndrome; often associated with situs inversus and evidence of bronchitis or bronchiectasis – see 6.12.8).
k. Primary ciliary dyskinesia (see 6.12.7).
l. Cryptococcosis* – especially cats.
m. Capillariasis* – may rarely cause rhinitis.
n. *Pneumonyssus caninum** – nasal mite.
o. Fibrous osteodystrophy secondary to hyperparathyroidism (see 1.16.4).

2. Increased radiopacity with loss of the underlying turbinate pattern – usually begins unilaterally (there may also be destruction of the vomer and/or surrounding bones). Note that inability to identify a turbinate pattern does not necessarily mean that lysis has occurred; intact turbinates may be obscured by adjacent tissue, especially in cats with nasal lymphoma.

a. Neoplasia (Fig. 4.14) – carcinoma most common; also sarcomas, including chondrosarcoma and lymphoma (especially cats). Nasal lymphoma in cats may be associated with renal lymphoma. Neoplasia may also extend into the nasal cavity from the frontal sinus or orbit. Nasal tumours are usually seen in middle-aged and older animals and are much less common in brachycephalic than mesati- or dolichocephalic dogs. They usually arise in the caudal or mid-third of the nasal cavity, often near the carnassial tooth. Initially unilateral but often extend into the contralateral nasal cavity with interruption of the intervening vomer or nasal septum. Nasal neoplasia is often associated with frontal sinus opacification due to trapped secretions, whereas this is unusual with rhinitis. Erosion of surrounding bones (nasal, maxilla, palate) occurs in severe cases.
b. Nasal polyp – cats > dogs. In cats, also known as ethmoturbinate polyps, as they are inflammatory polyps arising from the nasal ethmoturbinates; they usually follow a preceding upper respiratory infection and are mainly seen in cats 6–24 months old.

Unilateral or bilateral nasal cavity involvement. Most reported cases are from Italy.

c. Fungal rhinitis, especially aspergillosis*, usually overall decreased opacity but see patchy increased opacity if there is marked retention of necrotic material or a fungal granuloma – see below. Unilateral or bilateral, with variable involvement of the nasal septum or vomer and frontal sinuses, and osteomyelitis of surrounding bones in severe cases.

d. Other inflammatory rhinitides (e.g. lymphoplasmacytic rhinitis) may cause mild to moderate turbinate destruction; unilateral or bilateral.

e. Chronic nasal foreign body; unilateral.

f. Fibrous dysplasia; bilateral.

3. Mineralization within the nasal cavity.
a. Mineralization of neoplasia (e.g. osteosarcoma, chondrosarcoma).
b. Mineralization of a fungal granuloma.
c. Mineralized foreign body.
d. Displaced tooth – congenital, traumatic.

4.23 DECREASED RADIOPACITY OF THE NASAL CAVITY

1. Decreased radiopacity with retention of the underlying turbinate pattern – bilateral.
a. Overexposure.
b. Overdevelopment.
c. Severe fogging of the film.

2. Decreased radiopacity with destruction of the underlying turbinate pattern – unilateral or bilateral; may be interspersed with ill-defined patches of increased opacity. An ill-defined, rostrally directed lucent tract may be seen adjacent to the nasal septum; this is due to widening of the common nasal meatus as conchae are destroyed.
a. Fungal rhinitis (Fig. 4.15) – especially *Aspergillus** spp. but also *Penicillium*, *Cryptococcus** and other species; may also be present with a foreign body. Mainly young dogs of dolichocephalic and mesaticephalic breeds; less common in cats and in brachycephalic dogs. Unilateral or bilateral and usually starts in the rostral part of the nasal cavity, sparing the ethmoturbinates.

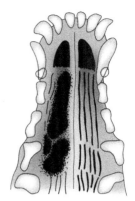

Figure 4.15 Destructive rhinitis (aspergillosis): loss of the turbinate pattern, with ill-defined and patchy increase in radiopacity rather than diffuse nasal opacification.

Nasal septum or vomer shadow may or may not be interrupted. In some cases, frontal sinus changes due to osteomyelitis or fungal granuloma may be seen.

b. Viral rhinitis, leading to chronic, destructive bacterial rhinitis (cats).
c. Lymphoplasmacytic rhinitis.
d. Nasal foreign body.
e. Destruction of the supporting palatine or maxillary bone if nasal neoplasia is eroding the surrounding bones; may be small, punctuate lucencies or larger areas.
f. Congenital defect of the hard palate.
g. Previous rhinotomy.
h. Nasal tumour that has fragmented and been sneezed out or displaced by nasal flushing.

FRONTAL SINUSES

Views

a. Rostrocaudal (vertical X-ray beam) or caudorostral (horizontal X-ray beam).
b. Lateral oblique.
c. Laterolateral (right and left frontal sinuses are superimposed).
d. Dorsoventral or ventrodorsal (frontal sinuses are partially superimposed by the caudal nasal cavity and rostral calvarium).

Normal appearance

The frontal sinuses should be filled with air, which outlines the smooth bony folds of the walls. The frontal sinuses are more prominent in larger breeds of dog and in cats than in smaller breeds of dog; they may be absent in some brachycephalic breeds. They are small at birth, enlarging with age. The sinuses are lined by mucoperiosteum.

Frontal sinus changes may arise secondary to nasal disease, and the radiographic protocol will usually need to include both areas.

4.24 VARIATIONS IN SHAPE OF THE FRONTAL SINUSES

1. Breed and conformational variations – the frontal sinuses may be extremely large and prominent in some giant breeds of dog, such as the St. Bernard, and small or absent in brachycephalic breeds.
2. Trauma.
   a. Fracture of the walls of the sinus, usually a depressed fracture leading to concavity of the sinus.
   b. Occlusion of drainage due to a nasofrontal fracture, leading to accumulation of frontal sinus secretions and an expanded sinus with thinning of the overlying frontal bones (frontal sinus mucocele).
3. Neoplasm involving the frontal bones; osteolysis and/or new bone production, usually with marked overlying soft tissue swelling.
4. Osteomyelitis involving the frontal bones; usually less severe than changes due to neoplasia; may produce a mottled radiopacity. Most often secondary to aspergillosis (see 4.23.2 and Fig. 4.15).
5. Craniomandibular osteopathy may affect the frontal bone, causing reduction in sinus volume internally and distortion externally, possibly leading to exophthalmos (see 4.11.1 and Fig. 4.6).
6. Aplasia – mucopolysaccharidosis in cats.

4.25 INCREASED RADIOPACITY OF THE FRONTAL SINUSES

Increased radiopacity of the frontal sinuses may be due to the presence of fluid or soft tissue within the sinus or to the superimposition of new bone or soft tissue swelling.

1. Sinusitis.
   a. Bacterial.

b. Fungal – especially *Aspergillus** spp.; some cases develop frontal bone osteomyelitis, which produces a mottled opacity to the bone; fungal granuloma may also occur. Nasal cavity changes usually predominate (see 4.23.2 and Fig. 4.15).
   c. Associated with rhinitis (e.g. idiopathic lymphoplasmacytic rhinitis).
   d. Allergic.
   e. Subsequent to viral respiratory disease.
   f. Kartagener's syndrome (see 6.12.8).
2. Occlusion of drainage of the frontal sinuses, leading to mucus retention.
   a. Trauma – occlusion of the frontonasal ostium due to a fracture, leading to accumulation of secretions and a frontal sinus mucocele.
   b. Mass in the caudal nasal cavity, usually neoplastic (see 4.22.2 and Fig. 4.14).
3. Neoplasia (note that neoplastic tissue and trapped fluid cannot be distinguished on radiographs, and both will cause increase in sinus opacity).
   a. Extension of nasal or orbital neoplasia into the frontal sinuses.
   b. Soft tissue or bone neoplasia arising within the frontal bone or sinus.
      – Carcinoma – soft tissue radiopacity; osteolytic.
      – Osteosarcoma – mixed bone lesion.
      – Osteoma or MLTB; mainly proliferative (see 4.6.3 and Fig. 4.3).
4. Haemorrhage following trauma (usually with bony changes as well).
5. Craniomandibular osteopathy – thickening of the frontal bones and reduction of sinus volume may occur, usually in conjunction with new bone in other typical locations (see 4.11.1 and Fig. 4.6) but occasionally in isolation.
6. Canine leucocyte adhesion deficiency – young Irish Setters (see 1.24.9).

4.26 VARIATIONS IN THICKNESS OF THE FRONTAL BONES

1. Increase in thickness of the frontal bones or bony mass.
   a. Healing or healed fracture.
   b. Secondary to fungal sinusitis.

c. Neoplasm involving the frontal bones (see above).

d. Craniomandibular osteopathy (see 4.11.1 and Fig. 4.6).

e. Calvarial hyperostosis of Bullmastiffs (see 4.6.2).

f. Canine leucocyte adhesion deficiency (young Irish Setters – see 1.24.9).

g. Acromegaly (cats).

2. Decrease in thickness or osteolysis of the frontal bones.

a. Neoplasm involving the frontal bones (see above).

b. Osteomyelitis involving the frontal bones.

c. Erosion by an adjacent mass.

d. Secondary to a frontal sinus mucocele – likely to be expansile.

3. Bony masses – see 4.6.3 (cranial bony masses), as the principles of interpretation are the same.

TEETH

Views

a. Lateral oblique.

b. Intraoral DV and VD views of the maxilla and mandible, respectively.

c. Bisecting angle technique (incisors, canines and upper premolars and molars).

d. Intraoral parallel technique (mandibular premolars and molars).

e. Near-parallel view for carnassial teeth (108, 208) in cats.

Normal appearance

Each normal tooth has a well-defined crown and one or more clearly defined roots (Fig. 4.16). Most

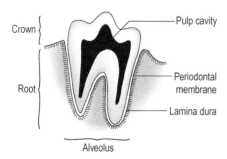

Figure 4.16 Anatomy of a normal tooth.

of the tooth consists of dentin, with a covering of enamel over the crown and cementum over the root. Blood vessels and nerves lie in the inner pulp cavity. Enamel, dentin and cementum are radiopaque, while the inner pulp cavity is relatively radiolucent. Occasionally, the enamel is seen to be more radiopaque than the underlying dentin. In the immature animal, the pulp cavity is wide with an open apical foramen; in the mature animal, the pulp cavity narrows and the apical foramina close. The tooth roots are embedded in the alveolar bone of the mandible, maxilla or premaxilla. They are surrounded by a radiolucent zone created by the periodontal membrane and outlined by a thin, radiopaque line – the lamina dura. Some permanent tooth germs already start forming in utero.

The normal dental formulae for the dog and cat are given below.

Immature (deciduous teeth)
- Dog: $2 \times I\,^3/_3\,C\,^1/_1\,PM\,^3/_3 = 28$
- Cat: $2 \times I\,^3/_3\,C\,^1/_1\,PM\,^3/_2 = 26$

Mature
- Dog: $2 \times I\,^3/_3\,C\,^1/_1\,PM\,^4/_4\,M\,^2/_3 = 42$
- Cat: $2 \times I\,^3/_3\,C\,^1/_1\,PM\,^3/_2\,M\,^1/_1 = 30$

The modified Triadan system for numbering teeth allows each tooth to be identified by a number: the right (pre)maxillary teeth being prefixed 1, left teeth (pre)maxillary 2, left mandibular 3 and right mandibular 4; for example, left maxillary PM4 in the adult dog is 208.

4.27 VARIATIONS IN THE NUMBER OF TEETH

1. Decrease in the number of teeth (hypodontia).
a. Congenital.
   - Anodontia (total absence of teeth) – very rare.
   - Isolated hypodontia (oligodontia) – reduction in the number of teeth; may be symmetrical or asymmetrical; common in Kerry Blue, Bull Terrier breeds, Labrador and Golden Retriever.
   - Ectodermal dysplasia – breeds deficient in structures that originate from ectoderm (e.g. Mexican Hairless dog, Chinese Crested).
b. Acquired.
   - Previous tooth extraction.

– Tooth loss due to severe periodontal disease or destructive neoplasia.
– Fusion of teeth.

2. Increase in the number of teeth (hyperdontia).
   a. Retained temporary teeth (pseudopolydontia).
   b. Congenital polydontia – usually unilateral and more common in the upper jaw than in the lower; mainly extra incisors or premolars; true extra teeth, referred to as supernumerary teeth.
   c. Germination – incomplete splitting of a tooth into two teeth may produce a single tooth with a double crown, which may be mistaken for two separate teeth.

4.28 VARIATIONS IN THE SHAPE OF TEETH

1. Change in shape of the crown.
   a. Fracture of the crown.
   b. Abnormal wear of the crown (e.g. stone chewing), resulting in flattening of the tooth tip.
   c. Crown removed; one or more roots retained.
   d. Gemination and/or fusion may create a tooth with an abnormal crown (see 4.27.2).
   e. Supernumerary mandibular fourth premolars may have a conical crown instead of the normal triangular shape.
2. Change in shape of the root.
   a. Periodontal disease leading to deformity or erosion of the root, especially feline odontoclastic resorptive lesions, which cause circumferential erosion just beneath the gum line that may lead to fracture of the crown.
   b. Deformation or displacement by an adjacent mass.
   c. Lysis due to adjacent malignant tumour.
   d. Dilaceration – the root shows a sudden change in direction, usually of about 90°.

4.29 VARIATIONS IN STRUCTURE OR RADIOPACITY OF THE TEETH

1. Fracture of the tooth.
2. Caries – radiolucent defects in the crown.
3. Wide pulp cavity.
   a. Immature tooth (all teeth appear similar).
   b. Dead tooth (other live teeth have a narrower pulp cavity).
   c. Inflammation of the pulp cavity.

– Secondary to fracture of the tooth.
– Secondary to periodontal disease.
– Associated with a dental abscess.

4. Dentinogenesis imperfecta – thinning of dentine layer leading to multiple fractures; sometimes seen with osteogenesis imperfecta (see 1.16.13).

4.30 PERIODONTAL RADIOLUCENCY

1. Periodontal disease – destruction of alveolar bone and resorption of the alveolar crest between the tooth and its neighbours; may extend to form a radiolucent halo around the tooth root, which in the mandible may result in pathological bone fracture.
2. Apical tooth root abscess – pulp necrosis causes inflammation and/or infection around the root apex (Fig. 4.17).
3. Neoplasia (see 4.9.1 and 4.9.2 and Figs 4.4 and 4.7).
4. Primary or secondary hyperparathyroidism (generalized loss of bone radiopacity, although changes due to renal secondary hyperparathyroidism are often most severe around tooth roots – see 4.9.5 and Fig. 4.5).

4.31 DISPLACEMENT OR ABNORMAL LOCATION OF TEETH

1. Normal crowding of premaxillary and maxillary teeth in brachycephalic animals – as the maxilla shortens, the premolars rotate in order to occupy less space; PM3 is affected first.
2. Supernumerary teeth may lie in an abnormal location (e.g. an extra incisor tooth on the palate).
3. Developmental – dentigerous or dental cysts; normal or slightly deformed tooth in an

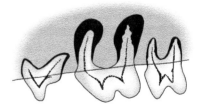

Figure 4.17 Apical tooth root abscess: radiolucent halo around the affected tooth (the carnassial tooth, upper PM4), with irregularity of one of the tooth roots. Dental abscessation at this site is sometimes called malar abscess, and there may be facial swelling ± a discharging sinus.

abnormal location; may be surrounded by a radiolucent cystic area.

4. Fibromatous epulis of periodontal ligament origin – dogs, rare in cats; mainly around canine and carnassial teeth in brachycephalic dogs. Tooth displacement but no osteolysis.

5. Neoplasia – teeth displaced by tumour mass; osteolysis is present and there may be tooth loss (see 4.9.1. and Fig. 4.4). Subtle displacement of tooth roots may be an early sign of jaw neoplasia.

6. Trauma (e.g. in the upper jaw, a tooth may be impacted into the nasal cavity).

PHARYNX AND LARYNX

Views

a. Laterolateral. A true lateral view, without an endotracheal tube in place, is essential for evaluation of the pharynx.

b. Ventrodorsal or dorsoventral: of limited value due to superimposition of the skull and spine.

Normal appearance

The pharynx is divided into the oro- and nasopharynx by the soft palate, which should extend to the tip of the epiglottis, and the area of the pharynx above the larynx is the laryngopharynx (Fig. 4.18). The larynx normally lies the length of C3 ventral to the cervical spine. Mineralization of the laryngeal cartilages in the dog is quite normal and usually begins at 2–3 years of age (or earlier in large or chondrodystrophic breeds).

4.32 VARIATIONS IN THE PHARYNX

1. Reduction or obliteration of the air-filled nasopharynx.
   a. Soft tissue mass in the nasopharynx.
      – Nasopharyngeal polyp (inflammatory, so may be associated with radiological evidence of otitis media, i.e. increased radiopacity of the bulla lumen and thickening of the bulla wall) (Fig. 4.19).
      – Neoplasia (most commonly carcinoma in dogs and lymphoma in cats).
      – Abscess or foreign body reaction.
      – Granuloma.
      – Cyst – nasopharyngeal epidermoid cyst or cystic remnant of Rathke's pouch (may have mineralized wall).
   b. Thickening of the soft palate.
      – Part of brachycephalic obstructive airway syndrome.
      – Palatine mass – tumour, cyst or granuloma.
   c. Excessive pharyngeal tissue – part of the brachycephalic obstructive airway syndrome.
   d. Foreign body in the nasopharynx – will be outlined by air.
   e. Retropharyngeal swelling.
      – Enlarged retropharyngeal lymph nodes (e.g. lymphoma).
      – Retropharyngeal abscess.
      – Retropharyngeal tumour (e.g. of thyroid gland).
   f. Nasopharyngeal stenosis; membranes or fibrotic web.

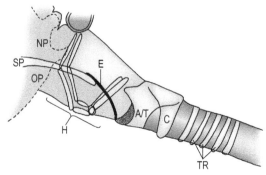

Figure 4.18 Normal lateral pharynx. A/T, arytenoid and thyroid cartilages of the larynx; C, cricoid cartilage of the larynx; E, epiglottis; H, hyoid apparatus; NP, nasopharynx; OP, oropharynx; SP, soft palate; TR, tracheal rings.

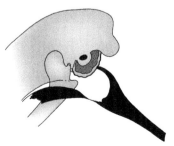

Figure 4.19 Nasopharyngeal polyp in a cat: a soft tissue mass is seen in the nasopharynx, depressing the soft palate. Bony changes are present in one of the tympanic bullae.

    – Congenital stenosis, usually affecting the rostral nasopharynx (e.g. choanal atresia).

    – Stenotic nasopharyngeal dysgenesis – especially Dachshunds; congenital thickening of the palatopharyngeal muscles reducing the intrapharyngeal ostium to a narrow slit. Lateral radiographs show a thick band of soft tissue extending from the terminal soft palate region to the caudodorsal laryngopharynx.

    – Acquired, secondary to trauma or to previous upper respiratory tract disease in cats; strand-like soft tissue opacity or slight dorsal deviation of the soft palate may be seen.

  g. Obesity.

2. Ballooning of the pharynx.
  a. Pharyngeal paralysis.
  b. Respiratory obstruction or air hunger.
  c. Pharyngeal diverticulum, presumably associated with trauma.

3. Radiopacities within the pharynx.
  a. Superimposed ear canal and pinna shadows.
  b. Hyoid bones (see 4.35 and Fig. 4.18).
  c. Mineralization of laryngeal cartilages (see 4.33.3 and Fig. 4.18).
  d. Radiopaque foreign body.
  e. Dystrophic calcification within a mass.
  f. Ossification within a mass.
  g. Superimposed salivary calculi.

4. Miscellaneous.
  a. Abscessation of the tongue in dogs has been reported, with soft tissue swelling of the root of the tongue ± gas-filled centre on radiography, and a fluid-filled cavity seen on ultrasonography.

4.33 VARIATIONS IN THE LARYNX

1. Ventral displacement of the larynx and proximal trachea.
  a. Normal in brachycephalic dogs.
  b. Flexion of the head and neck during radiography.
  c. Enlargement of one or both retropharyngeal lymph nodes.
  d. Enlargement of one or both thyroid glands.

  e. Cellulitis, abscessation or foreign body affecting the retropharyngeal tissues.
  f. Neoplasia involving the retropharyngeal tissues.

2. Caudal displacement of the larynx and proximal trachea.
  a. Normal in brachycephalic dogs.
  b. Extreme dyspnoea.
  c. Laryngeal paralysis.
  d. Disruption of the hyoid apparatus or of the muscles between hyoid and larynx due to trauma (e.g. bite wounds, choke chain injury) or neoplasia.

3. Mineralization of laryngeal cartilages.
  a. Normal ageing changes.
  b. Secondary to laryngeal neoplasia (mineralization is usually more extensive and less ordered).
  c. Secondary to laryngeal chondritis.

4. Reduction or obliteration of the laryngeal airway.
  a. Neoplasia – may show a discrete soft tissue opacity or reduction in margination of laryngeal structures.
    – Carcinoma is most common in the dog.
    – Lymphoma is most common in the cat.
  b. Inflammation.
  c. Lymphoid hyperplasia.
  d. Haemorrhage (e.g. trauma).
  e. Foreign body.
  f. Laryngeal cyst.
  g. Laryngeal granuloma.

4.34 ULTRASONOGRAPHY OF THE LARYNX

Examination from the ventral aspect of the larynx shows the thyroid and cricoid cartilages, with a central stream of reverberations from the air column within. The vocal folds and the cuneiform processes abduct and adduct during respiration.

1. Absence of motion of the cuneiform processes.
  a. Breathing at rest.
  b. Laryngeal paralysis (bilateral).

2. Asymmetry of motion of the cuneiform processes.
  a. Asymmetrical plane of section.
  b. Laryngeal paralysis (unilateral).

3. Distortion or displacement of the central air column.

a. Laryngeal tumour.

b. Laryngeal cyst.

c. Laryngeal collapse due to trauma or secondary to severe obstructive airway disease.

4. Thickening of the soft tissues of the larynx.

a. Laryngeal tumour.

b. Laryngeal cyst.

c. Inflammation.

d. Oedema.

4.35 CHANGES IN THE HYOID APPARATUS

1. Artefactual appearance of subluxation between hyoid bones due to positioning for radiography.
2. Caudal displacement of the hyoid apparatus by a soft tissue mass is normal in brachycephalic breeds (e.g. Bulldog and Pug), the mass being prominent masseter muscles.
3. Fracture – choke chain injuries or other direct trauma.
4. Disruption of relationship between individual hyoid bones – hanging injuries.
5. Bone proliferation and/or destruction.

a. Osteomyelitis.

b. Neoplasia (e.g. thyroid carcinoma).

6. Hyoid hypoplasia – mucopolysaccharidosis; mainly cats (see 5.4.9 and Fig. 5.8).

SOFT TISSUES OF THE HEAD AND NECK

4.36 THICKENING OF THE SOFT TISSUES OF THE HEAD AND NECK

Abnormality may be recognized by displacement of normal structures (e.g. trachea) or by displacement or loss of fascial planes. A barium swallow may be helpful to show the location of the oesophagus. If an area of swelling is identified, further information about its nature may be obtained using ultrasonography, and this will also allow ultrasound-guided fine needle aspiration or biopsy, avoiding vascular structures.

1. Focal thickening of the soft tissues of the head and neck.

a. Sialocele.

b. Soft tissue tumour; injection site sarcoma is seen in cats.

c. Abscess, sometimes secondary to foreign body penetration; bony changes may be seen on adjacent vertebrae.

d. Haematoma.

e. Granuloma.

f. Cyst.

g. Recent administration of subcutaneous fluids into the neck area.

2. Diffuse thickening of the soft tissues of the head and neck.

a. Obesity (fat is more radiolucent than other soft tissues).

b. Cellulitis.

c. Oedema.

d. Diffuse neoplasia.

4.37 VARIATIONS IN RADIOPACITY OF THE SOFT TISSUES OF THE HEAD AND NECK

1. Decreased radiopacity of soft tissues.

a. Gas within soft tissues.

– Oesophageal gas; a small amount of gas is commonly seen in the proximal oesophagus, especially if the animal is under general anaesthesia or is dyspnoeic.

– Secondary to pharyngeal or oesophageal perforation.

– Secondary to tracheal perforation.

– Discharging sinus or fistulous tract; most likely to be associated with a foreign body such as a stick. Geometric, linear gas shadows may outline the foreign body. Further investigation may include fistulography using water-soluble iodinated contrast medium and/or ultrasonography. Chronic cases may give rise to periosteal new bone or osteomyelitis affecting adjacent vertebrae.

– Secondary to pneumomediastinum (gas tracks cranially along cervical fascial planes from the thorax).

– Abscess cavity.

– Puncture or laceration of skin leading to subcutaneous emphysema.

b. Fat within soft tissues.

– Normal subcutaneous and fascial plane fat.

– Obesity.

– Lipoma or liposarcoma.

2. Increased radiopacity of soft tissues.

a. Artefactual (e.g. wet hair, dirty coat).

b. Mineralization.

- Calcinosis circumscripta (rounded deposits of amorphous mineralization) (see 12.2.2 and Fig. 12.1). Mainly young dogs of large breeds, especially the German Shepherd dog.
- Calcinosis cutis (secondary to hyperadrenocorticism; linear streaks in fascial planes or granular deposits near skin surface).
- Dystrophic calcification in a tumour, haematoma, abscess, granuloma or at the site of a previous depot injection.
  c. Radiopaque foreign body in oesophagus or soft tissues.
  d. Sialolithiasis, if in a location consistent with a salivary gland or duct.
  e. Microchip – characteristic appearance.
  f. Leakage of barium sulphate into soft tissues through a pharyngeal or oesophageal tear.

4.38 CONTRAST STUDIES OF THE NASOLACRIMAL DUCT (DACRYOCYSTORHINOGRAPHY)

Dacryocystorhinography is not often performed but may be used to demonstrate occlusion of the nasolacrimal duct in animals with chronic epiphora, to detect leakage from the duct, and to evaluate whether a known lesion is connected to or has an effect on the duct. Survey radiographs should be taken prior to the contrast study, with the patient anaesthetized. A fine catheter is then placed within either the upper or the lower punctum of the eyelids, and while digital pressure and a swab are used to occlude the other punctum, 1–1.5 mL of a water-soluble, iodinated contrast medium is slowly injected into the duct. Injection may also be made in a retrograde fashion from the rostral opening of the duct, caudal to the nares. A radiograph is then taken immediately, usually with the patient in lateral recumbency. The normal opacified nasolacrimal duct is seen on a lateral radiograph as a narrow, slightly undulating line crossing the maxilla approximately halfway between the hard palate and the dorsum of the nose. On a DV intraoral view, it lies immediately medial to the cheek teeth.

1. Contrast column does not fill the duct.
   a. Poor technique.
      - Leakage of contrast from one or both puncta.
      - Inadequate volume of contrast medium used.
   b. Nasolacrimal duct not patent.
      - Aplasia of a segment of the nasolacrimal duct.
      - Occlusion of the nasolacrimal duct by foreign material, mucus, purulent material, inflammation, stricture formation or neoplasia.
2. Irregular contrast column in the nasolacrimal duct.
   a. Contrast mixing with mucus or purulent material.
   b. Contrast outlining foreign material in the nasolacrimal duct.
   c. Inflammation of the nasolacrimal duct.
   d. Neoplasia involving the nasolacrimal duct.
3. Leakage of contrast medium from the nasolacrimal duct.
   a. Rupture of the nasolacrimal duct.
   b. Entry into a nasolacrimal duct cyst.
   c. Contrast exiting the rostral opening of the nasolacrimal duct may leak back into the nasal cavity, outlining the turbinates and mimicking rupture of the duct; this may be avoided by keeping the nose lower than the caudal aspect of the head.

4.39 ULTRASONOGRAPHY OF THE EYE AND ORBIT

Radiography of the eye is of limited value, so ultrasound is increasingly used to image this region when visual inspection is impaired, for example by eyelid swelling, opacity of the cornea or lens, or intraocular haemorrhage. It is usually best performed in the conscious animal, in which the eye is in a normal position; under anaesthesia, it often may retract and rotate ventrally. A high-frequency ($\geq$ 7.5 MHz) sector or curvilinear transducer is placed directly on the cornea or nictitating membrane following topical anaesthesia and using viscous contact gel. A stand-off is useful when examining the cornea and anterior chamber. The eye should be examined in both dorsal (horizontal) and sagittal (vertical) planes, taking care to sweep through the whole volume of the globe and the retrobulbar structures. Images obtained through closed eyelids are very inferior. Images may also be obtained in the transverse plane relative to the eye by scanning from the lateral aspect near the

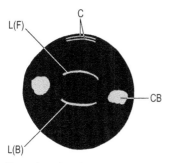

Figure 4.20 Normal ocular ultrasonogram. C, front and back of cornea; CB, ciliary body; L(B), back of lens; L(F), front of lens.

orbital ligament after clipping the hair (temporal approach).

The globe of the eye is approximately spherical and roughly 2 cm in diameter, with a smooth, thin, well-defined wall (Fig. 4.20). The aqueous and vitreous humours in the chambers of the eye are normally anechoic. With a stand-off, the front and back of the cornea are seen as a pair of short, parallel, echogenic lines. Separate layers of the sclera, retina and choroid are not normally recognized. A small depression or elevation may be seen at the back of the globe, representing the optic disc. The anterior and posterior surfaces of the lens are identified as short, curvilinear structures only at those points where the incident sound beam is perpendicular to the lens surface; at other points, the smooth curve of the lens surface scatters echoes away from the transducer. The substance of the lens is anechoic. The hyperechoic ciliary body and iris may be visible on either side of the lens.

Radiographic changes of orbital disease are seen only in cases of radiopaque foreign body and where orbital neoplasia is extensive and involving the nasal cavity and/or frontal sinus (see 4.22.2 and 4.25.3). Orbital ultrasonography is therefore a valuable technique, especially if MRI or CT is not readily available. Scanning is performed through the globe, which acts as an acoustic window. The retrobulbar tissues form an orderly cone behind the eye; retrobulbar muscles are hypoechoic, while the retrobulbar fat is hyperechoic. A temporal approach caudal to the orbital ligament can also be used to examine the retrobulbar structures, including the optic nerve.

1. Increased size of the globe (ultrasonography is helpful for differentiating increased globe size from exophthalmos, which may appear similar clinically).
   a. Breed-associated (bilaterally symmetrical).
   b. Glaucoma – hydrophthalmos.
2. Decreased size of the globe.
   a. Breed-associated (bilaterally symmetrical), for example Rough Collie.
   b. Congenital microphthalmos.
   c. Phthisis bulbi.
      - Following trauma.
      - Following inflammatory disease.
      - End-stage glaucoma.
3. Thickening of the wall of the globe.
   a. Generalized thickening.
      - Scleritis.
      - Chorioretinitis.
   b. Localized thickening.
      - Tumour.
      - Subretinal haemorrhage.
      - Granuloma (see below).
      - Optic neuritis – protrusion of the optic nerve head at the optic disc.
4. Echogenicities within the chambers of the eye.
   a. Generalized increase in echogenicity.
      - Gain settings inappropriately high.
      - Vitreal syneresis – degeneration that results in pockets of liquefaction and may be seen to move or swirl with eye motion; occurs as a natural ageing process in some dogs.
      - Haemorrhage (secondary to trauma, neoplasia, coagulopathy, hypertension, chronic glaucoma).
      - Inflammatory exudate (endophthalmitis).
      - Vitreous 'floaters'.
      - Asteroid hyalosis (calcium phospholipid particles suspended in relatively solid vitreous).
      - Synchysis scintillans (cholesterol particles suspended in liquefied vitreous).
   b. Localized mass effect.
      - Blood clot.
      - Sediment of inflammatory cells.
      - Intraocular tumour – melanoma (usually arise from ciliary body); ciliary body adenoma or adenocarcinoma; lymphoma (often bilateral, may be associated with intraocular haemorrhage); metastatic tumour.

- Intraocular granuloma – blastomycosis* (usually choroidal in origin); coccidioidomycosis*; cryptococcosis*; histoplasmosis*; feline infectious peritonitis; toxoplasmosis*.
- Subretinal haemorrhage.
- Iris cysts – attached to iris or free-floating; anechoic centre.
- Retinal detachment – occasionally gives rise to a mass effect but more often produces curvilinear echogenicities (see below).
- Intraocular foreign body – there may be acoustic shadowing, or if metallic, may see comet tail artefact.

c. Linear or curvilinear echogenicities.
- Retinal detachment (Fig. 4.21) – when complete, appears as 'seagull's wings', with attachments at optic disc and ciliary body. Partial detachments may also be visible as linear or curvilinear echoes within the vitreous. Retinal detachments often move with eye motion.
- Posterior vitreous detachment – similar in appearance to detached retina but not attached at the optic disc.
- Vitreous membranes or traction bands – fibrous strands that sometimes develop secondary to clot formation; can lead to tractional retinal detachment.
- Inflammatory tract from foreign body penetration.
- Persistent hyperplastic primary vitreous – linear structure running from posterior pole of lens to the optic nerve head; colour Doppler useful to detect patency of hyaloid artery.

5. Change in position of the lens – luxation or subluxation. The lens may move anteriorly or posteriorly.
a. Trauma.

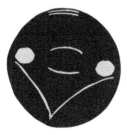

Figure 4.21 Total retinal detachment on ultrasonography.

b. Hereditary predisposition.
c. Displaced by an adjacent mass.
d. Glaucoma.

6. Increased echogenicity of the lens due to cataract formation. Increased echogenicity may be generalized or focal, and may be capsular and/or within the body of the lens.
a. Primary hereditary – many breeds, the appearance and age of onset being characteristic for the breed.
b. Secondary to another eye disease, which may be hereditary.
- Uveitis – various causes.
- Progressive retinal atrophy.
- Retinal dysplasia.
- Glaucoma.
- Lens luxation.
- Persistent hyaloid artery and persistent hyperplastic primary vitreous.
- Multilocular defects.
c. Other causes.
- Senile (age-related).
- Trauma.
- Diabetes mellitus.
- Toxins.
- Radiation.

7. Enlargement of the ciliary body.
a. Inflammation.
b. Neoplasia.
- Melanoma.
- Adenoma.
- Adenocarcinoma.
- Lymphoma – especially cats; may be bilateral.

8. Changes in the retrobulbar tissues.
a. Diffuse disturbance – heterogeneous in echogenicity and echotexture.
- Cellulitis.
- Extensive or diffuse neoplasia.
b. Solid mass – varying echogenicity but usually hypoechoic, often deforming the back of the globe.
- Neoplasia (lymphoma – often bilateral; other primary and metastatic neoplasms; extension from nasal or frontal sinus tumour).
- Myositis of the extraocular muscles, especially medial rectus muscle.
- Zygomatic sialadenitis.

c. Cavitary mass.
   - Retrobulbar abscess (bacterial, fungal, parasitic, secondary to foreign body).
   - Myxosarcoma – may produce pockets of viscous fluid that grossly mimic saliva.
   - Zygomatic mucocele.
d. Focal echogenicity (or echogenicities) ± acoustic shadowing.
   - Retrobulbar foreign body (NB: a metallic foreign body may give rise to a comet tail artefact).
   - Dystrophic calcification.
   - Bone proliferation arising from the bones of the orbit, suggesting aggressive neoplasia extending beyond the orbit.
e. Enlargement of the optic nerve ± protruding optic disc.
   - Optic neuritis (numerous causes including granulomatous meningoencephalitis, toxoplasmosis*, cryptococcosis*, canine distemper, blastomycosis*, feline infectious peritonitis, trauma).

4.40 CONTRAST STUDIES OF THE SALIVARY DUCTS AND GLANDS (SIALOGRAPHY)

Sialography is occasionally undertaken to characterize further the nature of swellings around the head and neck. A fine cannula is introduced into the appropriate duct opening:

- *parotid* (on the mucosal ridge opposite the caudal margin of the upper fourth premolar tooth)
- *zygomatic* (about 1 cm caudal to the parotid opening)
- *mandibular* (lateral surface of the lingual caruncle at the frenum linguae)
- *sublingual* (may be common with the mandibular opening or 1–2 mm caudal to it).

Between 1 and 2 mL of water-soluble iodinated contrast medium is injected carefully, taking care to avoid leakage back around the cannula, and radiographs of the appropriate region of the head and neck are taken immediately.

1. Salivary duct not filled.
   a. Inadequate technique.
      - Too little contrast medium used.
      - Leakage of contrast back around cannula.
   b. Occlusion of the salivary duct.
      - Sialolith; may be visible on a survey radiograph as a mineralized opacity, and sialography confirms its location within a salivary gland or duct.
      - Stricture.
      - Foreign body.
      - Compression of the salivary duct by an adjacent mass.
2. Extravasation of contrast medium into surrounding soft tissues.
   a. Rupture of the salivary duct.
   b. Salivary mucocele.
3. Irregular filling of the salivary duct.
   a. Inflammation.
   b. Neoplasia.
   c. Sialolith.
   d. Foreign material.
4. Uneven filling of the salivary gland.
   a. Insufficient contrast medium used.
   b. Abscessation of the salivary gland.
   c. Neoplasia of the salivary gland (e.g. adenocarcinoma).
   d. Salivary gland cyst.
   e. Infarction of the salivary gland.
   f. Compression of the salivary gland by an adjacent mass.

4.41 ULTRASONOGRAPHY OF THE SALIVARY GLANDS

The mandibular salivary gland is the only salivary gland that can be imaged consistently. It is located superficially, caudal to the angle of the mandible. Ultrasonographically, it appears well defined, oval and hypoechoic with a more echogenic capsule. There may be thin echogenic streaks within the substance of the gland.

1. Hypoechoic or anechoic foci in the salivary gland.
   a. Salivary gland cyst.
   b. Salivary gland abscess.
   c. Neoplasm.
2. Echogenic foci in the salivary gland – sialolith (often with acoustic shadowing).
3. Heterogeneous foci in the salivary gland.
   a. Neoplasm.
      - Benign papillomatous tumour.
      - Carcinoma.

b. Salivary gland abscess.

c. Foreign body reaction (e.g. grass seed in salivary duct).

4.42 ULTRASONOGRAPHY OF THE THYROID AND PARATHYROID GLANDS

A high-frequency transducer is required. The two lobes of the thyroid gland may be identified lying dorsolateral to each side of the trachea, caudal to the larynx and medial to the ipsilateral common carotid artery. Occasionally, especially in brachycephalic dogs, there is a narrow connection or isthmus between the caudal aspects of the two lobes, running ventral to the trachea. The lobes should be smooth, well defined and finely granular in texture. They are fusiform to elliptical in the longitudinal plane and round, oval or triangular in the transverse plane. They are usually hyperechoic to surrounding muscle but may also be isoechoic or hypoechoic. Each lobe of the normal thyroid gland in a medium-sized dog is around 2.5–3 cm long and 0.4–0.6 cm wide and correlates with body weight and surface area. In the cat, the normal dimensions are about 2 cm long and 0.2–0.3 cm wide. The normal parathyroids are sometimes seen as hypoechoic or anechoic foci 2–4.6 mm in diameter; there are two parathyroids within each thyroid gland, although they may not all be visible.

1. Nodules within the thyroid gland – may be of variable echogenicity.
   a. Thyroid tumour.
      – Adenoma.
      – Carcinoma.
   b. Parathyroid tumour.
      – Adenoma.
      – Carcinoma.
   c. Parathyroid hyperplasia.
   d. Thyroid cyst (irregularly marginated cysts with hyperechoic septations may be seen in hyperthyroid cats).
2. Enlargement of the thyroid gland.
   a. Well marginated, low echogenicity – thyroid adenoma.
   b. Poorly marginated, heterogeneous mass – thyroid carcinoma; may see invasion of common carotid artery and/or jugular vein, and involvement of regional lymph nodes.
3. Decrease in size of the thyroid gland.

a. Acquired hypothyroidism; may be associated with a decrease in echogenicity, irregular capsule delineation and abnormal shape.

4.43 ULTRASONOGRAPHY OF THE CAROTID ARTERY AND JUGULAR VEIN

The external jugular veins lie in a groove on the ventrolateral aspect of the neck. The common carotid arteries lie deep to the jugular veins, bifurcating near the head into external and internal carotid arteries. The vein is thin-walled and compressible, with anechoic contents, while the arteries have thicker walls and are less compressible. Doppler ultrasound may be used to confirm the arterial or venous nature of the blood flow.

1. Intraluminal mass in the carotid artery or jugular vein.
   a. Thrombus.
   b. Invasion by adjacent tumour.
2. Multiple abnormal vessels associated with the carotid artery or jugular vein.
   a. Collateral vessels.
      – Secondary to obstruction of normal vessels.
      – Supplying an abnormal mass.
   b. Arteriovenous malformation.
      – Secondary to trauma.
      – Secondary to neoplasia.
      – Congenital malformation.

4.44 ULTRASONOGRAPHY OF LYMPH NODES OF THE HEAD AND NECK

Most lymph nodes in the head and neck of the dog and cat are small (< 5 mm diameter) and are not consistently seen ultrasonographically. Based on work in humans, lymph nodes in the head and neck are considered enlarged if they exceed 1 cm in diameter. Enlarged lymph nodes usually remain hypoechoic but may become heterogeneous, especially if cavitation occurs. In humans, reactive lymph nodes tend to retain their oval or flat shape, while neoplastic lymph nodes are more likely to become round. It is not clear whether this applies to small animals.

1. Enlarged lymph nodes.
   a. Reactive.
   b. Neoplasia.
      – Lymphoma.
      – Metastases.

4.45 CERVICAL OESOPHAGUS

Disease of the cervical oesophagus is less common than that of the thoracic oesophagus, but the same principles of interpretation apply – see Chapter 8.

4.46 NASAL DERMOID SINUS CYST

A dermoid sinus is a neural tube defect resulting from incomplete separation of the skin and neural tube during embryonic development. In dogs, dermoid sinuses are typical in the cervical and dorsal midline, and the Rhodesian Ridgeback is predisposed. Nasal dermoid sinuses have recently been recognized, with extension into the nasal cavity from a midline dorsal opening. Plain radiographs are usually unremarkable, but the sinus tract can be demonstrated with sinography, allowing surgical planning.

Further reading

General

Dernell, W.S., Straw, R.C., Cooper, M. F., Powers, B.E., LaRue, S.M., Withrow, S.J., 1998. Multilobular osteochondrosarcoma in 39 dogs: 1979–1993. J. Am. Anim. Hosp. Assoc. 34, 11–18.

Gibbs, C., 1976. Radiological refresher: The head part I – Traumatic lesions of the skull. J. Small Anim. Pract. 17, 551–554.

Johnston, G.R., Feeney, D.A., 1980. Radiology in ophthalmic diagnosis. Vet. Clin. North Am. Small. Anim. Pract. 10, 317–337.

Konde, L.J., Thrall, M.A., Gasper, P., Dial, S.M., McBiles, K., Colgan, S., et al., 1987. Radiographically visualized skeletal changes associated with mucopoly-saccharidosis VI in cats. Vet. Radiol. 28, 223–228.

Cranial cavity

Garosi, L.S., Penderis, J.P., Brearley, M. J., Brearley, J.C., Dennis, R., Kirkpatrick, P., 2002. Intraventricular tension pneumocephalus as a complication of transfrontal craniectomy: diagnosis and surgical management. Vet. Surg. 31, 226–231.

Hudson, J.A., Cartee, R.E., Simpson, S. T., Buxton, D.F., 1989. Ultrasonographic anatomy of the canine brain. Vet. Radiol. 30, 13–21.

Hudson, J.A., Simpson, S.T., Buxton, D. F., Cartee, R.F., Steiss, J.E., 1990. Ultrasonographic diagnosis of canine hydrocephalus. Vet. Radiol. 31, 50–58.

McConnell, J.F., Hayes, A.M., Platt, S. R., Smith, K.C., 2006. Calvarial hyperostosis syndrome in two bullmastiffs. Vet. Radiol. Ultrasound 47, 72–77.

Muir, P., Dubielzig, R.R., Johnson, K. A., Shelton, D.G., 1996. Hypertrophic osteodystrophy and calvarial hyperostosis. Compend. Contin. Educ. Pract. Veterinarian (Small Animal) 18, 143–151.

Pastor, K.F., Boulay, J.P., Schelling, S. H., Carpenter, J.L., 2000. Idiopathic hyperostosis of the calvaria in five young bullmastiffs. J. Am. Anim. Hosp. Assoc. 36, 439–445.

Spaulding, K.A., Sharp, N.J.H., 1990. Ultrasonographic imaging of the lateral cerebral ventricles in the dog. Vet. Radiol. 31, 59–64.

Maxilla and premaxilla

Featherstone, H., Llabres Diaz, F., 2003. Maxillary bone epithelial cyst in a dog. J. Small Anim. Pract. 44, 541–545.

Frew, D.G., Dobson, J.M., 1992. Radiological assessment of 50 cases of incisive or maxillary neoplasia in the dog. J. Small Anim. Pract. 33, 11–18.

Mandible

Gibbs, C., 1977. Radiological refresher: The head part II – Traumatic lesions of the mandible. J. Small Anim. Pract. 18, 51–54.

Watson, A.D.J., Adams, W.M., Thomas, C.B., 1995.

Craniomandibular osteopathy in dogs. Compend. Contin. Educ. Pract. Veterinarian (Small Animal) 17, 911–921.

Temporomandibular joint

Gemmill, T., 2008. Conditions of the temporomandibular joint in dogs and cats. In Pract. 30, 36–43.

Lane, J.G., 1982. Disorders of the canine temporomandibular joint. Vet. Ann. 22, 175–187.

Meomartino, L., Fatone, G., Brunetti, A., Lamagna, F., Potena, A., 1999. Temporomandibular ankylosis in the cat: a review of seven cases. J. Small Anim. Pract. 40, 7–10.

Sullivan, M., 1989. Temporo-mandibular ankylosis in the cat. J. Small Anim. Pract. 30, 401–405.

Ear

Benigni, L., Lamb, C., 2006. Diagnostic imaging of ear disease in the dog and cat. In Pract. 28, 122–130.

Bischoff, M.G., Kneller, S.K., 2004. Diagnostic imaging of the canine and feline ear. Vet. Clin. North Am. Small. Anim. Pract. 34, 437–458.

Eom, K.D., Lee, H.C., Yoon, J.H., 2000. Canalographic evaluation of the external ear canal in dogs. Vet. Radiol. Ultrasound 41, 231–234.

Garosi, L.S., Dennis, R., Schwarz, T., 2003. Review of diagnostic imaging of ear diseases in the dog and cat. Vet. Radiol. Ultrasound 44, 137–146.

Gibbs, C., 1978. Radiological refresher: The head part III – Ear disease. J. Small Anim. Pract. 19, 539–545.

Hofer, P., Meisen, N., Bartholdi, S., Kaser-Hotz, B., 1995. Radiology corner – A new radiographic view of the feline tympanic bulla. Vet. Radiol. Ultrasound 36, 14–15.

Hoskinson, J.J., 1993. Imaging techniques in the diagnosis of middle ear disease. Semin. Vet. Med. Surg. 8, 10–16.

Trower, N.D., Gregory, S.P., Renfrew, C.R., Lamb, C.R., 1998. Evaluation of the canine tympanic membrane by positive contrast ear canalography. Vet. Rec. 142, 78–81.

Ziemer, L.S., Schwarz, T., Sullivan, M., 2003. Otolithiasis in three dogs. Vet. Radiol. Ultrasound 44, 28–31.

Nasal cavity and frontal sinuses

Coulson, A., 1988. Radiology as an aid to diagnosis of nasal disorders in the cat. Vet. Ann. 28, 150–158.

Galloway, P.E., Kyles, A., Henderson, J.P., 1997. Nasal polyps in a cat. J. Small Anim. Pract. 38, 78–80.

Gibbs, C., Lane, J.G., Denny, H.R., 1979. Radiological features of intra-nasal lesions in the dog: a review of 100 cases. J. Small Anim. Pract. 20, 515–535.

Goring, R.L., Ticer, J.W., Gross, T.L., 1984. Contrast rhinography in the radiographic evaluation of diseases affecting the nasal cavity, nasopharynx, and paranasal sinuses in the dog. Vet. Radiol. 25, 106–123.

Kirberger, R.M., Fourie, S.L., 2002. An investigation into the usefulness of a rostrocaudal nasal radiographic view in the dog. J. S. Afr. Vet. Assoc. 73, 171–176.

Lamb, C.R., Richbell, S., Mantis, P., 2003. Radiographic signs in cats with nasal disease. J. Feline. Med. Surg. 5, 227–235.

O'Brien, R.T., Evans, S.M., Wortman, J.A., Hendrick, M.J., 1996. Radiographic findings in cats with intranasal neoplasia or chronic rhinitis: 29 cases (1982–1988). J. Am. Vet. Med. Assoc. 208, 385–389.

Sturgeon, C., 2008. Nasal dermoid sinus cyst in a shih tzu. Vet. Rec. 163, 219–220.

Sullivan, M., Lee, R., Jakovljevic, S., Sharp, N.J.H., 1986. The radiological features of aspergillosis of the nasal cavity and frontal sinuses of the dog. J. Small Anim. Pract. 27, 167–180.

Sullivan, M., Lee, R., Skae, C.A., 1987. The radiological features of sixty cases of intra-nasal neoplasia in the dog. J. Small Anim. Pract. 28, 575–586.

Teeth

DeForge, D.H., Colmery, B.H. (Eds.), 2000. An Atlas of Veterinary Dental Radiology. Iowa, State University Press, Ames.

Eisner, E.R., 1998. Oral-dental radiographic examination technique. Vet. Clin. North Am. Small. Anim. Pract. 28, 1063–1087.

Gibbs, C., 1978. Radiological refresher: The head part IV – Dental disease. J. Small Anim. Pract. 19, 701–707.

Gorrel, C., 1998. Radiographic evaluation. Vet. Clin. North Am. Small. Anim. Pract. 28, 1089–1110.

Harvey, C.E., Flax, B.M., 1992. Feline oral-dental radiographic examination and interpretation. Vet. Clin. North Am. Small. Anim. Pract. 22, 1279–1295.

Hooft, J., Mattheeuws, D., van Bree, P., 1979. Radiology of deciduous teeth resorption and definitive teeth eruption in the dog. J. Small Anim. Pract. 20, 175–180.

Lommer, M.L., Verstraete, F.J.M., Terpak, C.H., 2000. Dental radiographic technique in cats. Compend. Contin. Educ. Pract. Veterinarian (Small Animal) 22, 107–117.

Zontine, W.J., 1975. Canine dental radiology: radiographic technique, development and anatomy. Vet. Radiol. 16, 75–83.

Pharynx, larynx and other soft tissues of the neck

Bray, J.P., Lipscombe, V.J., White, R.A.S., Rudorf, H., 1998. Ultrasonographic examination of the pharynx and larynx of the normal dog. Vet. Radiol. Ultrasound 39, 566–571.

Gallagher, J.G., Boudrieau, R.J., Schelling, S.H., Berg, J., 1995. Ultrasonography of the brain and vertebral canal in dogs and cats: 15 cases (1988–1993). J. Am. Vet. Med. Assoc. 207, 1320–1324.

Gelatt, K.N., Cure, T.H., Guffy, M.M., Jessen, C., 1972. Dacryocystorhinography in the dog and cat. J. Small Anim. Pract. 13, 381–397.

Gibbs, C., 1986. Radiographic examination of the pharynx, larynx and soft tissue structures of the neck in dogs and cats. Vet. Ann. 26, 227–241.

Glen, J.B., 1972. Canine salivary mucocoeles: results of sialographic examination and surgical treatment of fifty cases. J. Small Anim. Pract. 13, 515–526.

Harvey, C.E., 1969. Sialography in the dog. J. Am. Vet. Radiol. Soc. 10, 18–27.

Hudson, J.A., Finn-Bodner, S.T., Steiss, J.E., 1998. Neurosonography. Vet. Clin. North Am. Small Anim. Pract. 28, 943–972.

Kirberger, R.M., Steenkamp, G., Spotswood, T.C., Boy, S.C., Miller, D.B., van Zyl, M., 2006. Stenotic nasopharyngeal dysgenesis in the dachshund: seven cases (2002–2004). J. Am. Anim. Hosp. Assoc. 42, 290–297.

Llabres Diaz, F., 2006. Practical contrast radiography 5. Other techniques (for dacryocysto-rhinography). J. Small Anim. Pract. 28, 32–40.

Moore, D., Lamb, C., 2007. Ocular ultrasonography in companion animals: a pictorial review. In Pract 29, 603–610.

Rudorf, H., 1997. Ultrasonographic imaging of the tongue and larynx in normal dogs. J. Small Anim. Pract. 38, 439–444.

Rudorf, H., 1998. Ultrasonography of laryngeal masses in six cats and one dog. Vet. Radiol. Ultrasound 39, 430–434.

Rudorf, H., Herrtage, M.E., White, R. A.S., 1997. Use of ultrasonography in the diagnosis of tracheal collapse. J. Small Anim. Pract. 38, 513–518.

Solano, M., Penninck, D.G., 1996. Ultrasonography of the canine, feline and equine tongue: normal finding and case history reports.

Vet. Radiol. Ultrasound 37, 206–213.

Stuhr, S.M., Scagliotti, R.H., 1996. Retrobulbar ultrasound in the mesaticephalic and dolichocephalic dog using a temporal approach. Vet. Comp. Ophthalmol. 6, 91–99.

Von Doernberg, M.C., Peeters, M.E., Ter Haar, G., Kirpensteijn, J., 2008. Lingual asbcesses in three dogs. J. Small Anim. Pract. 49, 413–416.

Williams, J., Wilkie, D.A., 1996. Ultrasonography of the eye. Compend. Contin. Educ. Pract. Veterinarian (Small Animal) 18, 667–676.

Wisner, E.K., Nyland, T.G., 1998. Ultrasonography of the thyroid and para-thyroid glands. Vet. Clin. North Am. Small. Anim. Pract. 28, 973–992.

Wisner, E.R., Mattoon, J.S., Nyland, T.G., Baker, T.W., 1991. Normal ultrasonographic anatomy of the canine neck. Vet. Radiol. 32, 185–190.

Wisner, E.R., Nyland, T.G., Mattoon, J.S., 1994. Ultrasonographic examination of cervical masses in the dog and cat. Vet. Radiol. Ultrasound 35, 310–315.

Wisner, E.R., Penninck, D., Biller, D. S., Feldman, E.C., Drake, C., Nyland, T.G., 1997. High resolution parathyroid sonography. Vet. Radiol. Ultrasound 38, 462–466.

Yakely, W.L., Alexander, J.E., 1971. Dacryocystorhinography in the dog. J. Am. Vet. Med. Assoc. 159, 1417–1421.

Chapter 5

Spine

CHAPTER CONTENTS

5.1 Radiographic technique for the spine   115
5.2 Variations in vertebral number   116
5.3 Variations in vertebral size and shape: congenital or developmental   117
5.4 Variations in vertebral size and shape: acquired   119
5.5 Variations in vertebral alignment   122
5.6 Diffuse changes in vertebral opacity   124
5.7 Localized changes in vertebral opacity   124
5.8 Abnormalities of the intervertebral disc space   126
5.9 Irregularity of the vertebral endplates   127
5.10 Abnormalities of the intervertebral foramen   128
5.11 Abnormalities of the articular facets   129
5.12 Lesions in the paravertebral soft tissues   130
5.13 Ultrasonography of paravertebral soft tissues   130
5.14 Spinal contrast studies: technique and normal appearance   131
5.15 Technical errors during myelography   133
5.16 Extradural spinal cord compression on myelography   134
5.17 Intradural–extramedullary spinal cord compression on myelography   137
5.18 Intramedullary spinal cord enlargement on myelography   138
5.19 Miscellaneous myelographic findings   139

5.20 Changes on plain radiographs that are unlikely to be significant   140
5.21 Neurological deficits involving the spinal cord or proximal nerve roots with normal plain radiographs and myelogram   140

5.1 RADIOGRAPHIC TECHNIQUE FOR THE SPINE

Optimal radiographs are obtained with the patient under sedation or general anaesthesia to minimize motion blur and allow accurate positioning.

True lateral and ventrodorsal (VD) positioning should be ensured by the use of positioning aids (Fig. 5.1A–D). At the lumbosacral junction, a VD radiograph obtained with the area flexed may also be helpful. In the cervical spine, oblique views increase the visibility of the intervertebral foramina, the dens (odontoid peg) and the occipital condyles. Horizontal VD views are desirable when severe instability or spinal fractures are suspected to avoid additional injury on manipulation of the patient. Detail intensifying screens are preferred, and a grid should be used if the tissue thickness is greater than 10 cm. Close collimation will also improve image definition by reducing the production of scattered radiation. If neurological deficits are present or if disc disease is suspected, the primary beam must be centred at the level of the suspected lesion.

Myelography used to be the most commonly used contrast medium technique for the evaluation of the spinal cord or cauda equina but in many

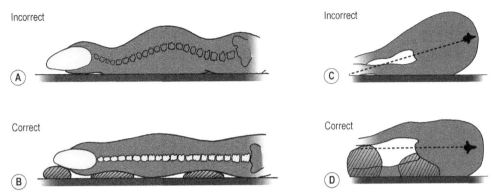

Figure 5.1 Achieving accurate positioning with the use of foam wedges.

establishments is being replaced by cross-sectional imaging techniques. Myelography is discussed further in Section 5.14. Epidurography, discography and lumbar sinus venography are additional techniques that are sometimes still used to evaluate the cauda equina but that are also becoming obsolete. Linear tomography is useful in the thoracic and lumbosacral regions to eliminate superimposition of the ribs and ilial wings, respectively. Cross-sectional images can be obtained by means of CT and MRI; CT provides better definition of bone and joint abnormalities, whereas MRI provides high soft tissue contrast and is ideal for cases with no survey film abnormalities, such as spinal tumours, early infection and ligamentous pathology. CT myelography can be performed to increase the information given about changes in cord size. Scintigraphy is occasionally used to identify the location of inflammatory or neoplastic processes but gives little anatomical detail.

Optimal interpretation of spinal radiographs requires a systematic evaluation that involves assessing radiographic quality and technique, extravertebral soft tissue structures, osseous vertebral structures, disc spaces and adjacent vertebral endplates, intervertebral foramina and articular facets. Each vertebra, disc space and intervertebral foramen should be compared with those adjacent to them. Disc spaces normally appear narrower towards the periphery of the film due to divergence of the primary X-ray beam.

Vertebral physes should be closed by 38 weeks, with cranial physes closing before caudal physes. The apex and body of the dens (odontoid peg) have separate ossification centres and are completely ossified by 25 weeks.

5.2 VARIATIONS IN VERTEBRAL NUMBER

The normal vertebral formula in the dog and cat is 7 cervical, 13 thoracic, 7 lumbar, 3 sacral and a variable number of caudal vertebrae. Numerical alterations may be genuine or may be accompanied by other congenital vertebral abnormalities, which may result in apparent vertebral number alterations (transitional vertebrae – see 5.3.2).

1. Six or eight lumbar vertebrae (especially Dachshund).
2. Four sacral vertebrae – vestigial disc spaces may be visible.
3. Twelve thoracic vertebrae.
   a. Twelve genuine thoracic vertebrae and seven lumbar vertebrae.
   b. T13 lacks ribs, giving the appearance of 12 thoracic and 8 lumbar vertebrae.
4. Fourteen thoracic vertebrae – usually due to the presence of rib-like structures on L1 rather than a genuine increase in number.
5. Inherited short tail (brachyury) in the Manx cat ('stumpies') and certain dog breeds, including the Pembroke Welsh Corgi, Brittany Spaniel, Bouvier des Flandres, Swedish Vallhund and Polish Lowland Sheepdog. In the Manx cat, other spinal deformities are often associated.
6. Inherited taillessness (anury); especially the Manx cat ('rumpies'), and associated with other spinal deformities (see 5.3.20).
7. Perosomus elumbis – rare neuroskeletal congenital defect in which there is agenesis of the lumbosacral spinal cord and vertebrae, with associated pelvic limb deformities; mainly cattle but has been reported in dogs.

5.3 VARIATIONS IN VERTEBRAL SIZE AND SHAPE: CONGENITAL OR DEVELOPMENTAL

More than one abnormality may be present.

1. Normal variants.
   a. The neural arch of C1 is often short in toy breeds of dog.
   b. C7 and L7 may be shorter than the adjacent vertebrae.
   c. The ventral margins of L3 and L4 vertebral bodies are often poorly defined due to bony roughening at the origins of the diaphragmatic crura.
2. Transitional vertebrae – these are vertebrae that have anatomical features of two adjacent regions. They are commonly seen and may accompany numerical abnormalities, but other than those at the lumbosacral junction they are not usually clinically significant. The transitional segment may show unilateral or bilateral changes.
   a. Sacralization of the last lumbar vertebra (Fig. 5.2A) – one or both transverse processes fuse to the wing of the sacrum and may also articulate with the ilium. Asymmetrical and symmetrical transitional vertebrae have roughly equal incidence. This may predispose to lumbosacral instability and disc degeneration with secondary cauda equina syndrome. If rotational malalignment is present, it may also predispose to unilateral hip dysplasia and result in an inability to obtain pelvic symmetry during positioning for hip dysplasia radiographs; this is more likely to occur with unilateral sacralization. Common in the German Shepherd dog but also in the Dobermann, Rhodesian Ridgeback, Greater Swiss Mountain dog and Brittany Spaniel.
   b. Lumbarization of S1 vertebra, which fails to fuse to the rest of the sacrum (Fig. 5.2A); appears similar to the above radiographically and may be differentiated only by counting the number of normal adjacent vertebral segments.
   c. Partial or complete fusion of S3 to Cd1; also common in cats, particularly Burmese. Pseudoarticulation of the transverse processes may be present. Often seen with (b) in an attempt to restore three sacral segments.

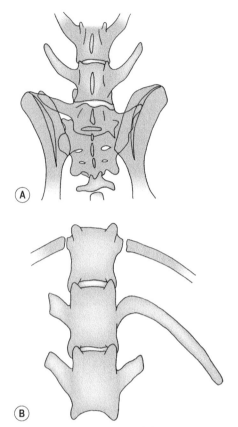

Figure 5.2 Transitional vertebrae: (A) at the lumbosacral junction, with a transverse process at one side and articulation with the ilium on the other; (B) at the thoracolumbar junction, with one rib and one transverse process.

   d. Transitional T13 vertebra (Fig. 5.2B) – a rib develops into a transverse process; a vestigial rib may be seen as a mineralized line in the soft tissues.
   e. Transitional L1 vertebra – a transverse process elongates and develops into a rib-like structure; also common in cats.
   f. Transitional C7 vertebra – a transverse process elongates and develops into a rib-like structure.
   g. Occipitalization of the atlas.
3. Hemivertebrae (Fig. 5.3) – malformation of the vertebral body; a common abnormality in the thoracic and tail regions, particularly in screw-tailed breeds and the German Short-haired Pointer. Rare in cats. Multiple vertebrae are often affected. Clinical signs (neurological deficits due to spinal cord compression) are

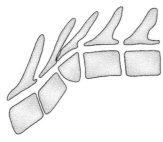

Figure 5.3 Typical mid-thoracic hemivertebra: a wedge-shaped vertebral body resulting in kyphosis and narrowing of the vertebral canal.

uncommon and usually occur in the first year of life during the growth phase.

   a. Dorsal hemivertebra – ventral half did not develop, producing kyphosis.

   b. Lateral hemivertebra – left or right half did not develop, producing scoliosis.

   c. Ventral hemivertebra – dorsal half did not develop, producing lordosis.

4. Block or fused vertebrae – usually only two and rarely three segments are fused – reduced or absent disc space with vertebrae of normal length. The degree of fusion varies. The increased stress on adjacent disc spaces predisposes to subsequent disc herniation. Differential diagnoses are old trauma, healed discospondylitis.

   a. Lumbar region.

   b. Cervical region.

5. Butterfly vertebrae (Fig. 5.4) – particularly brachycephalic breeds of dog; rare in cats. Unlikely to cause clinical signs. Seen on the VD view, particularly in the caudal thoracic and caudal lumbar regions as a cleft of the cranial and caudal vertebral endplates due to partial sagittal cleavage of the vertebral body.

6. Incomplete fusion of sacral segments.

7. C2 – dens (odontoid peg) abnormalities.

   a. Agenesis, hypoplasia or non-fusion leading to atlantoaxial instability (see 5.5.5).

   b. Dorsal angulation of the dens.

   c. Cats – aplasia, hypoplasia or irregular ossification may occur in mucopolysaccharidosis (see 5.4.9).

8. Cervical spondylopathy (wobbler syndrome; see 5.4.20 and Fig. 5.5) – especially Dobermann. Malformed caudal cervical vertebrae, often with a plough-share appearance of the centrum and wedge-shaped disc spaces; the neural arch may also be angled cranioventrally, and both of these result in vertebral canal stenosis. Spinal cord compression may be worsened on flexion of the neck due to vertebral instability, creating a dynamic lesion. However, neurological signs are seen in young animals only when stenosis is severe. See 5.4.14 for description of acquired changes.

9. Narrowed vertebral canal (spinal stenosis) – needs myelography or MRI to demonstrate the degree of cord compression.

   a. Secondary to hemivertebrae or block vertebrae.

   b. Cervical spondylopathy (wobbler syndrome; Fig. 5.5).

   c. Thoracic stenosis.

     – T3–6 usually with no cord compression – Dobermann.

     – Individual thoracic vertebrae – Bulldog.

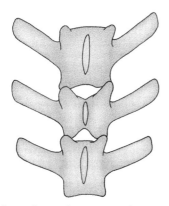

Figure 5.4 Butterfly vertebrae seen on the ventrodorsal view.

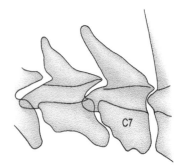

Figure 5.5 Typical vertebral malformation seen with cervical spondylopathy (wobbler syndrome): deformity and upward tilting of the vertebral body and low position of the neural arch resulting in vertebral canal stenosis. Subluxation may occur with neck flexion.

d. Congenital lumbosacral stenosis in small and medium-sized dogs.

10. Sacral osteochondrosis – clinical signs not usually apparent until skeletally mature (see 5.4.16 and Fig. 5.8).

11. Congenital metabolic disease affecting vertebrae at a young age.
    a. Pituitary dwarfism – especially German Shepherd dog; proportionate dwarfism ± epiphyseal dysgenesis.
    b. Congenital hypothyroidism – especially Boxer; disproportionate dwarfism with epiphyseal dysgenesis leading in the spine to delayed vertebral endplate ossification and growth plate closure; endplates may show characteristic ventral spikes. Pathological fracture through an unfused growth plate has been reported. Long bone changes also occur (see 1.22.9).

12. Fused dorsal spinous processes.

13. Spina bifida – results in a split or absent dorsal spinous process or absent lamina, most common in the caudal lumbar region; especially the Bulldog and rare in cats. A widened vertebral canal may be seen on the lateral view. May be accompanied by spinal dysraphism, a defective closure of the neural tube. Myelography is required to assess soft tissue changes.
    a. Spina bifida occulta – normal spinal cord and intact skin. Common in short-tailed breeds.
    b. Meningocele – herniated meninges, skin intact.
    c. Myelomeningocele – herniated spinal cord and meninges, skin intact.
    d. Spina bifida manifesta – herniated spinal cord and meninges exposed to the exterior.
    e. Spina bifida cystica – herniated spinal cord and meninges elevated above the skin.

14. Dermoid (pilonidal) sinus – occasionally associated with defects in the dorsal spinous process or neural arch, if the sinus tract extends to the dura (see 5.7.4).

15. Occipitoatlantoaxial malformations – combinations of abnormalities including occipital dysplasia, fusion of the occiput to the atlas, short atlas neural arch, deformities of the dens and atlantoaxial subluxation; clinical signs depend on the degree of resulting cord compression, and some may be clinically silent.

16. Other occasional complex vertebral anomalies, especially in the cervical area.

17. Articular facet aplasia.
    a. Cervical.
    b. Thoracolumbar, often with hyperplasia of the adjacent facet.

18. Idiopathic multifocal osteopathy of the Scottish Terrier (see 1.18.7); absence of parts of vertebrae may occur, particularly dorsally in the cervical spine.

19. Perocormus – severe shortening of the vertebral column.

20. Cats – sacrococcygeal (sacrocaudal) dysgenesis; varies from spina bifida to complete sacrococcygeal agenesis. Especially in Manx cats, in which it may be accompanied by other anomalies such as shortened cervical vertebrae, butterfly vertebrae, fusion of lumbar vertebrae and meningo(myelo)cele.

21. Cats – mucopolysaccharidosis – congenital lysosomal storage disease, although signs may not manifest until later in life (see 5.4.9).

5.4 VARIATIONS IN VERTEBRAL SIZE AND SHAPE: ACQUIRED

For articular facet variations, see 5.11.

Increased vertebral size

1. Spondylosis deformans – varying sizes of ventral and lateral bony spurs that may bridge the disc space (Fig. 5.6). Usually clinically insignificant unless so extensive as to result in nerve root involvement; at the lumbosacral junction it may be associated with other pathology and cauda equina syndrome.
    a. Initiated by degeneration of annulus fibrosus – an incidental finding that may start as young as 2 years, is very common and increases in incidence with age; less common and generally milder in cats.

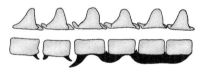

Figure 5.6 Varying degrees of spondylosis: small spurs of new bone progressing to ankylosis.

b. Secondary to:
- chronic disc herniation
- cervical spondylopathy (wobbler syndrome)
- disc fenestration
- discospondylitis
- hemivertebrae
- fracture or luxation injuries.

c. Syndesmitis ossificans – extensive ossification of the ventral longitudinal ligament – young Boxers.

2. Fracture and enlarged vertebra due to callus formation.
a. Trauma.
b. Pathological fracture (extensive callus unlikely).
   - Nutritional secondary hyperparathyroidism (juvenile osteoporosis – see 1.16.4).
   - Osteolytic tumour (e.g. plasma cell myeloma).
   - Bone cyst (see 1.19.2 and 3).

3. Neoplasia.
a. Benign neoplasia or disorder of skeletal development.
   - Single osteochondroma or multiple cartilaginous exostoses, often producing expansile lesions of the dorsal spinous processes in young animals. Growth ceases at skeletal maturity in dogs, but lesions may continue to grow after the active growth phase in cats (see 1.15.2). Malignant transformation to osteosarcoma or chondrosarcoma has been reported.
b. Malignant neoplasia.
   - Osteosarcoma.
   - Other primary or metastatic tumours.
c. Hindquarter soft tissue tumours resulting in ventral periosteal reaction on caudal lumbar and sacral vertebrae (Fig. 5.7; differential diagnosis is spondylitis – see below, but neoplastic changes are usually more caudal). The new bone is not necessarily neoplastic but is a reaction to local malignancy.
   - Prostatic tumour – the most common cause of such new bone.
   - Bladder or urethral tumour.
   - Perianal tumour.
   - Mammary tumour.

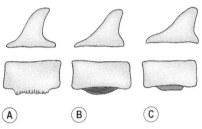

Figure 5.7 New bone on the ventral margins of vertebral bodies due to local neoplasia (usually L5–7) or spondylitis (usually L1–3). The new bone may be brushlike (A), lamellar (B) or solid (C). See 1.6 for further description of periosteal reactions.

4. Spondylitis (Fig. 5.7) – usually characterized by vertebral body periosteal reactions, particularly ventrally, and may progress to osteomyelitis of the vertebral body. Conversely, osteomyelitis may also originate haematogenously within the vertebra and extend peripherally. Note that the ventral margins of L3 and L4 are often poorly defined due to bony roughening at the origins of the diaphragmatic crura, and this should not be mistaken for spondylitis.
a. Bacterial.
   - Migrating plant material – especially ventral to L1–3 (T13–L4). Medium and large-sized dogs are thought to aspirate vegetation such as grass awns, which migrate through the lung and diaphragm to the origin of the crura at L3 and L4; an alternative proposed route is via penetration of the gastrointestinal tract. May be associated with paraspinal abscessation, and such changes may be visible with ultrasonography (see 5.13).
   - Other foreign bodies.
   - Haematogenous infection.
   - Bite wounds.
   - Iatrogenic due to surgical complications.
b. Parasitic.
   - Spirocerca lupi* – spondylitis of mid-thoracic vertebrae (T5–11); with caudal mediastinal (oesophageal) mass (see 8.19.5).
c. Fungal.
   - Actinomycosis*.
   - Coccidiodomycosis*.
   - Aspergillosis,* especially German Shepherd dogs.

d. Protozoal.
- Hepatozoonosis* – there may be extensive new bone formation, including other bones of the body (see 1.14.2).
5. Disseminated (diffuse) idiopathic skeletal hyperostosis – similar to the disease of the same name in humans and seen in large and giant dogs; the main changes are in the spine, with extensive, flowing new bone formation along the ventral and lateral margins of the vertebral bodies and at sites of ligamentous attachments; also extremital periarticular new bone and enthesiophyte formation. Aetiology unknown but appears to represent an exaggerated response to stimuli that would normally induce little, if any, new bone formation and may be considered to be an ossifying diathesis.
6. Baastrup's disease – bony proliferation between dorsal spinous processes. Larger dog breeds, especially Boxer.
7. Aneurysmal bone cyst (see 1.19.3).
8. Cats – hypervitaminosis A; extensive new bone formation on cervical and cranial thoracic vertebrae and rarely further caudally. Mainly ventrally, mimicking severe spondylosis, but may also involve the sides and dorsum of the vertebrae. Long bone joints may also be affected at sites of soft tissue attachments, especially the elbow and stifle. Ankylosis of the spine and affected limb joints may occur. Usually 2- to 9-year-old cats on raw liver diets; differential diagnosis is mucopolysaccharidosis.
9. Mucopolysaccharidosis; lysosomal storage diseases causing new bone on the vertebrae, which may lead to spinal fusion, and endplate dysplasia; also dwarfism, facial deformity, pectus excavatum, hip dysplasia and epiphyseal dysplasia leading to osteoarthrosis. More common in cats, especially those with Siamese ancestry; rare in the dog; differential diagnosis is hypervitaminosis A. Mucopolysaccharidosis type VII has been reported to cause shortened vertebral bodies and irregular vertebral epiphyses as well as disproportionate dwarfism in a German Shepherd dog.

Decreased vertebral size

10. Fractures – may result in shortened vertebra due to compression.
a. Trauma.

b. Pathological fracture.
- Nutritional secondary hyperparathyroidism (juvenile osteoporosis) (see 1.16.4).
- Osteolytic tumour (e.g. plasma cell myeloma); may be subtle, so compare with adjacent vertebrae.
- Severe spondylitis.
11. Discospondylitis – osteolysis of vertebral endplates eventually results in a shortened vertebral body, with secondary spondylosis deformans and even fusion in the later stages (see 5.9.1 and Fig. 5.10).
12. Indented vertebral endplates.
a. Intravertebral disc herniation (Schmorl's node) – particularly L7 and/or S1; medium and large breeds, especially German Shepherd dog.
b. Nutritional secondary hyperparathyroidism (juvenile osteoporosis) – the central part of the endplate is indented by the nucleus pulposus while the bones are soft and then remains for life.
13. Mucopolysaccharidosis; the vertebrae may be shortened or misshapen because dwarfism and epiphyseal dysplasia may be a feature (see 5.4.9).

Altered vertebral shape

14. Cervical spondylopathy (wobbler syndrome) – congenitally malformed ± unstable cervical vertebrae that may be accompanied at a later age by acquired changes such as remodelling of the centrum, endplate sclerosis, spondylosis and secondary disc herniation. Especially Dobermann (see 5.3.8 and Fig. 5.5). Most cases present in middle age due to secondary disc herniation, although in cases of severe deformity neurological signs are evident at a younger age. If MRI is not available, myelography is required to demonstrate acquired soft tissue changes and to quantify the degree of cord compression, which may be due to primary bony deformity or to secondary disc herniation, facet arthrosis or ligamentum flavum hypertrophy or redundancy (see also 5.16.3–5, 5.16.7 and 5.16.8).
15. Fractures – the vertebrae may be misshapen due to malunion or asymmetric compression.
a. Trauma.

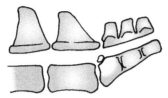

Figure 5.8 Sacral osteochondrosis: there is remodelling and sclerosis of the craniodorsal aspect of the sacral endplate with an overlying osteochondral fragment.

    b. Pathological fracture.
- Nutritional secondary hyperparathyroidism (juvenile osteoporosis).
- Osteolytic tumour (e.g. plasma cell myeloma).
- Bone cyst (see 1.19.2 and 1.19.3).
- Vertebral physitis.

16. Sacral osteochondrosis (Fig. 5.8) – remodelling (angulation, lipping, bone defect, subchondral sclerosis) of the craniodorsal aspect of S1 and rarely the caudodorsal aspect of L7 ± an osteochondral fragment; mainly young male German Shepherd dogs but also Boxers and Rottweilers. On the VD view, seen to be paramedian or bilateral rather than midline. Myelography may show deviation or compression of the dural sac. Although a developmental disease, clinical signs are not usually seen until > 18 months of age.
17. Neoplasia (see 5.4.3).
18. Mucopolysaccharidosis (see 5.4.9).

Vertebral canal changes

19. Widened vertebral canal.
    a. Normal at the level of the cervical (C5–T2) and lumbar (L2–5) intumescentia.
    b. Enlarged spinal cord due to chronic pathology.
       - Tumour (e.g. slow-growing astrocytoma, ependymoma, meningioma).
       - Syringohydromyelia, especially at the level of C2; common in the Cavalier King Charles Spaniel.
    c. Spinal arachnoid pseudocyst.
20. Narrowed vertebral canal.
    a. Cervical spondylopathy (wobbler syndrome).
       - Lateral view; dorsoventral narrowing at the cranial end of the affected vertebra.

- VD view; medially deviating pedicles of the caudal vertebral canal, particularly in the Great Dane and Boerboel.
b. Expansile or healing lesions of adjacent bone.
c. Lumbosacral stenosis.
d. Calcium phosphate deposition disease in Great Dane pups – dorsal displacement of C7 accompanied by deformation of the articular facets.

5.5 VARIATIONS IN VERTEBRAL ALIGNMENT

The floor of the vertebral canal of adjacent vertebrae should form a continuous straight to gently curved line. Malalignment may be constant and visible on survey radiographs, or intermittent and require radiographs made while the region is flexed or extended (stress radiography) to demonstrate instability.

1. Scoliosis (lateral curvature).
   a. Muscular spasm.
   b. Congenital vertebral abnormalities, for example hemivertebrae (see 5.3.3 and Fig. 5.3).
   c. Pathological fracture.
   d. Spinal cord abnormalities leading to functional scoliosis.
      - Dandy–Walker syndrome.
      - Spinal dysraphism – Weimaraner.
      - Syringohydromyelia; especially Cavalier King Charles Spaniel.
2. Lordosis (ventral curvature).
   a. Normal conformational variant.
   b. Muscular spasm.
   c. Congenital vertebral abnormalities, for example hemivertebrae (see 5.3.3 and Fig. 5.3), although kyphosis is more common.
   d. Loss of fibrotic vertebral support – old and heavy dogs.
   e. Pathological fracture.
   f. Nutritional secondary hyperparathyroidism (juvenile osteoporosis), especially caudal lumbar spine (see 1.16.4).
3. Kyphosis (dorsal curvature).
   a. Normal conformational variant.
   b. Muscular spasm.
   c. Congenital vertebral abnormalities, for example hemivertebrae (see 5.3.3 and Fig. 5.3).

d. Thoracolumbar disc disease.

e. Discospondylitis.

f. Pathological fracture.

g. Nutritional secondary hyperparathyroidism (juvenile osteoporosis) (see 1.16.4).

4. Trauma: a three-compartment model may be used to assess the stability of spinal fractures. Each vertebra is divided into a dorsal compartment (articular processes, spinous processes, laminae, pedicles, supporting soft tissues), a middle compartment (dorsal longitudinal ligament, dorsal part of annulus fibrosus, dorsal aspect of vertebral body) and a ventral compartment (remainder of vertebral body and annulus fibrosus, nucleus pulposus, ventral longitudinal ligament). If two of the three compartments are damaged, the fracture is considered to be unstable. CT is more reliable than radiography for determination of the extent of spinal fractures. Remember that bony displacement at the time of injury may have been greater than is recognized radiographically, having been reduced again by muscle spasm. Subsequent callus formation may cause worsening of neurological deficits some time after the injury. Small chip fractures may also be seen due to avulsion of soft tissue attachments.

a. Fracture.

b. Subluxation.

c. Luxation.

d. Salter–Harris type I or II fracture through vertebral physis in immature animal, with displacement of the epiphysis.

5. Atlantoaxial subluxation (Fig. 5.9) – abnormal alignment of C2 (axis) relative to C1 (atlas), which results in widening of the intervertebral space between the neural arch of C1 and the cranioventral aspect of the spine of C2, exacerbated by mild neck flexion (note that subtle widening of this space occurs in normal subjects on flexion). Dorsal subluxation of C2 may also occur. Marked flexion must be avoided, as it may cause spinal cord damage in the presence of instability. Usually due to defects of the dens (odontoid peg), evaluation of which is best achieved on oblique or VD views of the neck. The rostrocaudal open mouth view has been described for evaluation of the dens but in the presence of instability is likely to cause spinal cord damage. Clinical signs of neck

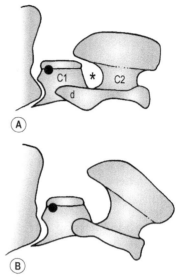

Figure 5.9 Atlantoaxial subluxation. (A) In the lateral view of a normal spine, the spinous process of C2 overhangs the arch of C1, producing a comma-shaped intervertebral foramen*; no significant alteration is seen on flexion. (B) In cases of atlantoaxial instability, abnormal flexion occurs at this joint and the intervertebral foramen is wide. In the case shown here, C2 lacks a dens.

pain and varying degrees of motor dysfunction result.

a. Congenital atlantoaxial instability – younger miniature and toy breeds (especially Yorkshire Terrier, Toy Poodle, Chihuahua, Pomeranian and Maltese), rarely large-breed dogs. May present clinically at a later age due to superimposed minor trauma.
   – Aplastic dens.
   – Hypoplastic dens.
   – Non-fusion of the dens to C2 (fusion normally completed at 6 months).
   – Absence of the dens ligaments.
   – Cats – dens agenesis resulting from mucopolysaccharidosis (see 5.4.9).

b. Acquired.
   – Fracture of the dens or cranial part of C2.
   – Rupture of the transverse ligament of the atlas, which normally holds the dens against the floor of that vertebra.

6. Cervical spondylopathy (wobbler syndrome) (see 5.3.8 and Fig. 5.5) – mainly Dobermann.

a. Static – malformed caudal cervical vertebrae with craniodorsal subluxation (tipping) of one or more vertebrae and a dorsoventrally narrowed cranial vertebral canal opening. Often accompanied by wedge-shaped or narrowed disc spaces and spondylosis.

b. Dynamic – malalignment worsens with ventroflexion of the neck.

7. Lumbosacral instability – step formation between the last lumbar and first sacral vertebrae. May be seen only on stress radiography of the region. Common in the German Shepherd dog, in which transitional lumbosacral vertebrae may predispose to instability; may progress to degenerative lumbosacral stenosis and cauda equina syndrome (see 5.16.6 and Fig. 5.17).

8. Calcium phosphate deposition disease in Great Dane pups – dorsal displacement of C7 accompanied by deformation of the articular facets.

5.6 DIFFUSE CHANGES IN VERTEBRAL OPACITY

Generalized decrease in radiopacity of the vertebrae (see also 1.16, *Osteopenia*)

1. Artefactual generalized decrease in vertebral radiopacity.
   a. Overexposure.
   b. Long-scale exposure techniques (high kV, low mAs).
   c. Obese or large patients creating large amounts of scattered radiation, especially if a grid was not used or with inadequate collimation.
   d. Overdevelopment.
   e. Fogging of the film (numerous causes).

2. Metabolic bone disease.
   a. Secondary hyperparathyroidism.
   b. Primary hyperparathyroidism.
   c. Corticosteroid excess.
      – Hyperadrenocorticism – Cushing's disease.
      – Iatrogenic – long-term corticosteroid administration.
   d. Hyperthyroidism.
   e. Diabetes mellitus.
   f. Congenital hypothyroidism – especially Boxer; delayed closure of vertebral physes and dysgenesis of endplates.

g. Pseudohyperparathyroidism; hypercalcaemia of malignancy.

h. Osteogenesis imperfecta – long bone changes usually predominate.

3. Senile osteoporosis – especially aged cats.

4. Neoplastic.
   a. Plasma cell myeloma (multiple myeloma) – genuine osteopenia as well as multiple osteolytic lesions (see 1.18.2).

5. Cats – hypervitaminosis A (raw liver diets); although proliferative bony changes predominate and mask the osteopenia (see 5.4.8).

6. Cats – mucopolysaccharidosis; likewise (see 5.4.9).

Generalized increase in radiopacity of the vertebrae (see also 1.13, *Increased radiopacity within bone*)

7. Artefactual generalized increase in vertebral radiopacity.
   a. Underexposure.
   b. Underdevelopment.

8. Osteopetrosis–osteosclerosis complex – hereditary in the Basenji.

9. Fluorosis.

10. Cats – feline leukaemia virus-associated medullary sclerosis.

5.7 LOCALIZED CHANGES IN VERTEBRAL OPACITY

Localized decrease in radiopacity of one or more vertebrae (see also 1.18, *Osteolytic lesions* and 1.19, *Expansile osteolytic lesions*)

1. Artefactual localized decrease in vertebral radiopacity.
   a. Superimposed skin defect, bowel or lung air on rotated lateral or VD views.
   b. Superimposed subcutaneous gas.

2. Decreased radiopacity of the vertebral endplate.
   a. Discospondylitis – endplate also irregular, and sclerotic in chronic cases (see 5.9.1 and Fig. 5.10).
   b. Neoplasia (see below).
   c. Intravertebral disc herniation (Schmorl's node) – particularly at L7 and/or S1;

medium and large breeds, especially
German Shepherd dog.

3. Irregular or discrete radiolucencies – single or
multiple radiolucent areas involving single or
multiple vertebrae and that may be
accompanied by bone production. Pathological
fracture may occur.
   a. Primary tumour – usually only one vertebra
   involved; less common than neoplasia in the
   appendicular skeleton; often primarily
   osteolytic.
      – Osteosarcoma.
      – Fibrosarcoma.
      – Chondrosarcoma.
      – Haemangiosarcoma.
      – Solitary plasma cell myeloma –
      characteristic punched-out appearance
      with little surrounding reaction.
      – Others.
   b. Metastatic or multifocal tumours – may
   involve multiple vertebrae or other bones;
   often primarily osteolytic.
      – Multiple myeloma (plasma cell
      myeloma).
      – Lymphoma.
      – Histiocytic sarcoma (malignant
      histiocytosis) – especially Rottweiler,
      Bernese Mountain dog, Golden Retriever,
      Flat-coated Retriever.
      – Metastases from, for example, prostatic,
      mammary, thyroid carcinomas;
      osteosarcoma.
   c. Infiltrative soft tissue tumours – may
   involve more than one vertebra, or a
   vertebra and adjacent bone (rib, pelvis);
   an adjacent soft tissue mass may be
   evident.
      – Haemangiosarcoma.
      – Lymphoma.
      – Fibrosarcoma.
      – Rhabdomyosarcoma.
      – Others.
   d. Benign tumours – osteochondroma or
   multiple cartilaginous exostoses may
   produce expansile osteolytic lesions
   (see 1.15.2).
   e. Severe spondylitis – osteolysis and
   pathological fracture are reported with
   systemic aspergillosis*.
   f. Aneurysmal bone cyst.

g. Dermoid or epidermoid cyst.
h. Post surgery (e.g. hemilaminectomy bone
defect).

4. Linear radiolucencies.
   a. Fractures.
   b. Widened vertebral physis.
      – Salter–Harris growth plate fractures
      in skeletally immature animals.
      – Vertebral physitis – haematogenous
      infection in young dogs, affecting
      mainly caudal lumbar physes, where
      blood flow is sluggish; may be
      associated with portosystemic shunts.
      – Congenital hypothyroidism – delayed
      closure of vertebral physes with
      dysgenesis of endplates; especially Boxer
      (see 1.22.9 and 5.3.11).
   c. Dermoid (pilonidal) sinus extending from
   the dorsal midline usually to cervical or
   cranial thoracic vertebrae; especially
   in young Rhodesian Ridgebacks, in which it
   shows autosomal recessive inheritance;
   sporadic in other breeds. Variable depth, in
   some cases extending to the dural sac either
   through the interarcuate space or via a
   neural arch defect, the latter appearing as a
   linear radiolucency. Clinical signs occur if
   the sinus involves the meninges and/or
   becomes infected. Sinography using non-
   ionic contrast medium may be used to detect
   the depth of the sinus.

Localized increase in radiopacity of one or more vertebrae

5. Artefactual localized increase in vertebral
radiopacity.
   a. Superimposed structures (e.g. extruded,
   mineralized disc material superimposed
   over neural arch).
   b. Underexposure of thicker areas of tissue.
6. Inflammation or osteomyelitis – it may not
be possible to differentiate periosteal new
bone superimposed over the vertebra from
increased density of the bone itself (sclerosis).
   a. Spondylosis.
   b. Discospondylitis.
   c. Spondylitis.
7. Neoplasia – although osteolysis usually
predominates, areas of increased radiopacity

may also be visible and some tumours are genuinely sclerotic.
a. Osteogenic osteosarcoma.
b. Chondrosarcoma.
c. Osteochondroma or multiple cartilaginous exostoses (see 1.15.2).
d. Chordoma has been reported as an intramedullary, mineralized spinal cord mass that mimicked disc extrusion on plain radiographs.

8. Fractures.
a. Compression fracture.
b. Healed fracture.

9. Vertebral endplate sclerosis.
a. With collapsed disc space.
   – Old disc herniation, especially at the lumbosacral junction.
   – Old surgically fenestrated disc.
b. Relative sclerosis compared with osteopenic vertebra (see 1.16 for causes).
c. Chronic discospondylitis (see 5.9.1 and Fig. 5.10).
d. Hemivertebra.
e. Adjacent to sacral osteochondrosis; especially German Shepherd dog (see 5.4.16 and Fig. 5.8).

10. Ossifying pachymeningitis (dural osseous metaplasia – see 5.10.1 and Fig. 5.11D).

11. Vertebral angiomatosis – cats 1–2 years old in thoracic vertebrae; rare condition in which a vascular malformation causes expansion and sclerosis of the pedicles.

12. Lead poisoning – metaphyseal sclerosis.

13. Mineral radiopacity in vertebrae.
a. Bullets and air gun pellets.
b. Incorrect microchip placement.
c. Surgical implants.

Mixed radiopacity of one or more vertebrae

14. Neoplasia.
a. Primary.
b. Metastatic.
c. Infiltration from adjacent soft tissue tumour.

15. Osteomyelitis or spondylitis.
a. Bacterial.
b. Fungal.

5.8 ABNORMALITIES OF THE INTERVERTEBRAL DISC SPACE

1. Disc space widened.
a. Normal variants.
   – Lumbar disc spaces are wider than thoracic disc spaces.
   – The lumbosacral disc space may be wider than adjacent lumbar disc spaces.
b. Artefactual widening – traction during stress radiography.
c. Apparent widening due to vertebral endplate erosion.
   – Discospondylitis (see 5.9.1 and Fig. 5.10).
   – Osteolytic tumour of adjacent vertebral body.
   – Intravertebral disc herniation (Schmorl's node) – particularly at L7 and/or S1; medium and large breeds, especially German Shepherd dog.
d. Trauma.
   – Subluxation.
   – Luxation.
e. Adjacent to hemivertebra.
f. Congenital hypothyroidism due to epiphyseal dysgenesis; especially Boxer (see 5.3.11 and 1.22.9).
g. Cats – mucopolysaccharidosis due to shortened vertebral bodies (see 5.4.9).

2. Disc space narrowed or of irregular width.
a. Normal at T10–11 (anticlinal junction; T11 is usually the anticlinal vertebra).
b. Artefactual narrowing.
   – Disc spaces appear to narrow towards the periphery of a radiograph due to divergence of the primary X-ray beam.
   – Spine not positioned parallel to cassette as result of muscular spasm or incorrect positioning; especially in the mid-cervical region due to sagging of this area when in lateral recumbency if not correctly supported with radiolucent foam wedges beneath (see Fig. 5.1A and B).
   – On VD views, where the disc space is not parallel to primary beam (e.g. cervical disc spaces and at the lumbosacral junction).
c. Ageing change in cats – multiple narrowed disc spaces and minor spondylosis often seen, especially in the thoracic spine.

d. Herniated disc – spondylosis may be seen with chronic lesions (note that survey radiography is unreliable for accurate localization of significant disc disease, as false positives and negatives are common and clinical signs may lateralize to the side contralateral to the compressive lesion; myelography, CT or MRI is required prior to surgery).

- Hansen type I disc disease – nucleus pulposus degeneration of chondroid metaplasia with calcification occurring in middle-aged chondrodystrophic dogs, especially the Dachshund; spinal pain or neurological signs tend to have an acute onset due to rupture of the annulus fibrosus and extrusion of calcified disc material into the vertebral canal. Rare in cats.
- Hansen type II disc disease – nucleus pulposus degeneration of fibrous metaplasia in older dogs of other breeds; clinical signs are often gradual in onset due to progressive hypertrophy and dorsal protrusion of the annulus fibrosus ± hypertrophy of the dorsal longitudinal ligament. A common incidental finding in older cats on post-mortem examination, although not usually associated with clinical signs.
- Combined type, in which a protruding annulus weakens and nuclear material then extrudes.
- Trauma – acute onset; usually extrusion of varying amounts of non-degenerate disc material.

e. Cervical spondylopathy (wobbler syndrome) with malformed caudal cervical vertebrae; disc space cranial to the malformed vertebra is usually wedge-shaped, apex ventrally.

f. After surgical fenestration.

g. Associated with advanced spondylosis.

h. Subluxation due to trauma (orthogonal view may show greater displacement).

i. Discospondylitis – (see 5.9.1 and Fig. 5.10).
- Early phase before vertebral endplate osteolysis.
- Healing phase.

j. Collapse of disc space due to adjacent vertebral neoplasm.

k. Narrow, vestigial disc space within a block or fused vertebra (see 5.3.4).

l. Adjacent to hemivertebra.

m. Intravertebral disc herniation (Schmorl's node) – particularly L7 and/or S1; medium and large breeds, especially German Shepherd dog.

3. Increased radiopacity of the disc space.

a. Artefactual increased radiopacity.
- Superimposed rib or transverse process on lateral radiographs.
- Vertebral endplate seen obliquely.

b. Mineralization of the nucleus pulposus in chondrodystrophic breeds, sometimes beginning at less than 1 year of age and mainly around the thoracolumbar junction; less often in older dogs of other breeds (usually an incidental finding, especially if *in situ* with a rounded dorsal margin).

c. Contrast medium deposition during a discogram.

4. Increased radiolucency of the disc space.

a. Gas due to vacuum phenomenon – indicative of disc degeneration.
- May be consistently present.
- May be present only during traction.

5.9 IRREGULARITY OF THE VERTEBRAL ENDPLATES

1. Discospondylitis (Fig. 5.10) – infection or inflammation of the intervertebral disc and adjacent vertebral endplates, sometimes with adjacent soft tissue swelling due to cellulitis or abscessation; dogs more than cats; especially male large breeds. Infection is usually haematogenous, and a source of infection should be sought (e.g. cystitis, prostatitis or vegetative endocarditis). Vertebral endplate osteolysis creates irregular margination of the disc space, which may be either narrowed or widened, and mild subluxation may occur. In the early stages, the endplates may show decreased radiopacity but later become sclerotic with surrounding spondylosis. At the lumbosacral junction, early discospondylitis must be distinguished from intravertebral disc herniation (Schmorl's nodes, see 5.9.6). Survey lateral radiographs of the rest of the spine

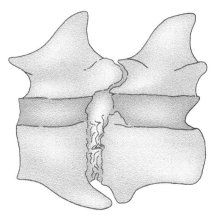

Figure 5.10 Discospondylitis: irregularity of the disc space due to erosion of adjacent vertebral endplates; secondary spondylotic new bone and facet arthropathy.

should be obtained, as multiple disc spaces may be involved. Mild spinal cord compression is sometimes present, demonstrable by myelography or MRI. In severe, healed cases, adjacent vertebrae may fuse together.

  a. Bacterial – *Staphylococcus aureus* most commonly; also *S. intermedius*, *Escherichia coli*, *Corynebacterium diphtheria*, *Pasteurella multocida*, *Brucella canis* (mainly USA), *Streptococcus* spp., *Nocardia asteroides*. May be secondary to transient immunosuppression with canine parvovirus infection.

  b. Fungal – especially *Aspergillus** spp. in immunocompromised German Shepherd dogs.

  c. Iatrogenic – complication of intervertebral disc surgery or discogram.

2. Old cats – indentation of multiple endplates is commonly seen, especially in the thoracic spine.

3. Congenital hypothyroidism – vertebral epiphyseal dysgenesis with characteristic ventral spikes of bone; especially Boxers (see 1.22.9).

4. Mucopolysaccharidosis due to epiphyseal dysplasia; especially cats (see 5.4.9).

5. Compression fractures.

  a. Trauma.

  b. Nutritional secondary hyperparathyroidism (juvenile osteoporosis) (see 1.16.4).

6. Schmorl's nodes – herniation of intervertebral disc material into the adjacent vertebral endplate; well recognized in humans, causing lower back pain rather than neurological signs.

Much less common in dogs, due to thicker subchondral bone; mainly at the lumbosacral junction. Seen as a sharply defined indentation of the vertebral endplate, sometimes with a sclerotic margin and vacuum phenomenon in the disc space (see 2.2.13). Speculatively a cause for fibrocartilaginous embolism. Not reported in cats but possibly the cause of 5.9.2 above. Differential diagnosis is discospondylitis, but more focal and well defined.

7. Remodelled vertebrae following nutritional secondary hyperparathyroidism.

8. Sacral osteochondrosis (see 5.4.16 and Fig. 5.8) – irregularity of craniodorsal sacral endplate.

5.10 ABNORMALITIES OF THE INTERVERTEBRAL FORAMEN

The lumbar intervertebral foramina are readily seen on the lateral views, although the thoracic ones are mostly obscured by the ribs. The cervical intervertebral foramina open ventrolaterally and are not seen on the routine lateral view except to a limited extent at C2–3. They are best evaluated by making a VD radiograph and tilting the spine 45° to the left and right sides.

1. Opacified intervertebral foramen.

  a. Normal – superimposition of accessory processes in the thoracolumbar region (Fig. 5.11A).

  b. Artefactual.

    – Superimposed bony rib nodules in the thoracic spine.

    – Superimposed skin opacities.

  c. Extrusion of mineralized disc material (Fig. 5.11B).

    – Dorsally into the vertebral canal and therefore superimposed over the foramen on lateral radiographs but difficult to see on the VD.

    – Laterally into the foramen itself, compressing the nerve roots; seen in the foramen on a VD radiograph.

  d. Dorsally bulging calcified annulus fibrosus (Fig. 5.11C).

  e. Osteochondral fragment from osteochondrosis dissecans at the lumbosacral junction (see 5.4.16 and Fig. 5.8).

  f. Ossifying pachymeningitis (dural osseous metaplasia) – fine, horizontal linear opacity

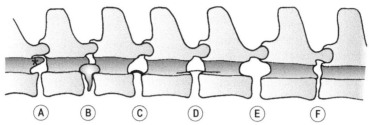

Figure 5.11 Intervertebral foramen abnormalities: (A) normal foramen with accessory process*; (B) extruded mineralized nucleus pulposus in or overlying the foramen; (C) dorsally bulging mineralized annulus fibrosus; (D) ossifying pachymeningitis; (E) enlarged foramen due to nerve root neoplasia; (F) small foramen secondary to disc herniation and collapse of disc space.

ventrally or dorsally, best seen over disc spaces; an incidental finding, usually older dogs of larger breeds (Fig. 5.11D).
  g. Proliferative bony lesions of adjacent vertebrae (e.g. dorsolateral spondyles, facet joint osteoarthrosis).
  h. Calcinosis circumscripta dorsal to the spinal cord at C1–2 and at T2–3 has been described in young dogs (see 12.2.2 and Fig. 12.1).
  i. Bullets, air gun pellets or other missiles.
2. Enlarged intervertebral foramen.
  a. Neoplasia of nerve root (Fig. 5.11E).
    – Neurofibrosarcoma.
    – Schwannoma.
    – Meningioma.
  b. After surgery.
    – Foraminotomy or pediculectomy.
  c. Trauma.
    – Fracture of adjacent vertebra.
    – Vertebral subluxation.
  d. Atlantoaxial subluxation (see 5.5.5 and Fig. 5.9) – widening of the normal comma-shaped foramen between C1 and C2.
  e. Vascular anomalies resulting in compensatory increased vertebral artery blood flow, which enlarges the foramen.
3. Reduced intervertebral foramen size.
  a. Artefactual due to opacification (see 5.10.1).
  b. Disc herniation with associated narrowing of the disc space (Fig. 5.11F).
  c. Bony proliferative tumour of adjacent vertebra.
  d. Facet joint osteoarthrosis (see 5.11.3).
  e. Trauma.
    – Fracture of adjacent vertebra.
    – Subluxation.

    – Callus of a healing or healed vertebral fracture.
  f. Block vertebra (see 5.3.4).

5.11 ABNORMALITIES OF THE ARTICULAR FACETS

1. Widened joint space.
  a. Normal with ventroflexion of spine.
  b. Subluxation.
  c. Joint effusion.
  d. Severe kyphosis.
  e. Aplasia of the facets (see below).
2. Narrowed joint space.
  a. Associated with narrowed disc space and intervertebral foramen.
    – Disc herniation.
    – Trauma with (sub)luxation.
  b. Spondylarthrosis (see below).
3. Irregular joint space.
  a. Facet joint osteoarthrosis (spondylarthrosis) – degenerative changes of the facetal synovial joint with osteophyte formation, subchondral sclerosis and occasionally bridging; associated synovial cysts have been reported. Most commonly seen in the thoracolumbar region, occasionally cervical. Bony changes are easily seen on lateral radiographs, but the VD view is needed to show whether one or both sides are affected. Associated soft tissue hypertrophy is not seen on plain radiographs. May cause pain due to arthropathy or nerve root compression; severe cases show neurological deficits with cord compression evident on myelography, MRI or CT.
    – Idiopathic – single or multiple joints in older dogs.

- Cervical spondylopathy (wobbler syndrome) – in young Great Danes, Boerboels and Mastiffs due to malformed and malpositioned articular facets, which often show secondary arthrosis.
    - Familial in young Shiloh Shepherd dogs T11–L2; Scottish Deerhounds C2–3.
  b. Secondary to trauma – usually a single joint.
  c. Infection – irregularity of facets is seen in some cases of discospondylitis.
  d. Mucopolysaccharidosis – especially cats. Fusion of the facets may eventually occur (see 5.4.9).
4. Enlarged and/or sclerotic facets – osteoarthrosis (see above).
5. Absent articular facets.
  a. Articular facet aplasia.
    - Cervical.
    - Thoracolumbar – absence of caudal articular facets with compensatory hypertrophy of the adjacent cranial facets and ligamentum flavum, secondary arthrosis and compressive myelopathy have been reported; German Shepherd dogs possibly predisposed. Facet hypoplasia may also occur and may be clinically silent.
  b. After spinal surgery.

5.12 LESIONS IN THE PARAVERTEBRAL SOFT TISSUES

Soft tissue changes in the tissues surrounding the spine may be indicative of trauma, neoplastic or infectious changes that could involve the spine.
1. Gas accumulation in paravertebral soft tissues.
  a. Trauma with an open wound.
  b. Gas-producing bacterial infection.
2. Metallic foreign bodies.
  a. Microchip.
  b. Bullets, air gun pellets and other missiles.
  c. Needles etc. that may have been ingested and exited the gut.
3. Swelling of paravertebral soft tissues – more likely in the sublumbar and lumbosacral region, often displacing the descending colon ventrally.
  a. Reactive lymph nodes.
  b. Neoplasia.

- Osseous.
    - Soft tissue.
  c. Abscess.
  d. Granuloma.
  e. Haematoma.
4. Mineralization in the paravertebral soft tissues.
  a. Dystrophic mineralization in a tumour.
  b. Calcinosis circumscripta – in soft tissues at the level of C1–2 and C5–6 regions and occasionally elsewhere near the spine. Especially affects young German Shepherd dogs (see 12.2.2 and Fig. 12.1).

5.13 ULTRASONOGRAPHY OF PARAVERTEBRAL SOFT TISSUES

Ultrasonographic examination of the paravertebral soft tissues is most readily performed from a dorsal or lateral approach. The ventral aspects of the vertebral bodies in the cervical and lumbar regions can be visualized if the transducer is placed laterally, just below the ventral margin of the sublumbar musculature, and angled dorsally, or via a transabdominal approach. Ultrasound guidance may be used to aspirate the caudal lumbar disc spaces if affected by discospondylitis.

1. Irregularity of the margins of the vertebral bodies.
  a. Spondylosis (see 5.4.1).
  b. Spondylitis (see 5.4.4).
  c. Neoplasia (see 5.4.3).
  d. Healed or healing bony trauma.
  e. Bone discontinuity associated with recent bony trauma.
  f. Disseminated skeletal hyperostosis (see 5.4.5).
  g. Hypervitaminosis A (especially cats – see 5.4.8).
  h. Mucopolysaccharidosis (see 5.4.9).
2. Disturbances of the normal fibre alignment of the paravertebral muscles.
  a. Trauma with contusion and/or muscle fibre tearing (e.g. iliopsoas strain).
  b. Previous surgery.
  c. Cellulitis and/or abscess formation, often suspected to be due to migrating foreign body.
  d. Neoplasia.
3. Echogenic foci within paravertebral soft tissues.

a. Foreign body (often surrounded by a small amount of fluid).
b. Bone fragments.
c. Mineralization within paravertebral soft tissues.
   – Within a focus of chronic inflammation.
   – Within a neoplasm.
   – Secondary to trauma.
   – Calcinosis cutis (see 12.2.2).
   – Calcinosis circumscripta (see 12.2.2).
d. Gas.
   – Subcutaneous emphysema.
   – Within a sinus tract.
4. Fluid accumulation within paravertebral soft tissues.
   a. Haematoma.
   b. Abscess ± foreign body.
   c. Retroperitoneal fluid, usually inflammatory, blood or urine.
   d. Ventral disc space in discospondylitis.
5. Sublumbar lymph nodes, especially medial iliac and hypogastric.

5.14 SPINAL CONTRAST STUDIES: TECHNIQUE AND NORMAL APPEARANCE

Myelography

Myelography involves injection of non-ionic, iodinated contrast medium into the subarachnoid space, and may be performed either via the cervical or the lumbar route. The latter is regarded as safer for the patient but is more difficult to perform. Reliability of results can be improved by injecting the contrast medium at the site closer to the suspected lesion.

The patient is anaesthetized and the site prepared for aseptic injection. The normal dosage rate is 0.3 mL/kg of iopamidol or iohexol at a concentration of 300 mg/mL, with a minimum of 2 mL for cats and small dogs. Cerebrospinal fluid (CSF) may be collected prior to injecting the contrast medium. The contrast medium should be warmed to reduce its viscosity.

Following contrast medium injection, lateral and VD radiographs are obtained routinely following the contrast medium along the spine; if any alteration in the contrast column is identified, oblique views should also be obtained, as these will skyline areas dorsolateral and ventrolateral to the cord.

Obtaining lateral radiographs in both right and left lateral recumbency may also be beneficial for lateralized lesions, which may be better outlined by contrast medium when dependent. In the cervicothoracic area, the DV view is preferred to the VD in order to encourage contrast medium to pool in the area rather than flowing away. In lateral recumbency, elevation of the body cranial and caudal to a lesion will likewise encourage pooling of contrast in the area of interest. Stressed views (flexed, extended and traction) of the cervical and lumbosacral areas may assist in recognizing dynamic lesions, although care should be taken if the stressed position may worsen neurological compression.

Cervical (cisterna magna) myelography
An assistant holds the dog's head at right angles to the neck, with the median plane of the nose and skull parallel to the table. The spinal needle must penetrate the skin at a point in the midline midway between the levels of the external occipital protuberance of the skull and the cranial edges of the wings of the atlas, these landmarks being palpated.

In small dogs and cats, a 4- to 5-cm 22-gauge spinal needle is used; once the skin has been penetrated, the stylet should be removed and the needle advanced slowly. In larger dogs, a 6- to 9-cm needle is required, and the stylet is left in the needle until the resistance offered by the strong dorsal atlanto-occipital ligament is felt or until the ligament has been perforated. When the needle enters the subarachnoid space, CSF will begin to flow from the needle and may be collected for analysis. The needle should be held firmly at its point of entrance through the skin to prevent movement of the needle when the syringe is attached. The contrast medium is injected slowly over about 1 min.

Lumbar myelography
Injection may be made with the patient in lateral or sternal recumbency, and many operators prefer the spine to be flexed to widen the interarcuate space through which the needle enters the vertebral canal. The site of injection is normally L5–6 in dogs and L6–7 in cats (Fig. 5.12). The dorsal spinous process of the caudal vertebra is located just cranial to a line through the wings of the ilium, and the spinal needle is introduced flush against its cranial edge in a direction perpendicular to the long axis of the spine and parallel or vertical to the table top (depending on the patient's position) until

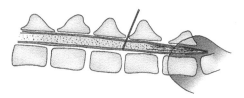

Figure 5.12 Normal lumbar myelogram with correct needle placement at L5–6.

solid resistance by the bony vertebral canal floor is felt. The spinal cord is deliberately penetrated to reach the more voluminous ventral subarachnoid space. Penetration of the cauda equina often results in a hindquarter jerk or anal twitch, indicating correct needle placement. If the needle will not enter the vertebral canal, it must be redirected slightly. The stylet is removed when the needle tip is the vertebral canal. Free flow of CSF confirms correct needle position, although the amount of CSF obtained is usually much less than with cervical puncture, and lack of CSF flow does not necessarily indicate wrong placement of the needle.

If severe spinal cord compression or swelling is suspected, the contrast medium must be injected rapidly over 10 s and exposures made immediately and again after 30 s. The first exposure will show the caudal edge of the lesion to best advantage and the slightly delayed one the cranial end.

Normal myelographic appearance
On the lateral radiograph, dorsal and ventral contrast columns are visible; on the VD or DV view, the lateral columns are seen. The columns are of even width along the vertebral canal except cranially, within C1 and C2, where they are dilated due to the cisterna magna. The dorsal contrast column is often slightly wider than the ventral column. The ventral contrast column is often slightly indented over the disc spaces (especially C2–3), without effect on the diameter of the spinal cord. The spinal cord creates a non-opacified band between the columns, with mild diffuse enlargement at the brachial (C5–7) and lumbar (L3–4) intumescentia. The cord is relatively large compared with the size of the vertebral canal in small dogs and cats, and appears relatively smaller in large breeds of dog. From the mid-lumbar area, the spinal cord tapers and is surrounded by the nerves forming the cauda equina, creating a converging, striated appearance. The shape of the caudal end of the dural sac is variable and may be sharply

pointed or blunted. The location of its termination is variable between dogs; in most dogs, the dural sac crosses the lumbosacral disc space and enters the sacrum, but in some it terminates more cranially. In cats, the spinal cord and dural sac extend more caudally than in dogs.

Changes in the contrast columns include thinning, interruption, obstruction, outward or inward displacement, dilation and splitting.

Complications of myelography
1. Seizures, especially if contrast medium enters the cranial cavity.
2. Aggravation of clinical signs may occur within the first day – these are related to manipulation during positioning.
3. Apnoea can occur if the injection is given too rapidly via the cisternal route.
4. Penetrating the spinal cord or brainstem with the needle during cisternal myelography – may result in death.
5. Penetrating the cerebellar vermis with the needle during cisternal myelography in dogs with caudal occipital malformation (Chiari-type abnormality; mainly Cavalier King Charles Spaniels).
6. Injection into the central canal of the spinal cord may cause severe paresis or paralysis, depending on the quantity of contrast medium injected. Such injections usually occur when lumbar puncture is performed cranial to L5–6 (Fig. 5.14).
7. Haematoma has been reported after lumbar puncture, presumably due to damage to the vertebral venous sinuses.

Epidurography

Epidurography is used mainly to investigate cauda equina syndrome. The dog may be positioned in sternal or lateral recumbency. A spinal needle is introduced into the epidural space via the sacrocaudal junction or between caudal vertebrae 1 and 2 or 2 and 3. The lumbosacral junction should normally be avoided, as pathology is often located at this site. In large-breed dogs, about 4–8 mL of contrast medium is injected and immediate lateral and DV or VD radiographs are made.

The normal epidurogram creates an undulating or scalloped appearance, with the ventral contrast column elevated over each disc space and draped more ventrally in between. It is much more difficult to interpret than a myelogram.

Discography

Discography is occasionally performed at the lumbosacral junction in order to detect disc degeneration. The normal nucleus pulposus is difficult to inject, while degenerate discs accommodate more contrast medium and may show dorsal leakage. Needle placement is facilitated by the use of fluoroscopy with image intensification. However, discography is being superseded by the use of CT and MRI.

5.15 TECHNICAL ERRORS DURING MYELOGRAPHY

General myelography: Technical errors (Figs 5.13 and 5.14)

1. Single or multiple 1–3 mm diameter radiolucent filling defects – air bubbles due to air in syringe during injection.
2. Contrast medium in soft tissues dorsal to injection site – leakage of contrast medium up the needle tract.

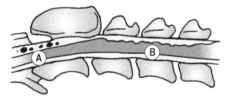

Figure 5.13 Cervical myelogram showing technical errors: (A) air bubbles in the contrast medium; (B) subdural contrast medium injection.

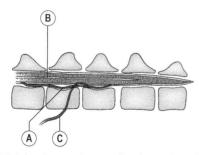

Figure 5.14 Lumbar myelogram showing technical errors: (A) epidural leakage of contrast medium; (B) contrast medium in the central canal of the spinal cord; and (C) leakage of contrast medium into blood vessels.

Cervical myelogram: Technical errors

3. Poor distribution of contrast medium in the subarachnoid space resulting in an uneven or bizarre myelographic appearance; differential diagnoses are severe meningitis, diffuse neoplasia (e.g. lymphoma).
   a. Inadequate subarachnoid volume of contrast medium.
      – Initial volume too small.
      – Marked extradural injection or leakage (see below).
   b. Contrast medium not warmed to body temperature; poor mixing with CSF may contribute.
   c. Injecting too slowly may contribute.
4. Subdural contrast medium injection or leakage – contrast medium lies mainly dorsally, is very dense and has an undulating, scalloped inner margin and a knife-shaped distal termination; differential diagnosis is spinal arachnoid pseudocyst.
5. Contrast medium in the central canal.
   a. Central canal > 2 mm wide.
      – Inadvertent injection into syringohydromyelic cord. Unlikely to result in additional neurological effects.
   b. Central canal 0.5–2 mm wide.
      – Reflux into the canal if the spinal needle accidentally penetrated the spinal cord and passed through or close to the canal.
6. Contrast medium accidentally injected into the spinal cord parenchyma – the prognosis for patient survival is volume-dependent.
7. Contrast medium does not pass an obstructive lesion (may enter cranium instead) – try elevating head and neck further to gravitate the contrast medium past the obstructive site.
   a. Lack of pressure of cisterna magna injection does not allow contrast medium to force its way past lesions totally obstructing the subarachnoid space. An additional lumbar puncture myelogram should be performed.
   b. Inadequate volume of contrast medium.
   c. If contrast medium does not outline the caudal cervical region on a VD radiograph, obtain a DV radiograph to encourage pooling of contrast medium in this area.

Lumbar myelogram: technical errors

8. Scalloped appearance of contrast medium.
   a. Epidural injection.
      - Needle tip too deep when in the ventral part of the vertebral canal.
      - Multiple dural punctures with contrast leaking out of the subarachnoid space.
      - Needle tip in an extradural mass lesion.
9. Subdural contrast medium injection or leakage – less common than with cisterna magna puncture.
10. Contrast medium pooling in the intervertebral foramina and around nerve roots – epidural injection.
11. Contrast medium in sublumbar vasculature, lymphatics and lymph nodes following epidural injection.
12. Contrast medium in the central canal – more likely to occur with needle placement cranial to the recommended L5–6 interarcuate space.
    a. Central canal 0.5–2 mm wide.
       - Reflux into the canal if the spinal needle passed through or close to the canal.
       - Aberrant communication between the subarachnoid space and the central canal due to tumour, herniated disc or malacic cord.
    b. Central canal > 2 mm wide.
       - Iatrogenic distension of the central canal due to direct injection. Depending on the extent, the dog may go into respiratory or cardiac arrest and will develop neurological deficits that may or may not improve over time.
       - Syringohydromyelia – usually with Chiari-like malformation in Cavalier King Charles Spaniels; inadvertent canalogram may occur during cisterna magna injection.
13. Contrast medium injected into the spinal cord parenchyma; differential diagnosis is leakage into an area of myelomalacia.

5.16 EXTRADURAL SPINAL CORD COMPRESSION ON MYELOGRAPHY

The spinal cord is usually narrowed on one view and widened on the orthogonal view (Fig. 5.15). The contrast columns are deviated and thinned or interrupted. Occasionally, an hourglass

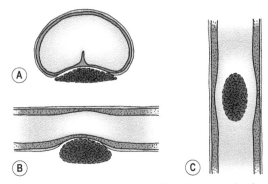

Figure 5.15 Schematic representation of an extradural lesion: (A) mass position, lying outside the meninges; (B) myelogram view tangential to the lesion shows spinal cord compression; and (C) the orthogonal view shows apparent spinal cord widening.

compression is seen with neoplasia, disc material or haematoma, which may encircle the cord. Focal extradural compressions may occasionally create the impression of contrast column splitting when imaged tangentially, and this can give an erroneous diagnosis of an intradural lesion.

1. Normal variants – slight compression of the subarachnoid space, with no attenuation of the opposite contrast medium column or spinal cord.
   a. Ventral contrast column over C2–3 disc space.
   b. Dorsal contrast column at the C3–4–5–6–7 articulations.
   c. Ventral contrast column over other disc spaces, especially in large breeds of dog.
2. Artefactual – contrast medium in the ventral epidural space following lumbar puncture; produces a thick, wavy line that is elevated over each disc space (see Fig. 5.14).
3. Disc extrusion (Hansen type I disc disease; Fig. 5.16). Spinal cord compression may be from any direction and may not necessarily be at the level of a disc space.

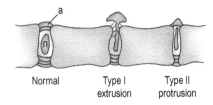

Figure 5.16 Normal disc (a, annulus fibrosus; n, nucleus pulposus), type I disc disease (extrusion) and type II disc disease (protrusion).

a. Thoracolumbar region (T11–L3), especially in chondrodystrophic breeds; more caudal lumbar disc spaces are less often affected. Extruded disc material, and thus spinal compression, may be ventral, ventrolateral, lateral, dorsolateral and occasionally dorsally, or in combinations of these locations. Oblique views are helpful to localize disc material, which is usually located at or cranial to the affected disc space. Disc lesions T1–10 are unusual due to the presence of the intercapital ligament between the heads of the ribs. Rare in cats.

b. Cervical region (C2–7) in any breed of dog, mainly smaller breeds. C2–3 is the commonest site in small breeds and C6–7 in larger breeds. The major clinical sign is often neck pain rather than a neurological deficit. The disc material usually lies ventrally or ventrolaterally. Rare in cats.

c. Cervical spondylopathy (wobbler syndrome) – caudal cervical region in large-breed dogs, especially Dobermann and Rottweiler. Mainly ventrally. Traction or ventroflexion of the neck has minimal effect on the compression. However, disc lesions secondary to caudal cervical vertebral malformation are more often protrusions than extrusions (see below).

d. Lumbosacral disc disease, especially larger breeds such as the German Shepherd dog (Fig. 5.17). Predisposed to by lumbosacral transitional vertebra. Disc material lies within the ventral part of the vertebral canal, causing compression of the cauda equina. Again, disc protrusions are more common than extrusions.

e. Adjacent to deformed vertebrae or rigid sections of the spine (e.g. hemivertebrae, block vertebra and areas of ankylosed spondylosis).

4. Hypertrophied annulus fibrosus or disc protrusion ± hypertrophy of the dorsal longitudinal ligament (Hansen type II disc disease; Fig. 5.16) – ventral or ventrolateral compression of the spinal cord (chronic compression may lead to spinal cord atrophy, seen on myelography as reduced cord diameter with visible surrounding subarachnoid space and no evidence of current compression).

a. Common in dogs, mainly caudal cervical and thoracolumbar spine in large breeds; may be multiple. Commonly found in older cats on post-mortem examination but rarely cause clinical signs.

b. Cervical spondylopathy (wobbler syndrome) – caudal cervical region, large-breed dogs, especially Dobermann, Rottweiler and Dalmatian. Traction or ventroflexion of the neck may reduce the compression by flattening the bulging soft tissue.

c. Cauda equina syndrome, especially larger breeds such as the German Shepherd dog (Fig. 5.17). Stressed views are helpful, as the degree of dural sac compression is often worse in extension than in flexion, reflecting the clinical signs, in which discomfort is more severe when the lumbosacral joint is extended.

5. Hypertrophied or redundant ligamentum flavum (interarcuate ligament) – dorsal compression of the spinal cord or cauda equina.

a. Cervical spondylopathy (wobbler syndrome) – large-breed dogs. Ventroflexion of the neck reduces the compression; dorsoflexion of the neck aggravates the compression. Especially C5–7 Great Dane, C2–3 Rottweiler; associated with other lesions of caudal cervical vertebral malformation.

b. Lumbosacral instability; degenerative lumbosacral stenosis.

6. Instability between adjacent vertebrae.

a. Atlantoaxial subluxation (see 5.5.5 and Fig. 5.9).

b. Caudal cervical spine, especially C6–7, in cervical spondylopathy (wobbler syndrome) (see 5.3.8 and Fig. 5.5).

c. Lumbosacral junction, predisposing to degenerative lumbosacral stenosis and cauda equina syndrome (Fig. 5.17).

d. Trauma and spinal fracture or subluxation.

7. Extradural neoplasia with or without bony changes.

a. Primary or metastatic tumour in surrounding bone – often osteolytic lesions and may be accompanied by pathological fractures.
   – Various histological types in adults, for example osteosarcoma, histiocytic sarcoma (especially Bernese Mountain dog and Rottweiler), articular facet myxosarcoma.

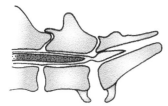

Figure 5.17 Compression of the cauda equina (cauda equina syndrome) on myelography: various combinations of lumbosacral instability, disc disease, bony stenosis and dorsal soft tissue hypertrophy causing degenerative lumbosacral stenosis.

- In young animals, consider osteochondroma or multiple cartilaginous exostoses (see 1.15.2).
- Osteosarcoma in older cats.
  b. Originating from soft tissues within the vertebral canal.
  - Neurofibroma.
  - Myxoma or myxosarcoma.
  - Meningioma.
  - Lymphoma.
  - Lipoma, angiolipoma or myelolipoma.
  - Haemangiosarcoma.
  c. Paraspinal tumour from the soft tissues surrounding the vertebral column.
  - Phaeochromocytoma, usually cranial lumbar region.
  - Spinal nerve tumour (may also produce intradural–extramedullary and intramedullary lesions).
  d. Cats – lymphoma from as young as 6 months, male preponderance. Test for feline leukaemia virus and look for lymphoma in other organs.
8. Extradural bony lesions.
  a. Neoplasia (see above).
  b. Congenital vertebral malformations (see 5.3).
  c. Trauma.
  - Fracture; acute fracture or fracture healing with callus formation.
  - Spinal luxation or subluxation.
  d. Cervical spondylopathy (wobbler syndrome).
  - Ventral or dorsal compression from vertebral canal stenosis – caudal cervical spine; especially Dobermann (see 5.3.8 and Fig. 5.5).

- Dorsal compression from vertebral canal stenosis – cranial cervical spine; especially Bassett Hound.
  - Dorsolateral compression – malformation of articular facets, mainly caudal cervical spine; especially Great Dane, Boerboel, Mastiff.
  - Lateral compression from medially converging caudal cervical pedicles, visible only on VD view; especially Great Dane, Boerboel.
  e. Lumbosacral malalignment or instability.
  f. Lumbosacral osteochondrosis; usually the craniodorsal margin of S1; especially German Shepherd dogs (see 5.4.16 and Fig. 5.8).
  g. Cats – hypervitaminosis A – occasionally causes spinal cord compression (see 5.4.8).
9. Articular facet lesions (see 5.11.3) – lateral or dorsolateral compression, best seen on VD or oblique views.
  a. Cervical spondylopathy (wobbler syndrome) – enlargement, malpositioning and arthrosis of articular facet joints mainly in the caudal cervical region, especially Great Dane and Mastiff.
  b. Facet arthrosis in older dogs; usually thoracolumbar area.
  c. Juxta-articular cysts.
  - Synovial cysts; cervical often multiple in younger dogs, especially Great Dane, Boerboel and Mastiff; thoracolumbar often single in older dogs, especially German Shepherd dog.
  - Ganglion cysts, usually in cervical or lumbosacral regions.
10. Extradural haematoma or haemorrhage.
  a. Trauma.
  - External trauma (e.g. road traffic accident).
  - Internal trauma due to acute disc herniation or dural tearing, especially if a vertebral venous sinus is lacerated; may be very extensive.
  - Post-surgical haemorrhage.
  - Iatrogenic haemorrhage caused by spinal needle.
  b. Coagulopathy.
  - Haemophilia A, especially young male German Shepherd dogs.
  - Anticoagulant poisoning.
  - Thrombocytopenia.

– Von Willebrand's disease; especially Dobermann.
c. Haemorrhage secondary to:
– tumour
– vascular malformation
– parasitic migration, especially *Spirocerca lupi**
– meningitis
– necrotizing vasculitis – Bernese Mountain Dog, German Short-haired Pointer and Beagle.
d. Subperiosteal vertebral haematoma.
11. Extradural infectious or inflammatory process, granuloma, focal abscess or more diffuse empyema.
a. Haematogenous infection.
– Bacterial.
– Fungal (e.g. histoplasmosis* in cats).
b. Direct extension from adjacent septic process in soft tissues.
c. Extension from discospondylitis (see 5.9.1 and Fig. 5.10).
– Bacterial.
– Fungal, especially cryptococcosis* in cats.
d. Extension from spondylitis (see 5.4.4 and Fig. 5.7).
– Bacterial.
– Fungal, especially cryptococcosis* in cats.
– Parasitic (e.g. *Spirocerca lupi**).
e. Steatitis – inflammation of epidural fat.
12. Membrane disease (epidural scarring) – weeks to months after laminectomy or hemilaminectomy.
13. Fibrosis of the interarcuate (yellow) ligament at C2–3 causing dorsal cord compression has been reported in two young Rottweilers.
14. Parasites.
a. Granuloma from aberrant migration of *Spirocerca lupi** larva in the caudal thoracic region; may present with acute pelvic limb paresis, mimicking disc extrusion.
b. Aberrant migration of heartworm (*Dirofilaria immitis**).
15. Vascular anomalies.
a. Aneurysm of venous sinus.
b. Aortocaval fistula with distension of vertebral venous plexus.
16. Calcinosis circumscripta – extradural location reported (e.g. at C1–2); especially young German Shepherd dogs.

17. Extradural foreign body (e.g. small fragments of wood following pharyngeal stick injuries); may be acute or months after the initial injury.
18. Post-operative seroma.
19. Extradural infiltrative lipoma.
20. Cyst of disc or associated intraspinal ligament.

5.17 INTRADURAL–EXTRAMEDULLARY SPINAL CORD COMPRESSION ON MYELOGRAPHY

The column of contrast medium splits (golf tee sign) or widens (teardrop shape) and often shows abrupt termination (Fig. 5.18). In the orthogonal plane, the spinal cord may appear widened due to compression caused by the intradural lesion.

1. Artefactual golf tee sign due to extradural contrast leakage outlining an extradural lesion.
2. Artefactual splitting of contrast column (usually on a lateral view) due to a focal central, ventral extradural lesion indenting the cord but allowing the subarachnoid space to drape back into place on either side, or a ventrolateral extradural lesion: differentiated from a true intradural lesion by utilizing oblique views.
3. Spinal arachnoid pseudocyst (leptomeningeal or meningeal cyst) – two distinct types are now recognized.
a. Bulbous or teardrop-shaped expansion of the dorsal subarachnoid space with attenuation of the subjacent spinal cord (Fig. 5.19A).

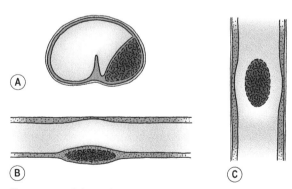

Figure 5.18 Schematic representation of an extramedullary, intradural lesion: (A) mass position, lying within the meninges but outside the spinal cord; (B) myelogram view tangential to the lesion shows spinal cord compression but splitting of the contrast column, which often terminates; (C) the orthogonal view shows apparent spinal cord widening due to spinal cord compression in the other plane.

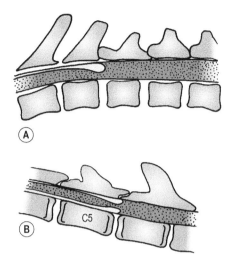

Figure 5.19 Spinal arachnoid pseudocyst: (A) dorsal lesion, typical of most breeds, directed caudally; (B) variant seen most often in Rottweilers and occasionally in other large dogs; in the cervical area and may be directed either cranially or caudally.

Usually at C2–3 (generally large dogs), T8–10 (generally small and medium-sized dogs) or the thoracolumbar area (cats). Tend to occur in young male animals, but the aetiology is unknown; possible causes include genetic factors, inflammation and trauma, probably giving rise to adhesive arachnoiditis, which alters CSF dynamics. These lesions are always directed caudally.

b. More recently, a different conformation of lesion has been recognized in the cervical spine at C2–3 or C5–6–7 for which Rottweilers are over-represented (Fig. 5.19B); there are both dorsal and ventral accumulations of contrast medium, and the cord adjacent to the lesion is focally swollen. These lesions are usually directed caudally, but some are directed the opposite way.

c. Erroneous pseudocyst diagnosis has been described in the lumbar area due to collapse of presumed lumbar syringomyelia from pressure due to a lumbar myelogram injection.

4. Neoplasia – tumours involving spinal nerve roots may cause enlargement of the intervertebral foramen visible on plain radiographs. They may also create extradural compression or intramedullary swelling on myelography rather than appearing as intradural–extramedullary lesions. However, if they do not enter the vertebral canal, radiographs are normal and MRI is needed for diagnosis.

a. Meningioma – mainly caudal cervical region and often near an intervertebral foramen.

b. Peripheral nerve sheath tumours (e.g. neurofibroma, neurofibrosarcoma and schwannoma) – mainly caudal cervical region.

c. Nephroblastoma (neuroepithelioma, Wilms' tumour) – caudal thoracic to cranial lumbar region (T10–L3) in dogs 6 months to 3 years of age; males and German Shepherd dogs are over-represented. May infiltrate the cord and appear intramedullary on myelography.

d. Myxoma or myxosarcoma.

e. Ependymoma.

f. Lymphoma – especially cats (although more often extradural or intramedullary). Test for feline leukaemia virus and look for lymphoma in other organs.

5. Herniated disc material that ruptures dural membranes.

6. Intradural haematoma or haemorrhage (see 5.16.10 for causes of spinal haemorrhage).

7. Intradural lipoma within a subcutaneous meningocele or myelomeningocele dorsal to the lumbosacral or sacrocaudal junction; especially Bulldogs and Manx cats with spina bifida or sacrocaudal dysgenesis.

5.18 INTRAMEDULLARY SPINAL CORD ENLARGEMENT ON MYELOGRAPHY

The spinal cord is widened on all views with divergence and attenuation of the contrast columns and general reduction of contrast opacity in the area (Fig. 5.20).

1. Normal spinal cord enlargement.
   a. Brachial intumescence – caudal cervical area.
   b. Lumbar intumescence – mid-lumbar area.
   c. The spinal cord to canal ratio is larger in cats and small-breed dogs than in large-breed dogs.
2. Neoplasia – most commonly seen at the cervicothoracic and thoracolumbar junctions.
   a. Primary spinal cord tumours.
      – Astrocytoma.
      – Oligodendroglioma.
      – Ependymoma.
      – Neurofibroma.

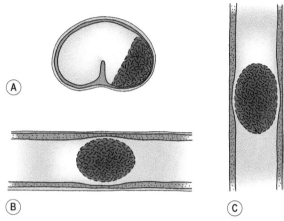

Figure 5.20 Schematic representation of an intramedullary lesion: (A) mass position, lying within the spinal cord; (B) and (C) myelogram views from any angle show spinal cord widening.

   - Lymphoma; especially young to middle-aged male cats; test for feline leukaemia virus and look for lymphoma in other organs.
   - Nephroblastoma (see 5.17.4).
   - Chordoma (see 5.7.7).
   b. Metastatic spinal cord tumours.
   c. Intradural–extramedullary tumour infiltrating the spinal cord (e.g. nerve root tumour).
3. Haemorrhage and/or oedema of the spinal cord.
   a. Acute spinal cord injury.
      - External trauma (e.g. road traffic accident).
      - Internal trauma due to acute disc herniation causing cord oedema or contusion; cord swelling may prevent contrast medium reaching and outlining the underlying lesion.
      - Myelomalacia subsequent to severe spinal cord damage; contrast medium enters the parenchyma.
      - Intramedullary disc extrusion – herniated disc material enters the cord parenchyma; rare.
      - Post-surgical effects on the spinal cord.
   b. Coagulopathy.
      - Haemophilia A, especially young male German Shepherd dogs.
      - Anticoagulant poisoning.
      - Thrombocytopenia.

   c. Haemorrhage secondary to:
      - tumour
      - vascular malformation
      - parasitic migration.
4. Fibrocartilaginous embolus or spinal infarct – occasionally causes mild spinal cord swelling, but the diagnosis is usually made based on typical peracute history and lack of myelographic findings, ruling out disc disease. Usually medium- and larger-sized dogs; rare in cats.
5. Granulomatous meningoencephalomyelitis – rarely causes spinal cord swelling; diagnosis often made based on clinical signs and analysis of CSF.
6. Syringohydromyelia – diffusely widened spinal cord, especially in the cervical area, usually associated with Chiari-like malformation in Cavalier King Charles Spaniels; inadvertent canalogram may occur during cisterna magna injection.
7. Dermoid or epidermoid cysts, usually in young animals; rare. Considered to be developmental malformations or teratomas.
8. Fungal granuloma.
9. Aberrant migration of *Spirocerca lupi** larva into the spinal cord.

5.19 MISCELLANEOUS MYELOGRAPHIC FINDINGS

1. Narrowed spinal cord with no external compression.
   a. Spinal cord atrophy due to chronic compression (e.g. at site of type II disc protrusion).
   b. Progressive haemorrhagic myelomalacia – often in non-responding acute disc herniation. Contrast medium is retained within damaged cord tissue.
   c. Spinal dysraphism – Weimaraner.
2. Myelomalacia – contrast medium leaks into liquefying cord tissue.
3. Spina bifida – contrast medium in the dural sac extends dorsal to the spine into a subcutaneous meningocele or myelomeningocele at the lumbosacral or sacrocaudal junction, and an intradural lipoma may also be present; especially Bulldogs and Manx cats (see 5.3.13).

4. Epidural contrast leakage.
   a. At the site of needle puncture through the dura.
   b. Meningeal trauma with dural tear, usually due to traumatic disc extrusion, vigorous exercise or other trauma.
   c. Increased meningeal permeability due to meningeal pathology.

5.20 CHANGES ON PLAIN RADIOGRAPHS THAT ARE UNLIKELY TO BE SIGNIFICANT

1. Spondylosis.
   a. Normal degeneration; Boxers often severely affected.
   b. Secondary to vertebral instability.
      – After disc fenestration.
      – Old disc herniation.
2. Mineralized intervertebral discs *in situ*.
3. Numerical variants.
4. Butterfly vertebrae.
5. Hemivertebrae in skeletally mature dogs.
6. Ossifying pachymeningitis (dural osseous metaplasia – see 5.10.1 and Fig. 5.11D).
7. Transitional vertebrae at the thoracolumbar or cervicothoracic junctions (at the lumbosacral junction, they may be associated with degenerative lumbosacral stenosis and cauda equina syndrome, and with unilateral hip dysplasia if asymmetrical).
8. Spina bifida in its simplest form with only a cleft of the dorsal spinous processes.

5.21 NEUROLOGICAL DEFICITS INVOLVING THE SPINAL CORD OR PROXIMAL NERVE ROOTS WITH NORMAL PLAIN RADIOGRAPHS AND MYELOGRAM

Ensure that the clinical signs are not due to an orthopaedic problem, myopathy, muscular dystrophy, neuromuscular transmission disorder, peripheral neuropathy or infectious agent such as distemper, toxoplasmosis or feline infectious peritonitis. Some of the conditions may produce changes that can be seen using MRI.

Congenital or hereditary diseases

Dogs

1. Neuroaxonal dystrophy – starts 1+ year in Rottweiler and 6+ weeks in Papillon.

2. Canine giant axonal neuropathy – starts 14+ months. Megaoesophagus may develop – German Shepherd dog.
3. Central peripheral neuropathy – starts 2+ months – Boxer.
4. Spinal muscular atrophy – starts 6+ weeks – Swedish Lapland dog, Brittany Spaniel, German Shepherd dog, Rottweiler and English Pointer.
5. Globoid cell leucodystrophy – starts 4+ months. West Highland White Terrier and Cairn Terrier, Poodle, Pomeranian, Beagle and Basset Hound.
6. Myelodysplasia, including spinal dysraphism – Weimaraner.
7. Hereditary myelopathy – 6–13 months – Afghan Hound.
8. Hereditary ataxia – 2–6 months – Fox Terrier and Jack Russell Terrier.
9. Progressive neuronopathy – 5+ months – Cairn Terrier.
10. Sensory neuropathy – 3–8 months – English Pointer.
11. Inherited hypertrophic neuropathy – 7–12 weeks – Tibetan Mastiff.
12. Syringohydromyelia.
13. Chiari-like malformation (caudal occipital malformation syndrome) with secondary syringohydromyelia; mainly the Cavalier King Charles Spaniel.
14. Non-mineralized foraminal (dorsolateral) disc extrusions causing nerve root compression.

Cats

15. Lysosomal storage diseases.
16. Distal polyneuropathy – 6+ weeks – Birman.
17. Globoid cell leucodystrophy – Domestic Short-haired cat.
18. Neuroaxonal dystrophy – 6 weeks.

Acquired diseases

Dogs

1. Degenerative myelopathy – 6+ years – especially German Shepherd dog and German Shepherd dog cross-breeds.
2. Fibrocartilaginous embolism (spinal infarct) with secondary necrotizing myelopathy – usually middle-aged medium and large breeds.

3. Acute idiopathic polyradiculoneuritis – adults of any breed.

4. Coonhound paralysis – acute polyradiculoneuritis after a racoon bite – adults of any breed.

5. Granulomatous meningoencephalomyelitis – 1+ years – smaller breeds, especially Poodle types.

6. Corticosteroid responsive meningitis (aseptic meningitis) – young medium- to large-breed dogs.

7. Secondary to modified live rabies vaccine – 7–10 days post vaccination.

8. Ischaemic neuromyopathy due to caudal aorta thromboembolism.

9. Leucoencephalomyelopathy – 1.5–4 years – Rottweiler.

10. Hound ataxia – 2–7 years – Fox Hound, Harrier Hound and Beagle.

11. Meningeal fibrosis with axonal degeneration secondary to necrotizing vasculitis –

5–13 months – Bernese Mountain Dog, German Short-haired Pointer and Beagle.

12. Chronic relapsing idiopathic polyradiculoneuritis.

13. Demyelinating myelopathy – 2–4 months – Miniature Poodles.

14. Syringohydromyelia.

Cats

15. Ischaemic neuromyopathy due to caudal aorta thromboembolism – secondary to cardiac disease.

16. Fibrocartilaginous embolism with secondary necrotizing myelopathy; rare.

17. Eosinophilic meningitis.

18. Secondary to modified live rabies vaccine – 7–10 days post vaccination.

19. Feline polioencephalomyelitis – 6+ months.

20. Degenerative myelopathy.

21. Chronic relapsing idiopathic polyradiculoneuritis.

22. Syringohydromyelia.

Further reading

General

Dennis, R., 1987. Radiographic examination of the canine spine. Vet. Rec. 121, 31–35.

Marioni-Henry, K., Vite, C.H., Newton, L., van Winkle, T.J, 2004. Prevalence of diseases of the spinal cord of cats. J Vet. Intern. Med. 18, 851–858.

McKee, M., 1993. Differential diagnosis of cauda equina syndrome. In Pract. 15, 243–250.

McKee, M., 1996. Cervical pain in small animals. In Pract. 18, 169–184.

McKee, M., Dennis, R., 2003. Radiology corner – Lumbosacral radiography. Vet. Radiol. Ultrasound 44, 655–657.

Morgan, J.P., Bailey, C.S., 1990. Cauda equina syndrome in the dog: radiographic evaluation. J. Small Anim. Pract. 31, 69–77.

Congenital and developmental diseases; diseases of young animals

Bailey, C.S., Morgan, J.P., 1992. Congenital spinal malformations.

Vet. Clin. North Am. Small Anim. Pract. 22, 985–1015.

Braund, K.G., 1994. Pediatric neuropathies. Semin. Vet. Med. Surg. (Small Animals) 9, 86–98.

Damur-Djuric, N., Steffen, F., Hassig, J.P., Morgan, J.P., Fluckiger, M.A., 2006. Lumbosacral transitional vertebrae in dogs: classification, prevalence and association with sacroiliac morphology. Vet. Radiol. Ultrasound 47, 32–38.

Drost, W.T., Lehenbauer, T.W., Reeves, J., 2002. Mensuration of cervical vertebral ratios in Doberman pinschers and Great Danes. Vet. Radiol. Ultrasound 43, 124–131.

Fluckiger, M.A., Damur-Djuric, N., Hassig, J.P., Morgan, J.P., Steffen, F., 2006. A lumbosacral transitional vertebra in the dog predisposes to cauda equina syndrome. Vet. Radiol. Ultrasound 47, 39–44.

Hanna, F.Y., 2001. Lumbosacral osteochondrosis: radiological features and surgical management in 34 dogs. J. Small Anim. Pract. 42, 272–278.

Hay, C.W., Dueland, R.T., Dubielzig, R.R., Bjorenson, J.E., 1999. Idiopathic multifocal osteopathy in four Scottish terriers (1991–1996). J. Am. Anim Hosp. Assoc. 35, 62–67.

James, C.C.M., Lassman, L.P., Tomlinson, B.E., 1969. Congenital anomalies of the lower spine and spinal cord in Manx cats. J. Pathol. 97, 269–276.

Kloc, P.A., Scrivani, P.V., Barr, S.C., Reese, C.J., Trotter, E.J., Forest, T.W., et al., 2001. Vertebral angiomatosis in a cat. Vet. Radiol. Ultrasound 42, 42–45.

Konde, L.J., Thrall, M.A., Gasper, P., Dial, S.M., McBiles, K., Colgan, S., et al., 1987. Radiographically visualized skeletal changes associated with mucopolysaccharidosis VI in cats. Vet. Radiol. 28, 223–228.

Lang, J., Haeni, H., Schawalder, P., 1992. A sacral lesion resembling osteochondrosis in the German Shepherd dog. Vet. Radiol. Ultrasound 33, 69–76.

Morgan, J.P., 1999. Transitional lumbosacral vertebral anomaly in the dog: a radiographic study. J. Small Anim. Pract. 40, 167–172.

Newitt, A., German, A.J., Barr, F.J., 2008. Congenital abnormalities of the feline vertebral column. Vet. Radiol. Ultrasound 49, 35–41.

Penderis, J., Schwarz, T., McConnell, J.F., Garosi, L.S., Thomson, C.E., Dennis, R., 2005. Dysplasia of the caudal vertebral articular facets in four dogs: results of radiographic, myelographic and magnetic resonance imaging investigations. Vet. Rec. 156, 601–605.

Sharp, N.J.H., Wheeler, S.J., Cofone, M., 1992. Radiological evaluation of 'wobbler' syndrome – caudal cervical spondylomyelopathy. J. Small Anim. Pract. 33, 491–499.

Werner, T., McNicholas, W.T., Kim, D.K., Baird, D.K., Breur, G.J., 2004. Aplastic articular facets in a dog with intervertebral disk rupture of the 12th to 13th thoracic vertebral space. J. Am. Anim. Hosp. Assoc. 40, 490–494.

Metabolic diseases (some overlap with above)

Konde, L.J., Thrall, M.A., Gasper, P., Dial, S.M., McBiles, K., Colgan, S., et al., 1987. Radiographically visualized skeletal changes associated with mucopolysaccharidosis VI in cats. Vet. Radiol. 28, 223–228.

Lieb, A.S., Grooters, A.M., Tyler, J. W., Partington, B.P., Pechman, R.D., 1997. Tetraparesis due to vertebral physeal fracture in an adult dog with congenital hypothyroidism. J. Small Anim. Pract. 38, 364–367.

Polizopoulou, Z.S., Kazakos, G., Patsikas, M.N., Roubies, N., 2005.

Hypervitaminosis A in the cat: a case report and review of the literature. J. Feline Med. Surg. 7, 363–368.

Infective and inflammatory conditions

Du Plessis, C.J., Keller, N., Millward, I.R., 2007. Aberrant extradural spinal migration of *Spirocerca lupi*: four dogs. J. Small Anim. Pract. 48, 275–278.

Dvir, E., Kirberger, R.M., Mallaczek, D., 2001. Radiographic and computed tomographic changes and clinical presentation of spirocercosis in the dog. Vet. Radiol. Ultrasound 42, 119–129.

Dvir, E., Perl, S., Loeb, E., Shklar-Hirsch, O., Chat, O., Mazaki-Tovi, M., et al., 2007. Spinal intramedullary aberrant *Spirocerca lupi* migration in 3 dogs. J Vet. Intern. Med. 21, 860–864.

Frendin, J., Funquist, B., Hansson, K., Lönnemark, J., Carlsten, J., 1999. Diagnostic imaging of foreign body reactions in dogs with diffuse back pain. J. Small Anim. Pract. 40, 278–285.

Jimenez, M.M., O'Callaghan, M.W., 1995. Vertebral physitis: a radiographic diagnosis to be separated from discospondylitis. Vet. Radiol. Ultrasound 36, 188–195.

Kornegay, J.N., Barber, D.L., 1980. Discospondylitis in dogs. J. Am. Vet. Med. Assoc. 177, 337–341.

Lavely, J.A., Vernau, K.M., Vernau, E.J., Herrgesell, E.J., Lecouteur, R.A., 2006. Spinal epidural empyema in seven dogs. Vet. Surg. 35, 176–185.

Neoplasia

Gilmore, D.R., 1983. Intraspinal tumours in the dog. Compend. Contin. Educ. Pract.Veterinarian 5, 55–64.

Green, E., Adams, W.M., Steinberg, H., 1999. Malignant transformation of solitary spinal osteochondroma in two mature

dogs. Vet. Radiol. Ultrasound 40, 634–637.

Levy, M.S., Kapatkin, A.S., Patnaik, A.K., Mauldin, G.E., 1997. Spinal tumours in 37 dogs: clinical outcome and long-term survival (1987–1994). J. Am. Anim. Hosp. Assoc. 33, 307–312.

Macri, N.P., Alstine, W.V., Coolman, R.A., 1997. Canine spinal nephroblastoma. J. Am. Anim. Hosp. Assoc. 33, 302–306.

Morgan, J.P., Ackerman, N., Bailey, C.S., Pool, R.R., 1980. Vertebral tumors in the dog: a clinical, radiologic, and pathologic study of 61 primary and secondary lesions. Vet. Radiol. 21, 197–212.

Pease, A.P., Berry, C.R., Mott, J.P., Peck, J.N., Calderwood, M.B., Hinton, D., 2002. Radiographic, computed tomographic and histopathologic appearance of a presumed spinal chordoma in a dog. Vet. Radiol. Ultrasound 43, 338–342.

Schultz, R.M., Puchalski, S.M., Kent, P.F., Moore, P.F., 2007. Skeletal lesions of histiocytic sarcoma in nineteen dogs. Vet. Radiol. Ultrasound 48, 539–543.

Trauma

Anderson, A., Coughlan, A.R., 1997. Sacral fractures in dogs and cats: a classification scheme and review of 51 cases. J. Small Anim. Pract. 38, 404–409.

Hay, C.W., Muir, P., 2000. Tearing of the dura mater in three dogs. Vet. Rec. 146, 279–282.

Kinns, J., Mai, W., Seiler, G., Zwingenberger, V., Johnson, V., Caceres, A., et al., 2006. Radiographic sensitivity and negative predictive value for acute canine spinal trauma. Vet. Radiol. Ultrasound 47, 563–570.

Roush, J.K., Douglass, J.P., Hertzke, G.A., Kennedy, G.A., 1992. Traumatic dural laceration

in a racing greyhound. Vet.
Radiol. Ultrasound 33, 22–24.

Yarrow, T.G., Jeffery, N.D., 2000.
Dura mater laceration
associated with acute paraplegia
in three dogs. Vet. Rec. 146,
138–139.

Disc disease and fibrocartilaginous embolism (spinal infarcts)

Cauzinille, L., Kornegay, J.N., 1996.
Fibrocartilagenous embolism of
the spinal cord in dogs: review of
36 histologically confirmed cases
and retrospective study of 26
suspected cases. J Vet. Intern.
Med. 10, 241–245.

Dyce, J., Houlton, J.E.F., 1993.
Fibrocartilaginous embolism in
the dog (review). J. Small Anim.
Pract. 34, 332–336.

Gaschen, L., Lang, J., Haeni, H., 1995.
Intravertebral disc herniation
(Schmorl's nodes) in five dogs.
Vet. Radiol. Ultrasound 36,
509–516.

Gibbons, S.E., Macias, C., de
Stefani, G.L., Pinchbeck, G.L.,
McKee, W.M., 2006. The value of
oblique *versus* ventrodorsal
myelographic views for lesion
lateralization in canine
thoracolumbar disc disease.
J. Small Anim. Pract. 47, 658–662.

Kirberger, R.M., Roos, C.J., Lubbe, A.
M., 1992. The radiological
diagnosis of thoracolumbar disc
disease in the dachshund. Vet.
Radiol. Ultrasound 33, 255–261.

Lamb, C.R., 1994. Common
difficulties with myelographic
diagnosis of acute intervertebral
disc prolapse in the dog. J. Small
Anim. Pract. 35, 549–558.

Lamb, C.R., Nicholls, A., Targett, M.,
Mannion, P., 2002. Accuracy of
survey radiographic diagnosis of
intervertebral disc protrusion in
dog. Vet. Radiol. Ultrasound 43,
222–228.

McKee, M., 2000. Intervertebral disc
disease in the dog 1.
Pathophysiology and diagnosis.
In Pract. 22, 355–369.

Munan, K.R., Olby, N.J., Sharp, N.J.H.,
Skeen, T.M., 2001. Intervertebral
disk disease in 10 cats. J. Am. Anim.
Hosp. Assoc. 37, 384–389.

Squires Bos, A., Brisson, B.A.,
Holmberg, D.L., Nykamp, S.,
2007. Use of the ventrodorsal
myelographic view to predict
lateralization of extruded disk
material in small-breed dogs with
throacolumbar intervertebral disk
extrusion: 104 cases (2004–2005).
J. Am. Vet. Med. Assoc. 230,
1860–1865.

Miscellaneous conditions

Chrisman, C.L., 1992. Neurological
diseases of Rottweilers:
neuroaxonal dystrophy and
leucoencephalomalacia. J. Small
Anim. Pract. 33, 500–504.

Dickinson, P.J., Sturges, B.K.,
Berry, W.L., Vernau, K.M.,
Koblik, P.D., Lecouteur, R.A.,
2001. Extradural spinal synovial
cysts in nine dogs. J. Small Anim.
Pract. 42, 502–509.

Dyce, J., Herrtage, M.E., Houlton, J.E.F.,
Palmer, A.C., 1991. Canine spinal
'arachnoid cysts'. J. Small Anim.
Pract. 32, 433–437.

Galloway, A.M., Curtis, N.C.,
Sommerland, S.F., Watt, P.R.,
1999. Correlative imaging
findings in seven dogs and one
cat with spinal arachnoid cysts.
Vet. Radiol. Ultrasound 40,
445–452.

Gnirs, K., Ruel, Y., Blot, S., Begon, D.,
Rault, F., Delisle, F., et al., 2003.
Spinal subarachnoid cysts in 13
dogs. Vet. Radiol. Ultrasound 44,
402–408.

Goncalves, R., Hammond, G.,
Penderis, J., 2008. Imaging
diagnosis: Erroneous
localization of spinal arachnoid
cyst. Vet. Radiol. Ultrasound 49,
460–463.

Hannel, R.M., Graham, J.P., Levy, J.K.,
Buergelt, C.D., Creamer, J., 2004.
Generalized osteosclerosis in a cat.
Vet. Radiol. Ultrasound 45,
318–324.

Jurina, K., Grevel, V., 2004. Spinal
arachnoid pseudocysts in 10
Rottweilers. J. Small Anim. Pract.
45, 9–15.

Kirberger, R.M., Jacobson, L.S.,
Davies, J.V., Engela, J., 1997.
Hydromyelia in the dog.
Vet. Radiol. Ultrasound 38,
30–38.

Lewis, D.G., Kelly, D.F., 1990.
Calcinosis circumscripta as a
cause of spinal ataxia. J. Small
Anim. Pract. 31, 36–38.

Morgan, J.P., Stavenborn, M., 1991.
Disseminated idiopathic
skeletal hyperostosis (DISH)
in a dog. Vet. Radiol. 32, 65–70.

Webb, A.A., Pharr, J.W., Lew, L.J.,
Tryon, K.A., 2001. MR imaging
findings in a dog with lumbar
ganglion cysts. Vet. Radiol.
Ultrasound 42, 9–13.

Contrast radiography of the spine

Kirberger, R.M., 1994. Recent
developments in canine lumbar
myelography. Compend. Contin.
Educ. Pract. Veterinarian (Small
Animal) 16, 847–854.

Kirberger, R.M., Wrigley, R.H., 1993.
Myelography in the dog: review
of patients with contrast medium
in the central canal. Vet. Radiol.
Ultrasound 34, 253–258.

Lang, J., 1988. Flexion–extension
myelography of the canine cauda
equina. Vet. Radiol. 29, 242–257.

Llabres Diaz, F., 2005. Practical
contrast radiography 4.
Myelography. In Pract. 27,
502–510.

Lu, D., Lamb, C.R., Targett, M.P.,
2002. Results of myelography in
seven dogs with myelomalacia.
Vet. Radiol. Ultrasound 43,
326–330.

Matteucci, M.L., Ramirez III, O.,
Thrall, D.E., 1999. Radiographic
diagnosis: Effect of right *versus*
left lateral recumbency on
myelographic appearance of a
lateralized extradural mass.
Vet. Radiol. Ultrasound 40,
351–352.

McKee, M., Penderis, J., Dennis, R., 2000. Radiology corner – Obstruction of contrast medium flow during cervical myelography. Vet. Radiol. Ultrasound 41, 342–343.

Penderis, J., Sullivan, M., Schwarz, T., Griffiths, I.R., 1999. Subdural injection of contrast medium as a complication of myelography. J. Small Anim. Pract. 40, 173–176.

Ramerez III, O., Thrall, D.E., 1998. A review of imaging techniques for cauda equina syndrome. Vet. Radiol. Ultrasound 39, 283–296.

Roberts, R.E., Selcer, B.A., 1993. Myelography and epidurography. Vet. Clin. North Am. Small Anim. Pract. 23, 307–328.

Scrivani, P.V., 2000. Myelographic artefacts. Vet. Clin. North Am. Small Anim. Pract. 30, 303–314.

Scrivani, P.V., Barthez, P.Y., Leveille, R., 1996. Radiology corner: The fallibility of the myelographic 'double line' sign. Vet. Radiol. Ultrasound 37, 264–265.

Stickle, R., Lowrie, C., Oakley, R., 1998. Radiology corner: Another example of the myelographic 'double line' sign. Vet. Radiol. Ultrasound 39, 543.

Weber, W.J., Berry, C.R., 1994. Radiology corner: Determining the location of contrast medium on the canine lumbar myelogram. Vet. Radiol. Ultrasound 35, 430–432.

Chapter 6

Lower respiratory tract

CHAPTER CONTENTS

6.1 Radiographic technique for the thorax and effect of positioning 145
6.2 Ultrasonographic technique for the thorax 146
6.3 Poor intrathoracic ultrasonographic visualization 147
6.4 Thoracic radiological changes associated with ageing 147
6.5 Border effacement in the thorax 148
6.6 Tracheal displacement 148
6.7 Tracheal diameter variations 150
6.8 Tracheal lumen opacification 151
6.9 Tracheal wall visibility variations 151
6.10 Tracheal ultrasonography 152
6.11 Changes of the main stem (principal) bronchi 152
6.12 Bronchial lung pattern 153
6.13 Artefactual increase in lung opacity 154
6.14 Alveolar lung pattern 154
6.15 Poorly marginated pulmonary opacities or areas of consolidation 157
6.16 Ultrasonography of areas of alveolar filling 159
6.17 Single radiopaque lung lobe 159
6.18 Ultrasonography of consolidated lung lobes 160
6.19 Solitary pulmonary nodules or masses 160
6.20 Nodular lung pattern 161
6.21 Ultrasonography of pulmonary nodules or masses 163

6.22 Interstitial lung pattern 163
6.23 Vascular lung pattern 165
6.24 Mixed lung pattern 167
6.25 Generalized pulmonary hyperlucency 168
6.26 Focal areas of pulmonary hyperlucency (including cavitary lesions) 169
6.27 Intrathoracic mineralized opacities 170
6.28 Hilar masses 171
6.29 Increased visibility of lung or lobar edges 171
6.30 Lower respiratory tract clinical signs but normal radiographs 171

6.1 RADIOGRAPHIC TECHNIQUE FOR THE THORAX AND EFFECT OF POSITIONING

Precise positioning using artificial aids is required, with the thoracic limbs pulled forwards to avoid overlay of the cranial thorax. True lateral and dorsoventral (DV) or ventrodorsal (VD) positioning should be ensured. In lateral recumbency, the upper lung lobes are seen better due to relatively increased aeration. The dependent lobes are poorly aerated due to pressure from mediastinal structures (especially the heart) and the dependent crus of the diaphragm, particularly in anaesthetized dogs, and this means that lesions in the dependent lobe are often not visible. Anaesthesia-induced atelectasis may arise quickly after induction, especially in large or fat dogs, and it may be wise to obtain the DV view first, because atelectasis arising in lateral recumbency may mimic aspiration pneumonia radiographically. In dorsal recumbency for the VD view, the cardiac silhouette tends to displace cranially, allowing greater visualization of the accessory lung lobe region; the divergence of the X-ray beam plus the shape of the diaphragm also mean that more of the caudal lung field will be visible. However, the VD view is often less helpful than the DV for assessment of cardiac size and shape.

A minimum of two orthogonal views are required to build up a three-dimensional image, i.e. a right or left lateral recumbent and a DV or VD radiograph. Some radiologists prefer left lateral recumbency (LLR) and VD for general thoracic evaluation and right lateral recumbency (RLR) and DV for assessment of the heart, but consistency of technique is probably more important. A combination of RLR and LLR ± VD views is recommended for suspected metastases or small, poorly defined pulmonary lesions. Dorsal recumbency for a VD view is contraindicated in patients with severe dyspnoea, and in such patients it may be wise to obtain horizontal beam radiographs with the patient non-recumbent first. Horizontal beam radiographs utilizing the effect of gravity may also be helpful to highlight certain types of pathology, such as mediastinal masses, fluid lines in cavitary masses and small amounts of free fluid or air. In the case of suspected emphysema, a horizontal beam view with the suspected affected lobe dependent will show whether or not it collapses under the weight of the overlying heart.

Routine views should be made at maximum inspiration. Additional expiratory views are indicated for suspected tracheal or bronchial collapse; incomplete bronchial obstruction; identification of occult bullae, blebs or emphysema; and detection of small-volume pneumothorax.

For digital radiography, an appropriate algorithm should be used to combine resolution and contrast. For conventional film radiography, a fast film–screen combination should be used to minimize motion blur, and a grid should be employed if the thorax is > 12 cm thick or in smaller, obese dogs. A long-scale contrast technique (high kV, low mAs) will reduce the naturally high contrast in the thorax and increase the lung detail visible, as well as reducing the exposure time. Exposure should be made at the end of inspiration to maximize lung aeration and optimize contrast, using manual inflation if necessary in anaesthetized patients (allowing for radiation safety).

Optimal evaluation of thoracic radiographs requires a systematic approach, which involves assessing radiographic technique, extrathoracic structures (soft tissues, osseous structures, thoracic inlet and diaphragm) and intrathoracic structures, and then re-evaluating abnormalities and areas indicated by clinical history. Intrathoracic evaluation is done on a system basis: respiratory, cardiovascular, lymphatic, pleural space and mediastinum (including the oesophagus). For viewing thoracic radiographs, the convention is that lateral views are examined with the thoracic inlet facing to the left and DV and VD views with the thoracic inlet uppermost and the left side of the patient on the right side of the computer screen or light box. Consider the effect that age, body condition, breed and respiratory phase may have on the image. (See Table 6.1, and 8.26 and Fig. 8.16.)

6.2 ULTRASONOGRAPHIC TECHNIQUE FOR THE THORAX

Normal, aerated lung does not transmit ultrasound, but in the presence of pulmonary disease or free thoracic fluid ultrasonography may be very useful. Sector or curvilinear transducers allow optimal access to intrathoracic structures. As high a frequency as possible should be selected while still achieving adequate tissue penetration (e.g. 7.5 MHz for cats and small dogs and 5 MHz for medium or large dogs). An acoustic window that overlies the area of interest is chosen, avoiding intervening skeletal structures and minimizing the amount of interposed air-filled lung. In general, this means placing the transducer in an appropriate intercostal space, but parts of the thorax may also be imaged from a cranial abdominal approach through the liver, or from the thoracic inlet. When the patient is in lateral recumbency, the dependent lung lobes become compressed, and less interference from air-filled lung then occurs if the thorax is imaged from beneath. The position of the animal can be altered if necessary to make use of the effects of gravity on the distribution of free fluid or free air in the thoracic cavity. Free fluid acts as an excellent acoustic window, and thoracic ultrasound should be performed before thoracocentesis.

The chosen acoustic window should be carefully prepared by clipping hair from the area, cleaning the skin with surgical spirit to remove dirt and grease, and applying liberal quantities of acoustic gel.

Table 6.1   Effect of positioning on thoracic structures in normal dogs

ANATOMICAL AREA	RIGHT LATERAL RECUMBENCY	LEFT LATERAL RECUMBENCY
Diaphragm	Right crus lies more cranially; crura are parallel	Left crus lies more cranially; crura diverge dorsally
Heart	More sternal contact	Less sternal contact: the apex may be elevated from the sternum and the heart appears more rounded
Lungs	Any pathology seen is likely to be in the left (uppermost) lung	Any pathology seen is likely to be in the right (uppermost) lung
Mediastinum	Cranioventral mediastinum is seen more clearly than on LLR	
	Extrapleural sign of sternal lymph node is seen more clearly than on LLR	
Aorta		More clearly seen than on RLR
Distal oesophagus	Not seen	Sometimes seen in larger dogs

	DORSOVENTRAL	VENTRODORSAL
Diaphragm	Seen as a single, rounded structure	Often seen as a three-domed structure (two crura and central cupola)
Heart	Usually contacts the diaphragm	Usually does not contact the diaphragm
	Constant location	Often tilts cranially and to the right
	Asymmetrical ovoid shape; right margin more curved	Right atrium may protrude, giving the heart a slightly angular outline
		1–2 o'clock bulge due to pulmonary artery
Caudal vena cava		Longer and seen more clearly
Lungs	Caudal lobe blood vessels are seen more clearly	
	Less divergence of the main stem (principal) bronchi	More divergence of the main stem (principal) bronchi
	Less visibility of the accessory lobe	More visibility of the accessory lobe
Thoracic disc spaces	Caudal disc spaces seen more clearly	Cranial disc spaces seen more clearly
Thoracic width	Wider	Narrower

Ultrasound-guided fine needle aspiration using a 22-gauge spinal needle may be performed on superficial lesions that are in contact with the thoracic wall.

6.3 POOR INTRATHORACIC ULTRASONOGRAPHIC VISUALIZATION

May be due to any combination of the following factors:

1. Poor preparation of the scanning site.
2. Poor skin–transducer contact.
3. Rib interposed between the transducer and the region of interest.
4. Too much aerated lung interposed between the transducer and the region of interest.
5. Free air in the thoracic cavity.
6. Subcutaneous emphysema.
7. Obesity.
8. Calcification of intra-thoracic structures sufficient to result in acoustic shadowing.

6.4 THORACIC RADIOLOGICAL CHANGES ASSOCIATED WITH AGEING

1. Calcification of costochondral junctions and chondral cartilages.
   a. Rosette appearance around costochondral junctions in old dogs.
   b. Appearance of fragmentation of calcified costal cartilages in old cats.
2. Tracheal ring calcification – especially chondrodystrophic breeds.
3. Bronchial wall calcification – especially chondrodystrophic breeds.
4. Spondylosis and sternal new bone.
5. Pleural thickening.
6. Pulmonary osteomata (heterotopic bone formation) and calcified pleural plaques in older, large-breed dogs; 2- to 4-mm diameter nodules of varying number and slightly irregular outline, very radiopaque and distributed randomly throughout the lungs,

although often in greatest numbers ventrally; differential diagnosis is miliary neoplasia when present in large numbers.

7. Fine, diffuse, reticular to reticulonodular interstitial lung pattern.
8. More horizontal orientation of the heart in aged cats, with exaggerated cranial curvature of the aortic arch and sometimes marked undulation of the descending aorta.

6.5 BORDER EFFACEMENT IN THE THORAX

Border effacement, previously referred to as the silhouette sign, occurs when pathological soft tissue or fluid opacity comes into direct contact with normal thoracic soft tissue structures (Fig. 6.1A). This eliminates the air usually present between the two structures, resulting in the creation of a single shadow with loss of visibility of the adjacent margins of the individual structures. This can affect the cardiac silhouette, vascular markings and diaphragmatic line and may be generalized or localized. Conversely, if the individual borders of two superimposing soft tissue structures are visible it implies that these two structures are not touching each other and that air-filled lung is interposed (Fig. 6.1B). Border effacement must not be confused with fat deposits (pleural, pericardial and epicardial) lying adjacent to soft tissues. Accumulations of fat are less radiopaque than soft tissue and can be differentiated on good-quality radiographs.

1. Artefactual border effacement due to technical factors.
   a. Underexposure due to inadequate penetration of tissues (kV too low).
   b. Underdevelopment of the film.
   c. Poor aeration of the lungs.
2. Pleural or mediastinal effusion.
3. Pleural masses.
4. Alveolar lung pattern.
5. Severe interstitial lung pattern.
6. Pulmonary masses.
7. Diaphragmatic rupture or hernia.
8. Large mediastinal masses.

6.6 TRACHEAL DISPLACEMENT

The normal position of the trachea is shown in Figure 6.2A and E.

1. Dorsal displacement of the trachea.
   a. Artefactual.
      – Expiration; cranial movement of intrathoracic structures.
      – Rotated lateral positioning.
   b. Conformation (e.g. Bulldog and Yorkshire Terrier).
   c. Whole trachea elevated (Fig. 6.2B).
      – Generalized cardiomegaly (see 7.5).
      – Right heart enlargement (see 7.11 and 7.12).
      – Left heart enlargement (see 7.8 and 7.9).
      – Large cranial mediastinal mass (see 8.11.1 and Fig. 8.10).
      – Large amount of mediastinal fluid.
      – Diaphragmatic rupture and displacement by herniated abdominal contents.
   d. Cranial thoracic trachea elevated, dipping ventrally towards the carina (Fig. 6.2C).
      – Artefactual, due to neck flexion.
      – Cranial mediastinal mass (see 8.11.1 and Fig. 8.10).
      – Cranial mediastinal and tracheobronchial lymphadenopathy (see 8.11.3 and Fig. 8.10).

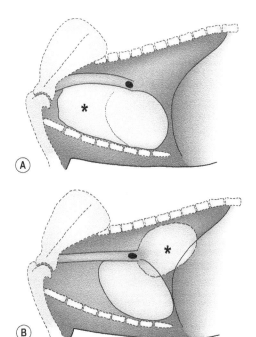

Figure 6.1 (A) Effacement of the cranial heart border due to a mediastinal mass (*); the mass is touching the heart and no air-filled lung lies between the two structures. (B) A large caudal lobe mass (*) with no border effacement of the heart or diaphragm, indicating that air-filled lung is interposed.

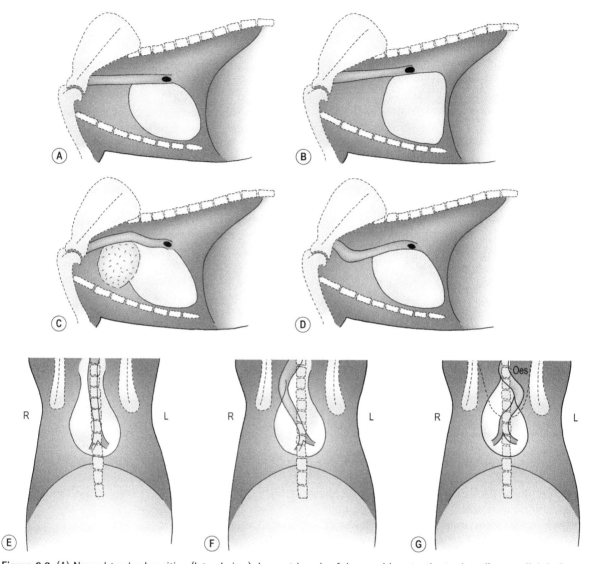

Figure 6.2 (A) Normal tracheal position (lateral view). In most breeds of dogs and in cats, the trachea diverges slightly from the spine. (B) The trachea is elevated throughout its length, in this case due to generalized cardiomegaly. (C) The trachea is elevated cranial to the heart, but the carina is in a normal position, in this case due to a cranial mediastinal mass. (D) Ventral tracheal displacement. (E) Normal tracheal position (dorsoventral view); slight curvature to the right through the thoracic inlet, especially in chondrodystrophic dogs. (F) Lateral displacement of the trachea, usually to the right. (G) Lateral displacement of the terminal trachea to the left; the cranial mediastinum is also widened due to the presence of a dilated oesophagus (Oes).

   – Right atrial enlargement (see 7.11 and Fig. 7.7).
   – Heart base tumour (see 7.16.2).
   – Lung lobe torsion (see 6.17.5 and Fig. 6.11).
2. Ventral displacement of the trachea (Fig. 6.2D).
  a. Oesophageal dilation (see 8.17 and Fig. 8.11).
  b. Oesophageal foreign body (see 8.20).

  c. Severe ventral displacement just cranial to the heart.
    – Persistent right aortic arch with retro-oesophageal subclavian artery.
    – Double aortic arch.
  d. Tracheobronchial lymphadenopathy (see 8.11.3 and Fig. 8.10).
  e. Craniodorsal mediastinal mass or loculated fluid (see 8.11.2 and Fig. 8.10).

f. Massive cervicothoracic spondylosis or other bony mass.

g. Post-stenotic aortic dilation distal to coarctation of the aorta (see 7.10.1).

3. Right lateral displacement of the trachea (Fig. 6.2F); displacement is usually to the right, as the aorta prevents displacement to the left.

a. Artefactual.
   – Ventral flexion of the head or neck.
   – Expiration; cranial movement of intrathoracic structures.
   – Rotated DV or VD positioning.

b. Normal in chondrodystrophic dogs, especially if obese.

c. Cranial mediastinal mass (see 8.11.1 and 8.11.2 and Fig. 8.10).

d. Oesophageal dilation (see 8.17).

e. Cranial mediastinal shift (see 8.8).

f. Diaphragmatic rupture and displacement by herniated abdominal contents.

g. Heart base tumour (see 7.16.2).

4. Left lateral displacement of the terminal trachea (Fig. 6.2G) – persistent right aortic arch; the cranial mediastinum will also be widened.

6.7 TRACHEAL DIAMETER VARIATIONS

The tracheal diameter as a ratio to the thoracic inlet, measured at the thoracic inlet on the lateral view, should be not less than 0.20 in normal, non-brachycephalic dogs (Fig. 6.3). In brachycephalic dogs, the ratio should be 0.16 or higher, although in Bulldogs the ratio may be as low as 0.13.

1. Narrowing of the trachea.

a. Artefactual.
   – Superimposition of the longus colli muscle or oesophagus at the level of and cranial to the thoracic inlet.
   – Hyperextension of the neck.
   – Intrathoracic structures superimposed on the thoracic trachea (e.g. dilated, post-stenotic pulmonary artery, cranial mediastinal blood vessels highlighted by pneumomediastinum, or pulmonary nodules).

b. Congenital hypoplasia – Bulldog and other brachycephalic breeds, Bullmastiff and occasionally the Labrador, German Shepherd dog, Weimaraner, Basset Hound and in cats. May be accompanied by other congenital abnormalities, megaoesophagus and secondary aspiration bronchopneumonia.

c. Tracheal collapse syndrome – due to deformed tracheal cartilage rings and invagination of the dorsal tracheal membrane. Often there is dynamic narrowing of the cervical trachea during inspiration and of the intrathoracic trachea during expiration. The tangential view of the thoracic inlet is more reliable for detection of collapse than lateral radiographs (Fig. 6.4). Fluoroscopy and endoscopy are useful ancillary diagnostic techniques.
   – Congenital – Yorkshire Terrier and Chihuahua; may not manifest until older age.

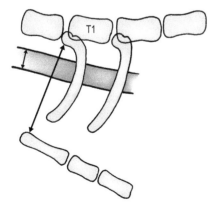

Figure 6.3 Measurement of the trachea at the thoracic inlet: the tracheal diameter is usually at least 20% of the thoracic inlet depth in non-chondrodystrophic breeds.

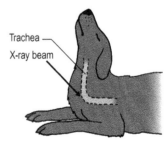

Figure 6.4 Tangential view of the thoracic inlet for demonstration of the trachea in cross-section. The normal trachea is round in cross-section or only slightly flattened dorsally. A collapsed trachea appears more markedly flattened dorsally, or crescentic, depending on the degree of collapse. Positioning is achieved using soft ties or a perspex frame; positioning aids are not shown.

– Acquired – obese, older, small and miniature breeds (Pomeranian and Toy Poodle), often secondary to chronic bronchitis; rare in large dog breeds and cats.

d. Mucosal thickening.
– Tracheitis due to respiratory viral infections; inhalation of gases; smoke and dust; allergies; bacterial and parasitic infections.
– Submucosal haemorrhage – anticoagulant poisoning or trauma.
– Cats – feline infectious peritonitis (FIP).

e. Extrinsic pressure – the tracheal rings are fairly rigid and tracheal displacement is more likely than narrowing.
– Cranial mediastinal mass (see 8.11.1 and Fig. 8.10).
– Hilar mass (see 8.11.3 and Fig. 8.10).
– Oesophageal foreign body (see 8.20).
– Oesophageal dilation (see 8.17).
– Vascular ring anomaly with oesophageal dilation cranial to the anomaly.

f. Tracheal stricture or segmental stenosis.
– Old traumatic injury.
– Prolonged intubation with excessive cuff pressure.
– Congenital.
– Cats – intrathoracic tracheal avulsion with stenosis of the separated tracheal ends; usually 2–3 weeks after blunt trauma. An air-filled tracheal pseudodiverticulum may also be seen as a circular gas lucency superimposed over the thoracic trachea.

g. Focal mass lesions of the tracheal wall (see 6.8.2–6).

h. Cats – dynamic tracheal collapse secondary to obstruction of the upper respiratory tract (e.g. nasal or laryngeal neoplasia).

2. Widening of the trachea.
a. Normal variant in chondrodystrophic breeds.
b. On inspiration, due to obstruction of airflow cranially resulting from a laryngeal or proximal tracheal lesion.
c. Adjacent to tracheal collapse or during the opposite phase of respiration.
d. Scarring adjacent to the trachea.
e. Cats – intrathoracic tracheal avulsion, with focal widening between the separated segments.

6.8 TRACHEAL LUMEN OPACIFICATION

1. Artefactual.
a. Intrathoracic structures superimposed on the thoracic trachea.
2. Aspirated foreign body.
3. *Oslerus osleri** (previously *Filaroides osleri*) – soft tissue nodules on the floor of the terminal trachea and main stem (principal) bronchi. More common in young dogs; does not occur in cats.
4. Abscess or granuloma involving the tracheal mucosa.
a. Infectious.
b. Eosinophilic.
c. Trauma.
d. Iatrogenic (e.g. post tracheotomy).
5. Neoplasia.
a. Osteochondroma – young large breeds, may mineralize.
b. Hamartoma – may mineralize.
c. Chondrosarcoma – may mineralize.
d. Osteosarcoma – may mineralize.
e. Mast cell tumour.
f. Leiomyoma.
g. Infiltrative tumour (e.g. thyroid carcinoma).
h. Fibrosarcoma.
i. Extramedullary plasmacytoma.
j. Lymphoma – especially cats.
k. Adenocarcinoma – especially cats.
6. Tracheal polyp.
7. Positive contrast agents – mineral opacity.
a. Inadvertent aspiration during gastrointestinal contrast studies.
b. Oral contrast studies in dysphagic animals.
c. Gastrointestinal contrast studies with a tracheo-oesophageal or broncho-oesophageal fistula present.

6.9 TRACHEAL WALL VISIBILITY VARIATIONS

The tracheal wall is a soft tissue opacity that contacts the surrounding cranial mediastinal structures and is therefore not usually visible.

1. Mineralization of cartilage rings – a normal ageing change, especially in chondrodystrophic dogs.
2. Tracheal stripe sign – the dorsal wall of the trachea and adjacent ventral oesophageal wall summate

and become visible due to the presence of air in the oesophagus – usually due to oesophageal dilation (see 8.17 and Figs 8.11 and 8.12).

3. Pneumomediastinum (see 8.9.1–6).

6.10 TRACHEAL ULTRASONOGRAPHY

Because the trachea is air-filled, ultrasonographic imaging is limited. However, the shape of the air column in the cervical trachea may be evaluated.

1. Flattening of the air column in the cervical trachea.
   a. Dynamic, on hyperextension of the neck.
      – Tracheal collapse syndrome.
   b. Static.
      – Traumatic stricture.
      – Congenital stenosis.
      – Mass lesions of the tracheal wall (see 6.8.2–5).

6.11 CHANGES OF THE MAIN STEM (PRINCIPAL) BRONCHI

The main stem bronchi are visible for a short distance caudal to the carina as superimposed air-filled structures on the lateral view and diverging at an angle of about 60–90° on the DV view (Fig. 6.5A–C).

1. Displacement of the main stem bronchi.
   a. Artefactual.
      – Rotated lateral view (Fig. 6.5B).
      – Wider main stem bronchi angle on VD than DV radiograph.
   b. Enlarged left atrium (see 7.8) (Fig. 6.5B and D).
   c. Hilar lymphadenopathy (see 8.12.1–6) (Fig. 6.5B and D).
   d. Large caudal oesophageal mass (e.g. *Spirocerca lupi** granuloma).

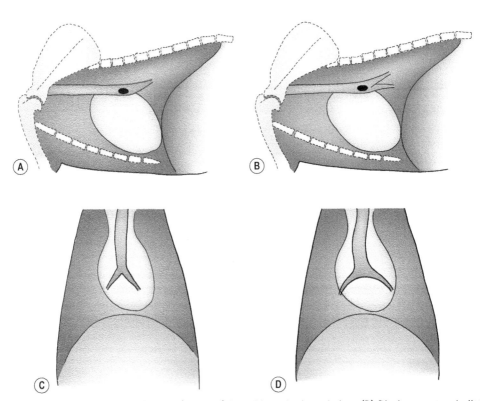

Figure 6.5 (A) Normal superimposed main stem (principal) bronchi on the lateral view. (B) Displacement or 'splitting' of the main stem bronchi on the lateral view. (C) Normal main stem bronchi on the dorsoventral (DV) view, diverging at 50–60°. (D) Widened angle of the main stem bronchi on the DV view.

e. Lung lobe torsion – may result in axial rotation of the tracheal bifurcation (see 6.17.5 and Fig. 6.11).

2. Narrowing of the main stem bronchi.
   a. External compression from enlarged left atrium, hilar lymphadenopathy or oesophageal mass, as above; may be displaced too.
   b. Loss of bronchial wall rigidity resulting in dynamic airway collapse and secondary chronic obstructive pulmonary disease is frequently observed in association with tracheal collapse syndrome (see 6.7.1).
   c. Severe mucosal thickening.
   d. Lung lobe torsion (see 6.17.5 and Fig. 6.11).

3. Opacification of the main stem bronchi – similar to the trachea and the rest of the bronchial tree (see 6.8 and 6.12).

6.12 BRONCHIAL LUNG PATTERN

In the normal lung, vessels are seen clearly but bronchial walls are usually seen only in the perihilar area, where the bronchi are relatively large (Fig. 6.6). A bronchial pattern implies increased visibility of the bronchial tree, which may be accompanied by changes in size and shape of the lumen and reduced visibility of adjacent vascular structures (Fig. 6.7). However, it is not necessarily due to primary airway disease. The bronchial pattern may be due to luminal exudate, thickened bronchial mucosa or peribronchial cuffing, and is often accompanied by an interstitial lung pattern. In young animals, only the mineralized wall of the main stem (principal) bronchi may be visible. As the animal ages, this mineralization may extend more peripherally along the bronchial tree and may be accompanied by pulmonary fibrosis.

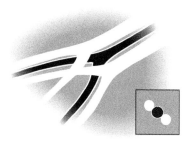

Figure 6.6 Normal lung pattern: the bronchus runs between the artery and vein and is barely visible (inset shows a cross-section).

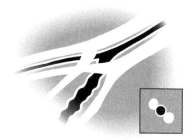

Figure 6.7 Bronchial lung pattern, producing 'tramline' and 'doughnut' markings. Bronchiectasis results in widened or irregular bronchi, as shown. (Compare with Fig. 6.6, *Normal lung pattern.*)

Increased bronchial wall visibility

1. Normal in aged and chondrodystrophic dogs – thin, mineralized wall.
2. Chronic bronchitis – mucosal inflammation and peribronchial cuffing produce thickened, soft tissue opacity walls (acute bronchitis usually lacks radiographic changes). Often a component of bronchopneumonia (see 6.14.2).
   a. Bacterial.
      – Non-specific bacterial infection.
      – Irish Wolfhound: hereditary rhinitis–bronchitis complex; young dogs with recurrent clinical signs due to primary immunodeficiency.
   b. Viral.
   c. Allergic.
      – Eosinophilic bronchopneumopathy (pulmonary infiltrate with eosinophils).
      – Cats – feline bronchial asthma.
   d. Fungal (see 6.15.5).
   e. Parasitic; usually a component of a pneumonic pattern, although sometimes the bronchial pattern may predominate (see 6.14.2e for list of parasites).
   f. Protozoal.
      – Toxoplasmosis*.
   g. Secondary to primary ciliary dyskinesia; mainly in young, purebred dogs, particularly Bichon Frise, Newfoundland and Rottweiler. May be accompanied by situs inversus (mirror image inversion of thoracic and abdominal structures).
   h. Severe small airway disease.

3. Neoplasia.
   a. Lymphoma, accompanied by a diffuse or reticulonodular interstitial lung pattern and mediastinal lymphadenopathy.
   b. Bronchogenic carcinoma, possibly accompanied by pulmonary nodules or masses.
4. Bronchial wall oedema – may be part of alveolar or interstitial oedema (see 6.14.1 and 6.14.7 for causes).
5. Bronchiectasis – see below.
6. Hyperadrenocorticism (Cushing's disease) or long-term corticosteroid administration; thin, mineralized bronchial walls, and may also see hepatomegaly, osteopenia and soft tissue mineralization.
7. Idiopathic pulmonary fibrosis – in combination with interstitial (dogs) or interstitial or alveolar (cats) pattern.

Bronchial dilation

8. Bronchiectasis – usually cranioventrally; uncommon in dogs and rare in cats. Saccular or cylindrical.
   a. Congenital predisposition.
      – Irish Wolfhound: hereditary rhinitis–bronchitis complex; young dogs with recurrent clinical signs due to primary immunodeficiency.
      – Primary ciliary dyskinesia – inherited abnormality of ciliary function leading to chronic rhinitis and severe pneumonia ± bronchiectasis; especially young Bichon Frise, Newfoundlands and Rottweilers.
      – Kartagener's syndrome – inherited condition as above but also associated with total situs inversus (mirror image transposition of heart and abdominal viscera) as well as rhinitis.
   b. Acquired bronchiectasis – usually middle-aged patients with chronic inflammatory airway disease.

Bronchial lumen opacification

9. Ill-defined opacities: mucus or exudate due to pneumonia (see 6.14.2) or bronchiectasis.
10. Single aspirated foreign body, especially grass awns in working dogs – mainly caudal lobes, often right bronchus. Chronic cases show secondary lobar bronchopneumonia.
11. *Oslerus osleri** (previously *Filaroides osleri*) – nodules in main stem (principal) bronchi, usually also with tracheal nodules. More common in young dogs; does not occur in cats.
12. Bronchiolitis obliterans – rare.
13. Cats – bronchial microlithiasis – rare.

6.13 ARTEFACTUAL INCREASE IN LUNG OPACITY

The following factors all contribute to an artefactual increase in lung opacity, which may result in false negative or false positive diagnoses.

1. Poorly inflated lungs.
   a. Exposure made on expiration.
   b. Preceding lateral recumbency, especially if anaesthetized.
   c. Laryngeal paralysis or other upper respiratory tract obstruction.
   d. Abdominal distension.
2. Obesity.
3. Motion blur.
4. Underexposure.
5. Underdevelopment.
6. Cranial thorax – overlying musculature if the thoracic limbs are not pulled cranially.
7. Bandages.
8. Wet or dirty hair coat.
9. Thymus in young animals (especially cats) – an ill-defined radiopacity blurring the cranial heart margin in the lateral view.

6.14 ALVEOLAR LUNG PATTERN

The alveoli lose air either by being filled with fluid and/or cells (alveolar consolidation) or by collapsing (atelectasis). The pattern is usually characterized by ill-defined, poorly demarcated infiltrates producing a patchy increase in lung opacity, although a more homogeneous infiltrate may give rise to a ground glass appearance. These patterns may progress to more severe lung opacification with air bronchograms and border effacement (see 6.5) in more advanced cases (Fig. 6.8). Changes may be widespread or lobar. A severe alveolar pattern may give rise to single or multiple poorly marginated apparent pulmonary masses or areas of

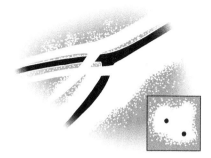

Figure 6.8 Alveolar lung pattern with blurring or loss of normal lung detail, patchy or diffuse increase in radiopacity and air bronchogram formation. (Compare with Fig. 6.6, *Normal lung pattern.*)

consolidation, which are described in Section 6.15. Alveolar changes are fairly labile, and frequent repeat radiography may be necessary to monitor the course of a disease. Alveolar lung patterns may arise from, or give rise to, interstitial lung patterns (see 6.22 and 6.24).

1. Cardiogenic pulmonary oedema – usually associated with cardiomegaly, especially left atrial dilation, and possibly a hypervascular pattern (see 6.23.1–4). However, with heart failure of rapid onset, the heart may appear unremarkable.
   a. Perihilar and symmetrical distribution in dogs.
   b. Perihilar to peripheral distribution in cats; the consolidations are often patchy and asymmetrical; may affect the right caudal lobe only.
2. Pneumonia.
   a. Bronchopneumonia – asymmetrical, mainly cranioventral lung lobes; starts peripherally and then spreads inwards. Often involves the right middle lobe. Usually initiated by viral infections (e.g. tracheobronchitis and distemper) or mycoplasma and then complicated by a bacterial infection. Usually also a pronounced bronchial lung pattern.
      – Irish Wolfhound: hereditary rhinitis–bronchitis complex; young dogs with recurrent clinical signs due to primary immunodeficiency.
      – Newfoundland and Rottweiler: ciliary dyskinesia (see 6.12.8).
      – Uncommon in cats.
   b. Aspiration pneumonia – observed along the bronchial tree, more commonly in ventral areas. Secondary to:
      – Regurgitation and vomiting, especially if oesophageal dilation is present.
      – Iatrogenic aspiration – force feeding, medication, anaesthesia and oral administration of contrast medium.
      – Swallowing disorders.
      – Weakness and debilitation.
      – Cleft palate.
      – Tracheo-oesophageal or broncho-oesophageal fistula.
      – Gastrobronchial fistula.
   c. Aspirated foreign body pneumonia, usually grass and barley awns in working dogs – caudodorsal segments of caudal lobes, usually affecting a single lobe. Focal alveolar or interstitial pattern, with a more widespread bronchial pattern too in chronic cases. May be accompanied by pneumothorax, pleural effusion or pleural thickening.
   d. Fungal pneumonia (see 6.15.5); often with mediastinal lymphadenopathy.
      – Also diffuse fungal pneumonia due to *Pneumocystis carinii** in immunocompromised dogs; especially in younger Miniature Dachshunds and Cavalier King Charles Spaniels.
   e. Parasitic pneumonia.
      – *Dirofilaria immitis** (heartworm); with right heart enlargement, prominence of the main pulmonary artery and an arterial hypervascular lung pattern; lung parenchymal changes are often most severe in the caudal lung lobes.
      – *Angiostrongylus vasorum** (French heartworm); younger dogs; often characteristic multifocal or peripheral lung involvement and usually no vascular changes; may present with coagulopathy rather than respiratory signs.
      – *Filaroides hirthi** and *F. milksi**: usually Beagles in breeding colonies.
      – *Crensoma vulpis** infection (fox lungworm) – bronchial pattern may predominate.
      – *Aelurostrongylus abstrusus** (feline lungworm) – usually younger cats but mostly asymptomatic; initial alveolar or

bronchoalveolar pattern progresses to a miliary nodular pattern.

f. Lipid or lipoid pneumonia (exogenous or endogenous) – especially cats.

g. Secondary to primary ciliary dyskinesia or as part of Kartagener's syndrome – especially Newfoundland and Rottweiler (see 6.12.8).

h. Radiation pneumonitis 1–2 months post radiation – localized to the irradiated area of the lung.

i. Tuberculosis – often also with cavitary lung lesions, mediastinal lymphadenopathy and/or pleural effusion.

j. *Francisella (Pasteurella) tularensis** (tularaemia) – very rare, potential contact with rodents.

3. Pulmonary haemorrhage – usually asymmetrical and less homogeneous than cardiogenic oedema.

a. Trauma – fractured ribs and subcutaneous emphysema may also be seen.

b. Coagulopathy.
   - Disseminated intravascular coagulation (DIC).
   - Anticoagulant poisoning.
   - Haemophilia, von Willebrand's disease (especially Dobermann) and other inherited coagulopathies.
   - Immune-mediated diseases.
   - Bone marrow depression.

4. Atelectasis (reduced aeration of a lung lobe) recognized by mediastinal shift on DV or VD views (see 8.8). Air bronchograms are observed only with moderate to severe lung collapse.

a. Peracute collapse of dependent lobes under gaseous anaesthesia; especially in the region of the heart (main differential diagnosis is aspiration pneumonia).

b. External compression of a lobe.
   - Extended periods in lateral recumbency.
   - Severe pneumothorax.
   - Severe pleural effusion.
   - Large pleural, rib or soft tissue mass.

c. Minor airway obstruction due to chronic bronchitis – especially middle and cranial lobes.

d. Major airway obstruction – any single lobe; usually no air bronchograms visible.
   - Intrinsic obstruction due to a foreign body or tumour blocking the bronchus.
   - Extrinsic obstruction due to compression.

e. Cicatrization due to chronic pleural and pulmonary disease.

f. Adhesive atelectasis – lack of surfactant; airways are patent.
   - Newborn animal.
   - Acute lung injury or acute respiratory distress syndrome (see 6.14.7 below).

g. Lung lobe torsion (see 6.17.5).

h. Cats – right middle lobe atelectasis often occurs in feline bronchial asthma; usually also with a bronchointerstitial pattern and pulmonary overinflation.

5. Allergic pulmonary disease – eosinophilic bronchopneumopathy (pulmonary infiltrate with eosinophils); occasionally see an alveolar pattern, more often interstitial or nodular ± bronchial.

6. Neoplasia.

a. Primary lung tumour – an alveolar or interstitial-type pattern is occasionally seen in cases of diffuse bronchiolar–alveolar carcinoma and may affect more than one lobe; air bronchograms are rare.

b. Histiocytic sarcoma (malignant histiocytosis) – middle-aged, large-breed dogs, with male preponderance; mainly Bernese Mountain Dog but also Rottweiler and Golden or Flat-coated Retrievers.

c. Pulmonary lymphomatoid granulomatosis – rare neoplastic disorder; often with pulmonary nodules or masses and hilar lymphadenopathy.

7. Non-cardiogenic pulmonary oedema.

a. Perihilar to peripheral – more likely in the caudodorsal area, often asymmetrical and more on the right side.
   - Airway obstruction (e.g. common in Bulldogs, also strangulation or laryngeal paralysis).
   - Neurogenic causes (e.g. post-ictal, electric shock, cranial trauma).
   - Near-drowning – more severe with salt water than fresh water.
   - Hypoalbuminaemia.
   - Multisystemic inflammatory and non-inflammatory diseases (e.g. uraemia, acute pancreatitis and sepsis).
   - Hunting dogs that bark continuously, especially in Sweden.
   - Anaphylactic reactions, including those to intravenous contrast media.

- Aspirated hyperosmolar contrast medium.
- Toxins (e.g. alphanapthylthiourea, snake venom and endotoxin, bee stings).
- Inhaled irritants (e.g. smoke and phosphorus).
- Re-expansion pulmonary oedema after treatment of pneumothorax, etc.

  b. Symmetrical – entire lung.
- Acute lung injury or acute respiratory distress syndrome (or shock lung). Causes include trauma, infection, anaphylaxis, severe babesiosis*, pancreatitis, inhalation, disseminated intravascular coagulation, ingested toxins and iatrogenic causes such as oxygen therapy, overhydration, cardioversion and drug reactions. Initial interstitial pattern progresses to a patchy alveolar pattern with reduced lung volume.

  c. One hemithorax.
- Hypostasis from extended lateral recumbency or anaesthesia.
- Hilar mass blocking pulmonary drainage mechanisms.

  d. Perihilar.
- Hilar mass blocking pulmonary drainage mechanisms.
- Iatrogenic overhydration with intravenous fluids.

8. Pulmonary contusion due to trauma; other signs of trauma are often present too (see 8.28).
   a. Road traffic accident.
   b. High-rise syndrome – triad of injuries: pulmonary contusion and/or pneumothorax, facial injuries and limb fractures.
9. Pulmonary thromboembolism – occasionally with a localized alveolar pattern (see 6.23.6).
10. Lung lobe torsion (see 6.17.5).
11. Pulmonary alveolar proteinosis (phospholipoproteinosis) – rare, young dogs.
12. Bronchiolitis obliterans, with bronchial and interstitial patterns too – rare.
13. Cats – idiopathic pulmonary fibrosis may give rise to an alveolar pattern.

6.15 POORLY MARGINATED PULMONARY OPACITIES OR AREAS OF CONSOLIDATION

Lesions may be single or multiple and are generally greater than 4 cm in diameter (see Fig. 6.9).

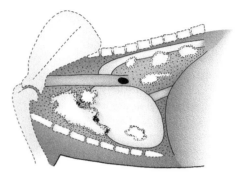

Figure 6.9 Poorly marginated pulmonary opacities or areas of consolidation.

For smaller lesions, see 6.14, *Alveolar lung pattern*; for well-defined lesions, see 6.19, *Solitary pulmonary nodules or masses* and 6.20, *Nodular lung pattern*.

1. Artefactual – food material in a distended oesophagus.
2. Pneumonia – a mixed bronchial–alveolar lung pattern ± larger areas of consolidation or poorly marginated opacities (see 6.14.2).
3. Neoplasia – may cavitate or calcify.
   a. Primary lung tumours.
      - Bronchogenic carcinoma most common – may be a solitary nodule or multicentric, although more often well-defined or lobar in shape than poorly marginated.
      - Adenocarcinoma and squamous cell carcinoma – especially cats (may be associated with multiple digital metastases – see 3.7.11 and Fig. 3.18).
   b. Metastatic lung tumours – a single metastatic nodule tends to be smaller than a single primary tumour; again, more likely to be well-defined, or ill-defined but small; usually multiple when diagnosed.
   c. Histiocytic sarcoma (malignant histiocytosis) – middle-aged, large-breed dogs, with male preponderance – mainly Bernese Mountain Dog but also Rottweiler and Golden and Flat-coated Retrievers.
4. Pulmonary oedema – usually produces an alveolar or interstitial lung pattern if cardiogenic in dogs, but in cats, cardiogenic pulmonary oedema can lead to patchy and asymmetric consolidations, especially in the right caudal lobe; oedema due to other causes may also produce poorly marginated areas of consolidation (see 6.14.7).

5. Pulmonary granulomatous diseases – cellular rather than exudative inflammatory reaction, often accompanied by thoracic lymphadenopathy. Granulomata may cavitate.
   a. Aspirated foreign body, especially grass awns in working dogs; usually solitary and in the caudal or intermediate lobes.
   b. Fungal and fungal-like diseases – in endemic areas and more likely in working and hunting dogs. No typical radiographic appearance; may also be a nodular to interstitial lung pattern. Additional foci of infection may be present elsewhere in the body (e.g. osteomyelitis, chorioretinitis, dermatitis and central nervous system involvement). There may also be a pleural effusion.

   Specific obligate pathogens
   – Histoplasmosis* – with moderate to marked lymphadenopathy that tends to calcify during healing; rare in cats.
   – Blastomycosis* – moderate lymphadenopathy occurs occasionally; rare in cats, in which a nodular pattern is more likely.
   – Coccidioidomycosis* – moderate to marked lymphadenopathy; rare in cats.
   – Cryptococcosis* – uncommon in dogs but the most common fungal infection in cats. Often associated with sternal lymphadenopathy.

   Opportunistic infections
   – Actinomycosis* – severe or mild pleural effusions. Pleural, mediastinal and pulmonary abscesses are more common; rare in cats.
   – Nocardiosis* – uncommon. Often younger dogs, also in cats; may be associated with migrating plant material. Severe or mild pleural effusions and moderate lymphadenopathy.
   – Aspergillosis* – most likely in immune-incompetent animals and a predisposition to the German Shepherd dog.
   – Sporotrichosis* – rare.
   c. Exogenous lipid or lipoid pneumonia – aspirated mineral or vegetable oil.
   d. Parasites.
   – Dirofilaria immitis* (heartworm); with right heart enlargement, prominence of the main

pulmonary artery and a hypervascular pattern.
   – Angiostrongylus vasorum* (French heartworm); younger dogs; often characteristic multifocal or peripheral lung involvement and usually no vascular changes.
   – Paragonimus kellicotti* (lung fluke); amorphous consolidations in the caudal lobes progressing to thin-walled cysts that may be septated.
   – Toxoplasmosis* – usually younger cats.
   – Larval migrans, changes very subtle.
   – Capillariasis* – rare.
   – Filaroides hirthi* and F. milksi*; usually Beagles in breeding colonies.
   – Cats – Aelurostrongylus abstrusus* (feline lungworm) – an initial bronchoalveolar pattern tends to become nodular with time.
   e. Eosinophilic pulmonary granulomatosis – often marked hilar lymphadenopathy.
   f. Lymphomatoid granulomatosis – rare neoplastic disease; often with an interstitial–alveolar lung pattern and hilar lymphadenopathy.
   g. Bacterial granulomatous diseases.
   – Tuberculosis, rare due to the reduction in incidence of bovine tuberculosis. The source of infection may include humans or birds. Pleural effusion and lymphadenopathy occur in dogs; pleural effusion is less common and milder in cats, in which a nodular pattern is more likely.
   – Corynebacterium.

6. Allergic lung disease – especially cats; although more usually a bronchointerstitial pattern with pulmonary overinflation.
7. Thromboembolic pneumonia – most likely peripherally in the caudal lobes.
   a. From a non-respiratory abscess or infection.
   b. In immune-compromised animals:
   – With lymphoma.
   – On immunosuppressive therapy.
   – Associated with autoimmune haemolytic anaemia.
   c. From bacterial endocarditis.
   d. In animals with fever of unknown origin.

e. From inflammatory joint disease.

8. Pulmonary embolism from other causes (see 6.23.6) – similar distribution to thromboembolic pneumonia.

9. Pulmonary alveolar proteinosis (phospholipoproteinosis) – rare, young dogs.

6.16 ULTRASONOGRAPHY OF AREAS OF ALVEOLAR FILLING

Regions of alveolar filling may be imaged ultrasonographically if they lie adjacent to the thoracic wall, the heart or the diaphragm. Bright echogenic specks indicate residual air. Anechoic tubes may represent pulmonary vessels or fluid-filled bronchi. The latter have more echogenic walls, but a better way to differentiate between these is to use colour or power Doppler. Ultrasound-guided fine needle aspiration of superficial lung lesions is possible (see 6.2). For differential diagnoses for alveolar filling, see 6.14 and 6.15.

6.17 SINGLE RADIOPAQUE LUNG LOBE

Increased radiopacity of the lobe with loss of visibility of the pulmonary vessels and border effacement of adjacent structures. Air bronchograms may be present (see 6.14 and Fig. 6.8). If the lobe is of normal size, consolidation is likely, whereas if it is reduced, collapse (atelectasis) is present. Increased size of a radiopaque lobe suggests neoplasia or torsion.

1. Artefactual.
   a. Mediastinal masses mimicking pulmonary lesions (e.g. *Spirocerca lupi** granuloma may mimic an accessory lobe mass).
   b. Diaphragmatic hernia, with herniated liver mimicking a caudal pulmonary mass.
2. Lobar pneumonia – often the right middle lobe; best seen on the DV or VD view (Fig. 6.10).
3. Atelectasis (collapse) – smaller lobe, possibly with concave borders; mediastinal shift towards the lobe. Especially cats with lower respiratory tract disease and usually the right middle lobe (Fig. 6.10).
4. Neoplasia – primary lung tumour; affected lobe may be enlarged with convex borders and mediastinal shift away from the lobe.
   a. Epithelial carcinomas are commonest.
      – Bronchiolar–alveolar.
      – Bronchogenic.

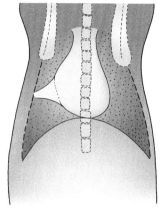

Figure 6.10 A single consolidated or collapsed lung lobe seen on the dorsoventral view; the right middle lobe is most often affected, especially in cats. Atelectasis (collapse) results in reduction in size of the lobe, whereas the size remains normal if the lobe is consolidated without collapse and may increase if neoplasia or torsion is present.

      – Epidermoid (squamous).
      – Bronchial gland carcinoma.
      – Anaplastic.
   b. Chondroma, chondrosarcoma, osteosarcoma – may mineralize.
      – Hamartoma – rare – may mineralize.
5. Lung lobe torsion (Fig. 6.11) – most commonly left or right cranial or right middle lobes; less likely to affect the caudal lobes; rarely affects the accessory lobe. The lobe is initially enlarged, with pulmonary vasculature or air bronchograms, if visible, running in an

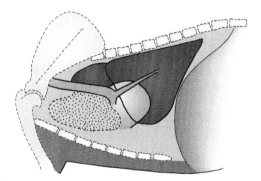

Figure 6.11 Lung lobe torsion, showing a consolidated and emphysematous cranial lung lobe and a marked pleural effusion. The terminal trachea is displaced ventrally, and the cranial lobe bronchus is occluded. The heart is partly obscured.

abnormal direction. The bronchus may be displaced, narrowed or seem to end abruptly. A characteristic vesicular gas pattern may be present within the consolidated lobe. Usually, there is concurrent pleural effusion. The diagnosis may be confirmed by means of bronchoscopy or thoracotomy.

a. Spontaneous – most commonly the right middle lobe in larger or deep-chested breeds and the cranial segment of the left cranial lobe in small, chondrodystrophic breeds such as Pugs.

b. Predisposed to by pleural effusion. Usually impossible to determine whether the effusion is primary or secondary. Cats often have a severe, bloody effusion.

c. Acute traumatic impact – rare; small breeds.

6. Occlusion of a bronchus.

a. Aspirated foreign body.

b. Mass within or compressing lumen.

c. Incorrectly placed endotracheal tube.

7. Pulmonary thromboembolism (see 6.23.6).

8. Fat embolism following a fracture.

6.18 ULTRASONOGRAPHY OF CONSOLIDATED LUNG LOBES

Consolidated lung lobes are usually seen as moderately echoic, well-demarcated structures that can be followed to the perihilar region. The main lobar blood vessels may be seen within the solid lung tissue in the perihilar region, with blood flow demonstrated by colour Doppler. Echogenic-walled, tubular structures with static anechoic contents are fluid-filled bronchi. Hyperechoic foci within the lobe, with or without acoustic shadowing, usually indicate areas of residual aeration.

1. Uniformly hypoechoic lung lobe, smoothly marginated with pointed tips; echotexture similar to that of liver.

a. Atelectasis due to:
   – Adjacent thoracic mass.
   – Pleural effusion.
   – Airway obstruction.

b. Lobar pneumonia.

c. Lobar haemorrhage.

d. Lung lobe torsion (usually associated with pleural fluid).

2. Variable echogenicity with loss of normal shape and lacking internal liver-like structure.

a. Lobar neoplasia.

b. Abscessation.

3. Abnormal orientation of a lung lobe.

a. Lung lobe torsion.

b. Displacement of lobe by adjacent mass or abdominal viscera.

6.19 SOLITARY PULMONARY NODULES OR MASSES

A nodule is a well-marginated, evenly rounded lesion measuring up to 4 cm in diameter. A mass is well marginated and larger than a nodule; it may be smooth or irregular in outline. The larger the nodule or mass, the more radiopaque it should be. Mineralized areas may be seen.

Solitary lesions are easily missed if they are small or in the perihilar region, cranial thorax, costophrenic recesses or paraspinal gutters. A solitary lesion should be differentiated from a composite mass consisting of multiple small coalescing or superimposed nodules. It is not possible to differentiate between causes radiologically, but repeat radiographs after 3–4 weeks are indicated. If the nodule or mass has enlarged, then biopsy is advised if possible. If no enlargement has occurred, repeat radiography should be performed after a further 3–4 months.

Nodules and masses may cavitate, especially if they are rapidly growing. In these cases, a radiolucent, gas-filled centre to the lesion is seen. For a fuller description and list of causes, see Section 6.27 and Figure 6.16.

1. Artefactual.

a. Overlying soft tissue structure, especially nipples, which lie ventrally and are often seen to be paired; ticks and warts may also be visible (see 8.21.4 and Fig. 6.12A). If a suspect external nodule can be identified clinically, repeating the radiograph after coating the structure with radiopaque contrast medium will identify it.

b. Costochondral junction (Fig. 6.12B).

c. Single blood vessel seen end on (Fig. 6.12C).

d. Healed rib fracture (Fig. 6.12D).

e. Adjacent pleural mass.

f. Small diaphragmatic rupture or hernia, often with incarcerated liver: between the heart and the diaphragm (Fig. 6.12E).

g. Diaphragmatic eventration (see 8.26.1).

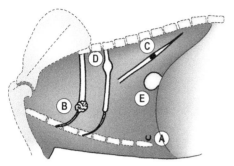

Figure 6.12 Artefactual lung nodules: (A) nipple, (B) prominent costochondral junction in an old dog, (C) blood vessel seen end on, (D) healed rib fracture, (E) small diaphragmatic rupture.

2. Neoplasia.
   a. Primary lung tumour – often arise in the perihilar region, tend to be large and may have partially irregular borders. Secondary changes include cavitation (becoming air-filled), calcification, spread to regional lymph nodes, compression of adjacent bronchi or pleural effusion. In dogs, metastasis tends to occur within the thorax, whereas in cats 75% metastasize elsewhere, for example the digits (see 3.7.13 and Fig. 3.18).
      – Adenocarcinoma.
      – Bronchogenic carcinoma.
      – Squamous cell carcinoma.
      – Histiocytic sarcoma (malignant histiocytosis) – middle-aged, large-breed dogs, with male preponderance; mainly Bernese Mountain Dog but also Rottweiler and Golden or Flat-coated Retrievers.
   b. Solitary lung metastasis – tend to involve the middle or periphery of the lung field and are usually nodular; additional metastases usually develop quickly.
3. Granuloma (see 6.15.5) – may cavitate.
   a. Foreign body – especially working dogs aspirating grass awns.
   b. Fungal – although more usually multiple, poorly defined and bizarrely shaped lesions; tend to be perihilar.
   c. Bacterial.
   d. Eosinophilic.
   e. Parasitic.
   f. Tuberculosis.

4. Abscess – often in younger patients and tend to occur in the perihilar or peripheral lung field; may cavitate.
5. Haematoma (haematocyst) – history of trauma, resolves with time.
6. Cyst.
7. Fluid-filled bulla.
8. Exudate- or mucus-filled bronchus or focal bronchiectasis.
9. Area of consolidation simulating a nodule (see 6.15).

6.20 NODULAR LUNG PATTERN

Nodules have to be at least 3 mm in diameter to be visible unless either they are mineralized or multiple nodules are summated on each other (Fig. 6.13). For differential diagnoses of cavitary nodules, see 6.26. A nodular pattern is sometimes associated with, and obscured by, an alveolar infiltrate, and high-definition images, lacking respiratory blur, are required to detect it.

1. Superimposition of nipples, costochondral junctions in older dogs or thoracic wall nodules (see 8.21.4).
2. Normal blood vessels seen end on (see Table 6.2) – these are more radiopaque, perfectly circular and well marginated, decrease in size towards the periphery and are associated with adjacent longitudinal blood vessels. If there is a hypervascular lung pattern (see 6.23), the end-on vessels will be larger and more numerous.
3. Severe bronchial disease with thickly cuffed ring markings or plugs of mucus or exudate in bronchi seen end on – especially in cats.

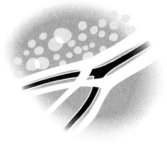

Figure 6.13 Nodular lung pattern. Apparent nodular opacities may be created by summation of two or more lesions. There may be an associated reticular interstitial pattern (see Fig. 6.14C). (Compare with Fig. 6.6, *Normal lung pattern*.)

Table 6.2	Distinguishing blood vessels seen end on from metastatic nodules	
CHARACTERISTIC	BLOOD VESSEL SEEN END ON	METASTATIC NODULE
Size	Become smaller peripherally; same size as other local blood vessels	Any size, unrelated to location in thorax
Location	May be superimposed over a longitudinal blood vessel	Not associated with blood vessels
Opacity	More radiopaque than a nodule	Less radiopaque than an end-on blood vessel
Margination	Well defined	Often indistinct

4. Nodules associated with ageing (incidental findings).
   a. Pulmonary osteomas (heterotopic bone formation) in older, large-breed dogs (see 6.4.6).
   b. Calcified pleural plaques – appear identical (see 6.4.6).
   c. Fibrotic nodules.
5. Multiple small lung nodules, 3–5 mm in diameter (see Table 6.2).
   a. Miliary nodules – a large number of smaller, diffusely distributed nodules that may have summating opacities, appearing to form larger conglomerates. They occur as a result of widespread haematogenous and/or lymphatic dissemination of pathogens or neoplastic cells and may be accompanied by hilar lymphadenopathy.
      – Metastatic tumours (e.g. mammary and thyroid carcinoma and haemangiosarcoma); has also been seen with multiple myeloma (rare).
      – Pulmonary lymphoma – usually with an interstitial lung pattern and mediastinal lymphadenopathy.
      – Haematogenous bacterial pneumonia.
      – Fungal pneumonia (see 6.15.5).
      – Disseminated intravascular coagulation.
      – Mycobacterial pneumonia – rare.
   b. Alveolar nodules due to aspiration or inhalation of radiopaque material.
      – Aspirated barium.
      – Pneumoconiosis.
   c. Eosinophilic bronchopneumopathy (pulmonary infiltrate with eosinophils) – there may be an ill-defined nodular pattern superimposed over the interstitial pattern.
   d. Parasitic – usually fewer nodules; may calcify (see 6.15.5).
      – Larval migrans.
      – Eosinophilic granulomatosis due to *Dirofilaria immitis** infection.

   – *Filaroides hirthi** and *F. milksi**.
   – Cats – *Aelurostrongylus abstrusus** infection (feline lungworm) – initial bronchoalvolear pattern, although older cats with resolving disease tend to show a more nodular pattern.
   e. Protozoal.
      – Toxoplasmosis*.
   f. Idiopathic mineralization (see 6.27.5).
   g. Leptospirosis – often a reticulonodular pattern.
   h. *Francisella (Pasteurella) tularensis** (tularaemia) – very rare, potential contact with rodents.
6. Multiple medium-sized lung nodules, 5–40 mm in diameter.
   a. Metastatic tumours – often 'cannon ball' nodules; randomly distributed, well-defined and do not coalesce although may summate; especially from primary osteosarcoma. Rapidly growing metastases may cavitate and become air-filled; main differential diagnosis is cavitating abscesses or granulomata.
   b. Pulmonary lymphoma – usually with an interstitial lung pattern and mediastinal lymphadenopathy.
   c. Fungal granulomata or abscesses (see 6.15.5).
      – Histoplasmosis nodules are often well circumscribed and may calcify.
   d. Multicentric primary tumours.
   e. Histiocytic sarcoma (malignant histiocytosis) – middle-aged large-breed dogs, with male preponderance; mainly Bernese Mountain Dog but also Rottweiler and Golden and Flat-coated Retrievers.
   f. Bacterial granulomata or abscesses.
   g. Foreign body granulomata.
      – Multiple small nodules due to mineral or vegetable oil aspiration.
   h. Enlarged blood vessels seen end on (see 6.23.1–4).
   i. Bronchi or bronchiectasis lesions filled with mucus or exudate.

j. Haematomata (haematocyst).

k. Fluid-filled cysts.
   – Congenital.
   – Hydatid.

l. Disseminated intravascular coagulation.

m. Pulmonary lymphomatoid granulomatosis – rare neoplastic disorder; often with an interstitial–alveolar lung pattern and hilar lymphadenopathy.

n. Parasitic.
   – *Paragonimus kellicotti** (lung fluke); nodules are rare in the dog and cystic lesions are more common (see 6.26.5), but the nodular granulomatous form is more common in the cat.
   – Cats – *Aelurostrongylus abstrusus** infection (feline lungworm – see 6.20.5).

o. Feline infectious peritonitis.

6.21 ULTRASONOGRAPHY OF PULMONARY NODULES OR MASSES

Pulmonary nodules or masses are visible ultrasonographically only if they lie adjacent to the thoracic wall, heart or diaphragm or are outlined by free thoracic fluid.

1. Well-defined, thin-walled nodule or mass with anechoic or hypoechoic contents (the presence of gas may result in hyperechoic foci within the anechoic or hypoechoic contents).
   a. Cyst.
   b. Haematoma.
   c. Abscess.

2. Variably well-defined, thick or irregular-walled nodule or mass with anechoic or hypoechoic contents (the presence of gas may result in hyperechoic foci within the anechoic or hypoechoic contents).
   a. Abscess.
   b. Cavitating tumour.
   c. Organizing haematoma.

3. Solid, homogeneous nodule or mass.
   a. Tumour of homogeneous cell type with little necrosis.
   b. Alveolar consolidation or collapse simulating a mass (see 6.14–6.18 for lists of differential diagnoses).

4. Solid, heterogeneous nodule or mass.
   a. Tumour of heterogeneous cell type and/or areas of necrosis, haemorrhage or calcification.

b. Organizing haematoma.

c. Abscess.

d. Granuloma.

6.22 INTERSTITIAL LUNG PATTERN

Changes occur primarily in the interstitial tissues (the alveolar walls and the connective tissue supporting airways and vessels) and not the air spaces, although the air content of the affected lung may be reduced as a result. It may be possible to recognize three types of interstitial lung pattern. A diffuse, unstructured interstitial pattern results in a semiopaque, generalized or regional pulmonary background opacity with reduced visibility of the pulmonary vasculature (Fig. 6.14A). Unlike the alveolar pattern, which is uneven and which may be most marked centrally, it is usually of a similar opacity throughout the affected area. There is no border effacement, but smudging or blurring of the outline of structures occurs. Air bronchograms may be seen in severe cases. A linear or reticular interstitial lung pattern is similar, but not all alveolar walls are affected. It consists of randomly arranged linear opacities that are more visible peripherally (Fig. 6.14B). This pattern is often described as being reticular (meshwork-like). It may also be accompanied by small nodules to form a reticulonodular interstitial pattern (Fig. 6.14C).

Other patterns may occur simultaneously; a bronchial component is often also present as well as an alveolar pattern.

1. Artefactual interstitial lung pattern (see 6.13).

2. Age-related interstitial lung pattern.
   a. In very young animals, due to increased water content of interstitial tissue.
   b. In old animals, due to ageing changes of interstitial fibrosis in the lung; usually reticular.

3. Infectious causes – pneumonia.
   a. Bacterial.
      – Irish Wolfhound: hereditary rhinitis–bronchitis complex; young dogs with recurrent clinical signs due to primary immunodeficiency.
   b. Viral (e.g. distemper) – often involves the caudodorsal lung lobes, but the changes are minimal unless complicated by bacterial infection.
   c. Fungal – often with mediastinal lymphadenopathy (see 6.15.5); may be reticular.

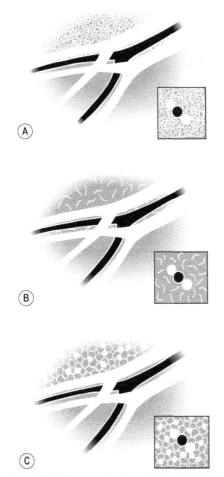

Figure 6.14 (A) Diffuse, unstructured interstitial lung pattern. (B) Linear or reticular interstitial lung pattern. (C) Reticulonodular interstitial lung pattern. (Compare with Fig. 6.6, *Normal lung pattern.*)

- Histoplasmosis*.
- Cryptococcosis*.
- Blastomycosis*.
- Coccidioidomycosis*.
- *Pneumocystis carinii** – immune-compromised patients, especially in younger miniature Dachshunds and Cavalier King Charles Spaniels.
d. *Mycoplasma* infection.
e. Rocky Mountain spotted fever (*Rickettsia rickettsii** infection).
f. Babesiosis*.
g. Toxoplasmosis* – caudal lobes; especially cats.
h. Leptospirosis – reticulonodular pattern.

i. Cats – *Aelurostrongylus abstrusus** infection (feline lungworm) – caudal lobes, often cats less than 1 year old; may also show a bronchoalveolar pattern progressing to a nodular pattern with time.
j. Cats – feline infectious peritonitis.
k. Cats – feline tuberculosis.

4. Oedema – interstitial oedema precedes alveolar oedema, and the aetiologies are similar (see 6.14.1 and 6.14.7).
   a. Cardiogenic – in dogs, symmetrically distributed in the perihilar region, extending peripherally, with progressing heart failure; in cats, more patchy or peripheral distribution; symmetrical, asymmetrical or right caudal lobe involvement.
   b. Non-cardiogenic – caudodorsal lobes, often asymmetrical (see 6.14.7).

5. Pulmonary haemorrhage.
   a. Trauma – fractured ribs and subcutaneous emphysema may also be seen.
   b. Coagulopathy.
      - Disseminated intravascular coagulation.
      - Anticoagulant poisoning.
      - Haemophilia, von Willebrand's disease (especially Dobermann) and other inherited coagulopathies.
      - Immune-mediated diseases.
      - Bone marrow depression.
   c. Metastatic haemangiosarcoma.
   d. Leptospirosis – due to vasculitis; often a reticulonodular pattern.

6. Neoplasia.
   a. Primary.
      - Pulmonary lymphoma (may be a reticulonodular pattern); usually also with marked mediastinal lymphadenopathy.
      - Bronchiolar–alveolar carcinoma; may affect multiple lobes, giving rise to a severe interstitial or alveolar pattern.
   b. Metastatic.
      - Pulmonary alveolar septal metastasis due to anaplastic scirrhous mammary carcinoma – rare; often reticular.
   c. Pulmonary lymphomatoid granulomatosis – rare neoplastic disorder; with pulmonary nodules or masses and hilar lymphadenopathy too.

7. Allergic – eosinophilic bronchopneumopathy (pulmonary infiltrate with eosinophils); an

ill-defined nodular pattern and bronchial markings may also be present.

8. Parasitic.

   a. *Dirofilaria immitis** (heartworm) – plus hypervascular and alveolar patterns (see 6.23.1), often worst in the caudal lung lobes; also right-sided cardiomegaly, pulmonary artery enlargement and arterial hypervascular pattern.

   b. *Angiostrongylus vasorum** (French heartworm) – plus multifocal or peripheral alveolar pattern (see 6.23.1).

   c. *Filaroides hirthi** and *F. milksi**.

   d. Cats – *Aelurostrongylus abstrusus** (feline lungworm) – caudal lobes, often cats less than 1 year old; may also show a bronchoalveolar pattern progressing to a nodular pattern with time.

9. Pulmonary thromboembolism (see 6.23.6).

10. Pulmonary fibrosis (usually reticular).

   a. Idiopathic – middle- to old-aged terriers, especially West Highland White and Staffordshire Bull Terrier and recently also described in cats; may also have a bronchial pattern.

   b. Chronic fibrosing interstitial pneumonia.

   c. Secondary to any chronic respiratory disease.

   d. Pneumoconiosis – see below.

11. Aspirated foreign body, especially grass or barley awns in working dogs; usually a focal alveolar or interstitial pattern in a caudal lobe. May be accompanied by pneumothorax, pleural effusion or pleural thickening.

12. Inhalation (toxic or irritant pneumonitis) – diffuse interstitial radiopacity in acute cases and pulmonary fibrosis (pneumoconiosis) in chronic cases.

   a. Smoke.

   b. Hydrocarbons (e.g. waterproofing spray).

   c. Dust.

     – Silica.

     – Asbestos.

     – Diesel exhaust fumes.

13. Hyperadrenocorticism (Cushing's disease) or long-term corticosteroid administration may rarely produce interstitial calcification, as well as calcification of the bronchial walls, hepatomegaly, osteopenia and soft tissue calcification.

14. Toxins – paraquat, diquat and morfamquat (herbicides) poisoning; often with pneumomediastinum too.

15. Lipid or lipoid pneumonia (exogenous or endogenous) – especially cats.

16. Acute lung injury or acute respiratory distress syndrome (shock lung) – initial interstitial pattern progresses to a patchy alveolar pattern with reduced lung volume (see 6.14.7 for causes).

17. Uraemia – rare.

18. Pancreatitis.

19. Radiation pneumonitis, 2–24 months following exposure – localized to the irradiated area of the lung; may be reticular.

20. Chronic antigen exposure.

21. Oxygen therapy.

22. Adverse drug reactions (e.g. to bleomycin).

6.23 VASCULAR LUNG PATTERN

The visibility of blood vessels depends on the amount of air in the lungs. Arteries and veins run adjacent to and on opposite sides of the associated bronchi and can be distinguished from each other by their location. On the lateral view, the cranial lobar arteries lie dorsal and parallel to the corresponding veins. On the DV or VD view, the caudal lobe arteries arise more cranial and lateral to the corresponding bronchi and veins. The veins run medial to the corresponding bronchus and lie within the bifurcation of the main stem (principal) bronchi. In dogs, arteries are normally the same size or slightly larger than veins. On lateral radiographs in dogs, the cranial lobe arteries should be 0.73 ± 0.24 times the diameter of the proximal third of the fourth rib where they cross this rib, and in cats the ratio is 0.70 ± 0.13. On DV or VD radiographs at the level of the tenth rib, the lobar artery width should not exceed that of the rib (see Fig. 6.15A and B).

An abnormal vascular pattern is recognized by a change in number, size, shape, or radiopacity of pulmonary blood vessels (Fig. 6.15C and D).

1. Arteries larger than veins (Fig. 6.15C).

   a. *Dirofilaria immitis** infection (heartworm) – the dilated arteries are often truncated and tortuous. May be accompanied by right heart enlargement and prominence of the main pulmonary artery with bronchopneumonia or

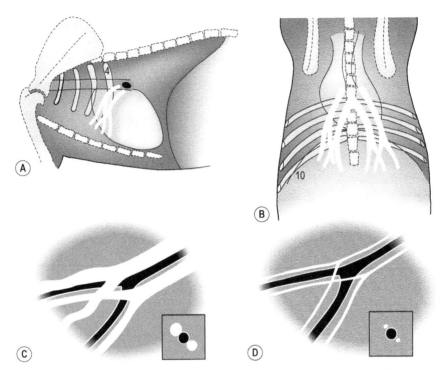

Figure 6.15 (A) Left cranial lobe blood vessels on the lateral view – approximately 75% of the diameter of the fourth rib. (B) Caudal lobe blood vessels on the dorsoventral view – no larger than the tenth rib. (C) Hypervascular lung pattern – affected vessels (in this case the artery) are enlarged and may become tortuous. (D) Hypovascular lung pattern – the blood vessels are thin and thread-like. (Compare with Fig. 6.6, *Normal lung pattern.*)

eosinophilic bronchopneumopathy (pulmonary infiltrate with eosinophils).
b. Large left to right shunts.
   – Patent ductus arteriosus.
   – Ventricular and atrial septal defect.
   – Endocardial cushion defect.
c. Pulmonary thromboembolism (see 6.23.6) – occasionally the affected artery may be mildly dilated proximal to abrupt attenuation.
d. Pulmonary hypertension, various causes – often accompanied by right heart enlargement (cor pulmonale).
e. Peripheral arteriovenous fistula.
f. *Angiostrongylus vasorum** (French heartworm) – changes are similar to those caused by *Dirofilaria immitis**, although the hypervascular pattern is often mild or absent and an alveolar or interstitial pattern predominates.
g. Cats – *Aelurostrongylus abstrusus** (feline lungworm) due to arteritis and arterial

hyperplasia; also an initial bronchoalveolar pattern becoming more nodular with time.
2. Veins larger than arteries.
   a. Left heart failure.
   b. Right to left shunts, due to relatively smaller arteries (e.g. tetralogy of Fallot).
   c. Left to right shunts – in some cases, the thin-walled veins show greater dilation than the arteries (e.g. ventricular and atrial septal defect).
   d. Lesions restricting pulmonary venous return (e.g. mitral valve stenosis, cor triatriatum sinister).
3. Generalized increased pulmonary vascularity – increased number and diameter of vessels, extending further to the periphery.
   a. Passive pulmonary congestion – left heart failure.
   b. Active pulmonary congestion – precedes pneumonia.

c. Left to right shunts.
- Patent ductus arteriosus.
- Ventricular and atrial septal defects.
- Endocardial cushion defect (large ventricular and atrial septal defects combined; complete atrioventricular canal).
- Aorticopulmonary septal defect (aorticopulmonary window or fenestration).
d. Iatrogenic overhydration.
4. Increased vascular radiopacity.
a. Left heart failure – the dilated veins may be more radiopaque than the arteries.
b. Vessel wall mineralization – rare and of uncertain aetiology.
- Hyperadrenocorticism (Cushing's disease) or long-term corticosteroid administration.
- Chronic renal failure.
- Cats – secondary to hypertension.
5. Generalized decreased pulmonary vascularity (Fig. 6.15D) – the lungs have an empty appearance, with thinner peripheral vessels that appear fewer in number and that do not reach the periphery.
a. Forced manual overinflation during anaesthesia.
b. Pulmonary hypoperfusion (may be accompanied by microcardia, small caudal vena cava and compensatory hyperinflation).
- Shock.
- Severe dehydration.
- Blood loss.
- Hypoadrenocorticism (Addison's disease).
c. Other causes of pulmonary overinflation (see 6.25.4–6).
d. Pericardial disease, reducing right heart output.
- Pericardial effusion with tamponade.
- Restrictive pericarditis.
e. Right heart failure.
f. Congenital cardiac disease with right to left shunts.
- Tetralogy of Fallot.
- Reverse-shunting patent ductus arteriosus.
- Reverse-shunting ventricular and atrial septal defect.
g. Severe pulmonic stenosis.

6. Localized decreased pulmonary vascular pattern.
a. Pulmonary thromboembolism; radiographs are frequently normal, despite severe dyspnoea, and this finding itself is suggestive of pulmonary thromboembolism;. If radiographic signs are present, the affected pulmonary artery may be irregular or abruptly attenuated; occasionally its central part is mildly dilated: DV view is best for assessment of vessels. May also see peripheral hypoperfusion, small or absent returning vein, patchy, wedge-shaped or lobar alveolar pattern and a small pleural effusion. Right lung affected more often than left, and especially caudal lobes.
- Autoimmune haemolytic anaemia.
- Renal amyloidosis, glomerular disease and nephrotic syndrome.
- Hyperadrenocorticism (Cushing's disease) or long-term corticosteroid administration.
- Diabetes mellitus.
- Polycythaemia.
- Post-operative thromboembolism.
- Thrombi from right-sided heart disease.
- *Dirofilaria immitis** and *Angiostrongylus vasorum** (see 6.23.1).
- Disseminated intravascular coagulation.
- Trauma.
- Septicaemia.
- Pancreatitis.
b. Lobar emphysema compressing blood vessels.

6.24 MIXED LUNG PATTERN

Many abnormal lung patterns consist of a combination of two, three or even four constituent patterns. Usually, however, one pattern is dominant and will help to elucidate the aetiology. The alveolar and interstitial patterns may be hard to distinguish and often coexist. The hypovascular pattern is often an incidental finding in a sick or dehydrated animal.

Some examples of common mixed patterns are given here.

1. Dominant pattern bronchial.
a. Bronchial pattern due to ageing changes, with an ageing interstitial pattern and/or other disease process superimposed.
b. Bronchial and alveolar ± interstitial.

- Various pneumonias, especially as they resolve.
- Irish Wolfhound: hereditary bronchitis–rhinitis complex.
- Cats – idiopathic pulmonary fibrosis.

  c. Bronchial pattern due to hyperadrenocorticism (Cushing's disease) or long-term corticosteroid administration, with other disease process superimposed – the bronchial pattern is clearly calcified.

2. Dominant pattern alveolar.
   a. Alveolar and bronchial ± interstitial.
      - Various pneumonias.
      - Cardiogenic oedema.
      - Pulmonary haemorrhage.
3. Dominant pattern hypervascular.
   a. Hypervascular and alveolar.
      - Cardiogenic oedema (congenital or acquired heart disease).
   b. Hypervascular, alveolar ± bronchial and interstitial.
      - *Dirofilaria immitis** (heartworm) and, to a lesser extent, *Angiostrongylus vasorum** (French heartworm).
4. Dominant pattern interstitial.
   a. Severe ageing interstitial pattern with other disease process superimposed.
   b. Interstitial and bronchial.
      - Severe chronic bronchitis.
      - Eosinophilic bronchopneumopathy (pulmonary infiltrate with eosinophils).
      - Severe small airway disease.
      - Idiopathic pulmonary fibrosis.
   c. Lymphoma; usually with mediastinal lymphadenopathy too.
   d. Paraquat poisoning; usually with pneumomediastinum too.
   e. Bronchiolar–alveolar carcinoma.
   f. Leptospirosis.

6.25 GENERALIZED PULMONARY HYPERLUCENCY

Two or more lung lobes are involved.

1. Artefactual pulmonary hyperlucency.
   a. Overexposure, overdevelopment or fogging of the film.
   b. Forced manual overinflation during anaesthesia.
   c. Deep inspiration (e.g. dyspnoea).
   d. Emaciation.
   e. Unilateral, due to thoracic rotation on DV or VD views.
2. Extrapulmonary hyperlucent areas that mimic increased pulmonary radiolucency.
   a. Pneumothorax.
   b. Air-filled megaoesophagus.
   c. Diaphragmatic rupture with distended, gas-filled gastrointestinal tract within the thoracic cavity.
   d. Subcutaneous emphysema.
   e. Pneumomediastinum.
3. Pulmonary hypoperfusion (hypovascular pattern, undercirculation – see 6.23.5).
   a. Shock.
   b. Severe dehydration.
   c. Hypoadrenocorticism (Addison's disease).
   d. Cardiac tamponade.
   e. Congenital cardiac disease with right to left shunts.
   f. Tetralogy of Fallot.
   g. Reverse-shunting patent ductus arteriosus.
   h. Reverse-shunting ventricular and atrial septal defect.
   i. Severe pulmonic stenosis.
4. Overinflation by air-trapping due to expiratory obstruction: the diaphragm is flattened, with little movement during respiration.
   a. Tracheal or bronchial foreign body.
   b. Chronic bronchitis.
   c. Allergic bronchitis, especially bronchial asthma in cats.
   d. Upper respiratory tract obstruction (e.g. nasopharyngeal polyp).
5. Compensatory overinflation.
   a. Following lobectomy.
   b. Secondary to atelectasis of another lobe or lobes.
   c. Secondary to congenital lobar atresia or agenesis.
6. Emphysema – the diaphragm may be caudally displaced and flattened, showing its costal attachments, the ribs positioned transversely and the cardiac silhouette small. Full inspiratory and expiratory radiographs should be made, and if there is little difference in pulmonary radiopacity and diaphragmatic position the diagnosis of emphysema is confirmed.

Alternatively, a DV or VD view using a horizontal beam and the animal in lateral recumbency with the affected lobe down will show that the affected lung does not collapse despite the weight of the heart above it.

   a. Acquired primary emphysema – rare.

   b. Congenital lobar emphysema – may involve one or more lobes; adjacent lobes may be compressed and mediastinal shift may occur (e.g. Shih Tzu and Jack Russell Terrier) – usually recognized in puppyhood.

6.26 FOCAL AREAS OF PULMONARY HYPERLUCENCY (INCLUDING CAVITARY LESIONS)

Improved visibility of focal areas of pulmonary hyperlucency occurs on expiratory radiographs and on radiographs with the affected area dependent, as the surrounding lung becomes more radiopaque. Fluid levels and wall thickness may be demonstrated in cysts and cavitary lesions by means of horizontal beam radiography; thin fluid contents will produce a flat, horizontal, gas–fluid interface, whereas thick contents will show a curved or irregular interface (Fig. 6.16).

1. Artefactual focal areas of pulmonary hyperlucency.

   a. Intrapulmonary.

     – Ring shadows may be mimicked by curved bronchial walls and pulmonary vessels and by lobar fissure lines, especially on DV or VD views.

   b. Extrapulmonary.

     – Gas-filled gastric fundus immediately caudal to the left crus, superimposed over

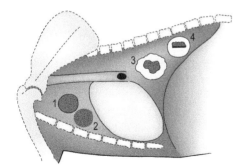

Figure 6.16 Focal areas of hyperlucency in the lungs: 1, cyst; 2, bulla; 3, cavitary lesion; and 4, cavitary lesion with fluid contents seen using horizontal beam radiography.

the caudodorsal lung on a left lateral recumbent radiograph.

   – Oesophageal air.

   – Gas-filled stomach or intestinal loop herniated into thorax or paracostally (see 8.2.3 and Fig. 8.3, for ruptured diaphragm).

   – Superimposed subcutaneous, pleural, subpleural or mediastinal air.

   – Foamy pneumothorax (concurrent pneumothorax and hydrothorax).

   – Pleural adhesions accompanied by pneumothorax.

   – Expansile rib osteolysis.

2. Normal – the tip of the left cranial lung lobe may be outlined just above the sternum on the lateral view and may appear more radiolucent than surrounding lung.

3. Bronchial structures seen end on.

   a. Prominent bronchi due to age.

   b. Chronic bronchitis.

   c. Bronchiectasis.

4. Radiolucent structure with absent or barely perceptible wall; may rupture and cause spontaneous and recurrent pneumothorax.

   a. Bulla – spherical, localized area of emphysema that is usually small but sometimes large; may be multiple. Usually traumatic in origin but can be congenital.

   b. Bleb – a subpleural bulla whose peripheral location makes it difficult to see unless it has resulted in pneumothorax, although often it will then have collapsed.

5. Radiolucent structure with a thin, regular wall – cysts and cyst-like structures; may rupture and cause spontaneous and recurrent pneumothorax. Congenital or acquired.

   a. Bronchogenic cyst – smooth, thin-walled; young animals.

   b. Pulmonary cyst or pseudocyst.

     – Pneumatocele (secondary to pneumonia or traumatized lung tissue) (note: *pneumatocele* and *bulla* are often used as synonyms, as they cannot be differentiated radiographically).

     – Pneumohaematocele – traumatic pneumatocele containing blood.

     – Thin-walled, healed abscess.

     – *Paragonimus kellicotti** (lung fluke) – septated or clustered, with a thin, smooth wall or an excentric, crescent-shaped wall

in dogs; cats are more likely to have a solid, nodular, granulomatous form.
  - Hydatid cyst.
6. Radiolucent structure with a thick and irregular wall, or cavitary lesion (an air-filled region within abnormal lung tissue); may develop from an apparently solid nodule or mass (see 6.19 for causes). Sometimes multiple cavities are present, especially in tumours. Rare in cats.
  a. Abscess or granuloma.
    - Bacterial.
    - Fungal – often thinner walls and associated hilar lymphadenopathy.
    - Parasitic.
    - Tuberculosis.
  b. Foreign body, especially aspirated grass awns in working dogs; usually caudal lobes. May be accompanied by pneumothorax, pleural effusion or pleural thickening.
  c. Neoplasia.
    - Primary – various carcinomas.
    - Metastatic – rapidly growing metastases (e.g. secondary to mammary and prostatic tumours and thyroid adenocarcinoma).
  d. Exogenous lipid or lipoid pneumonia (aspiration of mineral oil, etc.).
  e. Cavitary infarct – rare.
7. Emphysema (permanent enlargement of alveoli due to breakdown of their walls) – usually multiple radiolucent foci associated with overinflated lung: the affected lobe(s) may be markedly distended, displacing other structures.
    - Congenital lobar emphysema in young animals; right middle lobe most commonly affected.
    - Multifocal congenital bullous emphysema has also been described.
    - Acquired emphysema with diseases that cause pulmonary air-trapping (e.g. pneumonia, feline asthma).
8. Lobar vesicular gas pattern – lung lobe torsion (see 6.17.5 and Fig. 6.11).
9. Focal hyperlucent area peripheral to a pulmonary thromboembolism, without evidence of overinflation.
10. Dynamic cervical lung hernia just cranial to the thoracic inlet; secondary to increased respiratory rate and effort or chronic coughing.

6.27 INTRATHORACIC MINERALIZED OPACITIES

1. Artefactual superimposed opacities (see 8.20 and 8.21).
2. Incidental mineralization seen as an ageing change.
  a. Pulmonary osteomata (heterotopic bone formation) in older, larger-breed dogs (see 6.4.6).
  b. Calcified pleural plaques – appear identical to pulmonary osteomata (see 6.4.6).
  c. Calcified tracheal rings and bronchi, especially in chondrodystrophic breeds.
3. Oesophageal foreign body.
4. Aspirated contrast medium (barium) in alveoli or in hilar lymph nodes.
5. Pathological pulmonary mineralization.
  a. Healed fungal disease.
    - Histoplasmosis* – multiple small calcified nodules similar to pulmonary osteomata, accompanied by hilar lymph node calcification.
  b. Metastatic tumours from:
    - osteosarcoma
    - chondrosarcoma
    - bone-forming mammary tumours.
  c. Parasitic nodules.
  d. Primary lung tumours, especially in cats.
  e. Tracheal or bronchial hamartomas.
  f. Chronic infectious disease.
  g. Metastatic calcification.
    - Hyperadrenocorticism (Cushing's disease) or long-term corticosteroid administration; mainly calcification of bronchial walls but occasionally progresses to produce a calcified interstitial pattern.
    - Primary and secondary hyperparathyroidism.
    - Hypervitaminosis D.
    - Chronic uraemia.
  h. Idiopathic mineralization – tends to be diffuse and extensive.
    - Alveolar or bronchial microlithiasis.
    - Pulmonary calcification.
    - Pulmonary ossification.
  i. Cats – tuberculosis (may have skeletal lesions too – see 1.20.2).
  j. Cats – calcified peribronchial mucous glands are seen very occasionally with chronic bronchial disease.

6. Pathological mediastinal mineralization.
   a. Lymph nodes.
      – Histoplasmosis*, especially during healing phase.
      – Tuberculosis.
   b. Osteosarcoma transformation of oesophageal *Spirocerca lupi** granuloma.
   c. Thymic tumours.
   d. Metastatic mediastinal tumours.
7. Cardiovascular mineralization.
   a. Aorta (see 7.10.4).
   b. Coronary vessels (incidental finding) – tend to run caudoventrally from the aortic arch. Best seen on lateral views, as short, wavy lines of mineralization.
   c. Heart valves.
      – Idiopathic.
      – Bacterial endocarditis.
   d. Mineralized neoplasia (e.g. chondrosarcoma of pulmonary artery has been reported).

6.28 HILAR MASSES

Hilar masses usually result in poorly defined radiopacities near the base of the heart. The increased thickness of the lungs at this level means that diffuse pulmonary pathology may create a false impression of a hilar mass. Genuine hilar masses are usually within the mediastinum – see 8.11.3 for details.

6.29 INCREASED VISIBILITY OF LUNG OR LOBAR EDGES

The lungs normally extend to the periphery of the thoracic cavity, and individual lobe or lung edges are not seen except in two locations: (a) in the cranioventral thorax, where the mediastinum runs obliquely and outlines the cranial segment of the left cranial lung lobe on a lateral radiograph (see 8.7 and Fig. 8.7); and (b) along the ventral margins of the lungs, which may appear scalloped in some dogs on the lateral radiograph due to intrathoracic fat.

Increased visibility of the lung or lobar edges may be due to intrapulmonary disease, thickening of the pleura or diseases of the pleural space. See 8.2, 8.3 and 8.6 for further details.

6.30 LOWER RESPIRATORY TRACT CLINICAL SIGNS BUT NORMAL RADIOGRAPHS

Some animals may show dyspnoea or coughing without radiographic signs being apparent. If the condition does not resolve and structural lung disease remains a possibility, repeat radiography at 24 h intervals is recommended.

1. Lesions not apparent due to poor technique or overlooked during interpretation.
2. Respiratory signs arising from upper respiratory tract disease (e.g. nasal, nasopharyngeal or cranial tracheal disease).
3. Tracheitis.
4. Acute bronchitis or bronchospasm.
5. Acute pneumonia or pneumonitis (e.g. viral, mycoplasma).
6. Early idiopathic pulmonary fibrosis.
7. Pulmonary thromboembolism.
8. Early paraquat poisoning, prior to development of lung fibrosis (first 2–3 days).
9. Small or radiolucent foreign body in the early stages.
10. Anaemia.
11. Acidosis.
12. Central nervous system disease.
13. Pyrexia or heatstroke.
14. Weakness of respiratory muscles.
15. Anaphylaxis.
16. Pain.
17. Fear.

Further reading

Miscellaneous

Avner, A., Kirberger, R.M., 2005. The effect of the various thoracic views on the appearance of selected thoracic viscera. J. Small Anim. Pract. 46, 491–498.

Berry, C.R., Gallaway, A., Thrall, D. E., Carlisle, C., 1993. Thoracic radiographic features of anticoagulant rodenticide toxicity in fourteen dogs. Vet. Radiol. Ultrasound 34, 391–396.

Berry, C.R., Ackerman, N., Monce, K., 1994. Pulmonary mineralization in four dogs with Cushing's syndrome. Vet. Radiol. Ultrasound 35, 10–16.

Brinkman, L.E., Biller, D., Armbrust, L., 2006. The clinical usefulness of the ventrodorsal versus dorsoventral thoracic radiograph in dogs. J. Am. Anim. Hosp. Assoc. 42, 440–449.

Clerx, C., Reichler, I., Peeters, D., McEntee, A., German, A., Dubois, J., et al., 2003. Rhinitis/bronchopneumonia syndrome in Irish Wolfhounds. J. Vet. Intern. Med. 17, 843–849.

Cohn, L.A., Norris, C.R., Hawkins, E.C., Dye, J.A., Johnson, C.A., Williams, K.J., 2004. Identification and characterization of an idiopathic pulmonary fibrosis-like condition in cats. J. Vet. Intern. Med. 18, 632–641.

Coleman, M.G., Warman, C.G.A., Robson, M.C., 2005. Dynamic cervical lung hernia in a dog with chronic airway disease. J. Vet. Intern. Med. 19, 103–105.

Corcoran, B.M., Thoday, K.L., Henfrey, J.I., Simpson, J.W., Burnie, A.G., Mooney, C.T., 1991. Pulmonary infiltrate with eosinophils in 14 dogs. J. Small Anim. Pract. 32, 494–502.

D'Anjou, M., Tidwell, A.S., Hecht, S., 2005. Radiographic diagnosis of lung lobe torsion. Vet. Radiol. Ultrasound 46, 478–484.

Egenvall, A., Hansson, K., Säteri, H., Lord, P.F., Jönsson, L., 2003. Pulmonary oedema in Swedish hunting dogs. J. Small Anim. Pract. 44, 209–217.

Godshalk, C.P., 1994. Common pitfalls in radiographic interpretation of the thorax. Compend. Contin. Educ. Pract. Veterinarian (Small Animal) 16, 731–738.

Guglielmini, C., De Simone, A., Valbonetti, A., Diana, A., 2007. Intermittent cranial lung herniation in two dogs. Vet. Radiol. Ultrasound 48, 227–229.

Hayward, N.J., Baines, S.J., Baines, E.A., Herrtage, M.E., 2004. The radiographic appearance of the pulmonary vasculature in the cat. Vet. Radiol. Ultrasound 45, 501–504.

Jones, D.J., Norris, C.R., Samii, V.F., Griffey, S.M., 2000. Endogenous lipid pneumonia in cats: 24 cases (1985–1998). J. Am. Vet. Med. Assoc. 216, 1347–1440.

Kirberger, R.M., Avner, A., 2006. The effect of positioning on the appearance of selected cranial thoracic structures in the dog. Vet. Radiol. Ultrasound 47, 61–68.

Lobetti, R.G., Milner, R., Lane, E., 2001. Chronic idiopathic pulmonary fibrosis in five dogs. J. Am. Anim. Hosp. Assoc. 37, 119–127.

Lora-Michiels, M., Biller, D.S., Olsen, J.J., Hoskinson, J.J., Kraft, S.L., Jones, J.C., 2003. The accessory lung lobe in thoracic disease: a case series and anatomical review. J. Am. Anim. Hosp. Assoc. 39, 452–458.

Lord, P.F., Gomez, J.A., 1985. Lung lobe collapse: pathophysiology and radiologic significance. Vet. Radiol. 26, 187–195.

Norris, C.R., Griffey, S.M., Samii, V.F., 1999. Pulmonary thromboembolism in cats: 29 cases (1987–1997). J. Am. Vet. Med. Assoc. 215, 1650–1654.

Park, R.D., 1984. Bronchoesophageal fistula in the dog: literature survey, case presentations, and radiographic manifestations. Compend. Contin. Educ. Pract. Veterinarian (Small Animal) 6, 669–677.

Pechman, R.D., 1987. Effect of dependency versus nondependency on lung lesion visualization. Vet. Radiol. 28, 185–190.

Schultz, R.M., Zwingenberger, A., 2008. Radiographic, computed tomographic, and ultrasonographic findings with migrating intrathoracic grass awns in dogs and cats. Vet. Radiol. Ultrasound 49, 249–255.

Stafford-Johnson, M., Martin, M., 2008. Investigation of dyspnoea in dogs. In Pract. 30, 558–566.

Watson, P.J., Herrtage, M.E., Peacock, M.A., Sargan, D.R., 1999. Primary ciliary dyskinesia in Newfoundland dogs. Vet. Rec. 144, 718–725.

Winegardner, K., Scrivani, P.V., Gleed, R.D., 2008. Lung expansion in the diagnosis of lung disease. Compend. Contin. Educ. Veterinarians 30, 479–489.

Wood, E.F., O'Brien, R.T., Young, K.M., 1998. Ultrasound-guided fine-needle aspiration of focal parenchymal lesions of the lung in dogs and cats. J. Vet. Intern. Med. 12, 338–342.

Trachea

Buchanan, J.W., 2004. Tracheal signs and associated vascular anomalies in dogs with persistent right aortic arch. J. Vet. Intern. Med. 18, 510–514.

Coyne, B.E., Fingland, R.B., 1992. Hypoplasia of the trachea in dogs: 103 cases (1974–1990). J. Am. Vet. Med. Assoc. 201, 768–772.

Fujita, M., Miura, H., Yasuda, D., Orima, H., 2004. Tracheal narrowing secondary to airway obstruction in two cats. J. Small Anim. Pract. 45, 29–31.

Jakubiak, M.J., Siedleccki, C.T., Zenger, M.L., Matteucci, M.L., Bruskiewicz, K.A., Rohn, D.A., et al., 2005. Laryngeal, laryngotracheal, and tracheal masses in cats: 27 cases (1998–2003). J. Am. Anim. Hosp. Asoc. 41, 310–316.

Rudorf, H., Herrtage, M.E., White, R.A.S., 1997. Use of ultrasonography in the diagnosis of tracheal collapse. J. Small Anim. Pract. 38, 513–518.

White, R.N., Milner, H.R., 1995. Intrathoracic tracheal avulsion in three cats. J. Small Anim. Pract. 36, 343–347.

Lung patterns

Dennis, R., 2008. Radiological assessment of lung disease in small animals 1. Bronchial and vascular patterns. In Pract. 30, 182–189.

Dennis, R., 2008. Radiological assessment of lung disease in small animals 2. Alveolar, interstitial and mixed lung patterns. In Pract. 30, 262–270.

Gadbois, J., d'Anjou, M.A., Dunn, M., Alexander, G., Beauregard, G., D'Astous, J., et al., 2009. Radiographic abnormalities in cats with feline bronchial disease and intra- and interobserver variability in radiographic interpretation. J. Am. Vet. Med. Assoc. 234, 367–375.

Kramer, R.W., 1992. Radiology corner: The nodular pulmonary opacity – is it real? Vet. Radiol. Ultrasound 33, 187–188.

Myer, W., 1979. Radiography review: The alveolar pattern of pulmonary disease. J. Am. Vet. Radiol. Soc. 20, 10–14.

Myer, C.W., 1980. Radiography review: The vascular and bronchial patterns of pulmonary disease. Vet. Radiol. 21, 156–160.

Myer, W., 1980. Radiography review: The interstitial pattern of pulmonary disease. Vet. Radiol. 21, 18–23.

Myer, W., Burt, J.K., 1973. Bronchiectasis in the dog: its radiographic appearance. J. Am. Vet. Radiol. Soc. 14, 3–12.

Nykamp, S.G., Scrivani, P.V., Dykes, N.L., 2002. Radiographic signs of pulmonary disease: an alternative approach. Compend. Conin. Educ. Pract. Veterinarian (Small Animal) 24, 25–35.

Silverman, S., Poulos, P.W., Suter, P.F., 1976. Cavitary pulmonary lesions in animals. J. Am. Vet. Radiol. Soc. 17, 134–146.

Lung neoplasia

Ballegeer, E.A., Forrest, L.J., Stephen, R.L., 2002. Radiographic appearance of bronchoalveolar carcinoma in nine cats. Vet. Radiol. Ultrasound 43, 267–271.

Barr, F., Gruffydd-Jones, T.J., Brown, P.J., Gibbs, C., 1987. Primary lung tumours in the cat. J. Small Anim. Pract. 28, 1115–1125.

Forrest, L.J., Graybush, C.A., 1998. Radiographic patterns of pulmonary metastasis in 25 cats. Vet. Radiol. Ultrasound 39, 4–8.

Koblik, P.D., 1986. Radiographic appearance of primary lung tumours in cats: a review of 41 cases. Vet. Radiol. 27, 66–73.

Miles, K.G., 1988. A review of primary lung tumors in the dog, cat. Vet. Radiol. 29, 122–128.

Thrall, D.E., 1979. Radiographic diagnosis of metastatic pulmonary tumours. Compend. Contin. Educ. Pract. Veterinarian (Small Animal) 1, 131–139.

Infectious

Baumann, D., Flückiger, M., 2001. Radiographic findings in the thorax of dogs with leptospiral infection. Vet. Radiol. Ultrasound 42, 305–307.

Boag, A.G., Lamb, C.R., Chapman, P.S., Boswood, A., 2004. Radiographic findings in 16 dogs infected with *Angiostrongylus vasorum*. Vet. Rec. 154, 426–430.

Bolt, G., Monrad, J., Koch, J., Jensen, A.L., 1994. Canine angiostrongylosis: a review. Vet. Rec. 135, 447–452.

Burk, R.L., Corley, E.A., Corwin, A., 1978. The radiographic appearance of pulmonary histoplasmosis in the dog and cat: a review of 37 case histories. J. Am. Vet. Radiol. Soc. 9, 2–6.

Kirberger, R.M., Lobetti, R.G., 1998. Radiographic aspects of *Pneumocystis carinii* pneumonia in the miniature dachshund. Vet. Radiol. Ultrasound 39, 313–317.

Millman, T.M., O'Brien, T.R., Suter, P.F., Wolf, A.M., 1979. Coccidioidomycosis in the dog: its radiographic diagnosis. J. Am. Vet. Radiol. Soc. 20, 50–65.

Schmidt, M., Wolvekamp, P., 1991. Radiographic findings in ten dogs with thoracic actinomycosis. Vet. Radiol. 32, 301–306.

Shaiken, L.C., Evans, S.M., Goldschmidt, M.H., 1991. Radiographic findings in canine malignant histiocytosis. Vet. Radiol. 32, 237–242.

Walker, M.A., 1981. Thoracic blastomycosis: a review of its radiographic manifestations in 40 dogs. Vet. Radiol. 22, 22–26.

Chapter 7

Cardiovascular system

CHAPTER CONTENTS

7.1 Normal radiographic appearance of the heart 175
7.2 Normal cardiac silhouette with cardiac pathology 176
7.3 Cardiac malposition 177
7.4 Reduction in heart size: microcardia 178
7.5 Generalized enlargement of the cardiac silhouette 178
7.6 Pericardial disease 179
7.7 Ultrasonography of pericardial disease 181
7.8 Left atrial enlargement 181
7.9 Left ventricular enlargement 182
7.10 Aortic abnormalities 183
7.11 Right atrial enlargement 184
7.12 Right ventricular enlargement 185
7.13 Pulmonary artery trunk abnormalities 186
7.14 Changes in pulmonary arteries and veins 186
7.15 Caudal vena cava abnormalities 186
7.16 Cardiac neoplasia 187

Angiography 188
7.17 Angiography: left heart 188
7.18 Angiography: right heart 189

Cardiac ultrasonography 189
7.19 Two-dimensional and M-mode echocardiography: left heart 189
7.20 Two-dimensional and M-mode echocardiography: right heart 192

7.21 Contrast echocardiography: right heart 194
7.22 Doppler flow abnormalities: mitral valve 194
7.23 Doppler flow abnormalities: aortic valve 195
7.24 Doppler flow abnormalities: tricuspid valve 195
7.25 Doppler flow abnormalities: pulmonic valve 196

7.1 NORMAL RADIOGRAPHIC APPEARANCE OF THE HEART

The cardiac silhouette consists of pericardium, pericardial fluid, myocardium (including epicardium and endocardium), the origins of the major vessels and blood. Its size may change with the cardiac cycle, and it may be slightly larger during expiration than inspiration. Its appearance is slightly different between right and left lateral recumbency and between sternal and dorsal recumbency, and so a consistent technique should be adopted. Radiographic signs of heart disease include change in size or shape of the heart and evidence of right- or left-sided heart failure. Alteration in size or shape of the cardiac silhouette may be due to enlargement of any of its components and can often be distinguished only by angiography or ultrasonography; plain radiographs may be misleading. Conformation is the single

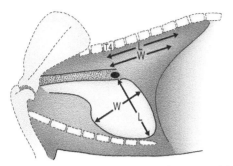

Figure 7.1 Cardiac measurement using the vertebral heart scale system. L, maximum length of heart; T4, fourth thoracic vertebra; W, maximum width of heart.

most important cause for apparent cardiomegaly in barrel-chested dogs such as the Bulldog, Yorkshire Terrier and Dachshund, which have a relatively large heart with elevated trachea on lateral radiographs. The Golden Retriever also has an apparently large and square-shaped heart on the lateral radiograph. Generalized cardiomegaly may be evaluated in dogs by means of the *vertebral heart scale measurement* (Fig. 7.1); on the lateral recumbent radiograph, the distance between the ventral aspect of the carina and the cardiac apex is taken as a length value, and the maximum width of the heart perpendicular to the length line is taken as the width of the heart. Starting at the cranial aspect of the fourth thoracic vertebra, the number of vertebral lengths is determined for each measurement. In 100 clinically normal adult dogs, the mean ($\pm$ SD) vertebral heart size was 9.7 $\pm$ 0.5. Cardiomegaly is usually considered present when the combined measurement exceeds 10.6 thoracic vertebrae, although in some breeds (e.g. Labrador, Golden Retriever, Boxer, Cavalier King Charles Spaniel, Greyhound, Whippet, Lurcher) this value is commonly exceeded in normal dogs. Reference ranges for some popular breeds have been published. In cats, the same technique can be used with a mean of 7.5 $\pm$ 0.3 and 8.1 being the cut-off point above which the heart is considered enlarged. Localized cardiac enlargement may be described according to the clock face analogy (Fig. 7.2).

It should be noted that radiography is an insensitive and relatively inaccurate method for diagnosis of heart diseases (especially congenital), and echocardiography is a much more efficient modality. Nevertheless, radiography is extremely important for assessment of signs of heart failure, especially in the lungs.

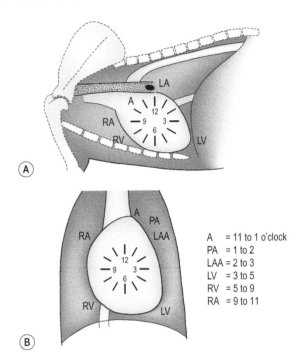

Figure 7.2 (A) Clock face analogy of cardiac anatomy (lateral view); (B) clock-face analogy of cardiac anatomy (dorsoventral view). A, aorta; LA, left atrium; LAA, left auricular appendage; LV, left ventricle; PA, pulmonary artery; RA, right atrium; RV, right ventricle.

7.2 NORMAL CARDIAC SILHOUETTE WITH CARDIAC PATHOLOGY

A normal cardiac silhouette may be present in spite of severe cardiac disease. Echocardiography and an electrocardiogram are essential diagnostic components of the cardiac examination for complete cardiac evaluation.

1. Conduction disturbances and arrhythmias.
2. Over-treated heart disease (e.g. excessive use of diuretics).
3. Concentric ventricular hypertrophy.
    a. Secondary to congenital heart disease.
       – (Sub)aortic stenosis (left ventricular hypertrophy).
       – Pulmonic stenosis (right ventricular hypertrophy).
    b. Acquired.
       – Idiopathic hypertrophic cardiomyopathy in cats and dogs.
       – Hypertrophic cardiomyopathy secondary to hyperthyroidism in older cats.
       – Systemic or pulmonary hypertension.

4. Small shunting lesions.
   a. Small atrial and ventricular septal defects (ASDs and VSDs).
   b. Small patent ductus arteriosus (PDA).
5. Endocarditis.
6. Acute myocardial failure.
7. Pericardial disease.
   a. Constrictive pericarditis.
   b. Acute traumatic haemopericardium.
8. Acute ruptured chordae tendineae.
9. Myocardial neoplasia.
10. Early or mild myocarditis.

7.3 CARDIAC MALPOSITION

Terminology

Levocardia – Heart lies in a normal left-sided position (Fig. 7.3A).
Dextrocardia – Heart lying predominantly in the right thorax with the cardiac apex pointing to the right (Fig. 7.3B).
Situs solitus – Normal position of thoracic and abdominal organs.
Situs inversus – Reversal of the normal thoracic and abdominal organs – mirror image (Fig. 7.3C).

Dextrocardia

1. Artefact – incorrectly labelled dorsoventral (DV) or ventrodorsal (VD) radiograph; check the position of the caudal vena cava (CdVC) and descending aorta, or the gastric air bubble and spleen in the cranial abdomen.
2. Normal variant in wide-chested dogs and occasionally in the cat.

3. Acquired causes of dextrocardia.
   a. Cardiac disease with left heart enlargement.
   b. Mediastinal shift (see 8.8).
4. Congenital extracardiac abnormalities.
   a. Pectus excavatum (see 8.23.1 and Fig. 8.15).
   b. Vertebral abnormalities resulting in an abnormally wide and shallow thorax.
5. Congenital cardiac abnormalities.
   a. Primary dextrocardia with situs inversus (see Fig. 7.3C) – the cardiac apex, left ventricle, aortic arch and gastric fundus all lie on the right side and the CdVC is on the left.
      – Part of Kartagener's syndrome (also includes rhinosinusitis and bronchiectasis due to ciliary dyskinesia).
   b. Dextrocardia with situs solitus – cardiac chambers normal but apex to right of midline.
   c. Levocardia with partial abdominal situs inversus has also been described.

Dorsal displacement of the heart

6. Fat in the pericardium or ventral mediastinum.
7. Sternal abnormalities (see 8.23).
8. Pneumothorax on a lateral recumbent radiograph (see 8.2.2).
9. Mediastinal shift (see 8.8).
10. Cranioventral thoracic masses (see 8.11.1).

The heart may also be displaced cranially, caudally, ventrally or further to the left by herniated abdominal viscera or by a variety of mass lesions or bony abnormalities.

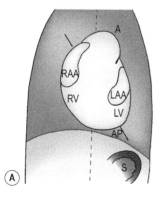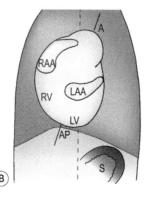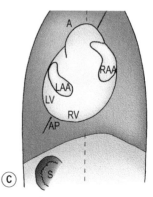

Figure 7.3 (A) Normal location of the heart (dorsoventral view); (B) dextrocardia; (C) dextrocardia with situs inversus. A, aorta; AP, apex; LAA, left auricular appendage; LV, left ventricle; RAA, right auricular appendage; RV, right ventricle; S, stomach.

7.4 REDUCTION IN HEART SIZE: MICROCARDIA

The heart silhouette is abnormally small and pointed, the ventricles appear narrower and the apex loses contact with the sternum. Thoracic blood vessels may appear smaller and the lungs hyperlucent (see hypovascular pattern, 6.23.5). The CdVC is also reduced in size (Fig. 7.4).

1. Artefactual reduction in heart size.
   a. Deep-chested dogs – narrow, upright heart with straight caudal border.
   b. Deep inspiration.
   c. Pulmonary overinflation (see 6.25.4 and 6.25.6).
   d. Heart displaced from the sternum.
      – Pneumothorax.
      – Mediastinal shift.
2. Hypovolaemia.
   a. Shock.
   b. Dehydration.
   c. Hypoadrenocorticism (Addison's disease) – may be accompanied by megaoesophagus.
3. Muscle mass loss.
   a. Emaciation.
      – Chronic systemic disease.
      – Malnutrition.
   b. Hypoadrenocorticism (Addison's disease).
   c. Atrophic myopathies.
4. Constrictive pericarditis.
5. Post thoracotomy.

7.5 GENERALIZED ENLARGEMENT OF THE CARDIAC SILHOUETTE

Some of the following diseases may only cause mild cardiomegaly or cardiomegaly only in advanced stages of the condition. Chamber lumen

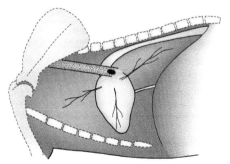

Figure 7.4 Microcardia, pulmonary hypoperfusion and small caudal vena cava.

dilation and heart wall hypertrophy cannot be distinguished radiographically, and myocardial pathology is much more readily diagnosed by means of two-dimensional and M-mode echocardiography.

Because it is hard to differentiate the left and right sides of the heart radiographically, disease that is confined to one side may nevertheless appear radiographically as generalized heart enlargement (see 7.8, 7.9, 7.11 and 7.12); the list below includes only diseases that genuinely affect both right and left sides. Assessment of pulmonary vasculature is also important in radiographic assessment of cardiac disease (see 6.23).

1. Normal.
   a. Athletic breeds (e.g. Greyhound and other sight hounds).
   b. Some young animals.
2. Artefactual.
   a. Intrapericardial and mediastinal fat (see 7.6.1).
   b. Expiratory radiograph.
3. Fluid overload.
4. Bradycardia (e.g. due to sedation), allowing increased diastolic filling.
5. End-stage, left-heart failure due to mitral valve insufficiency.
   a. Myxomatous atrioventricular valvular degeneration (endocardiosis).
   b. Valvular dysplasia.
   c. Bacterial endocarditis.
6. Congenital cardiac disease (see 7.8, 7.9, 7.11 and 7.12) – although specific chambers may be particularly enlarged, generalized cardiomegaly is often seen radiographically.
7. Non-inflammatory myocardial disease.
   a. Unknown aetiology.
      – Idiopathic dilated cardiomyopathy – large and giant breed mainly male dogs, 2–7 years old – especially Dobermann, Great Dane, Irish Wolfhound, Scottish Deerhound, Boxer, Dalmatian and Spaniels; juvenile dilated cardiomyopathy in Portuguese Water Dogs. Occasionally seen in cats.
      – Hypertrophic cardiomyopathy – rare in dogs (Rottweiler, Dalmatian and German Shepherd dogs may be predisposed); more common in adult male cats.
      – Restrictive cardiomyopathy – younger cats, rare; differential diagnosis

endocardial fibroelastosis, a congenital condition in Siamese and Burmese kittens and cats under 1 year old.

b. Secondary to a known aetiology.
- End-stage mitral valve insufficiency.
- Nutritional deficiency (e.g. carnitine).
- Toxic (e.g. cytotoxic drugs such as doxorubicin), heavy metals and toxaemia.
- Metabolic disorders, for example hypertrophic cardiomyopathy secondary to hyperthyroidism (especially in older cats) and hyperadrenocorticism.
- Arrhythmogenic right ventricular cardiomyopathy – Boxers, inherited; also cats: massively dilated right chambers.
- Cats – dilated cardiomyopathy; nutritional deficiency such as taurine, now rare due to dietary supplementation.
- Cats – dilated cardiomyopathy possibly genetic in Siamese, Burmese and Abyssinian.
- Cats – hypertrophic cardiomyopathy is genetic in Maine Coon cats.
- Cats – acromegaly (hypersomatotropism) may cause hypertrophic, occasionally dilated, cardiomyopathy.
- Cats – hypertrophic feline muscular dystrophy; also diaphragmatic changes.
- Neuromuscular disorders.
- Amyloidosis.
- Lipidosis.
- Mucopolysaccharidosis.
- Infiltrative disease (e.g. neoplasia and glycogen storage diseases).
- Physical agents (e.g. heat and trauma).
- Old age.

8. Concurrent left and right heart valvular insufficiency.
a. Myxomatous atrioventricular valvular degeneration (endocardiosis).
b. Valvular dysplasia.
c. Bacterial endocarditis.

9. Inflammatory myocardial disease.
a. Infectious.
- Viral (e.g. parvovirus in puppies).
- Bacterial.
- Mycoplasma.
- Protozoal (e.g. trypanosomiasis*).
- Parasitic.
- Fungal.
b. Non-infectious.
- Immune-mediated (e.g. rheumatoid arthritis).

10. Ischaemic myocardial disease.
a. Arteriosclerosis and thrombosis of large coronary artery branches.
b. Arteriosclerosis, amyloidosis or hyalinosis of intramural coronary arteries.
c. Angiopathies secondary to congenital heart disease.

11. Chronic anaemia.

12. Hyperviscosity syndrome (e.g. multiple myeloma).

13. Phaeochromocytoma – due to excessive catecholamine production.

14. Pericardial disease – see 7.6.

7.6 PERICARDIAL DISEASE

Pericardial disease may be difficult to distinguish from generalized cardiomegaly radiographically. The main difference is that most cases of cardiomegaly have left atrial enlargement, whereas pericardial effusion produces an enlarged, globular cardiac silhouette lacking specific chamber enlargement (Fig. 7.5). Its margins may be sharp due to reduced movement blur. Pericardial effusion may also often be differentiated from generalized cardiomegaly by the type of failure that results, which is right-sided, whereas left-sided or generalized failure is seen with the most common cause of generalized cardiomegaly, cardiomyopathy. Ultrasonography is the imaging modality of choice to evaluate pericardial pathology (see 7.7).

1. Artefactual appearance of pericardial effusion – obese animals may have large amounts of intrapericardial and mediastinal fat mimicking an enlarged cardiac silhouette and possible pericardial effusion. Fat is less radiopaque than soft tissue such as the myocardium, and on good-quality radiographs the pericardial fat can be distinguished from the myocardium; contrast can be enhanced by obtaining radiographs using lower kVp exposures. Normal pericardial fat often demonstrates the cardiac contour in animals with pleural effusion in which the heart is otherwise obscured.

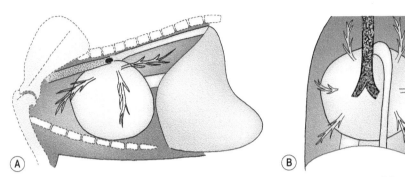

Figure 7.5 Pericardial effusion – the heart is enlarged and very rounded in shape: (A) lateral view; (B) dorsoventral view. In the case of pericardioperitoneal diaphragmatic hernia, gas-filled loops of the gastrointestinal tract may also be seen within the pericardial silhouette.

2. Pericardial effusion – usually male dogs over 6 years old and weighing more than 20 kg.
   a. Non-inflammatory pericardial effusions.
      – Idiopathic benign effusion, especially in the St Bernard and Golden Retriever; often haemorrhagic.
      – Hypoalbuminaemia.
      – Right-sided congestive heart failure, particularly feline hypertrophic cardiomyopathy.
      – Toxaemia.
      – Uraemia.
      – Trauma.
      – Neoplastic obstruction of lymph and blood vessels at the heart base.
      – Associated with a peritoneopericardial diaphragmatic hernia.
   b. Inflammatory pericardial effusions.
      – Idiopathic benign effusion.
      – Foreign body.
      – Septic, purulent process sometimes secondary to perforating wounds.
      – Tuberculosis.
      – Coccidioidomycosis*.
      – Steatitis.
      – Cats – feline infectious peritonitis is the most common cause.
   c. Neoplastic pericardial effusions – usually haemorrhagic (rare in the cat).
      – Right atrial haemangiosarcoma, especially in the German Shepherd dog and often associated with pulmonary, splenic or hepatic haemangiosarcoma.
      – Heart base tumours (see 7.16.2).
      – Mesothelioma.
      – Metastatic neoplasia.
      – Lymphoma, especially cats.
      – Thyroid carcinoma.
      – Rhabdomyosarcoma.
   d. Haemopericardium.
      – Bleeding tumour.
      – Trauma (e.g. gunshot, bite wound, sequel to pericardiocentesis).
      – Rupture of the left atrium by a severe jet lesion secondary to mitral valve insufficiency – especially Dachshund, Poodle and Cocker Spaniel.
      – Coagulopathy.
   e. Chylous pericardial effusion – very rare and of unknown aetiology.
3. Congenital peritoneopericardial diaphragmatic hernia (PPDH) – may be accompanied by sternal abnormalities and an umbilical hernia. Gas-filled intestinal loops or faecal material may be seen within the cardiac silhouette; sternal abnormalities may also be present. Often diagnosed only later in life.
4. Pneumopericardium – rare, usually due to trauma and not clinically significant; also reported secondary to positive-pressure ventilation and due to communication with lung bulla.
5. Intrapericardial cyst – rare. If large, mimics a pericardial effusion and may cause tamponade. Young animals; may be associated with a peritoneopericardial diaphragmatic hernia.
6. Pericardial neoplasia – rare; may extend externally (e.g. lipoma).

7.7 ULTRASONOGRAPHY OF PERICARDIAL DISEASE

1. Pericardial fluid (see 7.6.2 above). Usually anechoic or hypoechoic fluid. Swirling echoes within the fluid are suggestive of large numbers of cells, debris or gas bubbles. The pericardium may be thickened and distorted if the fluid is inflammatory. It is important to check for the presence of cardiac tamponade secondary to the fluid accumulation; in the early stages this is indicated by collapse of the right atrial wall during systole, and in more advanced cases by abnormal motion of the right ventricular free wall (Fig. 7.6). Right atrial collapse due to pericardial effusion may, however, be mimicked by severe pleural effusion.
2. Intrapericardial mass.
   a. Neoplasia.
      – Right atrial haemangiosarcoma; seen best on a right-sided long-axis four-chamber view, usually at the junction of the atrium and ventricle and extending into the pericardial sac (Fig. 7.6).
      – Heart base tumour; seen best on a right-sided short-axis view just dorsal to the aortic valve.
      – Others, listed in 7.6.2c.
   b. Thrombus.
   c. Abdominal organs in a peritoneopericardial diaphragmatic hernia.
   d. Intrapericardial cyst.

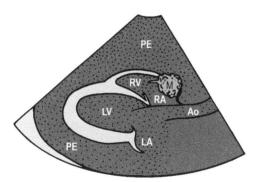

Figure 7.6 Right parasternal long-axis ultrasonogram of pericardial effusion, showing anechoic to hypoechoic fluid accumulation within the pericardial sac, with collapse of the right atrial wall during systole (cardiac tamponade). A mass is also seen at the junction of the right atrium and ventricle, most likely to be a haemangiosarcoma. Ao, aorta; LA, left atrium; LV, left ventricle; M, mass; PE, pericardial effusion; RA, right atrium; RV, right ventricle.

3. Thickening of the epicardium or pericardium – may lead to a restrictive state in which complete filling of the cardiac chambers is prevented.
   a. Mesothelioma.
   b. Reactive or inflammatory changes.

7.8 LEFT ATRIAL ENLARGEMENT

The lateral view shows bulging of the cardiac silhouette at 12–2 o'clock, with elevation and compression of the left main stem bronchus. The caudal border of the heart is abnormally straight and upright or even slopes caudodorsally, and the caudal cardiac waist is lost (Fig. 7.7A). On the DV view, atrial enlargement may push the main stem bronchi further apart (to > 60 °) and the enlarged left auricular appendage creates a bulge at 2–3 o'clock (Fig. 7.7B). The increased opacity of the dilated left atrium may be mistaken as lymphadenopathy or a lung mass on either view. Secondary pulmonary changes in the form of vascular congestion or pulmonary oedema may be present (see 6.14 and 6.24).

Volume overload

1. Mitral valve insufficiency.
   a. Myxomatous atrioventricular valvular degeneration (endocardiosis) – older, small-breed dogs.
   b. Secondary to left ventricular failure when the enlarging ventricle results in dilation of the annular ring (e.g. dilated cardiomyopathy).
   c. Bacterial endocarditis.
   d. Ruptured left ventricular chordae tendineae.
   e. Congenital mitral valve dysplasia – especially Great Dane, German Shepherd dog, Bull Terrier and cats.
   f. Ruptured papillary muscle.
2. Diastolic dysfunction of the left ventricle resulting in pooling of blood in the left atrium.
3. Patent ductus arteriosus with left to right shunting – especially German Shepherd dog, Spaniels, Border Collie, Keeshond, Pomeranian, Miniature Poodle and Irish Setter. About 25% of cases show a classic triad of aortic, pulmonary artery and left auricular appendage bulges on the DV view (Fig. 7.8).
4. Ventricular septal defect with left to right shunting – especially Border Collie, Springer Spaniel, West Highland White Terrier, Beagle, Bulldog, German Shepherd dog, Keeshond, Mastiff, Siberian Husky and cats.

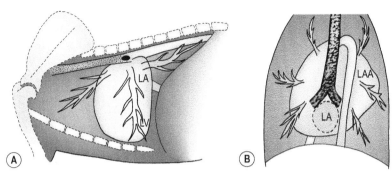

Figure 7.7 Left-sided cardiomegaly: (A) lateral view showing a tall heart and an enlarged left atrium; (B) dorsoventral view showing the enlarged left auricular appendage at 2–3 o'clock and the left atrium as a mass between the main stem bronchi. The heart apex is displaced to the right due to marked left ventricular enlargement. Signs of left-sided heart failure (pulmonary hyperperfusion and oedema) may also be present. LA, left atrium; LAA, left auricular appendage; LV, left ventricle.

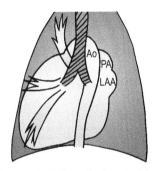

Figure 7.8 Dorsoventral view of a heart with patent ductus arteriosus, showing a classic triad of three bulges, representing an enlarged aortic arch (Ao, at 11–1 o'clock), an enlarged pulmonary artery (PA, at 1–2 o'clock) and an enlarged left auricular appendage (LAA, at 2–3 o'clock). Left ventricular enlargement causes the cardiac apex to lie on the right. There is also pulmonary hyperperfusion.

5. Aorticopulmonary septal defect with left to right shunting.
6. Endocardial fibroelastosis – Siamese and Burmese kittens.

Pressure overload

7. Left ventricular hypertrophy leading to mitral insufficiency.
   a. (Sub)aortic stenosis – especially Boxer, Golden Retriever, German Shepherd dog, Newfoundland, Pointer, Rottweiler, Bulldog and Bull Terriers.
   b. Hypertrophic cardiomyopathy – rare in dogs; in cats a 'valentine'-shaped heart is seen on the DV view due to atrial enlargement.

   – Idiopathic hypertrophic cardiomyopathy; cats and dogs.
   – Hypertrophic cardiomyopathy secondary to hyperthyroidism in older cats.
   c. Cats – restrictive cardiomyopathy – valentine heart on the DV view.
8. Congenital mitral valve stenosis – especially Newfoundland, Bull Terrier and cats – rare.
9. Cor triatriatum sinister – membranous septum in the left atrium.
10. Atrial or ventricular neoplasia interfering with transvalvular flow – rare.

7.9 LEFT VENTRICULAR ENLARGEMENT

On the lateral view, cardiac enlargement is seen at 2–5/6 o'clock, with increased height of the heart and elevation of the trachea (Fig. 7.7A). Left atrial enlargement is usually also present. On the DV view, the heart may appear elongated and enlargement is seen at 3–5 o'clock; in severe cases this displaces the cardiac apex to the right (Fig. 7.7B) (right heart enlargement due to, for example, pulmonic stenosis may displace the cardiac apex further to the left on the DV radiograph, mimicking left ventricular enlargement).

Volume overload

1. Mitral valve insufficiency (see 7.8.1).
2. Aortic insufficiency.
3. Patent ductus arteriosus with left to right shunting – the most common congenital cardiac condition in the dog but far less common in cats.

4. Ventricular septal defect with left to right shunting.
5. Endocardial cushion defects (persistent atrioventricular canal).
6. Aorticopulmonary septal defect.
7. Arteriovenous fistula.

Pressure overload

Results in concentric hypertrophy and often does not cause ventricular silhouette enlargement.

8. (Sub)aortic stenosis.
9. Systemic hypertension.
   a. Chronic renal failure, especially in cats.
   b. Hyperthyroidism.
   c. Hyperadrenocorticism (Cushing's disease).
10. Hypertrophic cardiomyopathy – rare in dogs. In cats, a valentine-shaped heart is seen on the DV view due to atrial enlargement.
    a. Idiopathic hypertrophic cardiomyopathy; cats and dogs.
    b. Hypertrophic cardiomyopathy secondary to hyperthyroidism in older cats.
    c. Acromegaly in cats.
11. Coarctation (narrowing) of the aorta – very rare.

Myocardial failure (see 7.5)

12. Dilated cardiomyopathy.
13. Myocarditis.
14. Myocardial neoplasia (see 7.16).

Miscellaneous

15. Ventricular aneurysm – localized protrusion of the left ventricle.
16. Thickened walls due to muscular dystrophy – Golden Retriever and cats.

7.10 AORTIC ABNORMALITIES

1. Enlargement of the aortic arch or descending aorta. On the lateral view, enlargement of the aortic arch may be seen at 11–12 o'clock, with reduction or possibly obliteration of the cranial cardiac waist (Fig. 7.9A). On the DV view, an aortic 'knuckle' is seen from 11 to 1 o'clock with mediastinal widening, and there is an apparent increase in the craniocaudal length of the heart (Fig. 7.9B).
   a. Post-aortic stenosis dilation – entire aortic arch.
   b. Large left to right shunting PDA due to increase in aortic circulating blood volume and inherent aortic wall weakness – predominantly descending part of aortic arch.
   c. Aneurysms.
      – Secondary to *Spirocerca lupi** migration or granulomas – seen as left-sided undulations of the descending aorta on a DV or VD view.
      – Idiopathic, with aortic dissection.
      – Ductus aneurysm or diverticulum.
      – Secondary to coarctation (narrowing of the aortic isthmus, between the left subclavian artery and the insertion of the ductus arteriosus).
   d. Aortic body tumour (chemodectoma).
   e. Systemic hypertension in cats.
   f. Coarctation (narrowing) of the aorta with post-stenotic dilation.
2. Redundant (tortuous or bulging) aorta.
   a. Brachycephalic breeds, especially the Bulldog.
   b. Some older dogs.
   c. Congenital hypothyroidism.

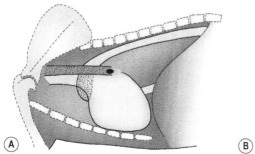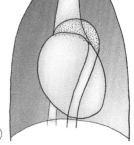

Figure 7.9 Location of an enlarged aortic arch: (A) lateral view; (B) dorsoventral view.

d. Systemic hypertension in cats.
e. Common in old cats, accompanied by a more horizontal heart – aorta bulges cranially and to the left.
3. Right-sided aorta.
   a. Congenital persistent right aortic arch; a vascular ring anomaly with secondary oesophageal dilation (see 8.17.6 and Fig. 8.12).
   b. Situs inversus (see Fig. 7.3C).
4. Calcification or mineralization of the aorta – uncommon and usually an incidental finding. Seen more easily on CT images.
   a. Idiopathic, of aortic bulb, aortic valves or coronary arteries; older dogs, especially Rottweilers.
   b. Lymphoma.
   c. Renal failure.
   d. Primary or secondary hyperparathyroidism.
   e. Arteriosclerosis.
   f. Hyperadrenocorticism (Cushing's disease).
   g. *Spirocerca lupi** larval migration – descending aorta.
   h. Hypervitaminosis D.

7.11 RIGHT ATRIAL ENLARGEMENT

On the lateral view, bulging of the cardiac silhouette occurs at 10–11 o'clock, with increased craniocaudal dimension of the heart and elevation of the terminal trachea and/or loss of the cranial cardiac waist in severe cases. There may be a widened CdVC as result of venous congestion (Fig. 7.10A). On the DV view, bulging is seen at 9–11 o'clock (Fig. 7.10B). In obese cats, the right atrial area outline may have a square or angular appearance on VD radiographs, due to pericardial fat rather than genuine chamber enlargement.

Volume overload

1. Tricuspid valve insufficiency.
   a. Myxomatous atrioventricular valvular degeneration (endocardiosis).
   b. Congenital tricuspid valve dysplasia – more common in cats than dogs; also Labrador and German Shepherd dog.
   c. Secondary to right ventricular failure when the enlarging ventricle results in dilation of the annular ring.
   d. Ebstein's anomaly – the valve leaflets are deformed and valvular insertions are displaced distally into the right ventricle; may be seen with tricuspid dysplasia.
   e. Bacterial endocarditis – more common in left heart.
   f. Ruptured right ventricular chordae tendineae.
   g. Anomalous pulmonary venous drainage.
   h. Chronic increased right ventricular pressure.
2. Atrial septal defect with left to right shunting – Old English Sheepdog, Samoyed and Boxer predisposed.
3. Arteriovenous fistula elsewhere in the body.

Pressure overload

4. Right ventricular hypertrophy leading to tricuspid insufficiency.
   a. Pulmonic stenosis – may result in secondary tricuspid valve insufficiency;

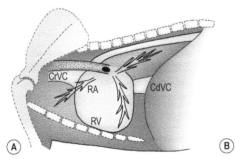
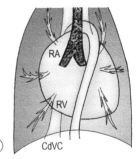

Figure 7.10 Right-sided cardiomegaly: (A) lateral view, showing rounding of the cranial heart margin and increase in sternal contact; (B) dorsoventral view, in which the heart has an inverted D shape due to rounding of the right heart border. Signs of right-sided heart failure (vena cava engorgement, hepatomegaly and ascites) may also be present. CdVC, caudal vena cava; CrVC, cranial vena cava; RA, right atrium; RV, right ventricle.

especially Boxer, Cavalier King Charles and Cocker Spaniel, Labrador, Bulldog, West Highland White Terrier, Yorkshire Terrier, Fox Terrier, Chihuahua, Miniature Schnauzer, Beagle and Keeshond; rare in cats.

b. Single right coronary artery giving rise to constricting circumpulmonary left coronary artery – Bulldogs.

c. Tetralogy of Fallot – especially the Keeshond.

5. Atrial or ventricular neoplasia interfering with transvalvular flow (see 7.16).

6. Cor pulmonale (see 7.12.9).

7. Congenital tricuspid valve stenosis – rare.

8. Cor triatriatum dexter – membranous septum in the right atrium.

Miscellaneous

9. Artefact – superimposed mediastinal, pulmonary or heart base mass.

10. Right atrial neoplasia – haemangiosarcoma, especially the German Shepherd dog and often associated with pulmonary, splenic or hepatic haemangiosarcoma.

11. Arrhythmogenic right ventricular cardiomyopathy (see 7.5.7).

12. Aneurysmal dilation of the right auricle though a pericardial defect.

13. Right atrial dilation has been reported in a Golden Retriever with polymyositis and myocarditis.

7.12 RIGHT VENTRICULAR ENLARGEMENT

Artefactual right ventricular enlargement may be seen on left lateral recumbent radiographs, in which there is increased sternal contact, rounding of the heart outline and elevation of the cardiac apex from the sternum. On the DV view, tilting of the chest with the sternum to the right may also create the false appearance of right-sided bulging. On the lateral view, right ventricular enlargement creates cardiac bulging at 5/6–9/10 o'clock, with increased craniocaudal dimension and increased sternal contact of more than 2.5 sternebrae in deep-chested dogs and 3.5 in broad-chested dogs. Accentuation of the cranial cardiac waist may occur (Fig. 7.10A). On the DV view, enlargement is at 5–9 o'clock, with excessive rounding of the right ventricle producing an inverted D-shaped heart (Fig. 7.10B). Puppies normally have a prominent right ventricle. Signs of right-sided failure include CdVC engorgement, hepatomegaly and ascites (pleural effusion is common in cats).

Volume overload

1. Tricuspid valve insufficiency (see 7.11.1).

2. Pulmonic valve insufficiency.

3. Ventricular septal defect.

4. Atrial septal defect.

5. Endocardial cushion defects (persistent atrioventricular canal) – more common in cats.

6. Arteriovenous fistula elsewhere in the body.

Pressure overload

Results in concentric hypertrophy and therefore may cause less cardiac silhouette enlargement than with volume overload.

7. Secondary to left heart failure or mitral valve disease (see 7.8).

8. Pulmonic stenosis.

9. Pulmonary hypertension (cor pulmonale).

a. *Dirofilaria immitis** (heartworm) or *Angiostrongylus vasorum** ('French' heartworm) infections – with hypervascular lung pattern and secondary bronchopneumonia.

b. Severe lung pathology; examples include:
  – Thromboembolism.
  – Primary pulmonary hypertension.
  – Chronic obstructive pulmonary disease.
  – High-altitude disease.
  – Pulmonary arteriovenous fistula.
  – Pulmonary vasculitis.

c. Various congenital heart diseases.
  – Ventricular septal defect.
  – Patent ductus arteriosus (left to right shunting with overcirculation; right to left shunting due to pulmonary hypertension).
  – Mitral valve dysplasia.
  – Aorticopulmonary septal defect.
  – Cor triatriatum sinister.

d. Secondary to chronic upper airway obstruction.

10. Eisenmenger's syndrome – pulmonary blood flow obstruction or pulmonary hypertension results in right to left shunting through a

congenital shunt (e.g. PDA or septal defect) and therefore cyanosis.

a. Defects combined with pulmonic stenosis.
  – Tetralogy of Fallot – the most common cyanotic heart disease of dogs; especially the Keeshond and English Bulldog, and cats.
  – Trilogy or pentalogy of Fallot.
  – Double outlet right ventricle – may be difficult to distinguish from tetralogy of Fallot.
  – Cats – persistent truncus arteriosus.

11. Single right coronary artery resulting in secondary constrictive pulmonic stenosis.
12. Congenital double-chambered right ventricle – especially in cats.
13. Primary infundibular stenosis – especially Golden Retriever and Alaskan Malamute.
14. Pulmonary artery neoplasia – haemangiosarcoma and chondrosarcoma described.

Myocardial failure

15. Dilated cardiomyopathy.
  a. Generalized together with left ventricular involvement.
  b. Arrhythmogenic right ventricular cardiomyopathy (see 7.5.7).
16. Myocarditis.
17. Myocardial neoplasia (see 7.16).

Miscellaneous

18. Ventricular aneurysm – localized protrusion of the right ventricle.

7.13 PULMONARY ARTERY TRUNK ABNORMALITIES

On the lateral view, enlargement may be difficult to see unless large, as the bulge may be superimposed over the terminal trachea. On the DV view, a pulmonary artery knuckle is seen at 1–2 o'clock (Fig. 7.11). On the VD view, a pulmonary artery knuckle is commonly seen in normal animals due to lateral tilting of the heart.

1. Artefactual.
  a. Radiograph made at the end of ventricular systole, especially in deep-chested dogs.
  b. Rotation of the thorax.
  c. Dorsal recumbency for VD view, resulting in tilting of the heart.

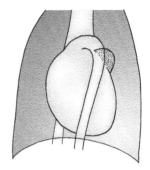

Figure 7.11 Location of an enlarged pulmonary artery segment; a knuckle is seen at 1–2 o'clock on the dorsoventral view.

2. Post-pulmonic stenosis dilation.
3. Increased circulating blood volume with large left to right shunts.
  a. Patent ductus arteriosus.
  b. Atrial septal defect.
  c. Ventricular septal defect.
4. Elevated pulmonary artery pressure secondary to pulmonary hypertension (cor pulmonale) (see 7.12.9).
5. Large collections of *Dirofilaria** or *Angiostrongylus** worms.
6. Pulmonary artery chondrosarcoma with mineralization.

7.14 CHANGES IN PULMONARY ARTERIES AND VEINS

See 6.23 (*Vascular lung pattern*).

7.15 CAUDAL VENA CAVA ABNORMALITIES

Temporary changes in the diameter of the CdVC are common incidental findings and may be due to thoracic and abdominal pressure changes and to differences in the cardiac or respiratory cycle. The ratio of the greatest CdVC diameter to the aortic diameter at the same intercostal space may be calculated. A ratio of < 1.0 indicates a normal CdVC; a ratio of > 1.5 indicates an abnormally widened CdVC.

Persistent widening of the caudal vena cava

Budd–Chiari syndrome is defined in humans as suprahepatic portal hypertension due to posterior (i.e. caudal) vena cava obstruction; the commonest causes are thrombosis, neoplasia or the presence of an obstructing membrane (e.g. due to cor triatriatum dexter). The condition has also been recognized in dogs and appears radiographically as a marked enlargement of the CdVC. Signs of right-sided heart failure may ensue.

1. Right heart failure.
2. Tricuspid valve insufficiency.
   a. Congenital dysplasia.
   b. Myxomatous atrioventricular valvular degeneration (endocardiosis).
   c. Endocarditis.
3. Cardiac tamponade due to pericardial effusion.
4. Constrictive pericarditis.
5. Obstruction of the right atrium or ventricle.
   a. Tumours (see 7.16).
   b. Thrombi.
6. Tumours infiltrating the CdVC.
   a. Phaeochromocytoma.
   b. Other invasive tumours from the right atrium, liver and kidney.
7. Large collections of *Dirofilaria** worms.
8. Pulmonary hypertension (see 7.12.9).
9. Cor triatriatum dexter – membranous septum in the right atrium.
10. Idiopathic CdVC stenosis.
11. Caudal vena cava thrombi.

Narrowed caudal vena cava

Often accompanied by microcardia, pulmonary undercirculation and in extreme cases a small aorta.

12. Shock.
13. Severe dehydration.
14. Pulmonary overinflation (see 6.25.4–6).
15. Hypoadrenocorticism (Addison's disease).

Absent caudal vena cava

16. Very rare congenital anomaly – abdominal blood flow returns via a greatly distended azygos vein.

Gas lucency in caudal vena cava

17. Air embolism (e.g. following dentistry with high-speed, air-driven drill) – gas also seen in cranial vena cava, right heart and abdominal veins; may cause cardiac arrest and sudden death.

7.16 CARDIAC NEOPLASIA

Uncommon; often there is little visible change to the cardiac silhouette unless the tumour is large or a pericardial effusion results (see 7.6). Heart base tumours may elevate the terminal trachea. Most clinically significant tumours are visible ultrasonographically.

Right atrial wall tumours

1. Haemangiosarcoma – especially the German Shepherd dog (primary or metastatic). May be accompanied by pericardial effusion and/or pulmonary, splenic or hepatic haemangiosarcoma.

Heart base tumours

2. Aortic body tumour (chemodectoma) – more common in older, male, brachycephalic dogs especially Boxers and Boston Terriers; very rare in the cat.
3. Ectopic thyroid tumour.
4. Ectopic parathyroid tumour.

Right chamber tumours

5. Myxoma.
6. Haemangiosarcoma – pericardial effusion common.
7. Fibroma.
8. Ectopic thyroid carcinoma.
9. Fibrosarcoma.
10. Myxosarcoma.
11. Chondrosarcoma.
12. Infiltrative chemodectoma.
13. Lipoma.
14. Metastatic tumours.

Left chamber tumours

Very rare in dogs and cats – types as for right chamber tumours.

Myocardial tumours

15. Metastatic tumours.
16. Haemangiosarcoma.
17. Rhabdomyosarcoma.
18. Lymphoma – especially cats.

Epicardial tumours

Pericardial effusion common.

19. Mesothelioma.
20. Metastatic neoplasia.

ANGIOGRAPHY

Many of the diagnoses previously made angiographically can now be made using echocardiography. *Selective angiography* is generally reserved for veterinary schools and specialist referral centres, as it requires high-pressure injectors and rapid cassette changers.

Non-selective angiography can readily be performed in private practice. The largest possible catheter is placed in a peripheral vein or passed to the right atrium or terminal cranial or CdVC. A water-soluble iodinated contrast medium is injected rapidly at a dose rate of 1–2 mL/kg and two to six radiographs are made immediately in lateral recumbency at 1 to 2 s intervals using a cassette tunnel. Sedation or general anaesthesia is necessary to prevent motion and avoid the need for manual restraint. Radiographs made within the first 4–5 s will generally demonstrate the right heart chambers, and those made after 5–6 s the left heart chambers.

7.17 ANGIOGRAPHY: LEFT HEART

Selective angiography with the catheter tip in the ascending aorta: abnormalities

1. Dilated aorta.
   a. Ascending aorta dilated.
      – Post stenotic dilation.
   b. Proximal descending aorta dilated.
      – Patent ductus arteriosus.
      – Patent ductus arteriosus ductus diverticulum; congenital or post surgically.
      – Dilation distal to coarctation (narrowing) of the aorta.
   c. Distal descending aorta dilated.
      – *Spirocerca lupi**.
2. Contrast crossing into the pulmonary vasculature – PDA with left to right shunting (usual).
3. Contrast refluxing into the left ventricle – aortic insufficiency.
4. Valvular defects.
5. Supravalvular stenosis.

6. Aortic interruption – absent initial descending aorta with a collateral vertebral artery supplying the caudal descending aorta.
7. Anomalous branching of the aortic arch.
8. Coronary artery anomalies.

Selective angiography with the catheter tip in the left ventricle: abnormalities

9. Contrast refluxing into the left atrium.
   a. Mitral valve insufficiency.
   b. Mechanical effect of the catheter.
   c. Premature ventricular contractions during the contrast injection.
10. Small left ventricular lumen with thick walls.
    a. Pressure overload (see 7.9.8–11).
    b. Hypertrophic cardiomyopathy.
       – Idiopathic hypertrophic cardiomyopathy; rare in dogs, commoner in cats.
       – Hypertrophic cardiomyopathy secondary to hyperthyroidism in older cats.
       – Acromegaly in cats.
11. Large left ventricular lumen with thin walls – volume overload (see 7.9.1–7).
12. (Sub)aortic stenosis.
13. Filling defects in the left ventricle.
    a. Thrombi.
    b. Papillary muscle hypertrophy in pressure overload (see 7.9.8–11).
    c. Tumours – rare.
14. Poor filling of the aorta – poor myocardial contractility.
15. Simultaneous filling of the right ventricle and pulmonary artery.
    a. Ventricular septal defect with left to right shunting.
    b. Tetralogy of Fallot.

Selective angiography with the catheter tip in the left atrium: abnormalities

16. Enlarged left atrium (see 7.8).
17. Simultaneous filling of the right atrium – ASD with left to right shunting.
18. Filling defects in the left atrium.
    a. Thrombi.
    b. Tumours – rare.
19. Mitral valve defects.

7.18 ANGIOGRAPHY: RIGHT HEART

Non-selective angiography with the catheter in a vein, or selective angiography with the catheter in the right atrium, ventricle or pulmonary artery: abnormalities

1. Filling defects in the right atrium, ventricle or pulmonary artery.
   a. Papillary muscle hypertrophy in pressure overload (see 7.12.7–14).
   b. *Dirofilaria** or *Angiostrongylus** worms.
   c. Thrombi.
   d. Lobar pulmonary artery thromboembolism.
   e. Tumours (see 7.16).
2. Small right ventricular lumen with thick walls – pressure overload (see 7.12.7–14).
3. Large right ventricular chamber with thin walls – volume overload (see 7.12.1–6).
4. Simultaneous filling of the left atrium – ASD with right to left shunting.
5. Simultaneous filling of the left ventricle.
   a. Ventricular septal defect with right to left shunting.
   b. Tetralogy of Fallot.
6. Contrast in the right atrium with ventricular catheter tip placement.
   a. Tricuspid insufficiency.
   b. Mechanical effect of the catheter.
   c. Premature ventricular contractions during the contrast injection.
7. Tricuspid and pulmonic valve defects.
8. Pulmonic stenosis.
9. Apparent thick atrial wall – restrictive pericarditis.
10. Eisenmenger's syndrome (see 7.12.10).
11. Dilated pulmonary arch – post-stenotic dilation.
12. Simultaneous filling of the pulmonary artery and aorta – PDA with right to left shunting (unusual).
13. Contrast in the right ventricle with pulmonary artery catheter tip placement.
   a. Pulmonic valve insufficiency.
   b. Mechanical effect of the catheter.

CARDIAC ULTRASONOGRAPHY

Two-dimensional echocardiography is the ideal diagnostic imaging modality for evaluation of the internal structure of the heart. The best images are obtained by scanning from the dependent side through a hole in a special table or platform. The heart falls to the dependent side and displaces the adjacent lung away from the heart, creating an acoustic window. Cardiac chamber and wall size are more accurately measured by means of M-mode echocardiography. Flow abnormalities may be detected using Doppler echocardiography or by identifying abnormalities of valvular motion in M-mode. Normal echocardiographic values are published, but as for the radiographic vertebral heart scale measurement, breed-specific differences need to be taken into account.

7.19 TWO-DIMENSIONAL AND M-MODE ECHOCARDIOGRAPHY: LEFT HEART

In the normal animal, the left heart chamber dimensions and ventricular wall thickness should be approximately 2–3 times those of the right ventricle, as seen from a right parasternal long-axis view.

Left atrial abnormalities

On a right parasternal long-axis M-mode view, atrial enlargement is present in the dog when the left atrium to aortic diameter ratio is > 0.95 and in the cat when the ratio is between 1 and 2 (Fig. 7.12A); alternatively, on a two-dimensional right parasternal short-axis view when the ratio is > 1.5 in the dog and > ≈ 1.6 in the cat (Fig. 7.12B).

1. Left atrial enlargement – volume overload (see 7.8.1–6).
   a. Mitral valve insufficiency – valvular abnormalities.
      – Incomplete closure during systole.
      – Valvular growths or nodules: myxomatous atrioventricular valvular degeneration (endocardiosis) and bacterial endocarditis.
      – Congenital valve deformity – mitral dysplasia.
      – Reverse doming (valve prolapses into the atrium) due to weak chordae tendineae.
      – Flail valve (valve prolapses into the atrium) due to chordae tendineae or papillary muscle rupture.
   b. Atrial septal defect – the adjacent edges of the septal walls are often thickened.
2. Left atrial enlargement – pressure overload (see 7.8.7–10).

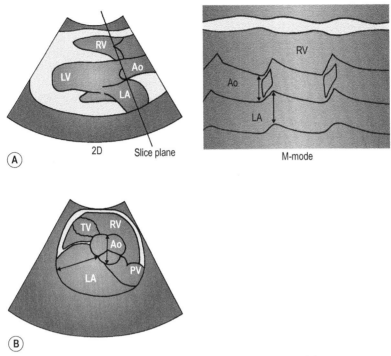

Figure 7.12 Left atrial measurement: (A) on right parasternal long-axis M-mode, and (B) on short-axis two-dimensional mode. Ao, aorta; LA, left atrium; LV, left ventricle; PV, pulmonic valve; RV, right ventricle; TV, tricuspid valve.

a. Mitral valve stenosis.
  – Doming of the valve leaflets.
  – Thickening of the valve leaflets.
  – Incomplete separation of the valve leaflets.
b. Cor triatriatum sinister – membranous septum in the left atrium.

3. Left atrial lumen abnormalities.
  a. Thrombi – hypoechoic; may float freely or be attached to the wall, particularly in the auricular appendage; may act as a ball valve.
  b. Tumours – very rare, hypo- to hyperechoic (see 7.16).
  c. Ruptured chordae tendineae – thin, linear streak in the region of the valve.
  d. Membranous septum in the atrium – cor triatriatum sinister.

Mitral valve abnormalities (Fig. 7.13)

4. Increased E point to septal separation (EPSS).
  a. With normal mitral valve movement.
    – Myocardial failure (e.g. dilated cardiomyopathy) due to decreased fractional shortening.
    – Volume overload (e.g. PDA) (see 7.8.1–6 and 7.9.1–7).

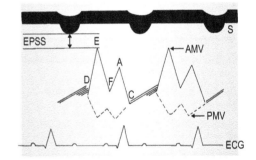

Figure 7.13 Schematic representation of normal M-mode mitral valve motion seen from the right parasternal long-axis view. A, peak mitral valve opening during atrial contraction; AMV, anterior mitral valve; C, complete closure of valve at the start of ventricular systole; D, end of ventricular systole; E, peak opening of mitral valve during early diastolic flow; ECG, electrocardiogram trace; EPSS, E point to septal separation; F, nadir of initial diastolic closing; PMV, posterior mitral valve; S, interventricular septum.

  b. Restricted mitral valve motion.
    – Aortic insufficiency.
    – Mitral valve stenosis.
  c. Reduced mitral valve motion.
    – Low cardiac output.

5. Decreased E point to septal separation.
   a. Increased fractional shortening.
      - Mitral valve insufficiency.
      - Aortic insufficiency.
      - Sympathetic over-stimulation.
      - High altitude.
      - Severe anaemia.
   b. Mitral valve growths.
      - Myxomatous atrioventricular valvular degeneration (endocardiosis).
      - Bacterial endocarditis.
   c. Pathological septal thickening.
      - (Sub)aortic stenosis.
      - Hypertrophic cardiomyopathy.
      - Hyperthyroidism.
      - Infiltrative cardiac disease.
      - Systemic hypertension.
   d. Physiological septal thickening.
      - Athletic dogs.
6. Thickened mitral valve leaflets.
   a. Myxomatous atrioventricular valvular degeneration (endocardiosis).
   b. Bacterial endocarditis.
   c. Valve dysplasia.
   d. Valve stenosis.
7. Lack of late diastolic (A peak) opening.
   a. Atrial fibrillation.
   b. Pulsus alternans – absent A peak every other beat; English Cocker Spaniels.
8. Diastolic anterior mitral valve flutter – aortic valve insufficiency.
9. Systolic mitral valve flutter – mitral valve insufficiency.
10. Abnormal systolic location of mitral valves.
    a. Valve prolapse.
       - Secondary to myxomatous atrioventricular valvular degeneration (endocardiosis).
       - Stretching of chordae tendineae.
       - Rupture of minor chordae tendineae.
       - Redundancy during hyperdynamic states.
    b. Systolic anterior motion of the mitral valve.
       - (Sub)aortic stenosis.
       - Hypertrophic cardiomyopathy.
       - Left ventricular hypertrophy.
       - Hyperkinesis.
    c. Flail valve – rupture of major chordae tendineae.

11. Abnormal diastolic location of mitral valves.
    a. Tips of valve leaflets pointing towards each other with doming of the valve – stenosis.
12. Decreased EF slope.
    a. Mitral valve stenosis (will include concordant anterior diastolic motion of the anterior and posterior mitral valve leaflets).
    b. Left ventricular diastolic dysfunction (e.g. hypertrophic cardiomyopathy).
    c. Decreased transmitral flow.
13. Normal E and A peaks followed by one or more A peaks only – second- and third-degree atrioventricular block.
14. E to A peak ratio changes – see 7.22.
15. Pulsus alternans – alternation of the pattern of mitral valve diastolic motion – English Cocker Spaniels with dilated cardiomyopathy.

Left ventricular abnormalities

16. Left ventricular chamber enlargement (see 7.9).
    a. Breed variation (e.g. Greyhound).
    b. Mitral valve insufficiency – valvular abnormalities.
       - See left atrium (7.19.1 and 7.19.2).
       - Displaced papillary muscles and chordae tendineae.
    c. Aortic valve insufficiency – valvular abnormalities.
       - Incomplete closure during diastole.
       - Valvular growths or nodules: myxomatous atrioventricular valvular degeneration (endocardiosis) and bacterial endocarditis.
       - Abnormally positioned valve.
    d. Ventricular septal defect seen in the proximal part of the septum.
17. Thickened left ventricular wall and/or septum as adjudged during diastole.
    a. Breed variation (e.g. Greyhound).
    b. Artefactual due to dehydration with relatively smaller chamber.
    c. Pressure overload with prominent papillary muscles and a small chamber (see 7.9.8–11).
    d. Hypertrophic cardiomyopathy.
       - Idiopathic hypertrophic cardiomyopathy; rare in dogs, commoner in cats. Hypertrophy may be generalized, or localized to certain areas of the ventricular wall, septum or papillary muscles. In cats, diastolic wall thickness > 6 mm on two-dimensional echocardiography confirms the diagnosis.

– Hypertrophic cardiomyopathy secondary to hyperthyroidism in older cats.
  – Acromegaly in cats.
  e. Boxer cardiomyopathy.
  f. Myocardial tumours (see 7.16).
  g. Hyperthyroidism.
  h. Cats – mild restrictive cardiomyopathy.
  i. Cats – hypertrophic muscular dystrophy.
18. Changes in echogenicity.
  a. Endocardium hyperechoic, possibly including papillary muscles.
    – (Sub)aortic stenosis.
    – Restrictive cardiomyopathy in the cat.
  b. Myocardium.
    – Chronic infarction – hyperechoic and thinner.
    – Neoplasia – hyperechoic and thicker.
    – Contusion – variable.
19. Altered fractional shortening of the left ventricle.
  a. Increased (hyperkinesis).
    – Mitral valve insufficiency.
    – (Sub)aortic stenosis and/or aortic insufficiency.
    – Volume overload with retained myocardial function – VSD or ASD.
    – Sympathetic stimulation.
    – Hyperthyroidism.
    – High altitude.
    – Severe anaemia.
  b. Decreased (hypo- or dyskinesia).
    – With myocardial failure (see 7.5).
    – End-stage left heart failure.
    – Drugs, including general anaesthesia.
20. Paradoxical septal motion – septum moves towards the right ventricle in systole, resulting in a flattened appearance on a right parasternal short-axis view.
  a. Right ventricle pressure overload – see 7.12.
  b. Right ventricle volume overload – see 7.12.
21. Lumen abnormalities.
  a. See left atrium (7.19.3).
  b. Linear transverse echogenic lines – moderator bands, rare in left ventricle.
22. Congenital membranous ventricular septal aneurysm – a thin membrane protruding into the right ventricle from the margins of a VSD, which may or may not be still patent.

Aortic and aortic valve abnormalities

23. Aortic stenosis.
  a. Thickening of the valve leaflets.
  b. Doming of the valve leaflets.
  c. Distorted or fused valves.
24. Thickened valve leaflets or valve growths.
  a. Myxomatous atrioventricular valvular degeneration (endocardiosis) – usually small.
  b. Bacterial endocarditis – may be large and can calcify.
25. M-mode systolic fluttering.
  a. Subvalvular or valvular aortic stenosis.
  b. Incidental.
  c. Hypertrophic obstructive cardiomyopathy.
26. M-mode diastolic flutter – aortic insufficiency.
27. Prolapse of the valve – high VSD.
28. Decreased aortic excursion.
  a. Advanced myocardial failure.
  b. Reduced cardiac output.
29. Normal opening followed by gradual closure.
  a. Myocardial failure.
  b. Severe mitral valve insufficiency.
30. Early systolic closure of valve.
  a. Aortic stenosis.
  b. Dynamic obstruction to flow.
31. Widened aortic root (sinus of Valsalva or beyond).
  a. Systemic hypertension in cats.
  b. Aneurysm.
32. Quadricuspid aortic valve (four leaflets).

7.20 TWO-DIMENSIONAL AND M-MODE ECHOCARDIOGRAPHY: RIGHT HEART

In the normal animal, the right heart chambers and ventricular wall thickness should be approximately one-third to one-half those of the left ventricle, as seen from a right parasternal long-axis view.

Right atrial abnormalities

1. Right atrial enlargement – volume overload (see 7.11.1–3).
  a. Tricuspid valve insufficiency – valvular abnormalities.
    – Incomplete closure during systole.

- Valvular growths or nodules: myxomatous atrioventricular valvular degeneration (endocardiosis) and bacterial endocarditis.
- Congenital valve deformity – tricuspid dysplasia.
- Reverse doming (valve prolapses into the atrium) due to weak chordae tendineae.
- Flail valve (valve prolapses into the atrium) due to chordae tendineae or papillary muscle rupture.
- Abnormally positioned valves: Ebstein's anomaly.
- Interference by *Dirofilaria** or *Angiostrongylus** worms.

  b. Atrial septal defect; the adjacent edges of the septal walls are often thickened.
  c. Arteriovenous fistula.

2. Right atrial enlargement – pressure overload (see 7.11.4–8).
   a. Tricuspid valve stenosis – rare.
   - Doming of the valve.
   - Thickening of the valve.
   - Incomplete separation of the valve leaflets.
   - Arrhythmogenic right ventricular cardiomyopathy (see 7.5.8); with right ventricular dilation, hypokinesia and paradoxical septal motion.
   b. Cor triatriatum dexter – membranous septum in the right atrium.

3. Right atrial wall abnormalities.
   a. Abnormal flapping motion of the right atrial wall – cardiac tamponade due to pericardial effusion or severe, bilateral pleural effusion; collapses inwards during diastole.
   b. Hypoechoic mass – haemangiosarcoma.

4. Right atrial lumen abnormalities.
   a. Thrombi – hypoechoic masses; may float freely or be attached to the wall, particularly in the auricular appendage.
   b. Tumours – hypo- to hyperechoic (see 7.16).
   c. Short, parallel echogenic lines 2 mm apart – *Dirofilaria** or *Angiostrongylus** worms.
   d. Membranous septum in the atrium – cor triatriatum dexter.
   e. Thin linear streak in the region of the valve – ruptured chordae tendineae.

Tricuspid valve abnormalities

5. Thickened tricuspid valves.
   a. Myxomatous atrioventricular valvular degeneration (endocardiosis).
   b. Bacterial endocarditis – less common than in the left heart.
   c. Tricuspid valve dysplasia.
   d. Tricuspid valve stenosis.

6. Diastolic tricuspid valve flutter – pulmonic valve insufficiency.

7. Systolic tricuspid valve flutter.
   a. Tricuspid valve insufficiency.
   b. Ventricular septal defect – accurate only in the absence of tricuspid insufficiency.

8. Abnormal systolic location of valves.
   a. Valve prolapse.
   - Secondary to myxomatous atrioventricular valvular degeneration (endocardiosis).
   - Stretching of chordae tendineae.
   - Rupture of minor chordae tendineae.
   b. Flail valve – rupture of major chordae tendineae.

9. Additional hyperechoic lines – *Dirofilaria** or *Angiostrongylus** worms.

Right ventricular abnormalities

10. Right ventricular chamber dilation (see 7.12).
    a. Tricuspid valve insufficiency – valvular abnormalities.
    - See right atrium (7.20.1 and 7.20.2).
    - Displaced papillary muscle and chordae tendineae.
    - Abnormally positioned tricuspid valve: Ebstein's anomaly.
    b. Pulmonic valve insufficiency – valvular abnormalities.
    - Incomplete closure during diastole.
    - Valvular growths or nodules: myxomatous atrioventricular valvular degeneration (endocardiosis) and bacterial endocarditis.
    - Abnormally positioned valve.
    c. Ventricular septal defect.
    d. Arrhythmogenic right ventricular cardiomyopathy (see 7.5.8); with right atrial dilation, hypokinesia and paradoxical septal motion.

11. Thickened right ventricular wall and septum with smaller chamber and often enlarged papillary muscles – pressure overload (see 7.12.7–14).
    a. Pulmonic stenosis.
    b. Pulmonary hypertension.
    c. Myocardial tumours (see 7.16).
12. Thickened right ventricular wall and enlarged right ventricle is seen in neonates.
13. Changes in echogenicity of the myocardium (see 7.19.18).
14. Abnormal flapping motion of the right ventricular wall – cardiac tamponade due to pericardial effusion.
15. Paradoxical septal motion – pressure overload (see 7.12.7–14).
16. Congenital membranous ventricular septal aneurysm – a thin membrane protruding into the right ventricle from the margins of a VSD, which may or may not be still patent.
17. Right ventricular lumen abnormalities.
    a. See right atrium (7.20.4).
    b. Linear transverse echogenic bands – moderator bands.
    c. Mid-ventricular muscular bundles from septum to free wall due to congenital double-chambered right ventricle, particularly in cats.
    d. Primary infundibular stenosis, especially Golden Retriever and Alaskan Malamute.
18. Transposed aorta – tetralogy of Fallot.

Pulmonic valve and pulmonary artery abnormalities

19. Pulmonic stenosis.
    a. Thickening of the valve leaflets.
    b. Doming of the valve leaflets.
    c. Distorted or fused valves.
20. Valve prolapse – PDA.
21. Distension of pulmonary artery – post-stenotic dilation.

7.21 CONTRAST ECHOCARDIOGRAPHY: RIGHT HEART

The anechoic blood may be temporarily replaced by multiple small echogenic specks. These are most readily created by rapid injections of agitated saline; 20 mL of saline is repeatedly transferred between two 20-mL syringes via a three-way stopcock and then injected into a peripheral vein. The echogenic specks should pass rapidly through the right heart and be absorbed in the pulmonary vasculature.

1. Pulsating filling defects within the echogenic cloud in the right atrium or ventricle adjacent to the septum – left to right shunting ASD or VSD, respectively.
2. Simultaneous specks in the left atrium or ventricle – right to left shunting (rare) ASD or VSD, respectively.
3. Persistence of echogenic specks in the right atrium and ventricle – tricuspid valve insufficiency.
4. Persistence of echogenic specks in the right ventricle – pulmonic valve insufficiency.
5. Echogenic specks in the abdominal aorta with normoechoic left heart and ascending aorta – PDA with right to left shunting (unusual).
6. Echogenic specks in the ascending aorta with normoechoic left heart – tetralogy of Fallot (overriding aortic arch).

7.22 DOPPLER FLOW ABNORMALITIES: MITRAL VALVE

1. Ventricular side increased forward diastolic flow.
    a. Laminar flow due to increased blood volume.
       – Mitral valve insufficiency.
       – Left to right shunting PDA.
       – Right to left shunting ASD.
    b. Turbulent flow – mitral stenosis – rare.
2. Ventricular side decreased forward diastolic flow.
    a. Left to right shunting ASD.
    b. Hypovolaemia.
       – Shock.
       – Dehydration.
    c. Drugs resulting in decreased blood pressure.
    d. Poor cardiac output.
    e. Left ventricular diastolic dysfunction; the A peak (active diastolic flow) is likely to be higher than the E peak (passive first diastolic flow).
       – (Sub)aortic stenosis.
       – Hypertrophic cardiomyopathy.
       – Systemic hypertension.
       – Restrictive cardiomyopathy.
    f. Lack of inflow every second cardiac cycle – pulsus alternans; English Cocker Spaniels with dilated cardiomyopathy.

3. Ventricular side E:A changes (normal ratio in the dog is > 1 and < 2).
    a. Decreased E:A.
        – Left ventricular diastolic dysfunction (see 7.22.2e above).
        – High altitude due to increased A peaks.
4. Atrial side increased forward diastolic flow – laminar flow due to increased blood volume (see 7.22.1 above).
5. Atrial side turbulent, high-velocity, reversed systolic flow – mitral insufficiency.
    a. Mild, detectable just behind the valve – physiological.
    b. Myxomatous atrioventricular valvular degeneration (endocardiosis).
    c. Bacterial endocarditis.
    d. Dilated left ventricle with secondary dilation of the annular ring.
    e. Mitral valve dysplasia.
6. Atrial side turbulent, low-velocity reversed diastolic flow – second- and third-degree atrioventricular block.
7. Pulsus alternans – alteration in regurgitant velocity; English Cocker Spaniels with dilated cardiomyopathy.

7.23 DOPPLER FLOW ABNORMALITIES: AORTIC VALVE

1. Aortic side increased forward systolic flow.
    a. Artefact – normally higher from a subcostal approach than from apical or right parasternal long-axis locations.
    b. Laminar flow due to increased blood volume.
        – Left to right shunting PDA.
        – Right to left shunting ASD or VSD.
        – Severe aortic insufficiency.
    c. Turbulent, high velocity.
        – Stenosis, usually subvalvular with peak velocity reached closer to mid systole, resulting in a more symmetric flow shape.
        – Hypertrophic cardiomyopathy – peak velocity usually reached later in systole with a concave, scimitar-shaped flow acceleration.
2. Aortic side decreased forward systolic flow.
    a. Left to right shunting ASD or VSD.
    b. Hypovolaemia.
        – Shock.
        – Dehydration.

c. Drugs resulting in decreased blood pressure.
    d. Poor cardiac output.
3. Ventricular side increased forward systolic flow – laminar flow due to increased blood volume (see 7.23.1 above).
4. Ventricular side reversed turbulent diastolic flow – aortic insufficiency.
    a. Mild, just behind the valve – physiological.
    b. Accompanying valvular stenosis.
    c. Bacterial endocarditis.
    d. Idiopathic.
    e. Flail aortic valve.
    f. Quadricuspid aortic valve (four leaflets).
5. Pulsus alternans – alternation in stroke volume in aortic outflow – English Cocker Spaniels with dilated cardiomyopathy.

7.24 DOPPLER FLOW ABNORMALITIES: TRICUSPID VALVE

1. Ventricular side increased forward diastolic flow.
    a. Laminar flow due to increased blood volume.
        – Tricuspid valve insufficiency.
        – Left to right shunting ASD.
    b. Turbulent flow – tricuspid stenosis – rare.
2. Ventricular side decreased forward diastolic flow.
    a. Right to left shunting ASD (rare).
    b. Hypovolaemia.
        – Shock.
        – Dehydration.
    c. Drugs resulting in decreased blood pressure.
    d. Poor cardiac output.
    e. Right ventricular diastolic dysfunction; the A peak (active diastolic flow) is likely to be higher than the E peak (passive first diastolic flow).
        – Pulmonic stenosis.
        – Pulmonary hypertension.
3. Atrial side increased forward diastolic flow – laminar flow due to increased blood volume (see 7.24.1 above).
4. Atrial side turbulent, high-velocity, reversed systolic flow – tricuspid insufficiency.
    a. Mild, detectable just behind the valve – physiological.
    b. Myxomatous atrioventricular valvular degeneration (endocardiosis).
    c. Bacterial endocarditis.

d. Dilated right ventricle with secondary dilation of the annular ring.

e. Secondary to pulmonic stenosis.

f. Tricuspid valve dysplasia.

7.25 DOPPLER FLOW ABNORMALITIES: PULMONIC VALVE

1. Pulmonary artery side increased forward systolic flow.
   a. Laminar flow due to increased blood volume.
      - Left to right shunting ASD or VSD.
      - Severe pulmonic valve insufficiency.
   b. Laminar flow due to high altitude.
   c. Turbulent, high velocity.
      - Adjacent to the valve due to valvular stenosis.
      - Starting further distally due to pulmonary artery atresia.
      - Compression of the outflow tract (e.g. heart base mass).
2. Pulmonary artery side increased forward or reversed (depending on cursor location) diastolic flow of turbulent, low to medium velocity – left to right shunting PDA, aorticopulmonary septal defect.
3. Pulmonary artery side decreased forward systolic flow.
   a. Right to left shunting ASD or VSD (rare).
   b. Hypovolaemia.
      - Shock.
      - Dehydration.
   c. Drugs resulting in decreased blood pressure.
   d. Poor cardiac output.
   e. Pulmonary hypertension.
4. Pulmonary peak systolic velocity reached within the first third of flow time (peak velocity is normally reached close to the middle of flow time; Fig. 7.14A): the acceleration time:flow time ratio is decreased (Fig. 7.14B).

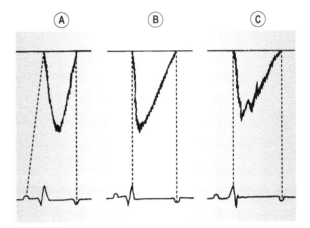

Figure 7.14 Doppler systolic flow patterns of the pulmonary artery: (A) dome-like flow in a dog with normal pulmonary artery pressure; (B) early peak of flow with increased pulmonary artery pressure; (C) early peak and notched decelerating flow seen with severely increased pulmonary artery pressure.

   a. Pulmonary hypertension.
   b. *Dirofilaria** or *Angiostrongylus** worms in the right heart.
5. Pulmonary peak systolic velocity reached within the first third of flow time with notched deceleration flow.
   a. Severe pulmonary hypertension (Fig. 7.14C).
6. Ventricular side increased forward systolic flow.
   a. Laminar flow due to increased blood volume (see 7.25.1).
   b. Turbulent flow due to dynamic right ventricular outflow obstruction in cats.
7. Ventricular side reversed, turbulent diastolic flow – pulmonic valve insufficiency.
   a. Mild, just behind the valve – physiological.
   b. Idiopathic.
   c. Accompanying valvular stenosis.

Further reading

Radiology and general

Brummitt, J.W., Essman, S.C., Kornegay, J.N., Graham, J.P., Webere, W.J., Berry, C.R., 2006. Radiographic features of golden retriever muscular dystrophy. Vet. Radiol. Ultrasound 47, 574–580.

Buchanan, J.W., 2000. Vertebral scale system to measure heart size in radiographs. Vet. Clin. North Am. Small Anim. Pract. 30, 379–394.

Buchanan, J.W., Bucheler, J., 1995. Vertebral scale system to measure canine heart size in radiographs. J. Am. Vet. Med. Assoc. 206, 194–199.

Cobb, M.A., Brownlie, S.E., 1992. Intrapericardial neoplasia in 14 dogs. J. Small Anim. Pract. 33, 309–316.

Douglass, J.P., Berry, C.R., Thrall, D.E., Malarkey, D.E., Spaulding, K.A., 2003. Radiographic features of aortic bulb/valve mineralization in 20 dogs. Vet. Radiol. Ultrasound 44, 20–27.

Godshalk, C.P., 1994. Common pitfalls in radiographic interpretation of the thorax. Compend. Contin. Educ. Pract. Veterinarian (Small Animal) 16, 731–738.

Guglielmini, C., Pietra, M., Cipone, M., 2001. Aorticopulmonary septal defect in a German shepherd dog. J. Am. Anim. Hosp. Assoc. 37, 433–437.

Herrtage, M.E., Gorman, N.T., Jefferies, A.R., 1992. Coarctation of the aorta in a dog. Vet. Radiol. Ultrasound 33, 25–30.

Lamb, C.R., Boswood, A., 2002. Role of survey radiography in diagnosing canine cardiac disease. Compend. Contin. Educ. Pract. Veterinarian (Small Animal) 24, 316–326.

Lamb, C.R., Wikeley, H., Boswood, D.U., Pfeiffer, D.U., 2001. Use of breed-specific ranges for the vertebral heart scale as an aid to the radiographic diagnosis of cardiac disease in dogs. Vet. Rec. 148, 707–711.

Lehmkuhl, L.B., Bonagura, J.D., Biller, D.S., Hartman, W.M., 1997. Radiographic evaluation of caudal vena cava size in dogs. Vet. Radiol. Ultrasound 38, 94–100.

Litster, A.L., Buchanan, J.W., 2000. Radiographic and echocardiographic measurement of the heart in obese cats. Vet. Radiol. Ultrasound 41, 320–325.

Litster, A.L., Buchanan, J.W., 2000. Vertebral scale system to measure heart size in radiographs of cats. J. Am. Vet. Med. Assoc. 216, 210–214.

Martin, M., 1999. Pericardial disease in the dog. In Pract. 21, 378–385.

Moon, M.L., Keene, B.W., Lessard, P., Lee, J., 1993. Age related changes in the feline cardiac silhouette. Vet. Radiol. Ultrasound 34, 315–320.

Myer, C.W., Bonagura, J.D., 1982. Survey radiography of the heart. Vet. Clin. North Am. Small Anim. Pract. 12, 213–237.

Rishniw, M., 2000. Radiography of feline cardiac disease. Vet. Clin. North Am. Small Anim. Pract. 30, 395–426.

Schwarz, T., Sullivan, M., Störk, C.K., Willis, R., Harley, R., Mellor, D.J., 2002. Aortic and cardiac mineralization in the dog. Vet. Radiol. Ultrasound 43, 419–427.

Schwarz, T., Willis, R., Summerfield, N.J., Doust, R., 2005. Aneurysmal dilatation of the right auricle in two dogs. J. Am. Vet. Med. Assoc. 226, 1512–1515.

Shaw, S.P., Rush, J.E., 2007. Canine pericardial effusion: pathophysiology and cause; diagnosis, treatment and prognosis. Compend. Contin. Educ. Vet. 29, 400–403 and 405–410.

Stafford-Johnson, M., 2006. Decision making in suspected congenital heart disease in dogs and cats. In Pract. 28, 538–543.

Thrall, D.E., Losonsky, J.M., 1979. Dyspnoea in the cat: Part 3 – radiographic aspects of intrathoracic causes involving the heart. Feline Pract. 9, 36–49.

Tilley, L.P., Bond, B., Patnaik, A.K., Liu, S.K., 1981. Cardiovascular tumors in the cat. J. Am. Anim. Hosp. Assoc. 17, 1009–1021.

Warman, S., Pearson, G., Barrett, E., Shelton, D.G., 2008. Dilatation of the right atrium in a dog with polymyositis and myocarditis. J. Small Anim. Pract. 49, 302–305.

Webster, N., Adams, V., Dennis, R., 2009. The effect of manual lung inflation vs. spontaneous inspiration on the cardiac silhouette in anesthetized dogs. Vet. Radiol. Ultrasound 50, 172–177.

Echocardiography

Bonagura, J.D., 1983. M-mode echocardiography: basic principles. Vet. Clin. North Am. Small Anim. Pract. 13, 299–319.

Bonagura, J.D., Herring, D.S., 1985. Echocardiography: congenital heart disease. Vet. Clin. North Am. Small Anim. Pract. 15, 1195–1208.

Bonagura, J.D., Herring, D.S., 1985. Echocardiography: acquired heart disease. Vet. Clin. North Am. Small Anim. Pract. 15, 1209–1224.

Bonagura, J.D., Pipers, F.S., 1981. Echocardiographic features of pericardial effusion in dogs. J. Am. Vet. Med. Assoc. 179, 49–56.

Bonagura, J.D., O'Grady, M.R., Herring, D.S., 1985. Echocardiography: principles of interpretation. Vet. Clin. North Am. Small Anim. Pract. 15, 1177–1194.

Boswood, A., Lamb, C., 2005. Doppler ultrasound examination in dogs and cats. 3. Assessment of cardiac disease. In Pract. 27, 286–292.

Darke, P.G.G., 1992. Doppler echocardiography. J. Small Anim. Pract. 33, 104–112.

Darke, P.G.G., 1993. Transducer orientation for Doppler echocardiography in dogs. J. Small Anim. Pract. 34, 208.

Jacobs, G., Knight, D.H., 1985. M-mode echocardiographic measurements in nonanesthetized healthy cats: effect of body weight, heart rate, and other variables. Am. J. Vet. Res. 46, 1705–1711.

Kirberger, R.M., 1991. Mitral valve E point to septal separation in the dog. J S Afr. Vet. Assoc. 62, 163–166.

Kirberger, R.M., Bland-van den Berg, B., Daraz, B., 1992. Doppler echocardiography in the normal dog. Part I, Velocity findings and flow patterns. Vet. Radiol. Ultrasound 33, 370–379.

Kirberger, R.M., Bland-van den Berg, R.J., Grimbeek, R.J., 1992. Doppler echocardiography in the normal dog. Part II, Factors influencing blood flow velocities and a comparison between left and right heart blood flow. Vet. Radiol. Ultrasound 33, 380–386.

Koffas, H., Luis Fuentes, V., Boswood, D.J., Connolly, D.J., Brockman, D.J., Bonagura, J.D., et al., 2007. Double chambered right ventricle in 9 cats. J. Vet. Intern. Med. 21, 76–80.

Lange, E., Beaudu-Lange, C., 2009. Septal myocardial abscess in a male great Anglo-French hound. J. Small Anim. Pract. 50, 311–316.

Lombard, C.W., 1984. Echocardiographic and clinical signs of canine dilated cardiomyopathy. J. Small Anim. Pract. 25, 59–70.

Luis Fuentes, V., 1992. Feline heart disease: an update. J. Small Anim. Pract. 33, 130–137.

Luis Fuentes, V., 1993. Cardiomyopathy in cats. In Pract. 15, 301–308.

Lusk, R.H., Ettinger, S.J., 1990. Echocardiographic techniques in the dog and cat. J. Am. Anim. Hosp. Assoc. 26, 473–488.

Miller, M.W., Knauer, K.W., Herring, D.S., 1989. Echocardiography: principles of interpretation. Semin. Vet. Med Surg. (Small Anim.) 4, 58–76.

Minors, S.L., O'Grady, M.R., Williams, R.M., O'Sullivan, M.L., 2006. Clinical and echocardiographic features of primary infundibular stenosis with intact ventricular septum in dogs. J. Vet. Intern. Med. 20, 1344–1350.

Moise, N.S., 1989. Doppler echocardiographic evaluation of congenital heart disease. J. Vet. Intern. Med. 3, 195–207.

Nelson, O.L., Reidesel, E., Ware, W.A., Christensen, W.F., 2002. Echocardiographic and radiographic changes associated with systemic hypertension in cats. J. Vet. Intern. Med. 16, 418–425.

O'Grady, M.R., Bonagura, J.D., Powers, J.D., Herring, D.S., 1986. Quantitative cross-sectional echocardiography in the normal dog. Vet. Radiol. 27, 34–49.

Rishniw, M., Thomas, W.P., 2002. Dynamic right ventricular outflow obstruction: a new cause of murmurs in cats. J. Vet. Intern. Med. 16, 547–552.

Shober, K.E., Baaded, H., 2006. Doppler echocardiographic prediction of pulmonary hypertension in West Highland white terriers with chronic pulmonary disease. J. Vet. Intern. Med. 20, 912–920.

Soderberg, S.F., Boon, J.A., Wingfield, W.E., Miller, C.W., 1983. M-mode echocardiography as a diagnostic aid for feline cardiomyopathy. Vet. Radiol. 24, 66–73.

Spotswood, T.C., Kirberger, R.M., Koma, L.M.P.K., Thompson, P.N., Miller, D.B., 2006. Changes in echocardiographic variables of left ventricular size and function in a model of canine normovolaemic anemia. Vet. Radiol. Ultrasound 47, 358–365.

Thomas, W.P., 1984. Two-dimensional, real-time echocardiography in the dog: technique and anatomic validation. Vet. Radiol. 25, 50–64.

Thomas, W.P., 2005. Echocardiographic diagnosis of congenital membranous ventricular septal aneurysm on the dog and cat. J. Am. Anim. Hosp. Assoc. 41, 215–220.

Thomas, W.P., Sisson, D., Bauer, T.G., Reed, J.R., 1984. Detection of cardiac masses in dogs by two-dimensional echocardiography. Vet. Radiol. 25, 65–72.

Thomas, W.P., Gaber, C.E., Jacobs, G.J., Kaplan, P.M., Lombard, C.W., Moise, N.S., Moses, B.L., 1993. Recommendation for standards in transthoracic two-dimensional echocardiography in the dog and cat. J. Vet. Med. 7, 247–252.

Chapter 8

Other thoracic structures: pleural cavity, mediastinum, thoracic oesophagus, thoracic wall

CHAPTER CONTENTS

Pleural cavity 199
8.1 Anatomy and radiography of the pleural cavity 199
8.2 Increased radiolucency of the pleural cavity 200
8.3 Increased radiopacity of the pleural cavity 202
8.4 Pleural and extrapleural nodules and masses 204
8.5 Ultrasonography of pleural and extrapleural lesions 205
8.6 Pleural thickening: increased visibility of lung lobe edges 205

Mediastinum 206
8.7 Anatomy and radiography of the mediastinum 206
8.8 Mediastinal shift 207
8.9 Variations in mediastinal radiopacity 208
8.10 Mediastinal widening 209
8.11 Mediastinal masses 210
8.12 Mediastinal lymphadenopathy 212
8.13 Ultrasonography of the mediastinum 212

Thoracic oesophagus 213
8.14 Normal radiographic appearance of the thoracic oesophagus 213
8.15 Oesophageal contrast studies: technique and normal appearance 214
8.16 Abnormalities on oesophageal contrast studies 214
8.17 Oesophageal dilation 215
8.18 Variations in radiopacity of the oesophagus 217

8.19 Oesophageal masses 217
8.20 Oesophageal foreign bodies 218

Thoracic wall 219
8.21 Variations in soft tissue components of the thoracic wall 219
8.22 Variations in the ribs 220
8.23 Variations in the sternum 221
8.24 Variations in thoracic vertebrae 222
8.25 Ultrasonography of the thoracic wall 222
8.26 Variations in the appearance of the diaphragm 222
8.27 Ultrasonography of the diaphragm 224

Miscellaneous 225
8.28 Thoracic trauma 225
8.29 Ultrasonography of thoracic trauma 225

PLEURAL CAVITY

8.1 ANATOMY AND RADIOGRAPHY OF THE PLEURAL CAVITY

The pleural cavity is a potential space between visceral and parietal pleura and surrounding each lung (Fig. 8.1). It contains only a small amount of serous fluid and is normally not visible. Visceral pleura is adherent to the lung surfaces; parietal pleura lines the thoracic wall and forms the mediastinum. In the dog, the caudoventral mediastinal pleura has fenestrations connecting the right and left pleural cavities, making bilateral pleural disease more likely. In the cat, the mediastinal pleura is often intact and unilateral pleural disease is more common. Unilateral or asymmetric pleural pathology may result in a

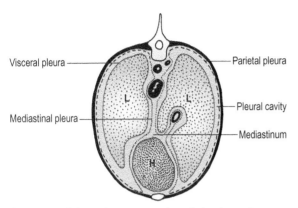

Figure 8.1 Schematic representation of the thorax in cross-section, showing the pleural and mediastinal spaces. H, heart; L, lung.

Visceral pleura — Parietal pleura — Pleural cavity — Mediastinum — Mediastinal pleura

mediastinal shift, with the heart and associated structures moving to the opposite side (see 8.8).

Radiography for suspected pleural disease should always include orthogonal views (lateral and dorsoventral, DV, or ventrodorsal, VD). Positional radiography (e.g. VD versus DV, horizontal beam views) may be helpful to distinguish pleural pathology from other thoracic pathology and to tell whether fluid is freely moving or trapped, provided that placing the animal in other positions does not compromise its well-being. Often, the cause of pleural pathology can be determined only after removal of pleural fluid or air, and follow-up radiographs should therefore always be made after thoracocentesis. Positive contrast peritoneography and gastrointestinal contrast studies may be of value in making a diagnosis when diaphragmatic rupture is present. Lymphangiography is a useful technique for planning thoracic duct ligation in animals with chylothorax: injection of contrast medium into mesenteric lymph nodes or lymphatics is described but requires laparotomy or laparoscopy; a less invasive technique is to inject contrast medium percutaneously into the popliteal lymph nodes, if necessary under ultrasound guidance. Pleurography is now rarely performed. If diagnostic ultrasound is available, it should be performed before draining any pleural fluid (see 8.5).

8.2 INCREASED RADIOLUCENCY OF THE PLEURAL CAVITY

Increased radiolucency results from air within the pleural cavity. The adjacent lung will collapse to a variable degree, making lung edges visible

because free air is more radiolucent than the air–interstitium content of the lung. The lungs show an increased radiopacity due to reduced air content.

1. Artefactual increased radiolucency of the pleural cavity – on careful examination, often requiring a hot light, pulmonary blood vessels will be seen in the area suspected of containing free air.
   a. Overexposure, overdevelopment or fogging of the film.
   b. Überschwinger (halo artefact, rebound effect) on digital radiographs (see Appendix).
   c. Lateral to superimposed axillary folds on the DV view, especially in deep-chested dogs; these can usually be followed outside the thoracic cavity (so-called false pneumothorax – Fig. 8.2A).
   d. Overinflation of the lungs (see 6.25).
   e. Deep inspiration.
   f. Hypovolaemia and pulmonary undercirculation.
   g. Subcutaneous emphysema.
   h. Lobar emphysema.
2. Pneumothorax – variable degrees of retraction of the lungs from the thoracic wall and spine, with surrounding gas lucency and corresponding increase in lung opacity (Fig. 8.2B); the cardiac apex will be separated

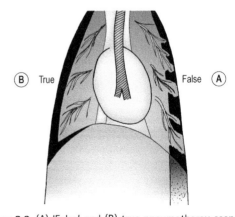

Figure 8.2 (A) 'False' and (B) true pneumothorax seen on the dorsoventral view. With false pneumothorax, the vascular markings are seen to extend to the periphery on hot light examination, and the skin folds continue beyond the thorax.

from the sternum on lateral recumbent radiographs, as support from the dependent lung is lost and the heart falls under gravity into the dependent hemithorax (differentiate from microcardia – see 7.4, and from pulmonary emphysema – see 6.25.6; in both of these, the heart apex may also be separated from the sternum for different reasons). Expiratory radiographs and left lateral recumbent views are more sensitive for the detection of small amounts of free air; alternatively, a standing lateral radiograph or a VD radiograph using a horizontal beam with the patient in lateral recumbency can be used – free air will collect beneath the uppermost part of the spine or rib cage, respectively. Pneumothorax is usually bilateral and symmetrical; focal areas of gas accumulation suggest underlying lung lobe pathology. Flattening and caudal displacement of the diaphragm together with outwardly bulging intercostal soft tissue suggest tension pneumothorax and prompt treatment is required.

a. Trauma with perforation of:
   - Lung and visceral pleura.
   - Thoracic wall and parietal pleura.
b. Spontaneous pneumothorax – tends to be recurring and may be life-threatening; especially large or deep-chested dogs. Classified as primary (rupture of a subpleural bulla or bleb without underlying lung pathology) or secondary (pre-existing lung disease). The underlying cause is usually very difficult to see radiographically and may be diagnosed only during surgery or post-mortem examination. CT is likely to be more rewarding.
   - Rupture of congenital or acquired bulla (between layers of visceral pleura) or bleb (beneath the internal layer of visceral pleura), most often in the apical area.
   - Bullous emphysema – the commonest underlying cause.
   - Rupture of pulmonary cyst.
   - Associated with small airway disease in cats.
   - Bacterial pneumonia.
   - Lung abscess.
   - Neoplasia.
   - Pleural adhesions.

   - Parasitic lesions (*Paragonimus**, *Oslerus**
     and *Dirofilaria**).
   - Migrating pulmonary foreign body (e.g.
     grass awn).
c. Perforations of:
   - Oesophagus.
   - Trachea.
   - Bronchi.
   - Cavitary mass.
d. Iatrogenic.
   - Lung aspirates.
   - Thoracotomy.
   - Thoracocentesis.
   - Neck surgery.
   - Vigorous cardiac massage.
   - Artificial ventilation with a respirator.
e. Secondary to lung lobe torsion; mechanism not known (see 6.17.5 and Fig. 6.11).
f. Infection with gas-producing organisms.
g. Extension of pneumomediastinum (see 8.9.1–6).

3. Diaphragmatic rupture – displaced, gas-filled gastrointestinal tract may result in localized areas of increased radiolucency in the pleural cavity (Fig. 8.3). The wall of the stomach or intestine is usually clearly seen because of enteric gas inside and pulmonic air outside the

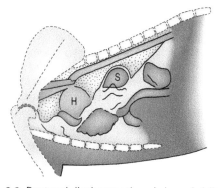

Figure 8.3 Ruptured diaphragm: there is loss of visibility of the heart and diaphragm, with heterogeneous increase in intrathoracic opacity, within which some gas-filled loops are seen. Abdominal organs are displaced cranially. Pericardioperitoneal diaphragmatic hernia may appear similar, but abdominal viscera are confined within the pericardial sac. On a dorsoventral view, similar changes with mediastinal shift to the contralateral side might be seen. H, heart (displaced dorsally and largely obscured); S, gas-filled fundus of stomach.

wall, and mineralized fragments in ingesta may also be visible.

  a. Large radiolucency on the left side of the thorax – herniated and dilated stomach.

  b. Small tubular radiolucencies – herniated small intestine; may enlarge with obstruction or incarceration (also seen with pericardioperitoneal hernia, in which intestine lies within the pericardial sac rather than the pleural cavity).

4. Hydropneumothorax – VD radiographs made with a horizontal beam and the patient in lateral recumbency may be required – usually more fluid than air is present.

  a. Pyopneumothorax – most common.

    – Ruptured pulmonary abscess with bronchopleural fistula.

    – Perforating oesophageal foreign body or *Spirocerca lupi** granuloma.

  b. Haemopneumothorax.

    – Following trauma.

    – Iatrogenic following thoracocentesis.

8.3 INCREASED RADIOPACITY OF THE PLEURAL CAVITY

Lung edges are displaced from the thoracic wall and become visible due to the difference between soft tissue opacity peripherally and air-filled lung centrally (Fig. 8.4A–C). Increased opacity of the pleural cavity must be distinguished from artefactual or genuine increases in lung opacity (see 6.13, 6.14 and 6.22). With severe effusions the heart is obscured, especially on lateral views, due to border effacement. However, in some animals a pericardial fat line is still visible, which suggests the location and size of the heart and may help in deciding whether cardiomegaly is present.

1. Fat opacity – in obese patients, a large sternal fat pad and a thinner layer of subpleural fat may be seen mimicking effusion. Fat may also accumulate in the pericardial sac. On careful examination, the fat will be seen to be less radiopaque than the adjacent cardiac and diaphragmatic silhouettes and no fissure lines will be seen.

2. Pleural effusion – pleural fluid creates interlobar fissure lines (see 8.6.2 and Fig. 8.4A), scalloping of the ventral lung margins, retraction of the lungs from the thoracic wall and border effacement of the heart and diaphragm. On DV

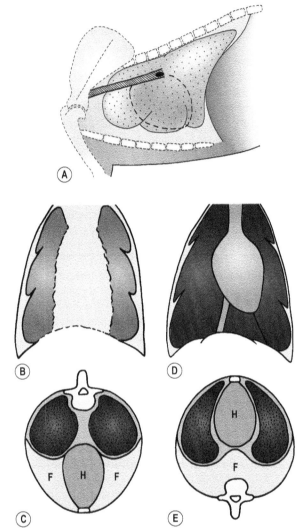

Figure 8.4 Pleural effusion and the effect of positioning on visibility of the heart. (A) Lateral view: the heart outline is obscured and the lungs are partly collapsed, being surrounded by a diffuse soft tissue radiopacity. (B) DV view, resulting in fluid accumulation in the narrow ventral aspect of the thorax, effacing the border of the cardiac silhouette. (C) Diagrammatic cross-section of thorax for dorsoventral (DV) view. (D) Ventrodorsal (VD) view, resulting in fluid accumulation in the wider paraspinal gutter area: the cardiac silhouette is now visible, as air-filled lung surrounds it. (E) Diagrammatic cross-section of thorax for VD view. F, pleural fluid; H, heart; L, lung.

views fissure lines, and border effacement of the heart and diaphragm are seen (Fig. 8.4B, C) whereas on VD views the lung edges are rounded at the costophrenic angle and the heart may still be visible, as the fluid drains into the dorsal (dependent) part of the thorax (Fig. 8.4D and E). Small amounts of fluid are best seen on expiratory radiographs when the thoracic volume is smaller, or on horizontal beam VD views with the affected side down and the beam centred on the lower rib cage. Increasing volumes of fluid result in greater border effacement of the heart and diaphragm, with pulmonary opacity approaching that of the fluid as the lungs collapse and contain less air. Fluid may be free and move with gravity or may be encapsulated or trapped. Fluid collecting around a single lung lobe suggests underlying lobar pathology. All fluids have the same radiographic opacity, and thoracocentesis is required to establish the type of fluid present; repeat radiographic examinations should be made after draining the fluid, to evaluate degree of success of fluid removal and to evaluate the lungs, mediastinum and thoracic wall more completely. The presence of simultaneous pleural and peritoneal effusions carries a poorer prognosis.

a. Artefactual increased radiopacity of the pleural cavity.
   - In obese dogs and cats, due to fat; see above.
   - In normal cats, the caudodorsal lung margins are separated from the thoracic spine on the lateral view by the intrathoracic psoas muscle.
   - In chondrodystrophic breeds, the costochondral junctions are indented medially, which may mimic pleural effusion on the DV or VD radiograph.

b. Transudate or modified transudate; likely to be bilateral.
   - Heart failure (especially in cats).
   - Neoplasia, especially lymphoma and mesothelioma; also may occur in association with ovarian tumours in dogs.
   - Liver lobe incarcerated in a diaphragmatic rupture.
   - Idiopathic effusion.
   - Sterile foreign body.
   - Pneumonia.
   - Hypoalbuminaemia (nephrotic syndrome, protein-losing enteropathy, chronic liver failure).
   - Lung lobe torsion.
   - Glomerulonephritis.
   - Pulmonary thromboembolism – mild.
   - Subarachnoid–pleural fistula (rare).
   - Urothorax (urine) secondary to kidney displaced through a ruptured diaphragm.
   - Cats – hyperthyroidism with or without heart failure.
   - Cats – secondary to perinephric pseudocyst.

c. Exudate; more likely to be unilateral or asymmetrical, as often inflammatory.
   - Pyothorax.
   - Pulmonary abscess.
   - Foreign body (e.g. migrating grass awn).
   - Nocardiosis*.
   - Actinomycosis* – often in combination with mediastinal or pulmonary masses ± rib osteomyelitis.
   - Tuberculosis.
   - Pneumonia.
   - Fungal effusions.
   - Autoimmune disorders (e.g. systemic lupus erythematosus and rheumatoid arthritis) – usually small volumes.
   - Neoplasia; mesothelioma most likely (rib and sternal lesions may also be seen).
   - Bilothorax – trauma (e.g. gunshot) or secondary to cholecystitis, although mechanism for the latter unknown; secondary to biloperitoneum in presence of ruptured diaphragm.
   - Cats – feline infectious peritonitis (FIP).

d. Chyle – conditions that cause increased right-sided venous pressure or obstruction of flow of lymph into the venous system; provokes an exudative response too.
   - Right heart failure, especially cats (may result in constrictive pleuritis).
   - Cardiomyopathy.
   - Congenital heart disease.
   - Pericardial effusion.
   - Trauma, rupturing thoracic duct.
   - Cranial mediastinal mass.
   - Neoplasia.
   - Lung lobe torsion.
   - Thrombosis.
   - Fibrosis.
   - Congenital (e.g. abnormal termination of the thoracic duct).

e. Haemorrhage.
   - Trauma with rupture of a blood vessel, often with cranial rib fractures.
   - Coagulopathy.
   - Bleeding haemangiosarcoma or erosion of blood vessel by other tumour.
   - Autoimmune disorders.
   - Complication of previous thoracic surgery.
   - Lung lobe torsion.
   - Ruptured aortic aneurysm – usually fatal.
   - Blood vessel perforation by aberrant migration of *Spirocerca lupi** larvae – usually fatal.
   - Thromboarteritis in *Dirofilaria immitis** infection.
   - Associated with *Angiostrongylus vasorum** infection, due to coagulopathy or lung rupture.
   - Spontaneous haemorrhage of the involuting thymus gland in young dogs.
   f. Pleural fluid may also arise secondary to abdominal effusion, crossing the diaphragm via lymphatics, for example.
      - Transudate secondary to liver disease.
      - Exudate secondary to pancreatitis.
3. Diaphragmatic rupture – herniation of liver, spleen, fluid-filled gastrointestinal tract or uterus all result in increased pleural opacity (see 8.2.3 and Fig. 8.3).

8.4 PLEURAL AND EXTRAPLEURAL NODULES AND MASSES

1. Artefactual lesions due to overlying soft tissue or osseous changes (see 8.21 and 8.22).
2. Extrapleural masses – these bulge into the pleural cavity from the parietal side of the chest wall, creating an extrapleural sign characterized by a well-demarcated, convex contour with tapering cranial and caudal edges (Fig. 8.5) Such lesions have a tendency to grow inwards rather than outwards and may widen the adjacent intercostal spaces and involve the ribs. They do not move with respiratory motion of the lung on fluoroscopy or ultrasonography. There is no (or minimal) pleural effusion unless the disease process has extended into the pleural cavity. Special

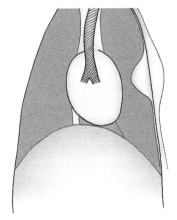

Figure 8.5 The extrapleural sign seen on the dorsoventral view, indicative of a mass lesion arising outside the pleura and not within the lung. See also Figure 8.14 (rib tumour).

oblique radiographs may be required to skyline the pathology.
   a. Rib tumours (see 8.22.5).
   b. Inflammatory conditions.
      - Osteomyelitis of the osseous thoracic wall structures.
      - Abscess.
      - Granuloma.
      - Foreign body reaction.
   c. Soft tissue tumours.
      - Lipoma – fat radiopacity usually obvious.
      - Haemangiosarcoma.
      - Fibrosarcoma.
      - Rhabdomyosarcoma.
   d. Sternal lymphadenopathy (see 8.12.7–11).
   e. Haematoma – as result of trauma and associated rib fractures.
3. Small diaphragmatic ruptures, hernias and eventration – sometimes incidental findings (see 8.26.1).
4. Pleural tumours – visible only after pleural drainage and if large enough.
   a. Mesothelioma – usually multiple or diffuse.
   b. Metastatic carcinomatosis – also diffuse.
5. Pleural abscess or granuloma (e.g. secondary to foreign body).
6. Encapsulated or loculated pleural fluid – does not move with gravity.
7. Pleural fluid collecting around a diseased lung lobe.
8. Fibrin remnants after pleural drainage.

8.5 ULTRASONOGRAPHY OF PLEURAL AND EXTRAPLEURAL LESIONS

Ultrasonography complements radiography in the investigation of pleural disease, especially when free fluid is present, and also allows ultrasound-guided aspiration of pockets of fluid or small lesions. Intercostal, parasternal, transhepatic and thoracic inlet approaches may be used. It may be helpful to scan the patient from different approaches, including the ventral aspect in which the effect of gravity may cause fluid to pool and create a useful acoustic window.

1. Pleural effusion – the ultrasonographic appearance of pleural fluid is variable but is usually anechoic to hypoechoic. Fluid surrounds and separates the lung lobes from each other and the thoracic wall, and acts as a useful acoustic window to examine other parts of the thorax. Many echoes within the fluid usually signify the presence of clumps of cells, debris and/or gas bubbles, although thoracocentesis is required to determine the nature of the fluid. It also facilitates imaging of intrathoracic structures that are not usually seen, such as the great vessels in the cranial mediastinum. The identification of echogenic tags and deposits on pleural surfaces is suggestive of the presence of an exudate, blood or chyle or a diffuse tumour such as mesothelioma. Mesothelioma may also produce cauliflower-like masses, especially in the dorsal part of the thoracic cavity. Inflammatory effusions may result in a septated appearance. For possible causes of pleural effusion, see 8.3.2. Severe pleural effusion may cause right atrial collapse, mimicking cardiac tamponade secondary to pericardial effusion.
2. Hypoechoic or anechoic, well-circumscribed areas.
   a. Encapsulated or trapped fluid.
   b. Pleural abscess.
   c. Haematoma.
   d. Sternal lymphadenopathy.
   e. Soft tissue tumour of homogeneous cellularity and with little haemorrhage or necrosis.
   f. Ectopic liver or a small portion of liver prolapsed through a diaphragmatic tear.
3. Heterogeneous area.
   a. Rib or sternal tumour.
   b. Soft tissue tumour of heterogeneous cellularity and/or fibrosis, calcification, necrosis or haemorrhage.
   c. Inflammatory conditions.
      – Abscess.
      – Granuloma.
      – Foreign body reaction.
4. Viscera within the thorax – the identification of abdominal viscera (e.g. liver, spleen, gastrointestinal tract) within the thoracic cavity is a more certain ultrasonographic indicator of diaphragmatic rupture than identification of the diaphragmatic defect. Variable quantities of thoracic fluid may also be seen.
   a. Artefactual due to mirror image artefact, giving the impression of liver tissue within the thorax when scanning transhepatically (see Appendix).
   b. Viscera not contained within the pericardium – traumatic diaphragmatic rupture.
   c. Viscera apparently contained within the pericardium – congenital peritoneopericardial diaphragmatic hernia.

8.6 PLEURAL THICKENING: INCREASED VISIBILITY OF LUNG LOBE EDGES

Lungs normally extend to the periphery of the thoracic cavity, and individual lobar edges are not seen except in two locations:

- In the cranioventral thorax, where the mediastinum runs obliquely and outlines the cranial segment of the left cranial lobe on a lateral radiograph (see 8.7 and Fig. 8.7A).
- Along the ventral margins of the lungs, which may appear scalloped in some dogs on the lateral radiograph due to intrathoracic fat.

1. Retracted lung borders making the edges visible.
   a. Artefactual.
      – Axillary skin folds or skin folds created by a foam wedge placed under the sternum – the line extends beyond the thorax, and pulmonary vasculature is visible peripheral to the line.
      – Inwardly displaced costochondral junctions in chondrodystrophic breeds, especially the Dachshund and Bassett Hound, creating a false impression of pleural fluid on the DV view.

b. Incidental intrathoracic fat.

c. Pneumothorax.

d. Pleural effusion.

e. Constrictive pleuritis secondary to pyo- or chylothorax (cortication).

f. Atelectasis.

2. Fissure lines – thin, radiopaque lines along the lobar borders (Fig. 8.6A and B).

a. Artefactual.
   – Thin, mineralized costal cartilages (on the DV view these tend to be concave cranially, whereas fissure lines are concave caudally).
   – Scapular spine or edges.

b. Incidental – a fine fissure line is occasionally seen over the heart on left lateral radiographs of larger dogs.

c. Mild pleural effusion – fissure lines are wider peripherally than centrally.

d. Fibrinous pleuritis (cortication) secondary to pyo- or chylothorax – especially in cats. Rounded lung borders outlined by fine, radiopaque lines are seen as the lungs fail to re-expand fully after thoracocentesis.

e. Pleural fibrosis or scarring – fine lines of uniform width.
   – Old age and healed disease.
   – Fungal disease (e.g. coccidioidomycosis* and nocardiosis*).
   – Parasitic disease (e.g. *Filaroides hirthi* and *F. milksi**).

f. Pleural oedema in left heart failure.

g. Dry pleuritis (e.g. migrating intrathoracic grass awns in working dogs).

h. Mediastinal fluid accumulation – fissure lines are seen on the DV or VD view and are wider centrally than peripherally (see 8.10 and Fig. 8.9).

3. Peripheral lobar consolidation or collapse highlighting interfaces with adjacent air-filled lobes.

MEDIASTINUM

8.7 ANATOMY AND RADIOGRAPHY OF THE MEDIASTINUM

The mediastinum is the space between the two pleural sacs and consists of two layers of mediastinal pleura, which separate the thorax into two pleural cavities. It accommodates a large number of structures, including the heart, large blood vessels, trachea, oesophagus and lymph nodes, and lies roughly in the midline (Figs 8.1 and 8.7A and B). Anatomically, it may be divided into cranial (precardiac), middle (cardiac) and caudal (post-cardiac) parts. The cranial part lies between the thoracic inlet and the heart and contains major blood vessels, trachea, oesophagus, lymph nodes, vagus nerve and thymus gland. The middle part contains the heart and major vessels, the terminal trachea and tracheobronchial lymph nodes. The caudal part lies between the heart and the diaphragm and contains the descending aorta, caudal vena cava (CdVC) and oesophagus. The mediastinum communicates cranially with fascial planes of the neck and caudally with the retroperitoneal space via the aortic hiatus. Cranial to the heart, the large dorsal and central soft tissue radiopacity is formed from the cranial thoracic blood vessels, oesophagus, trachea and lymph nodes. On DV or VD radiographs, the width of the cranial mediastinum in dogs should not normally exceed twice the

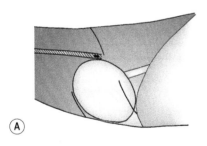

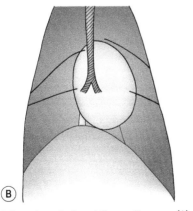

Figure 8.6 Location of pleural fissure lines on: (A) right lateral and (B) dorsoventral view.

width of the vertebral bodies. Ventrally, the cranial mediastinum forms a thin soft tissue fold running obliquely from craniodorsal to caudoventral on the lateral view. On DV or VD radiographs, it extends from craniomedial in a caudolateral direction to the left side, separating the right and left cranial lung lobes. This fold contains the sternal lymph node ventrally, and the thymus in young animals. Caudally, the ventral mediastinum is seen on DV or VD radiographs as a fold displaced into the left hemithorax by the accessory lung lobe. In cats, the width of the craniodorsal mediastinum is less than the width of the superimposed thoracic vertebrae on the DV or VD view and the cranioventral fold is difficult to see.

Apart from the heart, aorta, CdVC and trachea, which are surrounded by air, mediastinal structures cannot be identified separately, as they have similar soft tissue opacity and are in contact with each other. Surprisingly, the caudal oesophagus is rarely visible. The DV or VD view is usually more informative than the lateral for the investigation of mediastinal disease, with the exception of pneumomediastinum, although both views should be obtained. As for pleural disease, it is important to obtain orthogonal radiographs, and positional radiography as described in Section 8.1 may also be helpful when mediastinal and/or pleural fluid are present.

8.8 MEDIASTINAL SHIFT

Mediastinal shift is diagnosed by evaluating the position of the heart, trachea, main stem bronchi, aortic arch and vena cava on well-positioned DV or VD views.

1. Artefactual.
   a. Oblique DV or VD views.
2. Uneven inflation of the two hemithoraces due to unilateral pathology.

Mediastinal movement towards the affected hemithorax

a. Unilateral atelectasis of the lung.
   – General anaesthesia and lateral recumbency (may occur within a few minutes of induction, especially in large dogs).
   – Prolonged lateral recumbency with severe illness.
   – Faulty intubation – endotracheal tube in one bronchus.
   – Mass or foreign body obstructing a bronchus.
   – Cats – feline bronchial asthma with lobar bronchus obstruction.
b. Lung lobe torsion.
c. Lobectomy.
d. Lobar aplasia or hypoplasia.
e. Radiation-induced fibrosis and atelectasis.

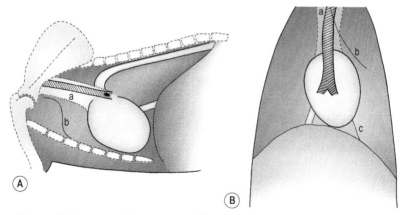

Figure 8.7 Location of the mediastinum on: (A) lateral and (B) dorsoventral or ventrodorsal views. a, Cranial mediastinal structures (blood vessels, oesophagus, trachea and lymph nodes); b, cranioventral fold of the mediastinum; c, caudoventral fold of the mediastinum.

f. Adhesions.

g. Unilateral phrenic nerve paralysis.

Mediastinal movement away from the affected hemithorax

h. Unilateral or asymmetric pneumothorax and tension pneumothorax.

i. Unilateral or asymmetric pleural effusion.

j. Diaphragmatic rupture or hernia (see 8.2.3 and Fig. 8.3).

k. Large lung, pleural or thoracic wall mass.

l. Lobar or unequal emphysema.

3. Chronic pleural disease with adhesions.

4. Contralateral thoracic wall pathology with mass effect (see 8.21 and 8.22).

5. Sternal and vertebral deformities (see 8.23 and 8.24 and Fig. 8.15).

6. Situs inversus – heart apex and caudal mediastinum to right of midline on DV view (see 7.3.5 and Fig. 7.3C).

8.9 VARIATIONS IN MEDIASTINAL RADIOPACITY

Most mediastinal changes are of soft tissue opacity, but the mediastinum may also be less radiopaque due to the presence of fat or air, or more radiopaque due to mineralization.

Reduced mediastinal radiopacity due to air: pneumomediastinum

Generalized pneumomediastinum with dissecting radiolucencies results in increased visibility of mediastinal structures such as blood vessels, tracheal walls and oesophagus (Fig. 8.8). Air may extend into the fascial planes of the neck and progress to subcutaneous emphysema, into the retroperitoneum and into the pericardium (rare). Occasionally, localized pneumomediastinum is seen as pockets of mediastinal air. An air-filled megaoesophagus will also produce mediastinal widening of air lucency and will increase the visibility of the dorsal tracheal wall (see 8.17) and should not be mistaken for pneumomediastinum. Pneumomediastinum may lead to pneumothorax, but the reverse does not occur. Compression of venous structures may cause circulatory collapse.

1. Artefact – gas-filled megaoesophagus superimposed over cranial mediastinal vessels.

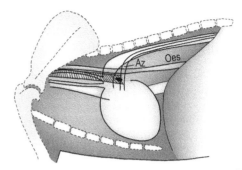

Figure 8.8 Pneumomediastinum: increased visibility of mediastinal structures. The azygos vein (Az) and oesophagus (Oes), which are not normally visible, are evident. Cranial mediastinal blood vessels are also apparent, and the tracheal walls are more obvious than normal.

2. Iatrogenic pneumomediastinum.

a. Post transtracheal aspiration.

b. Post lung aspirate.

c. Overinflation of the lungs during positive pressure ventilation.

d. Post endoscopy.

e. Trauma from endotracheal intubation.

f. In cats, following overinflation of the cuff of an endotracheal tube.

3. Extension of air from the neck.

a. Soft tissue trauma of the head or neck, with an open wound.

b. Cervical tracheal perforation.

c. Cervical oesophageal perforation.

d. Pharyngeal perforation.

e. Jugular venepuncture.

f. Soft tissue infection with gas formation.

4. Extension of air from the bronchi or lungs; air dissecting along perivascular or peribronchial adventitia.

a. Rupture of the bronchi or lungs.

– Rupture of pulmonary bulla, bleb or cyst.

– Bronchial parasitism.

– Compressive trauma.

– Lung lobe torsion.

– Lobar emphysema.

b. Spontaneous pneumomediastinum – racing Greyhounds.

5. Tracheal perforation within the thorax.

6. Oesophageal perforation within the thorax.

7. Secondary to severe dyspnoea – especially paraquat poisoning, with an interstitial lung pattern (see 6.22.14).
8. Emphysematous mediastinitis.
9. Extension from pneumoretroperitoneum.

Reduced mediastinal radiopacity: fat

10. Obesity – especially in chondrodystrophic dogs.

Increased mediastinal radiopacity, greater than soft tissue

11. Iatrogenic.
    a. Intravenous or intra-arterial catheter.
    b. Endotracheal tube.
    c. Feeding tube.
    d. Oesophageal stethoscope.
12. Food material in distended oesophagus – see 8.18.
13. Mineralization.
    a. Mineralized oesophageal foreign bodies (see 8.20).
    b. Mineralized fragments of ingesta accumulating in a dilated oesophagus (e.g. secondary to vascular ring anomaly).
    c. Neoplastic mass.
       – Osteosarcoma transformation of *Spirocerca lupi** granuloma.
       – Thymic tumour.
       – Lymphoma.
       – Metastatic mediastinal tumour.
    d. Chronic infectious lymph node involvement (see 8.12) (e.g. histoplasmosis* or tuberculosis).
    e. Cardiovascular mineralization – aorta, coronary vessels and heart valves (see 6.27.7).
14. Metal.
    a. Bullets and other metallic foreign bodies.
    b. Contrast media.
       – Leaking from a perforated oesophagus.
       – Positive contrast peritoneography with ruptured diaphragm.
       – Previously aspirated barium accumulating in hilar lymph nodes.

8.10 MEDIASTINAL WIDENING

Generalized mediastinal widening may be caused by accumulation of fat or fluid. Mediastinal fluid may result in reverse fissure lines as fluid dissects into the interlobar fissures from the hilar region. The reverse fissure lines are wider centrally and narrower peripherally (Fig. 8.9) and should not be confused with atelectatic lung lobes, especially a collapsed right middle lobe, which may appear small and triangular (see 6.17.3 and Fig. 6.10). Reverse fissures may also arise with pleural effusions but in these animals are likely to be obscured by the fact that the fluid is distributed over a larger area. Localized or walled-off accumulations of fluid mimic mediastinal masses (see 8.11). Mediastinal fluid may extend into the pleural space, but the reverse does not occur.

1. Incidental mediastinal widening.
   a. A widened cranial mediastinum is routinely seen on DV or VD radiographs of Bulldogs. The trachea is in its normal position, slightly to the right of the midline.
   b. In obese patients, especially in small and miniature breeds, large fat deposits result in a widened, smoothly margined cranial mediastinum. The trachea is in its normal position, slightly to the right of the midline.
   c. Thymic 'sail' on DV or VD view in young animals, between the right and left cranial lung lobes.
2. Mediastinal masses (see 8.11).
3. Oesophageal dilation (see 8.17).
4. Haemorrhage (for list of causes, see 8.3.2).
5. Mediastinitis or mediastinal abscess secondary to:
   a. oesophageal or tracheal perforation

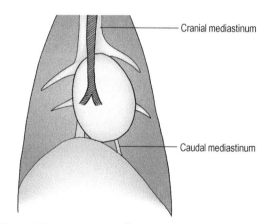

Figure 8.9 Reverse fissure lines due to mediastinal fluid, seen on the dorsoventral view. The mediastinum is also widened.

b. extension of lymphadenitis, pleuritis, pericarditis, pneumonia, or a deep neck wound

c. *Spirocerca lupi**

d. cats – mediastinal feline infectious peritonitis.

6. Oedema or transudate (often with pleural fluid too).
   a. Acute systemic disease.
   b. Trauma.
   c. Hypoproteinaemia.
   d. Right heart failure.
   e. Neoplasia, especially with cranial mediastinal masses in cats.

7. Chylomediastinum.

8. Azygos vein dilation secondary to azygos continuation of the CdVC ($\pm$ portocaval shunting) – widened caudal mediastinum on the VD view.

8.11 MEDIASTINAL MASSES

Mediastinal masses will displace adjacent structures, particularly the trachea, and cranial mediastinal masses may cause secondary oesophageal obstruction. Oesophageal contrast studies, angiography, horizontal beam radiography, pleurography, ultrasonography and CT may provide additional information about the location and nature of the mass (Fig. 8.10). Mediastinal masses may be mimicked by localized fluid accumulations (see 8.10) and by some pulmonary and thoracic wall masses.

1. Cranioventral mediastinal masses (precardiac) – may elevate $\pm$ compress the trachea and oesophagus.

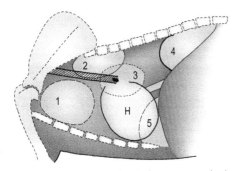

Figure 8.10 Location of mediastinal masses on the lateral view. H, heart; 1, cranioventral masses; 2, craniodorsal masses; 3, hilar and perihilar masses; 4, caudodorsal masses; 5, caudoventral masses.

a. Artefactual.
   – Flexion of the neck causes dorsal curvature of the intrathoracic trachea (see Fig. 6.2C).
   – Curvature of the intrathoracic trachea to the right on a DV or VD view is a normal feature of chondrodystrophic dogs (see Fig. 6.2F).
   – Masses in the tip of the cranial lung lobe may be in contact with the mediastinum, and the resultant border effacement may mimic a cranial mediastinal mass.
   – Pleural fluid often collects around the cranial lung lobes, effacing the heart outline and mimicking a mediastinal mass, especially in cats.
   – Mediastinal fat in obese animals, especially chondrodystrophic dogs.

b. Normal thymus – in immature dogs, a thymic 'sail' is seen in the cranioventral mediastinal fold, pointing caudolaterally to the left on the DV or VD view, and should not be confused with a reverse fissure line.

c. Neoplasia – often accompanied by a pleural effusion, and ultrasonography or repeat radiographs after thoracocentesis are needed for diagnosis. Occasionally may cause cranial vena cava syndrome, obstructing the cranial vena cava by compression, invasion and thrombus formation and causing oedema of the head, neck and forelimbs – demonstrated with non-selective angiography or ultrasonography.
   – Lymphoma; the most common cause in cats – especially feline leukaemia virus-positive, young, oriental breed cats.
   – Thymoma – may be accompanied by myasthenia gravis and megaoesophagus, especially in German Shepherd dogs.
   – Malignant histiocytosis – middle-aged, large-breed dogs, with male preponderance; mainly Bernese Mountain Dog but also Rottweiler and Golden and Flat-coated Retrievers.
   – Ectopic thyroid or parathyroid tumour.
   – Rib tumour – look for bony changes too (see 8.22.5 and Fig. 8.14).
   – Sternal tumour.
   – Other tumours (e.g. lipoma and fibrosarcoma).

d. Oesophageal dilation secondary to a vascular ring anomaly (see 8.17.6 and Fig. 8.12).

e. Sternal lymphadenopathy (see 8.12.7–11); note that enlargement of the sternal lymph node can signal pathology within the abdominal cavity. If due to lymphoma, other lymphadenopathy or abdominal organomegaly may be present too.

f. Mediastinal abscess or granuloma.
   - Foreign body reaction (e.g. sharp object penetrating via sternum).
   - Nocardiosis*.
   - Actinomycosis*.

g. Mediastinal haematoma.

h. Mediastinal cyst – especially older cats, and often an incidental finding.
   - Thymic branchial cyst.
   - Parathyroid cyst.
   - Thyroglossal cyst.
   - Pleural cyst.
   - Idiopathic cyst.

i. Aneurysmal dilation of the right auricle through a pericardial defect.

2. Craniodorsal mediastinal masses (precardiac) – may depress ± compress the trachea and oesophagus.
   a. Oesophageal pathology.
      - Dilation (see 8.17).
      - Foreign bodies (see 8.20).
      - Food in megaoesophagus.
      - Oesophageal abscess or granuloma.
      - Oesophageal neoplasia – rare (see 8.19.6).
   b. Aortic dilation, for example post stenotic dilation, aneurysm (see 7.10.1).
   c. Heart base tumour (see 7.16.2).
   d. Associated with vertebral lesions.
      - Neoplasia.
      - Severe spondylosis.
      - Osteomyelitis.
   e. Mediastinal abscess, granuloma or cellulitis.
      - After penetration of oesophagus by foreign body.
      - Reaction to migrating foreign body (e.g. grass awn).
      - Nocardiosis*.
      - Actinomycosis*.
      - Secondary to cervical trauma (e.g. bite wound, stick injury).
   f. Proximal rib tumour.
   g. Thymoma.
   h. Lymphadenopathy.
   i. Haematoma.

   - Blood vessel perforation by aberrant *Spirocerca lupi** larvae.
   - Coagulopathy (e.g. secondary to *Angiostrongylus vasorum** infection, haemophilia).
   j. Paraspinal nerve sheath tumour.

3. Hilar and perihilar masses – usually poorly defined masses at the base of the heart. The adjacent trachea and main stem bronchi may be displaced or compressed (see Fig. 6.5B and D).
   a. Tracheobronchial (hilar) lymphadenopathy – usually with associated pulmonary or pleural pathology and other systemic signs (see 8.12.1–6).
   b. Lymph node neoplasia (e.g. lymphoma, malignant histiocytosis).
   c. Oesophageal pathology.
      - Oesophageal foreign body (see 8.20).
      - *Spirocerca lupi** granuloma.
      - Oesophageal tumour, often secondary to *S. lupi** granuloma.
      - Food in megaoesophagus.
   d. Heart base tumour (see 7.16.2).
   e. Cardiovascular structure mimicking a mass (see 7.8, 7.10, 7.11 and 7.13).
      - Left or right atrial enlargement.
      - Perihilar pulmonary oedema.
      - Post stenotic dilation of the aorta or pulmonary artery.
      - Pulmonary artery enlargement.
      - Aortic aneurysm.
   f. Mediastinal abscess or granuloma.
   g. Ectopic thyroid mass.
   h. Adjacent pulmonary or bronchial mass.

4. Caudal mediastinal masses (post-cardiac).
   a. Artefactual – accessory lung lobe mass; mid- to dorsal thorax.
   b. Oesophageal pathology (see 8.19 and 8.20); mid- to dorsal thorax.
      - Foreign body.
      - Oesophageal granuloma or abscess (e.g. due to *S. lupi** or previous foreign body).
      - Oesophageal neoplasia (e.g. osteosarcoma or fibrosarcoma secondary to *S. lupi** granuloma, leiomyoma or leiomyosarcoma).
      - Hiatal hernia – may be associated with severe respiratory effort; can occur with tetanus.
      - Paraoesophageal hernia.

- Gastro-oesophageal intussusception.
- Oesophageal diverticulum or focal dilation.
- Food in megaoesophagus.

c. Mediastinal granuloma or abscess (e.g. migrating foreign body).
d. Mediastinal haematoma.
e. Associated with vertebral lesions.
f. Peritoneopericardial diaphragmatic hernia; ventral thorax (see 7.6.3).
g. True diaphragmatic hernia.
h. Diaphragmatic eventration (see 8.26.1).
i. Diaphragmatic abscess or granulomas (e.g. migrating foreign body).
j. Diaphragmatic neoplasia.
k. Mediastinal cyst – less common than cranial mediastinum.
l. Aortic aneurysm.
m. Herniation of liver:
  - Through diaphragmatic rupture.
  - Through CdVC hiatus.
n. Intrathoracic gall bladder.
o. Ectopic kidney.
  - Congenital.
  - Displaced through diaphragmatic rupture; reported in cats.
p. Azygos vein dilation secondary to azygos continuation of the CdVC (± portocaval shunting) – widened caudal mediastinum on the DV or VD view.

8.12 MEDIASTINAL LYMPHADENOPATHY

Enlargement of the tracheobronchial (hilar), bronchial and mediastinal lymph nodes results in poorly defined hilar masses (Fig. 8.10). These are often associated with pulmonary and pleural pathology and other systemic signs. An extrapleural sign may be a normal finding in the region of the sternal lymph node in right lateral recumbent radiographs, especially in larger dogs. It should not be mistaken for sternal lymphadenopathy, particularly if it is not seen on left lateral recumbent radiographs.

Hilar region lymphadenopathy

1. Fungal infections.
   a. Coccidioidomycosis* – younger dogs; rare in cats.
   b. Histoplasmosis* – mainly dogs and rare in cats; may calcify on recovery.
   c. Blastomycosis* – mainly dogs, rare in cats.
   d. Cryptococcosis* – more often in cats; uncommon in dogs.
2. Neoplasia.
   a. Lymphoma – often with an interstitial lung pattern too (see 6.22.6).
   b. Malignant histiocytosis – middle-aged, large-breed dogs, with male preponderance; mainly Bernese Mountain Dog but also Rottweiler and Golden and Flat-coated Retrievers.
   c. Metastatic neoplasia from the lungs and other body regions.
3. Bacterial infection or granuloma.
   a. Tuberculosis.
   b. Nocardiosis* – mainly younger dogs.
   c. Actinomycosis*.
4. Eosinophilic pulmonary granulomatosis.
5. Pulmonary lymphomatoid granulomatosis – with alveolar lung pattern and pulmonary nodules or masses too.
6. After resolved pleural or pulmonary infections.

Sternal lymphadenopathy

7. Artefactual, especially if seen only in right lateral recumbent radiographs in larger dogs.
8. Neoplasia.
   a. Lymphoma – often with an interstitial lung pattern too (see 6.22.6).
   b. Malignant histiocytosis (see 8.12.2).
   c. Metastatic neoplasia from:
     - Mammary tumour.
     - Cranial abdominal tumour.
9. Bacterial infection (see 8.12.3).
10. Fungal infection (see 8.12.1); especially cryptococcosis* in cats.
11. After resolved pleural or pulmonary infections.
12. Secondary to inflammatory or neoplastic abdominal disease, as sternal lymph nodes drain the peritoneal cavity.

8.13 ULTRASONOGRAPHY OF THE MEDIASTINUM

As for pleural disease, ultrasonography and radiography are often complementary tools in investigation of mediastinal pathology (see 8.5). Ultrasonography is particularly valuable for the investigation of a possible underlying mediastinal mass when radiographs show free pleural fluid, and for differentiating mediastinal cysts from solid soft tissue masses. When pleural fluid is present, the mediastinal pleura may be seen as an echogenic band, and mediastinal blood vessels and lymph nodes may also be seen. The presence of hyperechoic foci with ring-down or reverberation artefacts within a mass suggests small pockets of air and should arouse the suspicion of a pulmonary rather than a mediastinal mass.

1. Cranial mediastinal mass – evaluation of the cranial mediastinum may be carried out from either a right or left cranial intercostal approach, from the thoracic inlet or via a transoesophageal approach if endoscopic ultrasonography is available.
   a. Hypoechoic to anechoic; homogeneous.
      – Mediastinal fluid.
      – Abscess or granuloma; may have a thick, echogenic wall.
      – Cyst or cystic neoplasm – simple or multiloculated; cysts have a thin, regular wall.
      – Haematoma.
      – Lymphadenopathy.
      – Tumour of homogeneous cellularity (e.g. lymphoma).
      – Ectopic thyroid tissue.
   b. Heterogeneous in echogenicity or echotexture.
      – Abscess or granuloma.
      – Haematoma.
      – Tumour of heterogeneous cellularity and/ or fibrosis, calcification, cystic areas, necrosis or haemorrhage.

2. Caudal mediastinal mass – the caudal mediastinum is often most clearly imaged from a cranial abdominal approach, through the liver. If the lungs are well aerated and there is no pleural or mediastinal fluid, small mediastinal masses may, however, be difficult to image.
   a. Hypoechoic to anechoic, homogeneous.
      – Mediastinal fluid.
      – Abscess or granuloma.
      – Cyst.
      – Haematoma.
      – Tumour of homogeneous cellularity.
      – Liver within a peritoneopericardial hernia.
      – Ectopic liver.
   b. Heterogeneous in echogenicity and echotexture.
      – Abscess or granuloma.
      – Haematoma.
      – Tumour of heterogeneous cellularity and/ or fibrosis, calcification, necrosis or haemorrhage.

      – Abdominal viscera (within a peritoneopericardial diaphragmatic hernia or via a traumatic rupture of the diaphragm).
      – Oesophageal mass (see 8.19), including *Spirocerca lupi** granulomas.

3. Hilar and perihilar masses – if transoesophageal ultrasonography is not available, hilar masses are often best imaged through the heart. The heart is imaged in a short-axis view and the transducer angled dorsally to image the heart base. The heart is then imaged in a long-axis view, paying particular attention to the great vessels as they enter and exit the heart and atria.
   a. Enlargement of cardiac chambers or great vessels.
      – Left atrial enlargement (see 7.19.1 and 7.19.2).
      – Post stenotic dilation of the aorta or pulmonary artery.
      – Right atrial enlargement (see 7.20.1 and 7.20.2).
   b. Solid mass involving the cardiac chambers or great vessels (may be associated with pericardial effusions).
      – Heart base tumour – a hypo- to hyperechoic mass usually adjacent to, or surrounding, the aortic outflow tract.
      – Haemangiosarcoma – usually a hypoechoic mass involving the wall of the right atrium.
   c. Solid mass dorsal to the heart base (imaged either using the heart as a window or via the transoesophageal route).
      – Lymphadenopathy (see 8.12).
      – Pulmonary mass (see 6.19).
      – Oesophageal mass (see 8.19).
      – Oesophageal foreign body (see 8.20).

THORACIC OESOPHAGUS

8.14 NORMAL RADIOGRAPHIC APPEARANCE OF THE THORACIC OESOPHAGUS

A normal empty oesophagus is rarely visible on survey radiographs. Occasionally in dogs and cats, it is seen caudally as a poorly defined band of soft tissue opacity dorsal to the CdVC on a left lateral radiograph. A small amount of luminal air may often be observed cranial to the heart in conscious dogs, especially if they are dyspnoeic or struggling. Generalized oesophageal dilation is a common finding under anaesthesia. The oesophagus may also become visible in animals with pneumomediastinum (see Fig. 8.8).

8.15 OESOPHAGEAL CONTRAST STUDIES: TECHNIQUE AND NORMAL APPEARANCE

Contrast studies of the oesophagus may be performed for investigation of either suspected oesophageal disease or the nature of cervical and thoracic masses. No specific patient preparation is required. The patient must be conscious, although light sedation may be needed in fractious patients. Barium sulphate liquid or paste is usually indicated, but a 'barium burger' (barium mixed with food) is required for cases of suspected oesophageal dilation or stricture, in which paste or liquid may give false negative results. Lateral radiographs are usually more informative than DV or VD views, and fluoroscopic screening with recording facility is required for assessment of functional disorders.

Barium paste or liquid oesophagram

If only a small quantity is required, it can be administered with a syringe to which a short piece of stout rubber tubing is attached. The contrast medium is deposited between the molar teeth and the cheek and the patient given sufficient time to swallow between squirts. Aspiration of the barium should be avoided. Alternatively, a stomach tube or catheter can be passed through the opening in a spacer gag positioned transversely across the mouth just behind the canine teeth, so that its tip reaches the mid-cervical oesophagus. The barium liquid is then injected slowly via the tube or catheter.

Barium burger

One part of barium liquid is mixed with three parts of meat, which the patient is required to eat, although hand-feeding may be necessary. Fortunately, many dogs in need of such studies are hungry because of persistent regurgitation. Cats will not usually eat barium burgers, although intravenous administration of diazepam may encourage them to eat.

Iodine oesophagram

If there is a possibility that the oesophagus may be perforated (e.g. after removal of an oesophageal foreign body), 5–10 mL of a low-osmolarity water-soluble iodine preparation must be given to avoid complications arising from barium leaking into the mediastinum (adhesions and granuloma formation).

The canine oesophagus consists of striated muscle and after barium administration will be visible as a longitudinal linear pattern of barium trapped between the mucosal folds. In the cat, the terminal third of the oesophagus is smooth muscle and has a striated herringbone appearance on positive contrast studies.

8.16 ABNORMALITIES ON OESOPHAGEAL CONTRAST STUDIES

1. Deviation of the oesophageal lumen.
   a. Normal – the oesophagus lies dorsal to the trachea in the neck but drapes ventrally over its right side through the thoracic inlet before rising dorsal to it again within the thorax.
   b. Redundancy or folding at the thoracic inlet – normal variant, especially in Bulldogs.
   c. Displacement by cervical or intrathoracic masses.
   d. Displacement of lumen by a mural mass (see 8.19.5 and 8.19.6).
   e. Hiatal hernia (see 8.19.3).
2. Dilation (megaoesophagus) – generalized or localized (see 8.17).
3. Narrowing of the oesophageal lumen; may require barium burger for demonstration.
   a. Normal; mucosa smooth.
      – Peristalsis – use fluoroscopy or repeat the exposure.
      – Dorsal to the heart base.
   b. Apparent luminal narrowing around a foreign body (see 8.20).
   c. Inflammatory stricture; mucosal irregularity may also be seen; differential diagnosis is diffuse neoplasia.
      – After reflux of gastric acid during general anaesthesia.
      – After swallowing hot or caustic material.
      – Other causes of oesophagitis.
   d. Neoplasia; mucosal irregularity may also be seen – an associated mass lesion may not necessarily be present if the tumour is diffuse; differential diagnosis is oesophagitis.
   e. Granuloma, for example *Spirocerca lupi** (see 8.19.5 and Fig. 8.13).

f. Vascular ring anomaly – over heart base (see 8.17.6 and Fig. 8.12).

g. Abscess, for example post foreign body (see 8.20).

h. Gastro-oesophageal intussusception (see 8.19.2).

4. Filling defect.
   a. Artefact.
      – Food material if barium burger given.
      – Air bubble, especially if barium liquid given.
   b. Oesophageal mass (see 8.19).
   c. Oesophageal foreign body (see 8.20).

5. Mucosal irregularity.
   a. Normal herringbone pattern in caudal third of cat oesophagus.
   b. Artefact – food mixed with barium.
   c. Oesophagitis.
   d. Neoplasia.

6. Contrast medium extravasation.
   a. Artefact – contrast medium on hair of patient, cassette or table.
   b. Aspiration (e.g. due to dysphagia); contrast medium probably also seen in larynx.
   c. Oesophageal perforation (e.g. secondary to foreign body) – usually with pneumomediastinum and/or mediastinitis (Figs 8.8 and 8.9).
   d. Broncho-oesophageal or tracheo-oesophageal fistula.

7. Oesophageal dysmotility – reduced motility of all or part of the oesophagus seen on

fluoroscopy but without evidence of megaoesophagus on radiographs; especially young terriers; may regurgitate or be asymptomatic.

8.17 OESOPHAGEAL DILATION

A dilated oesophagus may be filled with food, fluid or (most commonly) air. When air-filled, the oesophageal wall becomes visible due to the presence of air inside the oesophagus and air outside the wall in the adjacent lungs or trachea. With the latter, the combined visibility of the tracheal and oesophageal wall is known as a tracheal stripe sign. The trachea may be displaced ventrally by the weight of the distended oesophagus (Fig. 8.11A and B). Chronic oesophageal dilation with regurgitation may lead to aspiration bronchopneumonia (see 6.14.2).

Generalized oesophageal dilation (Fig. 8.11)

Megaoesophagus results from a motility disorder due to central nervous system disease or neuromuscular disorders. Megaoesophagus is less common in cats than in dogs.

1. Transient megaoesophagus.
   a. Heavy sedation or general anaesthesia.
   b. Severe respiratory infections (e.g. acute tracheobronchitis).
   c. Sliding hiatal hernia.
   d. Following repair of ruptured diaphragm.
2. Congenital or hereditary megaoesophagus.

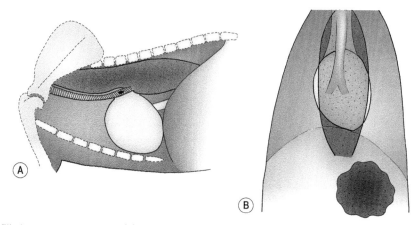

Figure 8.11 Air-filled megaoesophagus on (A) lateral and (B) dorsoventral or ventrodorsal views. On the lateral view, the oesophageal and tracheal walls summate, producing the tracheal stripe sign. The trachea is displaced ventrally.

a. Vascular ring anomaly (mainly persistent right aortic arch) – results in localized dilation cranial to the constriction, but a small percentage of these cases also have oesophageal dilation caudal to the constriction, resulting in generalized dilation. If air-filled, the constriction may be seen. German Shepherd dog, Labrador and Irish Setter.

b. Hereditary megaoesophagus – Wirehaired Fox Terrier and Miniature Schnauzer.

c. Familial predisposition – German Shepherd dog, Great Dane, Newfoundland, Shar Pei and Golden Retriever; Siamese cats.

d. Congenital myasthenia gravis – Jack Russell Terrier, Springer Spaniel and Smooth-haired Fox Terrier.

e. Canine glycogen storage disease – young Lapland dogs.

f. Hereditary myopathy – young Labradors.

g. Canine giant axonal neuropathy – young German Shepherd dogs.

3. Acquired megaoesophagus.

a. Idiopathic.

b. Immune-mediated myopathies and neuropathies.
   - Polymyositis – large breeds.
   - Acquired myasthenia gravis; generalized muscle disease or selective oesophageal involvement – may be associated with thymoma.
   - Acute polyradiculoneuritis.
   - Systemic lupus erythematosus.
   - Polyneuritis.
   - Dermatomyositis.

c. Metabolic neuropathies and myelopathies.
   - Hypoadrenocorticism (Addison's disease) often accompanied by microcardia.
   - Hypothyroidism.
   - Corticosteroid-induced polymyopathy.
   - Diabetes mellitus.
   - Hyperinsulinism.
   - Uraemia.

d. Toxic neuropathies.
   - Organophosphates.
   - Heavy metals, particularly lead but also zinc, cadmium and thallium.
   - Chlorinated hydrocarbons.
   - Anticholinesterase.
   - Herbicides.
   - Acrylamide.
   - Botulism.
   - Tetanus.

e. Secondary to:
   - Reflux oesophagitis, particularly as result of axial oesophageal hiatal hernias (see 8.19.3).
   - Distal oesophageal foreign body.
   - Acute gastric dilation and volvulus syndrome.
   - Brainstem disease (e.g. neoplasia).
   - Cats – pyloric dysfunction.
   - Snake bite.

f. Canine dysautonomia.

g. Cats – feline dysautonomia (Key–Gaskell syndrome).

h. Hypertrophic muscular dystrophy.

i. Thiamine deficiency.

Localized oesophageal dilation

4. Transient, localized oesophageal dilation.

a. Dyspnoea.

b. Aerophagia.

c. Normal swallowing.

5. Redundant oesophagus, seen particularly on contrast studies as a ventral oesophageal deviation at the thoracic inlet. Mainly brachycephalic breeds (e.g. Bulldog) but also described in the cat. Usually clinically insignificant.

6. Congenital localized oesophageal dilation.

a. Usually a vascular ring anomaly (Fig. 8.12) with oesophageal dilation cranial to the heart; uncommon in cats.
   - Ninety-five per cent are due to a persistent right aortic arch with terminal trachea displaced to the left on DV or VD views (Fig. 6.2G) – particularly German Shepherd dog, Boston Terrier and Irish Setter; main type in cats.
   - Double aortic arch – often accompanied by tracheal compression and coughing.
   - Right aortic arch with aberrant right subclavian artery.
   - Normal aorta with aberrant right subclavian artery.
   - Persistent right ductus arteriosus or ligamentum arteriosum.

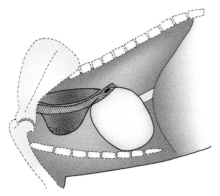

Figure 8.12 Vascular ring anomaly: severe oesophageal dilation cranial to the heart base, within which fragments of retained ingesta are often seen. The trachea is displaced ventrally and shows a tracheal stripe sign. The distal oesophagus may also be dilated in some cases.

    b. Dilation cranial to a congenital focal stenosis.
    c. Segmental oesophageal hypomotility – may be congenital; Shar Pei and Newfoundland.
    d. Congenital oesophageal diverticulum.
7. Dilation cranial to an oesophageal hiatal hernia or gastro-oesophageal intussusception.
8. Dilation adjacent to an oesophageal foreign body.
9. Iatrogenic segmental stenosis (peptic oesophageal stricture) following general anaesthesia; dilation forms cranial to the stenosis.
10. Cranial to a stricture or narrowing caused by:
    a. Compression of the oesophagus by a large external mass (e.g. a cranial mediastinal tumour).
    b. Scar tissue (e.g. after foreign body removal or ingestion of hot or caustic substances).
    c. Granuloma.
    d. Mucosal adhesion.
    e. Congenital focal stenosis.
    f. Oesophageal neoplasia.
11. Focal myasthenia gravis.
12. Severe oesophagitis.
13. Oesophageal diverticulum – often medium- to small-breed dogs.
    a. Pulsion diverticulum – usually with motility disturbances.
    b. Traction diverticulum – usually secondary to perioesophageal inflammation.

8.18 VARIATIONS IN RADIOPACITY OF THE OESOPHAGUS

1. Reduced oesophageal radiopacity – air.
    a. Small amounts.
       – Normal swallowed air, especially if animal struggling or dyspnoeic.
       – Localized dilation.
       – Redundant oesophagus at the thoracic inlet.
    b. Large amounts.
       – General anaesthesia.
       – Megaoesophagus (see 8.17).
2. Soft tissue oesophageal radiopacity.
    a. Non-distended soft tissue opacity of the distal oesophagus on left lateral recumbent views or superimposed on the dorsal aspect of the cervicothoracic trachea – normal.
    b. Small amounts on single radiograph and absent on follow-up radiographs – normal, transient fluid in oesophagus.
    c. Large amounts – fluid and food in a megaoesophagus (see 8.17).
    d. Non-mineralized foreign body (see 8.20).
    e. Oesophageal soft tissue mass (see 8.19).
3. Mineralized oesophageal radiopacity.
    a. Bone – oesophageal foreign body (see 8.20).
    b. Osteosarcoma transformation of *Spirocerca lupi** granuloma.
    c. Precardiac ingesta accumulation in an amotile distended oesophagus with vascular ring anomaly; usually cranial to the heart (see 8.17.6 and Fig. 8.12).
    d. Delayed transit of solid medications containing elements of high atomic number such as bismuth given *per os* (e.g. antacids or enteric-coated tablets).

8.19 OESOPHAGEAL MASSES

Oesophageal masses may be intraluminal, intramural or extraluminal.

Intraluminal oesophageal masses

1. Foreign body (see 8.20).
2. Gastro-oesophageal intussusception – the stomach and possibly other abdominal organs invaginate into oesophagus, usually secondary

to megaoesophagus; especially German Shepherd dog puppies.
3. Axial oesophageal hiatal hernia – the herniated stomach mimics an oesophageal mass on plain radiographs, but a barium study reveals that this is part of the stomach; often sliding, with secondary reflux oesophagitis and megaoesophagus.
   a. Congenital in the Shar Pei; concurrent herniation of liver with compression of the CdVC and Budd–Chiari-like syndrome also reported.
   b. Severe respiratory distress, particularly of upper respiratory tract origin or with tetanus.
   c. Congenital Golden Retriever muscular dystrophy, with diaphragmatic and pelvic changes.
   d. Sequel to repair of chronic diaphragmatic rupture.
4. Oesophageal diverticulum containing fluid or food.

Intramural oesophageal masses

5. Oesophageal granuloma.
   a. *Spirocerca lupi** – the granuloma arises out of the dorsal oesophageal wall, and barium will therefore pass only ventral to the mass (Fig. 8.13). May contain ill-defined foci of mineralization due to transformation to osteosarcoma, and pulmonary metastasis may be present; thoracic spondylitis is seen, and aortic aneurysm and hypertrophic osteopathy may also occur (see 7.10.1 and 1.14.6).
   b. Mural foreign body or infection.
6. Oesophageal neoplasia.
   a. Secondary to *S. lupi** granuloma.

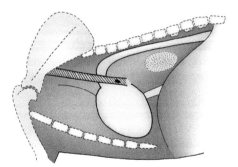

Figure 8.13 *Spirocerca lupi* granuloma in the distal oesophagus. Typical vertebral changes are also present.

   – Osteosarcoma.
   – Fibrosarcoma.
   b. Metastatic or infiltrative oesophageal tumour – rare; usually from thyroid carcinoma.
   c. Primary oesophageal tumour – rare.
      – Leiomyoma or leiomyosarcoma.
      – Squamous cell carcinoma.

Extraluminal oesophageal masses

7. Paraoesophageal hiatal hernia – the gastric fundus ± other organs are displaced through a diaphragmatic defect adjacent to the oesophageal hiatus.
8. Paraoesophageal abscess (e.g. following oesophageal perforation).

8.20 OESOPHAGEAL FOREIGN BODIES

Oesophageal foreign bodies may be radiopaque (such as bone and fishing hooks) or soft tissue opacity (such as gristle). The latter may require oesophageal contrast studies for visualization; air may be sufficient and is safer than positive contrast media if oesophageal perforation is present. Foreign bodies lodge most commonly at the thoracic inlet, over the base of the heart and just cranial to the diaphragm. Those in the caudal oesophagus may mimic *Spirocerca lupi** granuloma except that contrast medium will probably pass all around an intraluminal foreign body. The mass effect from a *S. lupi** granuloma may also result in secondary oesophageal foreign body accumulation. Oesophageal foreign bodies may displace adjacent structures, particularly the trachea, and a small amount of air may be seen cranial to or around them. In cats, fish bones and needles with thread occur commonly.

Complications usually occur in long-standing cases.

1. Aspiration pneumonia secondary to regurgitation.
2. Localized inflammatory reaction.
   a. Oesophagitis.
   b. Perioesophagitis.
   c. Focal mediastinitis.
3. Oesophageal perforation – should be confirmed by administering small amounts of water-soluble iodine contrast agents and not barium, as this leads to granulomatous reactions if it enters the mediastinum. Leakage may not be

evident on the oesophagram if the perforation has been partially or totally sealed by adhesions or fibrosis. Complications of oesophageal perforation include:

a. Pneumothorax.
b. Pneumomediastinum.
c. Mediastinitis or mediastinal abscess.
d. Pleuritis and pleural effusion.
e. Oesophagobronchial fistula.
f. Oesophagotracheal fistula.

4. Subsequent oesophageal stricture.
a. Mucosal scarring and oesophageal stenosis.
b. Perioesophageal fibrosis resulting in stenosis.

THORACIC WALL

A thorough radiological examination of the thorax always includes evaluation of the extrathoracic structures. By examining both orthogonal views, the extrathoracic location of the suspect pathology can usually be determined.

8.21 VARIATIONS IN SOFT TISSUE COMPONENTS OF THE THORACIC WALL

1. Widened thoracic wall – soft tissue radiopacity.
a. Diffuse widening.
  – Cellulitis.
  – Oedema.
  – Injected electrolyte solutions.
b. Localized widening.
  – Soft tissue neoplasia.
  – Rib lesion with bony changes subtle or overlooked.
  – Abscess or granuloma.
  – Cyst.
  – Haematoma.
  – Paracostal hernia.
  – Pleural and extrapleural nodules and masses (see 8.4).

2. Widened thoracic wall – fat radiopacity. Fat in fascial planes should not be mistaken for subcutaneous emphysema; it is slightly less radiopaque than soft tissue and highlights the muscles and fascial planes.
a. Obesity.
b. Chest wall lipoma.

3. Widened thoracic wall – gas radiolucency. Subcutaneous air due to:
a. Post trauma (e.g. bites and rib fractures).
b. Infection.
c. Pneumomediastinum – extension via fascial planes.
d. Paracostal hernia with gas-filled bowel loops – more common in cats.

4. Nodular, linear and other localized radiopacities.
a. Soft tissue opacities – these may easily be confused with pulmonary and pleural or extrapleural nodules. If there is doubt as to whether or not an apparent pulmonary nodule is due to a superficial structure such as a nipple, the radiograph should be repeated after painting the nipple with a small amount of barium.
  – Artefactual from dirty cassettes and intensifying screens or wet and/or dirty foam positioning wedges.
  – Muscle attachments to ribs – seen in obese animals on the DV or VD views, separated by fat; linear soft tissue radiopacities that are symmetrical on the two sides of the chest.
  – Nipples.
  – Skin masses.
  – Engorged female ticks.
  – Wet hair, particularly in long-haired breeds with matted blood.
  – Skin folds running caudally from the axilla.
  – Superimposed foot pads – poorly positioned pelvic limbs on DV radiographs.
  – Superimposed fingers during manual restraint without adequate radiation safety procedures.
  – Bandages, catheters, electrocardiogram pads.
b. Mineralized opacities.
  – Artefactual, from dirty cassettes and intensifying screens.
  – Mineralization around the costochondral junctions in older dogs.
  – Wide costochondral junctions in chondrodystrophic breeds.
  – Fractures of adjacent bony structures.
  – Embedded tooth after dog fight.
  – Sand, dirt or glass debris.

- Mineralized tumours (e.g. of ribs or mammary glands).
- Calcification of nipples.
- Dystrophic calcification of soft tissue lesions.
- Paracostal hernias containing mineralized fetus or gastrointestinal contents.
- Calcified cyst walls – eggshell appearance.
- Calcinosis cutis with hyperadrenocorticism (Cushing's disease).
  c. Metal opacity.
- Microchip identification markers.
- Spilt contrast medium on patient or cassette.
- Bandage clips, electrocardiogram attachments.
- Bullets and pellets.
- Needles, pins, arrow heads, etc.

8.22 VARIATIONS IN THE RIBS

Normal thoracic radiography may result in inappropriate exposure or contrast of bony structures, and if pathology is suspected a further radiograph of the affected region should be made using appropriate exposures, positioning and centring.

1. Mineralization of costal cartilages – normal from a few months of age onwards – starts caudally and often has a granular pattern in the young dog, becoming more sclerotic and irregular with age. Rosettes of mineralization may form around the costochondral junctions in older dogs. In older cats, the costal cartilages may be densely mineralized in short segments, giving the appearance of fractures.
2. Rib fractures – may be associated with pneumothorax, subcutaneous emphysema, etc. (see 8.28).
   a. Direct trauma; often multiple.
   b. Associated with severe respiratory distress (e.g. asthma in cats) – often proximal aspect of ribs 8–12; may also have acquired pectus excavatum.
3. Altered width of intercostal spaces.
   a. Artefactual – poor positioning, with a curved spine.
   b. Rib or spinal fractures.
   c. Rib or soft tissue tumours.
   d. Intercostal muscle tearing.
   e. Uneven pulmonary inflation.

f. Tension pneumothorax.
g. Thoracic wall pain.
h. Post thoracotomy.
i. Congenital rib or vertebral abnormalities, especially hemivertebrae, resulting in crowding of rib heads.
j. Pleural disease.
k. Large thoracic masses.

4. Altered rib cage conformation.
   a. Barrel-chested conformation.
      - Breed characteristic (e.g. Basset, Bulldog, Boston Terrier).
      - Severe pleural disease.
      - Large intrathoracic tumours.
      - Tension pneumothorax.
      - Pulmonary overinflation.
   b. Flat-chested conformation ('swimmers' and flat-chested puppies or kittens, especially Burmese) – reduction in height of thorax, with sharp angulation at costochondral junctions; may be associated with pectus excavatum (see 8.23.1 and Fig. 8.15).
5. Osteolysis ± bone production affecting the ribs (Fig. 8.14).
   a. Primary tumours – usually a mixed, aggressive bone lesion.
      - Osteosarcoma – most common; usually distal rib.
      - Chondrosarcoma.

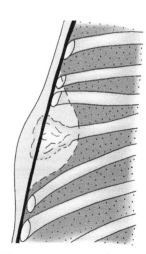

Figure 8.14 Rib tumour seen on a dorsoventral or lesion-oriented oblique view. There is a mixed, osteolytic and proliferative bone lesion, with displacement of the adjacent ribs and associated soft tissue swelling. Internally, the extrapleural sign is seen (see 8.4.2 and Fig. 8.5).

– Haemangiosarcoma.
– Fibrosarcoma.
– Multiple myeloma – usually osteolytic, may be multiple.
– Osteochondroma (cartilaginous exostosis) – young dogs; may be single or multiple.
– Osteoma.
– Multilobular tumour of bone.

b. Osteomyelitis.
c. Metastatic tumours – often smaller and multiple, and mainly osteolytic.
d. Soft tissue tumour involving bone, including mesothelioma (pleural effusion also present).

6. New bone on the ribs.
   a. Healed fractures – new bone smooth and solid.
   b. Hypertrophic non-union fractures – common, due to continual respiratory movement. May arise spontaneously in cats with allergic bronchitis (asthma), due to dyspnoea together with acquired pectus excavatum.
   c. Osteochondroma (cartilaginous exostosis) – young dogs; may be single or multiple (see 1.15.2 and Fig. 1.19).
   d. Periosteal reaction stimulated by adjacent rib or soft tissue mass, for example mesothelioma (pleural effusion also present).
   e. Aberrant migration of *Spirocerca lupi** larvae.

7. Congenital rib variants – uni- or bilateral; on transitional vertebrae (see 5.3.2 and Fig. 5.2B).
   a. Vestigial ribs.
      – L1.
      – C7.
   b. Abnormal rib curvature due to pectus excavatum (see 8.23.1 and Fig. 8.15).
   c. Flared ribs 1 and/or 2.
   d. Fusion of distal ribs 1 and 2.

8. Notching of the proximal parts of the caudal borders of ribs 4–8 secondary to dilated intercostal arteries supplying collateral circulation in animals with coarctation of the aorta – very rare.

8.23 VARIATIONS IN THE STERNUM

1. Changes in sternebral number and/or alignment.
   a. Malalignment of sternebrae is often seen, and the xiphisternum especially may appear

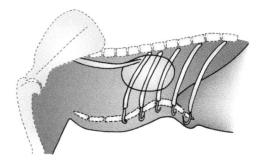

Figure 8.15 Pectus excavatum: the caudal portion of the sternum is displaced dorsally, elevating the heart and severely reducing the depth of the thorax. The ribs, costal cartilages and ventral diaphragm are distorted as a result of the sternal deformity.

subluxated or luxated; usually of little clinical significance.
   b. Pectus excavatum (funnel chest, congenital chondrosternal depression – Fig. 8.15) – the sternum deviates dorsally into the thorax, displacing the heart, lungs and ribs; brachycephalic breeds are over-represented; tracheal hypoplasia and pulmonary pathology may also be seen. The deformity may be quantified using the vertebral index or the frontosagittal index ratio. Pectus excavatum may also be seen in 'swimmer' puppies and kittens (flat chest syndrome).
   c. Pectus carinatum (pigeon breast) – the sternum is excessively angled caudoventrally – may be associated with cardiomegaly due to congenital cardiac pathology (e.g. patent ductus arteriosus).
   d. Sternebral absence, splitting (sternal dysraphism) or malformation may be associated with peritoneopericardial diaphragmatic hernia (see 7.6.3).

2. Mineralized intersternebral cartilages and sternal spondylosis – a normal ageing variant, especially in large dogs.

3. Osteolytic and/or productive sternebral lesion ± pathological fracture and adjacent soft tissue swelling.
   a. Osteomyelitis due to a penetrating foreign body, post trauma or sternotomy, haematogenous spread or of unknown origin.
   b. Neoplasia.
      – Chondrosarcoma.

- Osteosarcoma.
- Fibrosarcoma.
- Metastasis.
- Plasma cell (multiple) myeloma – osteolytic (see 1.18.2 and Fig. 1.24).
- Mesothelioma (pleural effusion also present; multiple sternebrae and ribs likely to be affected).

8.24 VARIATIONS IN THORACIC VERTEBRAE

See also Chapter 5, *Spine*. Only conditions that may affect the thorax are listed here.

1. Congenital vertebral malformations.
2. Vertebral fractures, luxations and subluxations associated with thoracic trauma.
3. Vertebral neoplasia with extension into the thorax or lung metastases.
4. Spondylitis of caudal thoracic vertebra – pathognomonic for *Spirocerca lupi** granuloma of the distal oesophagus. New bone along the entire ventral margins of the affected vertebrae differentiates this from spondylosis and discospondylitis.

8.25 ULTRASONOGRAPHY OF THE THORACIC WALL

1. Diffuse thickening of the thoracic wall on ultrasonography.
   a. Increased echogenicity or poor image quality.
      - Obesity.
      - Subcutaneous emphysema.
   b. Normal or decreased echogenicity.
      - Obesity.
      - Subcutaneous oedema.
      - Haemorrhage.
      - Cellulitis.
      - Electrolyte solutions injected subcutaneously and dispersed.
2. Localized swelling of the thoracic wall on ultrasonography.
   a. Fluid accumulation (anechoic to hypoechoic).
      - Abscess.
      - Haematoma.
      - Cyst.
      - Seroma post surgery.

- Recently injected electrolyte solutions.
   b. Soft tissue (hypoechoic to hyperechoic).
      - Abscess.
      - Granuloma.
      - Neoplasia.
3. Hyperechoic areas with acoustic shadowing.
   a. Normal ribs – multiple, regularly spaced.
   b. Subcutaneous emphysema.
   c. Foreign body.
   d. Paracostal hernia with gas-filled bowel loops.
   e. Dystrophic calcification.
   f. Rib tumour.

8.26 VARIATIONS IN THE APPEARANCE OF THE DIAPHRAGM

The diaphragm consists of a right and left crus dorsally and a cranioventral cupola. The CdVC passes through the caval hiatus in the right crus. On recumbent lateral radiographs in dogs, the dependent crus is pushed cranially by the abdominal contents (Fig. 8.16A–D). If the CdVC passes through the cranial crus and the crura are parallel, then the dog is lying on its right side; if the CdVC passes through the caudal crus and over the cranial crus and the crura diverge, the dog is lying on its left side. On the DV and VD views, the cupola and two crural silhouettes normally vary markedly due to X-ray beam direction and the pressure of abdominal contents influenced by gravity. On the DV view, the cupola is clearly visualized as a single dome with the right hemidiaphragm normally more cranial than the left. On the VD view, three bulges may be seen: a central cupola and two adjacent more caudal crura. The variations in diaphragm shape with posture are less obvious in small dogs and in cats.

1. Cranially displaced diaphragm – unilateral or bilateral.
   a. Abdominal causes.
      - Obesity.
      - Gastric distension with gas or food.
      - Severe abdominal effusion.
      - Severe organomegaly (especially liver and spleen).
      - Large abdominal mass.
      - Advanced pregnancy or pyometra.
      - Severe pain.
      - Severe pneumoperitoneum.
   b. Thoracic causes.

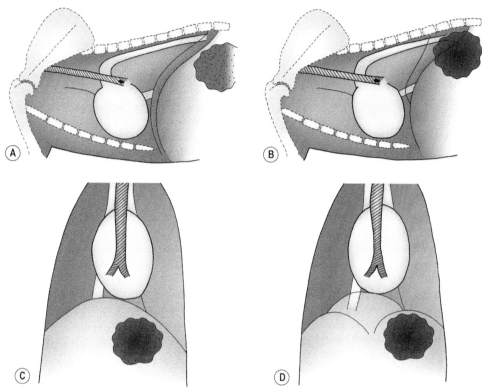

Figure 8.16 Diaphragm shape changes with posture. (A) Right lateral recumbency: the crura are parallel with the right crus lying more cranially. (B) Left lateral recumbency: the crura diverge dorsally and the gas-filled gastric fundus may overlie the caudodorsal lung field. (C) Sternal recumbency for the dorsoventral view: the diaphragm is smoothly curved, with the apex to the right of the midline. (D) Dorsal recumbency for the ventrodorsal view: the crura and cupola produce separate bulges.

- Expiration.
- Pulmonary fibrosis in aged patients.
- Pleural adhesions.
- Atelectasis.
- Severe pain.
- Radiation-therapy-induced fibrosis or atelectasis.
- Lung lobectomy.
- Diaphragmatic paralysis – confirm with fluoroscopy or ultrasonography; may be transient if due to trauma.
- Diaphragmatic neoplasia.
- Pectus excavatum (see 8.23.1 and Fig. 8.15).

c. Diaphragmatic rupture with a displaced, loose diaphragmatic flap (see 8.2.3 and Fig. 8.3).

d. Diaphragmatic eventration – thinning and weakening of one hemidiaphragm, with absence or atrophy of the muscles and cranial protrusion into the thorax; differential diagnosis is true diaphragmatic hernia, thoracic mass touching the diaphragm, diaphragmatic or liver mass, diaphragmatic paralysis. Usually no associated clinical signs.

e. Muscular dystrophy – unilateral.

2. Caudally displaced diaphragm – unilateral or bilateral.

a. Abdominal causes.
- Emaciation.
- Viscera displaced ventrally or caudally through a large body wall hernia or rupture.

b. Thoracic causes – may be accompanied by 'tenting', which represents the diaphragmatic attachments to the thoracic wall and is seen on the DV or VD view as pointed projections emanating from the diaphragmatic silhouette.
- Forced or deep inspiration.
- Dyspnoea (e.g. metabolic acidosis).
- Intrathoracic masses.

- Pleural effusion.
- Severe closed pneumothorax.
- Tension pneumothorax.
- Chronic bronchitis.
- Chronic obstructive lung disease.
- Acquired emphysema.
- Congenital lobar emphysema.
- Cats – feline bronchial asthma.

3. Diaphragm border effacement.
   a. Pleural effusion.
   b. Acquired diaphragmatic rupture – usually ventrally (see 8.2.3 and Fig. 8.3). Additional studies, including ultrasonography, positional radiography, oral positive contrast agents and positive contrast peritoneography, may be required for diagnosis. In obese animals, loss of the actual diaphragm line may be seen, cranial to falciform fat.
   c. Diaphragmatic hernia – displacement of viscera through an enlarged anatomical opening, usually the oesophageal hiatus.
      - Hiatal hernia, which includes sliding oesophageal hiatal, paraoesophageal, paravenous and para-aortic hernias; oral positive contrast studies are helpful in diagnosis (see 8.19.2 and 8.19.3).
      - Peritoneopericardial diaphragmatic hernia – continuous with an enlarged 'cardiac' silhouette; additional studies as above may be useful; may be associated with abdominal hernias and sternal abnormalities.
   d. Alveolar pattern of adjacent lung.
   e. Caudal mediastinal masses (see 8.11.4 and Fig. 8.10).
   f. Extrapleural masses in contact with the diaphragm.
4. Visibility of isolated portion of diaphragm.
   a. Normal – dorsal part of left crus if adjacent gastric fundus is gas-filled, resulting in a diaphragm–gastric wall stripe sign (Fig. 8.16B).
   b. Pneumoperitoneum (see 9.7).
   c. Pneumoretroperitoneum; usually an extension from pneumomediastinum – dorsal part of diaphragm outlined (see 9.11).
5. Altered diaphragmatic contour.
   a. Tenting of the diaphragm (see 8.26.2).
   b. Small diaphragmatic ruptures and hernias.

c. Diaphragmatic neoplasia (e.g. rhabdomyosarcoma).
d. Golden Retriever muscular dystrophy – diaphragmatic asymmetry and undulation, ± hiatal hernia and pelvic shape changes.
e. Feline hypertrophic muscular dystrophy – scalloping of the ventral diaphragm.
f. Pleural and extrapleural nodules and masses (see also 8.4).
   - Metastatic or invasive mediastinal or pleural tumours.
   - Granuloma.

8.27 ULTRASONOGRAPHY OF THE DIAPHRAGM

A transhepatic approach in which a large part of the diaphragm is roughly perpendicular to the ultrasound beam is recommended, as this will give the best visualization of the diaphragm.

1. Enhanced visibility of the diaphragm.
   a. Fluid in the pleural cavity or mediastinum.
   b. Fluid in the abdominal cavity.
   c. Caudal thoracic mass enhancing sound passage.
   d. Consolidation of caudal lung lobes enhancing sound passage.
2. Irregular diaphragmatic outline.
   a. Nodular hepatic disease.
   b. Irregular caudal thoracic mass.
   c. Small diaphragmatic hernia.
   d. Diaphragmatic inflammatory deposits (fibrin deposition, granulomata).
   e. Diaphragmatic neoplastic deposits (metastases, or mediastinal or pleural tumours).
   f. Feline hypertrophic muscular dystrophy.
3. Thickened, echogenic diaphragm.
   a. Congenital Golden Retriever muscular dystrophy.
4. Loss of integrity of the diaphragmatic outline.
   a. Diaphragmatic rupture; also see displacement of the liver ± abdominal viscera in the thoracic cavity; differential diagnosis is mirror image artefact giving the appearance of liver within the thoracic cavity (see Appendix).
   b. Congenital peritoneopericardial diaphragmatic hernia – may have coexisting cardiac defects.

MISCELLANEOUS

8.28 THORACIC TRAUMA

Multiple lesions may be present following thoracic trauma, and systematic radiographic evaluation is vital to recognize the cause and extent of possible life-threatening conditions and to prioritize them for treatment. Follow-up radiographs should be made to check the effectiveness of treatment and in patients that were initially radiologically normal but that fail to recover as expected or deteriorate. Refer to specific organ systems for more detail.

1. Soft tissues of the thoracic wall.
   a. Gas accumulation – subcutaneous emphysema.
   b. Swelling – oedema or haemorrhage.
   c. Foreign bodies.
   d. Paracostal hernia – more common in cats.
2. Skeletal structures.
   a. Single or multiple rib fractures, often with associated pneumothorax, haematoma, pleural effusion or pulmonary contusion. Flail chest occurs when two or more adjacent ribs have multiple fractures, or in young dogs in which the costochondral junctions are loose.
   b. Widened intercostal spaces due to intercostal muscle tearing.
   c. Sternal, vertebral, scapular and long bone fractures and/or luxations.
   d. Triad of facial, extremital and thoracic injuries (pulmonary contusion and pneumothorax) in cats and dogs with high-rise syndrome.
3. Cranial abdomen – organ trauma resulting from caudal thoracic injuries; clinical and radiographic changes may have a delayed onset (e.g. organs incarcerated in a diaphragmatic rupture – see 8.2.3 and Fig. 8.3).
4. Pleural cavity – accumulation or asymmetrical distribution of pleural air or fluid around a specific lobe suggest that the lobe is abnormal and has collapsed more than other lobes.
   a. Pneumothorax.
      – Closed.
      – Open.
      – Tension; diaphragm caudally displaced and flattened.
   b. Diaphragmatic rupture.
   c. Haemothorax.
   d. Subpleural haematoma.
   e. Haemopneumothorax.
   f. Pyothorax – delayed onset.
   g. Chylothorax – delayed onset.
   h. Bilothorax – very rare.
5. Lungs.
   a. Contusions – poorly defined interstitial or alveolar infiltrates; resolve in a few days.
   b. Haematomas – appear after contusions, rounded and take weeks to resolve.
   c. Cysts and bullae.
   d. Lacerations.
   e. Atelectasis.
   f. Oedema – post head trauma.
   g. Pneumonia – delayed onset.
   h. Acute respiratory distress syndrome (shock lung) – usually delayed onset (see 6.14.7).
6. Cardiovascular system.
   a. Evidence of shock.
      – Microcardia.
      – Hypovascular lung field.
      – Small CdVC and aorta.
   b. Haemopericardium with cardiac tamponade.
      – Acute, difficult to see radiologically if only a small volume change.
      – May be delayed days or weeks, often after bullet or air gun pellet wounds.
   c. Pneumopericardium – auricles become visible; generally not clinically significant.
   d. Traumatic cardiac displacement.
      – Rupture of cardiac ligaments.
      – Rupture of pericardium with heart displaced outside pericardium.
      – Secondary to mediastinal shift (see 8.8).
7. Mediastinum.
   a. Pneumomediastinum.
   b. Mediastinal haemorrhage.
   c. Mediastinal oedema.
   d. Chylomediastinum.

8.29 ULTRASONOGRAPHY OF THORACIC TRAUMA

Ultrasonography is generally used to evaluate further abnormal or suspicious areas identified on thoracic radiographs. Refer to specific organ systems for more detail.

1. Soft tissues of the thoracic wall.
   a. Fluid accumulation (haematoma).
   b. Foreign bodies.
   c. Subcutaneous location of abdominal viscera.
2. Pleural cavity.
   a. Free fluid in thoracic cavity.
   b. Diaphragmatic rupture.
3. Lungs – moderate or extensive areas of lung collapse or consolidation.
4. Heart.

   a. Evidence of shock (tachycardia).
   b. Displacement of the heart (e.g. by abdominal viscera in diaphragmatic rupture).
   c. Pericardial haemorrhage ± tamponade.
   d. Dysfunctional myocardium (e.g. due to ischaemia, contusion).
5. Mediastinum – fluid accumulation (e.g. haemorrhage).
6. Diaphragm – see 8.27.

Further reading

General

Avner, A., Kirberger, R.M., 2005. Effect of various thoracic radiographic projections on the appearance of selected throacic viscera. J. Small Anim. Pract. 46, 491–498.

Berry, C.R., Gallaway, A., Thrall, D.E., Carlisle, C., 1993. Thoracic radiographic features of anticoagulant rodenticide toxicity in fourteen dogs. Vet. Radiol. Ultrasound 34, 391–396.

Blackwood, L., Sullivan, M., Lawson, H., 1997. Radiographic abnormalities in canine multicentric lymphoma: a review of 84 cases. J. Small Anim. Pract. 38, 62–69.

Brinkman, E.L., Biller, D., Armbrust, L., 2006. The clinical usefulness of the ventrodorsal versus dorsoventral thoracic radiograph in dogs. J. Am. Anim. Hosp. Assoc. 42, 440–449.

Brumitt, J.W., Essman, S.C., Kornegay, J.N., Graham, J.P., Webere, W.J., Berry, C.R., 2006. Radiographic features of golden retriever muscular dystrophy. Vet. Radiol. Ultrasound 47, 574–580.

Godshalk, C.P., 1994. Common pitfalls in radiographic interpretation of the thorax. Compend. Contin. Educ. Pract. Veterinarian (Small Animal) 16, 731–738.

Gordon, L.E., Thacher, C., Kapatkin, A., 1993. High-rise syndrome in dogs: 81 cases (1985–1991). J. Am. Anim. Hosp. Assoc. 202, 118–122.

Kirberger, R.M., Avner, A., 2006. The effect of positioning on the appearance of selected cranial thoracic structures in the dog. Vet. Radiol. Ultrasound 47, 61–68.

Schmidt, M., Wolvekamp, P., 1991. Radiographic findings in ten dogs with thoracic actinomycosis. Vet. Radiol. 32, 301–306.

Vignoli, M., Toniato, M., Rossi, F., Terragni, M., Manzini, M., Franchi, A., et al., 2002. Transient post-traumatic hemidiaphragmatic paralysis in two cats. J. Small Anim. Pract. 43, 312–316.

Whitney, W.O., Mehlhaff, C.J., 1987. High-rise syndrome in cats. J. Am. Anim. Hosp. Assoc. 191, 1399–1403.

Pleural cavity

Aronson, E., 1995. Radiology corner: Pneumothorax: ventrodorsal or dorsoventral view – does it make a difference? Vet. Radiol. Ultrasound 36, 109–110.

Holtsinger, R.H., Beale, B.S., Bellah, J.R., King, R.R., 1993. Spontaneous pneumothorax in the dog: a retrospective analysis of 21 cases. J. Am. Anim. Hosp. Assoc. 29, 195–210.

Lipscomb, V.J., Hardie, R.J., Dubielzig, R.R., 2003. Spontaneous pneumothorax caused by pulmonary blebs and bullae in 12 dogs. J. Am. Anim. Hosp. Assoc. 39, 435–445.

Naganobu, K., Ohigashi, Y., Akiyoshi, M., Hagio, M., Miyamoto, I., Yamaguchi, I., 2006. Lymphangiography of the thoracic duct by percutaneous injection of iohexol into the popliteal lymph node of dogs: experimental study and clinical application. Vet. Surg. 35, 377–381.

Packer, R.A., Frank, P.M., Chambers, J.N., 2004. Traumatic subarachnoid fistula in a dog. Vet. Radiol. Ultrasound 45, 523–527.

Stork, C.K., Hamaide, A.J., Schwedes, C.M., Clercx, C.M., Snaps, F.R., Balligand, M.H., 2003. Hemiurothorax following diaphragmatic hernia and kidney prolapse in a cat. J. Feline Med. Surg. 5, 91–96.

Thrall, D.E., 1993. Radiology corner: Misidentification of a skin fold as pneumothorax. Vet. Radiol. Ultrasound 34, 242–243.

Mediastinum

Fischetti, A.J., Kovak, J., 2008. Imaging diagnosis: Azygous continuation of the caudal vena cava with and without portacaval shunting. Vet. Radiol. Ultrasound 49, 573–576.

Griffiths, L.G., Sullivan, M., Lerche, P., 1998. Intrathoracic tracheal avulsion and pseudodiverticulum following pneumomediastinum in a cat. Vet. Rec. 142, 693–696.

Kirberger, R.M., Dvir, E., van de Merwe, L.L., 2009. The effect of positioning on the radiographic appearance of caudodorsal mediastinal masses in the dog. Vet. Radiol. Ultrasound 50, 630–634.

Myer, W., 1978. Radiography review: The mediastinum. J. Am. Vet. Radiol. Soc. 19, 197–202.

Rossi, F., Gaschen, L., Lang, J., 2003. Radiographic diagnosis: Intrathoracic gall bladder in a dog. Vet. Radiol. Ultrasound 44, 652–654.

Scrivani, P.V., Burt, J.K., Bruns, D., 1996. Radiology corner: Sternal lymphadenopathy. Vet. Radiol. Ultrasound 37, 183–184.

Van den Broek, A., 1986. Pneumomediastinum in seventeen dogs: aetiology and radiographic signs. J. Small Anim. Pract. 27, 747–757.

Zekas, L.J., Adams, W.M., 2002. Cranial mediastinal cysts in nine cats. Vet. Radiol. Ultrasound 43, 413–416.

Oesophagus

Bexfield, N.H., Watson, P.J., Herrtage, M.E., 2006. Esophageal dysmotility in young dogs. J. Vet. Intern. Medic. 20, 1314–1318.

Buchanan, J.W., 2004. Tracheal signs and associated vascular anomalies in dogs with persistent right aortic arch. J. Vet. Intern Med. 18, 510–514.

Detweiler, D.A., Biller, D.S., Hoskinson, J.J., Harkin, K.R., 2001. Radiographic findings of canine dysautonomia in twenty-

four dogs. Vet. Radiol. Ultrasound 42, 108–112.

Dvir, E., Kirberger, R.M., Malleczek, D., 2001. Radiographic and computed tomographic changes and clinical presentation of spirocercosis in the dog. Vet. Radiol. Ultrasound 42, 119–129.

Elwood, C., 2006. Diagnosis and management of canine oesophageal disease and regurgitation. In Pract. 28, 14–21.

Galatos, A.D., Rallis, T., Raptopoulos, D., 1994. Post anaesthetic oesophageal stricture formation in three cats. J. Small Anim. Pract. 35, 638–642.

Hardie, E.M., Ramirez III, O., Clary, E.M., Kornegay, K.N., Corea, M.T., Feimster, R.A., et al., 1998. Abnormalities of the thoracic bellows: stress fractures of the ribs and hiatal hernia. J. Vet. Intern. Med. 12, 279–287.

Mears, E.A., Jenkins, C.C., 1997. Canine and feline megaesophagus. Compend. Contin. Educ. Pract. Veterinarian (Small Animal) 19, 313–326.

Pearson, H., Gaskell, C.J., Gibbs, C., Waterman, A., 1974. Pyloric and oesophageal dysfunction in the cat. J. Small Anim. Pract. 15, 487–504.

Pratschke, K.M., Hughes, J.M.L., Skelly, C.R., Bellenger, C.R., 1998. Hiatal herniation as a complication of chronic diaphragmatic herniation. J. Small Anim. Pract. 39, 33–38.

Sickle, R.L., Love, N.E., 1989. Radiographic diagnosis of esophageal disease in dogs and cats. Semin. Vet. Med. Surg. (Small Animal) 4, 179–187.

van der Merwe, L.L., Kirberger, R.M., Clift, M., Williams, M., Keller, N., Naidoo, V., 2008. *Spirocerca lupi* infection in the dog: a review. Vet. J. 176, 294–309.

van Gundy, T., 1989. Vascular ring anomalies. Compend. Contin.

Educ. Pract. Vet. (Small Animal) 11, 35–45.

Thoracic wall

Berry, C.R., Koblik, P.D., Ticer, J.W., 1990. Dorsal peritoneopericardial mesothelial remnant as an aid to the diagnosis of feline congenital peritoneopericardial diaphragmatic hernia. Vet. Radiol. 31, 239–245.

Brumitt, J.W., Essman, S.C., Kornegay, J.N., Graham, J.P., Weber, W.J., Berry, C.R., 2006. Radiographic features of golden retriever muscular dystrophy. Vet. Radiol. Ultrasound 47, 574–580.

Choi, J., Kim, H., Kim, M., Yoon, J., 2009. Imaging diagnosis – Positive contrast peritoneographic features of true diaphragmatic hernia. Vet. Radiol. Ultrasound 50, 185–187.

Dennis, R., 1993. Radiographic diagnosis of rib lesions in dogs and cats. Vet. Annu. 33, 173–192.

Fagin, B., 1989. Using radiography to diagnose diaphragmatic hernia. Vet. Med. 7, 662–672.

Fossum, T.W., Boudrieu, R.J., Hobson, H.P., 1989. Pectus excavatum in eight dogs and six cats. J. Am. Anim. Hosp. Assoc. 25, 595–605.

Hardie, E.M., Ramirez III, O., Clary, E.M., Kornegay, K.N., Corea, M.T., Feimster, R.A., et al., 1998. Abnormalities of the thoracic bellows: stress fractures of the ribs and hiatal hernia. J. Vet. Intern. Med. 12, 279–287.

Sullivan, M., Lee, R., 1989. Radiological features of 80 cases of diaphragmatic rupture. J. Small Anim. Pract. 30, 561–566.

Williams, J., Leveille, R., Myer, C.W., 1998. Imaging modalities used to confirm diaphragmatic hernia in small animals. Compend. Contin. Educ. Pract. Veterinarian (Small Animal) 20, 1199–1208.

Ultrasonography

Barrett, R.J., Mann, F.A., Aronson, E., 1993. Use of ultrasonography and secondary wound closure to facilitate diagnosis and treatment of a cranial mediastinal abscess in a dog. J. Am. Vet. Med. Assoc. 203, 1293–1295.

Reichle, J.K., Wisner, E.R., 2000. Non-cardiac thoracic ultrasound in 75 feline and canine patients. Vet. Radiol. Ultrasound 41, 154–162.

Spattini, G., Rossi, F., Vignoli, M., Lamb, C.R., 2003. Use of ultrasound to diagnose diaphragmatic rupture in dogs and cats. Vet. Radiol. Ultrasound 44, 226–230.

Tidwell, A.S., 1998. Ultrasonography of the thorax (excluding the heart). Vet. Clin North Am. Small Anim. Pract. 28 (4), 993–1016.

Chapter 9

Other abdominal structures: abdominal wall, peritoneal and retroperitoneal cavities, parenchymal organs

CHAPTER CONTENTS

9.1 Radiographic technique for the abdomen and effect of positioning   230

9.2 Ultrasonographic technique for the abdomen   231

Abdominal wall   232

9.3 Variations in shape of the abdominal wall   232

9.4 Variations in radiopacity of the abdominal wall   233

9.5 Ultrasonography of the abdominal wall   233

Peritoneal cavity   233

9.6 Increased radiopacity of the peritoneal cavity and/or loss of visualization of abdominal organs   233

9.7 Decreased radiopacity of the peritoneal cavity   235

9.8 Ultrasonography of the peritoneal cavity   235

Retroperitoneal space   236

9.9 Enlargement of the retroperitoneal space   236

9.10 Increased radiopacity of the retroperitoneal space and/or loss of visualization of the retroperitoneal structures   237

9.11 Decreased radiopacity of the retroperitoneal space   238

9.12 Ultrasonography of the retroperitoneal space   238

9.13 Ultrasonography of the lymph nodes in the retroperitoneal space   238

9.14 Ultrasonography of the abdominal aorta and caudal vena cava   238

Liver   239

9.15 Displacement of the liver   239

9.16 Variations in liver size   239

9.17 Variations in liver shape   241

9.18 Variations in liver radiopacity   242

9.19 Hepatic contrast studies   242

9.20 Ultrasonographic technique for the liver   245

9.21 Normal ultrasonographic appearance of the liver   245

9.22 Ultrasonographic abnormalities of the hepatic parenchyma   245

9.23 Ultrasonographic abnormalities of the biliary tract   247

9.24 Ultrasonographic abnormalities of the hepatic vascular system   247

Spleen   248

9.25 Absence of the splenic shadow   248

9.26 Variations in location of the spleen   248

9.27 Variations in splenic size and shape   249

9.28 Variations in splenic radiopacity   250

9.29 Ultrasonographic technique for the spleen   250

9.30 Normal ultrasonographic appearance of the spleen   250

9.31 Ultrasonographic abnormalities of the spleen   250

Pancreas 252
9.32 Pancreatic radiology 252
9.33 Ultrasonographic technique for the pancreas 252
9.34 Normal ultrasonographic appearance of the pancreas 252
9.35 Ultrasonographic abnormalities of the pancreas 253

Adrenal glands 253
9.36 Adrenal gland radiology 253
9.37 Ultrasonography of the adrenal glands 254

Abdominal masses 255
9.38 Cranial abdominal masses (largely within the costal arch) 255
9.39 Mid-abdominal masses 257
9.40 Caudal abdominal masses 259

Miscellaneous 260
9.41 Mineralization on abdominal radiographs 260

Table 9.1 Effect of positioning on abdominal structures in normal dogs

ANATOMICAL AREA	RIGHT LATERAL RECUMBENCY	LEFT LATERAL RECUMBENCY
Gas in stomach	Gas in the fundus and body; fluid gravitates to the dependent pylorus, where it may mimic a round soft tissue opacity, foreign body or mass	Gas in the pylorus
Gas in proximal duodenum	Not seen	Often seen
Kidneys	Less superimposition	More superimposition
Liver	Appears smaller than on left lateral recumbency	Appears larger than on right lateral recumbency
Spleen	Often seen	Rarely seen

9.1 RADIOGRAPHIC TECHNIQUE FOR THE ABDOMEN AND EFFECT OF POSITIONING

Radiography should be performed when possible as an elective procedure to ensure an empty gastrointestinal tract, as a food-filled stomach or faeces-filled colon may severely hamper interpretation. Lateral and ventrodorsal (VD) positions are the standard. The choice between right lateral recumbent (RLR) and left lateral recumbent (LLR) is a personal one, but whichever is chosen it should be used consistently to familiarize the user with its normal appearance. The differences between the two lateral views are described in Table 9.1. Collimation should include the whole diaphragm and the pelvic inlet. In animals with urinary obstruction, the radiograph should extend caudally to include the whole perineal and urethral area; in large dogs, this may require two separate radiographs. Exposure should be made on expiration to avoid motion blur. Left lateral decubitus views can be used to detect free abdominal gas (see 9.7).

For digital radiography, an appropriate algorithm should be used to combine resolution and contrast. For conventional film radiography, a fast film–screen combination should be used to minimize motion blur, and a grid should be employed if the abdomen is > 10 cm thick or in smaller, obese dogs. A short-scale contrast technique (low kV, high mAs) will improve the naturally low contrast of the abdominal organs. Increased abdominal detail can be obtained by trying to maximize organ separation. This can be achieved by placing the dog in dorsal rather than sternal recumbency, positioning the pelvic limbs perpendicular to the spine and making the exposure on expiration.

Optimal evaluation of abdominal radiographs requires a systematic approach, which involves assessing radiographic technique, signalment (breed type, age, sex, body condition), extra-abdominal structures (superficial soft tissues, osseous structures, caudal thorax and diaphragm) and intra-abdominal structures, and then re-evaluating abnormalities and areas in the light of the history and clinical examination. Intra-abdominal evaluation may be done on a system basis: gastrointestinal, urinary tract, reproductive tract, parenchymatous organs (liver and spleen), endocrine organs (adrenals and pancreas), peritoneal cavity and retroperitoneal space, and lymphatic system (sublumbar lymph nodes). Alternatively, a quadrant approach can be used. For viewing abdominal radiographs, the convention is that lateral radiographs are examined with the diaphragm facing to the left, and VD radiographs with the diaphragm uppermost and the left side of the patient on the right side of the computer screen or light box. Abdominal fat in smaller dogs and in cats helps to outline abdominal structures, as the lower fat opacity contrasts well with the soft tissue opacity of the majority of abdominal organs. However, in large obese dogs this advantage is lost, as the large amounts of fat result in excessive amounts of scatter, which degrades the image despite the use of a grid.

If an organ that is normally visible is not seen despite good-quality radiographs, pathology is implied. Similarly, if an organ that is normally not seen becomes partly or completely visible, disease is also likely. Structures normally visible and not visible on abdominal radiograph are listed in Box 9.1. There are some radiographic anatomical differences between the dog and cat, and these are given in Table 9.2.

BOX 9.1   Abdominal structures normally visible and not visible in the dog

Normally visible

- Ventral liver lobes.
- Spleen on right lateral recumbent view.
- Stomach.
- Small intestines.
- Caecum.
- Colon.
- Kidneys.
- Bladder.
- Prostate (not young dogs).
- Peritoneal cavity.
- Retroperitoneal space.

Normally not visible

- Pancreas.
- Adrenals.
- Gall bladder.
- Ureters.
- Urethra.
- Ovaries.
- Non-gravid uterus.
- Lymph nodes.
- Blood vessels.

Table 9.2   Differences between the abdomen of the normal dog and cat

ANATOMICAL AREA	DOG	CAT
Gastric and duodenal position on the ventrodorsal view	Lies transversely within the costal arch, and the descending duodenum is adjacent to the right body wall	Pylorus is in the midline with an acute angular incisure, and descending duodenum lies slightly to the right of the midline
Gastric layering	Not seen	May be seen due to fat deposition in wall
Kidneys	Whole left and caudal pole of right usually seen	Both kidneys seen; fat may be seen in the renal pelvis in obese cats
Bladder location	Bladder neck prepubic	Due to long urethra, lies more cranially in the abdomen
Spleen	Readily seen on right lateral recumbent views	Not usually seen in the ventral abdomen on lateral views
Caecum	Seen in the right mid-abdomen as gas-filled structure	Not seen
Adrenals	Not seen	Mineralized adrenals are occasionally seen as an incidental finding
Abdominal fat	May be present	Often large amounts, which provides good abdominal contrast

---

9.2 ULTRASONOGRAPHIC TECHNIQUE FOR THE ABDOMEN

Curvilinear or sector transducers allow optimal access to intra-abdominal structures, although linear array transducers may also be used. As high a frequency as possible should be selected while still achieving adequate tissue penetration (e.g. 7.5 MHz for cats or small dogs and 5 MHz for medium or large dogs).

The chosen acoustic window should be carefully prepared by clipping hair from the area, cleaning the skin with surgical spirit to remove dirt and grease, and applying liberal quantities of acoustic gel. In general, it is preferable to do a complete abdominal examination in each patient rather than restricting the examination to an individual organ system. It is essential to follow a systematic approach to the examination to ensure that no organ is missed. The precise order of the examination is not important, but it can be helpful to image the easier organs first to allow the patient to settle into the procedure. The patient may be in lateral or dorsal recumbency depending on personal preference. The position of the animal can be altered if necessary to make use of the effects of gravity on the distribution of intestine filled with large amounts of gas, or evaluating the mobility of suspect hyperechoic structures within fluid-filled structures.

Ultrasound-guided fine needle aspiration using a 22-gauge needle or spinal needle for deeper structures can be readily performed. With increasing expertise, the needle can be guided into small pathological areas. Alternatively, a tissue core biopsy can be performed under ultrasound guidance after ensuring that clotting factors are normal.

The selected acoustic window should be prepared aseptically and the transducer carefully cleaned. A sterile transducer sleeve can be used to cover the transducer if desired. The tissue or organ of interest should be imaged, and the position of the transducer adjusted until the region to be sampled is clearly seen and there is space to introduce the needle safely at an appropriate angle adjacent to the transducer.

In order to aspirate fluid, the needle is introduced until the tip is seen clearly within the fluid. If necessary, the transducer may be rocked gently from side to side to identify the needle. When positioning is confirmed, fluid is aspirated then the needle is withdrawn.

For fine needle aspiration of a solid organ, the needle is introduced as described above into the tissue of interest. When the needle tip is in position, a gentle in and out movement of the needle is made, and it is then withdrawn. If this does not yield a sample, the procedure may be repeated, applying gentle suction when the needle is in position.

For a tissue core biopsy, the needle is introduced as above and samples of tissue are collected from both the centre and the periphery of the lesion.

ABDOMINAL WALL

The abdominal wall is formed by the diaphragm and rib cage cranially, abdominal muscles ventrally and laterally, sublumbar muscles dorsally and peritoneum caudally.

9.3 VARIATIONS IN SHAPE OF THE ABDOMINAL WALL

1. Generalized distension of the abdominal wall.
   a. Obesity – abdominal viscera well outlined by fat; large falciform fat pad.
   b. Loss of muscle tone, resulting in sagging of abdominal structures.
      – Old age.
      – Cushing's syndrome (hyperadrenocorticism) – naturally occurring or iatrogenic.
   c. Large abdominal mass, especially splenic.
   d. Gastric distension by food or gas (see 10.3.4 and 10.3.5 and Fig. 10.2).
   e. Small intestinal distension (see 10.21.3 and Fig. 10.10, e.g. low obstruction).
   f. Severe faecal retention (see 10.40 and 10.41.4).
   g. Uterine distension in female animals.
      – Mid- to late-term pregnancy.
      – Large pyometra.
      – Large mucometra, haemometra or hydrometra.
   h. Severe peritoneal effusion.
      – Right heart failure.
      – Liver disease.
      – Nephrotic syndrome.
      – Other causes of hypoproteinaemia.
      – Obstruction of the caudal vena cava (CdVC).
      – Ruptured urinary bladder.
      – Intra-abdominal haemorrhage.
      – Cats – feline infectious peritonitis (FIP).
   i. Severe pneumoperitoneum.
2. Focal distension of the abdominal wall.
   a. Umbilical hernia.
   b. Inguinal hernia (Fig. 9.1).
   c. Traumatic rupture of abdominal or paracostal muscles.
   d. Surgical wound breakdown.
      In (a)–(d), viscera may be contained within the focal distension (a contrast study or ultrasonography may be helpful if this is unclear on plain radiographs).

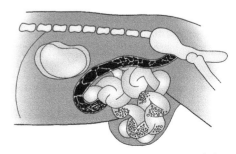

Figure 9.1 Inguinal hernia: viscera extend beyond the normal abdominal boundary and the line of the abdominal wall is lost.

e. Abdominal wall abscess.

f. Abdominal wall haematoma.

g. Abdominal wall seroma.

h. Abdominal wall neoplasm.

i. Lipoma – fat opacity.

3. Inward displacement of the abdominal wall.

a. Emaciation.

b. Diaphragmatic rupture with herniation of abdominal viscera into the thoracic cavity.

c. Peritoneopericardial diaphragmatic hernia, with movement of abdominal viscera into the pericardial sac.

d. Severe inspiratory dyspnoea.

4. Thickening of the abdominal wall.

a. After laparotomy.

b. Trauma – contusion, haemorrhage or rupture.

9.4 VARIATIONS IN RADIOPACITY OF THE ABDOMINAL WALL

In a well-nourished adult animal, fat interspersed between the fascial planes allows visualization of the various muscle layers.

1. Increased soft tissue radiopacity and loss of distinction of muscle layers of the abdominal wall.

a. Trauma with oedema or haemorrhage of the soft tissues.

b. Abdominal wall neoplasia.

c. Large volumes of fluid administered subcutaneously.

d. Cellulitis.

e. Healing laparotomy.

2. Mineralized radiopacity of the abdominal wall.

a. Overlying wire skin sutures or staples.

b. Overlying wet or dirty hair coat or ultrasound gel mimicking mineralized radiopacity.

c. Calcinosis cutis associated with hyperadrenocorticism (Cushing's disease).

d. Mineralization of superficial skin masses.

e. Foreign material (e.g. ballistics, dirt in the hair coat).

f. Ointments or lotions containing radiopaque compounds (e.g. iodine, zinc) applied to the skin surface.

3. Decreased radiopacity of the abdominal wall.

a. Fat – lipoma or liposarcoma.

b. Gas.

– Local skin lacerations or defects.

– Subcutaneous emphysema extending from a wound elsewhere.

– Gas dissecting along fascial planes from a pneumomediastinum or pneumoretroperitoneum.

– Recent surgical incision.

– Gas within a hernia that contains small intestine.

9.5 ULTRASONOGRAPHY OF THE ABDOMINAL WALL

Interpretation is similar to that of ultrasonography of the soft tissues of the thoracic wall (see 8.24).

PERITONEAL CAVITY

The abdominal cavity is lined by peritoneum, and the areas between the major organs and the intestine are known as the peritoneal cavity (Fig. 9.2). In the normal adult animal, serosal detail of abdominal viscera is demonstrated by intra-abdominal fat.

9.6 INCREASED RADIOPACITY OF THE PERITONEAL CAVITY AND/OR LOSS OF VISUALIZATION OF ABDOMINAL ORGANS

All causes of increased intra-abdominal radiopacity result in loss of serosal detail by obscuring intra-abdominal fat, which normally provides contrast with soft tissues. A diffuse and homogeneous increase in

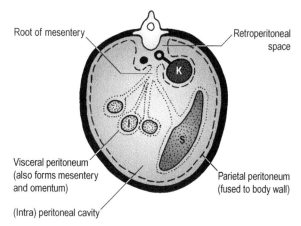

Figure 9.2 Schematic representation of the mid-abdomen in cross-section, showing the peritoneal cavity and retroperitoneal space. I, small intestine; K, kidney; S, spleen.

intra-abdominal opacity and loss of serosal detail is sometimes referred to as a ground glass appearance and is usually due to free abdominal fluid. Increase in opacity may also be patchy or mottled.

1. Generalized and homogeneous increase in radiopacity of the peritoneal cavity.
    a. Normal animal – suboptimal radiograph.
       – Underexposure.
       – Underdevelopment.
       – kVp setting too high, leading to reduced contrast.
       – Scattered radiation if no grid has been used with a large abdomen.
    b. Diffusely wet hair coat.
    c. Normal puppy or kitten – lack of abdominal fat due to young age.
    d. Emaciation and lack of abdominal fat – abdominal wall tucked inwards.
    e. Peritoneal effusion – often abdominal distension too.
       – Ascites (hydroperitoneum; Fig. 9.3): right heart failure, liver disease, portal hypertension, hypoproteinaemia, obstruction of the CdVC (see 9.16.1), neoplasia (specific organ, mesothelioma or carcinomatosis), other causes.
       – Haemoperitoneum: ruptured abdominal tumour, particularly splenic haemangiosarcoma (especially German Shepherd dogs); coagulopathy (warfarin poisoning, thrombocytopenia, disseminated intravascular coagulation, congenital bleeding disorders, angiostrongylosis*); trauma, ruptured vascular anomaly, spontaneous liver

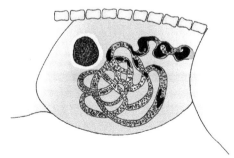

Figure 9.3 Ascites: loss of abdominal serosal detail and diffuse soft tissue (fluid) radiopacity, with only enteric gas, ingesta and faeces being visible. The abdomen is usually distended (cf. emaciation).

rupture with amyloidosis (especially oriental cats).
       – Uroabdomen – ruptured urinary bladder or urethra.
       – Bile peritonitis – ruptured gall bladder or bile duct.
       – Chylous effusion – may be due to neoplasia or hepatic portal vein obstruction.
       – Cats – feline infectious peritonitis.
    f. After peritoneal dialysis or other intraperitoneal fluid administration.
2. Generalized but heterogeneous increase in radiopacity of the peritoneal cavity.
    a. Artefactual due to overlying wet or dirty hair coat.
    b. Peritonitis.
       – Recent laparotomy.
       – Intestinal rupture – dilated intestinal loops and free gas in the peritoneal cavity are also likely; these findings warrant immediate surgical exploration.
       – Trauma (e.g. penetrating wounds).
       – Migrating gastrointestinal foreign body (e.g. wooden skewer).
       – Pancreatitis.
       – Bile or urine peritonitis.
    c. Small peritoneal effusion – see above for list of possible causes (ultrasonography is more sensitive than radiography for the detection of small effusions).
    d. Peritoneal carcinomatosis (usually metastatic) – due to neoplastic nodules and free fluid.
    e. Cats – steatitis – large amounts of intra-abdominal fat of mottled, increased opacity.
       – Vitamin E deficiency.
       – Fish diet.
3. Localized increase in radiopacity of the peritoneal cavity – often heterogeneous.
    a. Artefact – superimposed wet or dirty hair; ultrasound gel on coat; lotions or ointments containing radiopaque compounds.
    b. Abdominal lymphadenopathy, usually neoplastic.
    c. Localized abdominal trauma.
    d. Intestinal perforation walled off by mesentery.
    e. Pancreatitis – right cranial quadrant of abdomen.

f. Ruptured gall bladder – right cranial quadrant of abdomen.
g. Peritoneal spread from adjacent neoplastic mass.
h. Walled-off abscess.
i. Prostatitis.
j. Retained surgical swab.
4. Mineralized opacity in the peritoneal cavity – commoner causes (see 9.41 for a more comprehensive list).
a. Mineralized ingesta in the bowel.
b. Mineralized foreign bodies in the bowel.
c. Foreign body free in the peritoneal cavity.
d. Urolithiasis.
e. Pregnancy.
f. Cholelithiasis.
g. Paraprostatic cyst; wall often mineralized, with an eggshell appearance.
h. Dystrophic or metastatic mineralization of soft tissues (see 12.2.2).
   – Neoplasia.
   – Chronic haematoma or abscess.
   – Hyperparathyroidism.
   – Associated with retained surgical swab.
   – Nodular fat necrosis – usually old, obese cats.
i. Barium or iodinated contrast medium leaking from perforated gastrointestinal or urogenital tract.

9.7 DECREASED RADIOPACITY OF THE PERITONEAL CAVITY

1. Fat opacity – intra-abdominal lipoma; viscera will be displaced by the lipoma.
2. Gas opacity – a small volume of free gas is detected most accurately by taking a standing lateral radiograph or an LLR VD view with a horizontal beam. With both views, gas will rise to the highest part of the peritoneal cavity once the patient has maintained the position for a few minutes. With larger amounts of free gas, the liver and diaphragm will be separated, outlining the diaphragm, and there will be increased visibility of the serosal surface of intestines and other organs.
a. Iatrogenic.
   – Post laparotomy.
   – Post peritoneal dialysis.
   – Post paracentesis (small amounts of gas).
   – Overdistension of bladder during pneumocystography, especially in cats with feline idiopathic cystitis.
   – Retained surgical swab – small gas foci.
   – Air embolism – gas in blood vessels.
   – Pneumocoeliography.
b. Perforated hollow viscus (trauma, neoplasia, ulceration) – increased radiopacity may also be present due to peritonitis or free fluid.
   – Perforated stomach – large volume of gas causing abdominal distension and spontaneous pneumoperitoneum.
   – Perforated small or large intestine.
   – Ruptured bladder with pneumocystogram performed.
c. Leakage of gas from emphysematous organ (e.g. stomach, bladder, colon or uterus).
d. Leakage of gas through an intact, distended stomach wall (e.g. gastric dilation and volvulus, GDV).
e. Entry of air through the abdominal wall.
   – Penetrating wound.
   – Around an abdominal drain or feeding tube.
f. Infection with gas-producing organisms.
g. Gas in an abscess (may see fluid line with a horizontal beam).
h. Pneumothorax with a diaphragmatic rupture.
i. Post-mortem change in major vessels, occurring within 12 h of death.

9.8 ULTRASONOGRAPHY OF THE PERITONEAL CAVITY

1. Peritoneal fluid – fluid (transudate or modified transudate) is generally anechoic but may contain echoes (exudate) depending on its cellular content or the presence of debris or small gas bubbles. Fluid surrounds and separates the abdominal organs, often enhancing visibility of these structures. In order to detect small quantities of fluid, the dependent portions of the abdomen should be examined. In particular, small accumulations of fluid may be found between the liver lobes, between the liver and the diaphragm, and around the urinary bladder. Ultrasonography is more sensitive than

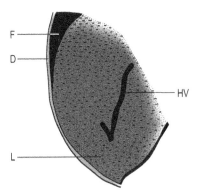

Figure 9.4 Mild ascites on ultrasound: a small amount of anechoic fluid is seen between the liver and diaphragm. D, diaphragm; F, free abdominal fluid trapped between the liver and the diaphragm; HV, hepatic vein; L, liver parenchyma.

radiography for detecting small quantities of free fluid (Fig. 9.4). For differential diagnoses for the causes of peritoneal effusions, see 9.6.1.

2. Free gas – this results in a poor-quality image and multiple artefacts (shadowing and reverberation). The effect of free gas on image quality can be reduced by altering the position of the patient and imaging from the dependent aspect. Radiography is more sensitive than ultrasound for the detection of small quantities of free gas in the peritoneal cavity; the gas rises to the uppermost portion of the abdomen and in dorsal recumbency will be found in the sternal region. For differential diagnoses for the causes of free gas, see 9.7.2.

3. Peritoneal masses.
   a. Carcinomatosis – parietal and visceral peritoneal masses and free fluid; may also see primary or metastatic masses in abdominal organs and enlarged abdominal lymph nodes.
   b. Granuloma – may occur around a retained surgical sponge or swab, non-absorbable sutures or other foreign material; hypoechoic mass with central strong acoustic shadowing.
   c. Abscess – wall of variable thickness and contents of variable echogenicity.
   d. Cyst – thin-walled, mostly septated cysts are seen on the peritoneal surface of abdominal organs and omentum in peritoneal cestodiasis in dogs and cats; in the later stages, there may be abdominal fluid and peritoneal thickening.

RETROPERITONEAL SPACE

The retroperitoneal space (retroperitoneum) is the region of the abdomen ventral to the spine and dorsal to the intestines, lying outside the peritoneal cavity (see Fig. 9.2). The kidneys and prostate protrude into the peritoneal cavity from the retroperitoneal space and are partly covered by peritoneum. Retroperitoneal fat outlines the kidneys and ventral musculature of the spine. In fat animals, the deep circumflex arteries seen end on ventral to the caudal lumbar vertebrae may simulate the appearance of mineral opacities such as ureteric calculi. The aorta, CdVC and ureters are occasionally seen running through the retroperitoneal space in obese animals, but other retroperitoneal structures such as the adrenal glands and lymph nodes are not detectable when normal. The overall radiopacity of the retroperitoneal space should be similar to that of the peritoneal cavity.

9.9 ENLARGEMENT OF THE RETROPERITONEAL SPACE

1. Generalized retroperitoneal enlargement of fat opacity; normal visualization of the kidneys and sublumbar musculature; ventral displacement of the intestines.
   a. Normal, obese animal; the kidneys are clearly seen, and occasionally blood vessels and ureters are visible.
   b. Retroperitoneal lipoma.
2. Generalized retroperitoneal enlargement of soft tissue opacity; loss of visualization of the kidneys and sublumbar musculature; ventral displacement of the intestines (Fig. 9.5).
   a. Retroperitoneal haemorrhage.

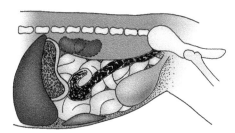

Figure 9.5 Generalized enlargement of the retroperitoneal space: loss of kidney outline (represented by dotted lines) and ventral displacement of intraperitoneal viscera.

- Trauma to the kidneys or retroperitoneal blood vessels (ensure renal artery and vasculature are intact using colour flow Doppler).
- Coagulopathy.
- Bleeding from retroperitoneal neoplasm (especially adrenal).
- Ruptured vascular anomaly.

b. Retroperitoneal urine.
- Trauma to the ureters (rupture, or avulsion from the kidneys or bladder); intravenous urography will demonstrate urine leakage, although the site of leakage may not be identified.

c. Inflammation or abscessation.
- Migrating foreign body (e.g. grass awn); a periosteal reaction may be present along the ventral margins of lumbar vertebrae, especially L3 and L4 (differential diagnosis is normal ill-defined ventral margins of these vertebrae where the diaphragmatic crura attach – see 5.4.4 and Fig. 5.7).
- Penetrating wounds (e.g. bites).
- Post-operative complication of ovariohysterectomy.
- Fat necrosis secondary to pancreatitis.

d. Neoplasia.
- Secondary to neoplasia of lumbar vertebrae (for bony changes, see 5.4.3 and Fig. 5.7).
- Sublumbar muscle.
- Other retroperitoneal organs or soft tissues.

3. Focal retroperitoneal enlargement of soft tissue opacity.
a. Renal mass (see 10.2.3, 10.2.4 and 9.39.3 and Fig. 9.18).
b. Enlargement of the medial iliac (sublumbar) lymph nodes ventral to L6–7; ventral displacement ± compression of the descending colon.
- Lymphoma (often with hepatosplenomegaly).
- Metastasis from malignant neoplasia in the hindquarters: prostate, urinary bladder, rectum and perianal region, pelvic canal, pelvic bones, pelvic limbs, tail.
- Reactive, secondary to inflammatory process in the hindquarters.

c. Urinoma (paraureteral or uriniferous pseudocyst) following ureteric trauma and encapsulated urine leakage.
d. Adrenal mass; mass medial or craniomedial to ipsilateral kidney; may show wispy mineralization.
- Adenocarcinoma.
- Adenoma.
- Phaeochromocytoma.
e. Abscess or focal inflammation of retroperitoneal soft tissue or sublumbar muscle.
f. Primary or metastatic neoplasia of retroperitoneal soft tissue or sublumbar muscle.
g. Soft tissue swelling associated with a lumbar or sacral vertebral lesion – look for bone changes too.
- Spondylitis.
- Spinal trauma.
- Neoplasia.

9.10 INCREASED RADIOPACITY OF THE RETROPERITONEAL SPACE AND/OR LOSS OF VISUALIZATION OF THE RETROPERITONEAL STRUCTURES

1. Soft tissue opacity of the retroperitoneal space, with loss of visualization of the kidneys and sublumbar musculature.
a. Overlying severe peritoneal effusion.
b. Retroperitoneal haemorrhage (see 9.9.2).
c. Retroperitoneal urine (see 9.9.2).
d. Inflammation or abscessation (see 9.9.2).
e. Neoplasia of lumbar vertebrae or sublumbar muscle (see 9.9.2).
2. Focal mineralized opacity of the retroperitoneal space.
a. Artefactual due to blood vessels seen end on.
b. Overlying intestinal contents.
c. Incidental mineralization of adrenals in aged animals, more often in cats (bilateral, dumb-bell-shaped).
d. Ureteral calculus; intravenous urography needed to demonstrate its ureteral location, although the osmotic diuresis induced may flush the calculus into the bladder.
e. Mineralization of a tumour (e.g. adrenal tumour); especially in dogs (unilateral, wispy or patchy mineralization).

f. Vertebral pathology with new bone extending into the sublumbar soft tissues.

g. Mineralization of major arteries.
   - Chronic renal failure.
   - Vitamin D toxicosis.
   - Primary hyperparathyroidism.
   - Hypercalcaemia of malignancy.
   - Cats – hypertension and secondary arteriosclerosis.

9.11 DECREASED RADIOPACITY OF THE RETROPERITONEAL SPACE

The dorsal part of the diaphragm and the retroperitoneal structures will be outlined.

1. Fat opacity in the retroperitoneal space.
   a. Excessive sublumbar fat in an obese animal.
   b. Retroperitoneal lipoma.
2. Gas lucency in the retroperitoneal space (pneumoretroperitoneum).
   a. Extension of pneumomediastinum through the aortic hiatus of the diaphragm.
   b. Following perineal urethrostomy or perforation of urethra during catheterization.
   c. Penetrating wound.

9.12 ULTRASONOGRAPHY OF THE RETROPERITONEAL SPACE

The retroperitoneal space may be imaged from a ventral abdominal or flank approach. A high-frequency (≥ 7.5 MHz) transducer should be used.

1. Retroperitoneal fluid – fluid is generally anechoic but may contain a variable number of echoes depending on the presence of cells, debris and/or gas bubbles. Fluid accumulations may be throughout the retroperitoneal space or localized. Small volumes of fluid will tend to spread along the natural planes in the retroperitoneum, giving a lacy appearance. For differential diagnoses for the causes of retroperitoneal fluid accumulation, see 9.9.2 and 9.9.3. A migrating foreign body may be seen as a hyperechoic structure, with or without acoustic shadowing, within an accumulation of fluid (see 12.6.3. and Fig. 12.5).
2. Retroperitoneal mass.
   a. Neoplasm.
      - Renal.
      - Adrenal.
      - Other.
   b. Granuloma.
   c. Abscess.
   d. Haematoma.
      - Traumatic.
      - Coagulopathy.
      - Bleeding from a retroperitoneal tumour or vascular anomaly.
   e. Enlarged lymph nodes (see 9.13).

9.13 ULTRASONOGRAPHY OF THE LYMPH NODES IN THE RETROPERITONEAL SPACE

The medial iliac lymph nodes lie close to the abdominal aorta and CdVC at their caudal bifurcation. They may be visible in normal animals as well-defined, elongated, hypoechoic structures. The lumbar lymph nodes extend along the paralumbar tissues but are usually recognized ultrasonographically only when enlarged. It is difficult to differentiate malignant from reactive lymph nodes. Neoplastic lymph nodes are usually rounded and hypoechoic but can be heterogeneous. Doppler blood flow patterns can be helpful, with predominantly hilar flow strongly suggestive of a benign process.

1. Enlargement of lymph nodes – tend to become more rounded as they enlarge, but they may also become irregular in shape and heterogeneous in echogenicity.
   a. Reactive enlargement in response to an inflammatory lesion in the hindquarters.
   b. Multicentric lymphoma or other myeloproliferative disorders.
   c. Metastasis from malignant neoplasia in the hindquarters.

9.14 ULTRASONOGRAPHY OF THE ABDOMINAL AORTA AND CAUDAL VENA CAVA

The aorta lies dorsal and to the left of the CdVC in the retroperitoneal space. Pulsations of both vessels may be evident, due to referred aortic pulsation affecting the CdVC. The CdVC is more easily compressed by pressure from the transducer. Doppler ultrasound allows definitive differentiation between the two.

1. Vascular intraluminal mass.
   a. Thrombus or embolus secondary to:

– Cardiac disease.
– Neoplastic invasion.
– Aortic aneurysm from *Spirocerca lupi** larval migration.
  b. Neoplastic invasion from an adjacent mass, especially adrenal.
2. Vascular narrowing.
  a. Caudal vena cava, due to transducer pressure.
  b. Extrinsic compression by a mass.
3. Vascular anomalies.
  a. Portosystemic shunts (see 9.24).
  b. Arteriovenous fistula.
  c. Other anomalies (e.g. azygos continuation of the CdVC).

LIVER

Radiographic examination of the liver is often unrewarding, because the gall bladder, bile ducts and hepatic vessels are not normally detectable on plain (survey) radiographs and parenchymal changes can be suspected only when obvious focal or generalized hepatomegaly or reduction in liver size is present. Ultrasonography is of value for assessing architecture, and scintigraphy can be used for functional testing including detection of portosystemic shunts.

Assessment of liver size is best made on an RLR radiograph by noting the position of the stomach axis and the thickness of the liver between the diaphragm and abdominal structures caudal to the liver. In most breeds of dog and in cats, the gastric axis lies parallel to the 10th rib, although in deep-chested dogs it lies vertically or may even slope cranioventrally. The caudoventral edge of the left lateral liver lobe is well visualized on lateral radiographs, forming a sharp and acute angle (the hepatic angle) near the costal arch. In deep-chested dogs, the hepatic angle lies cranial to the costal arch, and in other breeds and in cats it protrudes a variable distance beyond the costal arch (up to about twice the length of L2). In dogs with a pendulous abdomen or if there is caudal displacement of the liver due to thoracic expansion, the hepatic angle will be located more caudally.

9.15 DISPLACEMENT OF THE LIVER

1. Cranial displacement of the liver.
  a. Loss of integrity of the diaphragm.

– Diaphragmatic rupture or hernia.
– Peritoneopericardial hernia.
  b. Enlargement of other abdominal organs, including advanced pregnancy.
  c. Severe ascites.
2. Caudal displacement of the liver – expansion of thorax.
  a. Iatrogenic overinflation of lungs for thoracic radiography.
  b. Dyspnoea.
  c. Pulmonary emphysema.
  d. Large pleural effusion.
  e. Large intrathoracic mass.
3. Displacement of a single liver lobe – may be obscured by abdominal effusion.
  a. Lobar rupture.
  b. Lobar torsion – usually larger dogs.

9.16 VARIATIONS IN LIVER SIZE

Generalized changes in liver size may be inferred from the position of the stomach (see 10.2). Liver enlargement may be due to primary liver disease or secondary to disease in another organ system; it usually has to be severe and/or extensive before changes can be detected radiographically. On lateral radiographs, generalized hepatomegaly leads to projection of the ventral part of the liver further beyond the costal arch, caudodorsal displacement of the gastric axis and an increase in the hepatic angle with rounding of the liver margins. The position of the diaphragm, stomach and spleen allows evaluation of the size of the left side of the liver. Assessment of the right side is more difficult on the lateral radiograph, although gross enlargement will displace the pylorus, cranial duodenum and right kidney caudally. Right-sided hepatomegaly is better seen on VD radiographs, displacing the stomach to the left.

Reduction in liver size may be hard to differentiate from normal deep-chested canine conformation. Signs of reduced liver size include cranial displacement of the gastric axis and transverse colon, reduced distance between the stomach and diaphragm and loss of the hepatic angle.

Normal radiographic liver size does not preclude significant liver disease.

1. Generalized liver enlargement – hepatomegaly (usually causes left-sided and caudal gastric displacement) (Fig. 9.6).

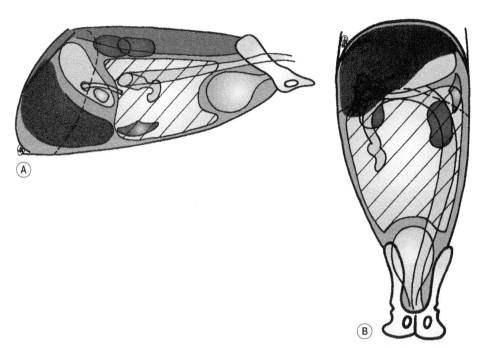

Figure 9.6 Generalized liver enlargement: (A) lateral and (B) ventrodorsal view. The body and pylorus of the stomach are displaced dorsally, caudally and to the left, and the ventral hepatic angle is rounded. In severe cases, other viscera may also be displaced caudally. *(From Thrall, D.E. (ed.) (1998)* Textbook of Veterinary Diagnostic Radiology, *4th edition. Philadelphia: Saunders, with permission.)*

a. Artefact.
  – Obese animal, pendulous abdomen.
  – Thoracic expansion displacing liver caudally.
  – Shallow-chested dogs, with liver extending further beyond costal arch.
  – Left lateral recumbent radiograph.
  – Spleen contacting hepatic angle, mimicking liver.
b. Young animal – liver is larger relative to body weight than in adult.
c. Venous congestion.
  – Right-sided heart failure (see 7.12 and Fig. 7.10).
  – Pericardial effusion or constrictive pericarditis reducing right atrial filling (cardiac tamponade) (see 7.6.2 and Fig. 7.5).
  – Budd–Chiari-like syndrome (post caval syndrome); mechanical obstruction of the post-sinusoidal hepatic veins, post-hepatic CdVC or right atrium causing hepatomegaly and high-protein ascites. CdVC occlusion has various causes,

including the following: compression by a diaphragmatic rupture or hernia, adhesions or kinking of the CdVC cranial to the liver (e.g. following trauma), CdVC thrombosis or invasion by neoplasia, heartworms, compression by thoracic masses, cardiac neoplasia, congenital cardiac anomalies, pericardial diseases and migrating foreign bodies.
d. Hyperadrenocorticism (Cushing's disease) – naturally occurring or iatrogenic; may also see any or all of bronchial mineralization, pot-bellied abdomen due to muscle weakness, osteopenia, calcinosis cutis and adrenal mass.
e. Diabetes mellitus.
f. Neoplasia.
  – Lymphoma (often with enlarged spleen ± lymph nodes, especially sublumbar; may also see interstitial lung pattern and thoracic lymphadenopathy).
  – Mast cell infiltration (often with enlarged spleen and lymph nodes).

- Haemangiosarcoma (may be also enlarged spleen ± free fluid).
- Other primary and metastatic tumours.
- Malignant histiocytosis – especially Bernese Mountain Dogs, Golden and Flat-coated Retrievers and Rottweilers, ± pulmonary and hepatic masses and lymphadenopathy.

g. Severe nodular hyperplasia.

h. Hepatitis.

i. Cirrhosis – in the early stages, hepatomegaly may be seen.

j. Cholestasis.

k. Storage diseases.

l. Amyloidosis.

m. Fungal infection*.

n. Alveolar echinococcosis*.

o. Cats – hepatic lipidosis.

p. Cats – feline infectious peritonitis.

q. Cats – lymphocytic cholangitis.

r. Cats – acromegaly.

s. Cats – hypertrophic feline muscular dystrophy.

2. Focal liver enlargement (Figs 9.14 and 9.15).

a. Focal neoplasia.
- Hepatoma – may be pedunculated and lie caudal to stomach.
- Various carcinomas (e.g. hepatocellular, cholangiocellular, adenocarcinoma).
- Haemangiosarcoma.
- Lymphoma.
- Malignant histiocytosis – especially Bernese Mountain Dogs, Golden and Flat-coated Retrievers and Rottweilers; changes in other organs too, as with lymphoma.
- Metastatic neoplasia.
- Biliary cystadenoma; especially in cats.

b. Intrahepatic abscess.

c. Biliary or parenchymal cyst(s) – may be associated with polycystic kidney disease in cats.

d. Large area of hyperplastic or regenerative nodule formation.

e. Haematoma.

f. Granuloma.

g. Alveolar echinococcosis* (dogs).

h. Liver lobe torsion.

i. Biloma (biliary pseudocyst) – usually secondary to trauma or iatrogenic injury to the hepatic parenchyma.

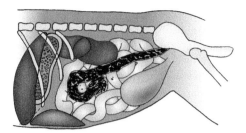

Figure 9.7 Reduced liver size: the gastric axis is displaced cranially and may slope cranioventrally. Other viscera also lie more cranially than normal, especially the spleen and small intestine.

j. Hepatic arteriovenous fistula.

3. Reduced liver size – microhepatica (Fig. 9.7).

a. Normal radiographic appearance in deep-chested dogs.

b. Artefactual.
- Elevation of liver on large falciform fat pad in obese cats.
- Diaphragmatic rupture or hernia with liver entering the thorax.

c. Portosystemic shunt (see 9.19.1 and Figs 9.8 and 9.9) – usually diagnosed in young animals due to anomalous development of vessels associated with the hepatic portal vein; less often acquired due to portal hypertension as a result of chronic liver disease. Renomegaly, urinary tract calculi and osteomyelitis may also be present. NB: cats with portosystemic shunts often have a normal-sized liver.

d. Hepatic microvascular dysplasia.

e. Chronic hepatitis – various causes.

f. Chronic cirrhosis – concurrent ascites is common.

g. Idiopathic hepatic fibrosis – young dogs, especially German Shepherd dogs – ascites common.

h. Hypovolaemia (e.g. Addison's disease).

9.17 VARIATIONS IN LIVER SHAPE

1. Rounding of the caudoventral liver margin (the hepatic angle).

a. Lateral rotation of the patient.

b. Any disease causing generalized liver enlargement (see 9.16.1 and Fig. 9.6).

2. Irregularity of the liver margins.
   a. In normal cats, a full gall bladder may protrude ventral to the liver margin and be highlighted against falciform fat as a smooth, rounded structure.
   b. Any disease causing focal liver enlargement (see 9.16.2).
   c. Any lesion near the liver surface.
   d. Cirrhosis and regenerative nodules (hobnail liver).
   e. Amyloidosis.

9.18 VARIATIONS IN LIVER RADIOPACITY

1. Branching mineralized radiopacities in the liver.
   a. Choledocholithiasis (biliary tree mineralization).
   b. Incidental hepatic mineralization – mainly in older, obese dogs, especially the Yorkshire Terrier (possibly due to chronic hepatopathy).
2. Focal, unstructured or shell-like mineralized radiopacities in the liver.
   a. Cholelithiasis (gallstones) – right cranioventral liver shadow; those in the common bile duct are located near the pyloroduodenal junction.
   b. Chronic cholecystitis, gall bladder neoplasia or cystic hyperplasia of the gall bladder wall.
   c. Chronic hepatopathy.
   d. Mineralized neoplasia (e.g. extraskeletal osteosarcoma).
   e. Chronic abscess, granuloma or haematoma.
   f. Mineralized regenerative nodules.
   g. Cyst (parasitic or developmental).
   h. Alveolar echincoccosis* – cavitary masses.
3. Metallic radiopacities in the liver – swallowed needles and wires may perforate the gastric wall and become embedded in the liver; usually incidental findings.
4. Fat radiopacity in the liver.
   a. Lipoma forming between liver lobes or around the gall bladder.
5. Branching, linear or circular gas lucencies in the liver.
   a. Gas in the biliary tree (pneumobilia).
      – Previous gall bladder surgery.
      – Reflux of gas from the duodenum due to an incompetent sphincter of Oddi.
      – Chronic bile duct obstruction with erosion into the duodenum.
      – Emphysematous cholecystitis or cholangitis secondary to diabetes mellitus or clostridial infections.
   b. Gas in the hepatic portal venous system (warrants a grave prognosis).
      – Secondary to GDV.
      – Necrotizing gastroenteritis.
      – Clostridial infections.
      – Secondary to functional ileus.
      – Secondary to air embolization during pneumocystography or pneumoperitoneography.
      – Post-mortem change occurring within 12 h of death.
6. Focal, patchy or streaky gas lucencies in the liver (emphysematous hepatitis).
   a. Hepatic abscess.
      – Penetrating injury.
      – Haematogenous infection.
   b. Infection with gas-producing organisms.
      – Emphysematous cholecystitis – in the region of the gall bladder.
      – Haematogenous infection.
      – Spread from an adjacent organ.
      – Vascular compromise due to liver lobe entrapment or torsion.

9.19 HEPATIC CONTRAST STUDIES

Contrast studies for the liver have largely been replaced by ultrasonography. Screening for porto-systemic shunts can also be performed using scintigraphy; computed tomography (CT) and magnetic resonance imaging (MRI) angiography may also be used. Portal venography for the diagnosis of shunts remains the most widely performed hepatic contrast technique. Digital subtraction is useful for contrast studies.

Portal venography (operative mesenteric portovenography)

This technique is used for the detection of porto-systemic shunts (anomalous vascular communications that bypass the liver). After laparotomy, a sterile intravenous catheter is placed into the splenic vein or a large mesenteric vein and directed towards the liver. An LLR abdominal radiograph is exposed at the end of a bolus injection of iodinated contrast medium at a dose of 1 mL/kg of body weight. Shunting vessels are usually well outlined, with sparse or absent opacification of normal hepatic vessels. An additional injection for a VD radiograph enables more accurate localization of the shunt. Shunts whose caudal limit lies cranial to the T12–13 disc space are usually intrahepatic, while those whose caudal limit extends caudal to this are likely to be extrahepatic. Surgical partial ligation of a single extrahepatic shunt is usually straightforward; surgical correction of intrahepatic shunts is much more difficult. Following partial or complete ligation of a shunting vessel, a repeated contrast study can be performed to assess changes in intrahepatic portal vessel blood flow, which can help in predicting outcome. A post-ligation study also confirms that the correct vessel has been ligated and rules out the possibility of more than one shunt. Reduced hepatic portal circulation (portal vein hypoplasia) may be seen secondary to the diminished blood flow that results from congenital shunting. Cirrhosis and diffuse hepatic vascular diseases also result in attenuation of intrahepatic portal circulation and eventually the formation of numerous tortuous collateral mesenteric vessels.

Types of portosystemic shunt (Fig. 9.8)

1. Intrahepatic portosystemic shunt (see Fig. 9.9) – most of the blood entering the liver in the hepatic portal vein passes directly to the CdVC through the shunting vessel; usually larger dog breeds (e.g. Irish Wolfhound and Golden Retriever); uncommon in cats.
   a. Left divisional – usually persistent ductus venosus.
   b. Central divisional.
   c. Right divisional.

2. Extrahepatic portosystemic shunt – an anomalous vessel carries blood from the extrahepatic portal vein or one of its contributors (usually gastroduodenal, splenic or colonic) directly into the CdVC, bypassing the intrahepatic portal vein and liver; usually smaller dog breeds (e.g. Yorkshire Terrier, Miniature Schnauzer), and cats. Differential diagnosis is retrograde flow of contrast medium into a tributary vein.

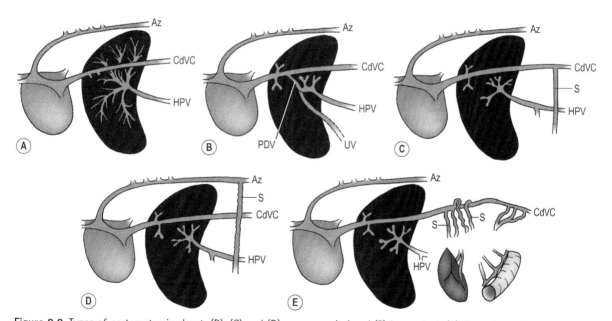

Figure 9.8 Types of portosystemic shunt: (B), (C) and (D) are congenital and (E) is acquired. (A) Normal portal venogram: the hepatic portal vein enters the liver and branches extensively within the parenchyma. (B) Intrahepatic portosystemic shunt, in this case patent ductus venosus. The position of the fetal umbilical vein that gave rise to the ductus venosus is indicated. (C) Extrahepatic portosystemic shunt. (D) Portoazygos shunt. (E) Multiple acquired extrahepatic portosystemic shunts, usually close to the kidneys. (Az, azygos vein, CdVC, caudal vena cava; HPV, hepatic portal vein; PDV, patent ductus venosus; S, shunting vessel; UV, fetal umbilical vein, which atrophies after birth.)

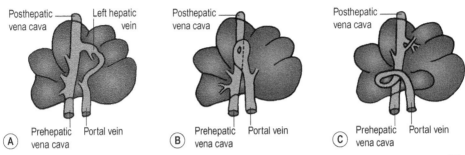

Figure 9.9 Conformation of types of intrahepatic portosystemic shunt as seen on ventrodorsal radiographs. (A) Typical left divisional intrahepatic shunt entering the left hepatic vein (persistent ductus venosus). (B) The most common conformation of a central divisional shunt in the right medial lobe; communication with the vena cava is via a foramen within a dilatation. (C) Typical right divisional shunt, passing as a broad loop through the right lateral lobe. *(From White, R.N., Burton, C.A. and McEvoy, F.J. (1998) Surgical treatment of intrahepatic portosystemic shunts in 45 dogs. Veterinary Record **142**, 358–365, with permission.)*

3. Portoazygos shunt – the anomalous vessel arises from the extrahepatic portal vein and enters the azygos vein rather than the CdVC; a prominent azygos vein may be visible on a lateral thoracic radiograph.
   a. With normal CdVC.
   b. With discontinuation of the post-hepatic CdVC.
4. Multiple, acquired extrahepatic shunts – persistent portal hypertension (usually due to liver disease) encourages the opening up of normally non-functional portocaval and portoazygos connections in the mesentery, which are now the path of least resistance, thus bypassing the liver. Ascites is often seen. Animals may present at a young age due to congenital or developmental liver disease, or at an older age due to acquired liver disease. Acquired shunts are less common than congenital types and are rare in cats. Simultaneous congenital and acquired shunts have been described.
   a. Congenital portal vein hypoplasia or atresia.
   b. Hepatic arteriovenous fistula.
   c. Juvenile or idiopathic hepatic fibrosis.
   d. Breed-related hepatopathies.
   e. Cirrhosis.
   f. Other hepatic diseases causing portal hypertension.
   g. Obstruction of the post-hepatic CdVC (e.g. Budd–Chiari syndrome).

Splenoportography

An alternative approach for the detection of portosystemic shunts. Injection of contrast medium is made directly into the splenic parenchyma either via laparotomy or percutaneously (preferably ultrasound-guided); however, this technique is associated with greater patient morbidity than portal venography. Poor opacification of portal vessels may occur, especially if contrast is not entirely injected into the splenic parenchyma.

Cholecystography

Cholecystography allows visualization of the gall bladder and common bile duct and assessment of patency of the latter. Contrast medium may be administered orally, intravenously or injected percutaneously into the gall bladder using ultrasound guidance but is rarely performed nowadays.

Coeliography (peritoneography)

The main indications of this technique are for assessment of the liver when abdominal detail is poor, and for the integrity of the diaphragm. Coeliography uses negative or positive contrast medium with conventional radiographic positioning and erect, horizontal beam radiography. Administration of a large volume of air is contraindicated if the diaphragm may not be intact.

Coeliac or cranial mesenteric arteriography

Mainly for investigation of arteriovenous malformations.

9.20 ULTRASONOGRAPHIC TECHNIQUE FOR THE LIVER

The patient should be fasted prior to ultrasonographic examination of the liver, although free access to water may be given. The liver is usually imaged from a ventral abdominal approach; the transducer is placed just caudal to the xiphisternum and angled craniodorsally to image the liver. Sweeps of the sound beam are made throughout the organ in at least two planes of section. If the liver is very small, it may be preferable to examine it from a lateral intercostal approach, although it is then more difficult to ensure that the entire organ is inspected. A right dorsal flank approach can be particularly useful for evaluation of the CdVC and portal vein, and for the detection of any anomalous shunting vessels. Ultrasonography is poorer than radiography for assessment of liver size, especially as falciform fat appears similar to liver.

Contrast ultrasonography

Ultrasound contrast techniques rely on the injection of suspensions of tiny microbubbles of inert gas protected by a stabilizing shell that allows them to survive passage through capillaries. Most bubbles in commercially available ultrasound contrast media are < 10 μm in diameter. The bubbles are mildly echogenic. However, when subjected to low-frequency sound (1–3 MHz), they rhythmically change in diameter and generate both fundamental and harmonic signals. The harmonic component strongly increases the backscattered signal.

When ultrasound contrast medium is injected intravenously, peak contrast enhancement of the liver in the normal dog occurs 15–60 s later, coinciding with peak portal flow. Most contrast agents remain in the blood vessels, but some generate a late phase of contrast enhancement due to intracellular contrast uptake; this late phase lasts from under an hour up to several days, depending on the contrast agent.

Contrast ultrasound can be used to improve visibility of nodules in the liver and improve differentiation between benign and malignant nodules. Malignant nodules tend to be hypoechoic when the surrounding normal liver is at peak contrast enhancement. Benign nodules tend to be isoechoic and thus less conspicuous.

9.21 NORMAL ULTRASONOGRAPHIC APPEARANCE OF THE LIVER

The normal liver is moderately echoic, with an even, granular texture (Fig. 9.10). The lobes should be smooth in outline and sharply pointed. The gall bladder appears rounded or pear-shaped, depending on the plane of section, and lies just to the right of midline. The walls of the gall bladder should be thin and smooth, and the contents are usually anechoic. The cystic duct may be seen leading from the gall bladder, especially in cats. The common bile duct runs caudally, ventral to the portal vein, but is often not visible in normal animals. If visible, the common bile duct may be up to 3 mm in diameter in normal dogs and up to 4 mm in normal cats. Intrahepatic bile ducts are not generally seen in the normal animal.

The portal vein enters the liver at the porta hepatis, where it branches laterally. Intrahepatic veins are seen as anechoic tubes; the portal veins have echogenic borders, while the hepatic veins for the most part do not. The larger hepatic veins may be followed to their junction with the CdVC, located dorsally. Intrahepatic arteries are not usually seen in the normal animal unless colour flow Doppler is used.

9.22 ULTRASONOGRAPHIC ABNORMALITIES OF THE HEPATIC PARENCHYMA

1. Irregular hepatic margins on ultrasonography.
   a. Any disease causing focal liver enlargement (see 9.16.2).

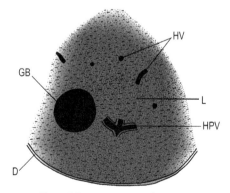

Figure 9.10 Normal liver ultrasound (see text for description). D, diaphragm; GB, gall bladder; HPV, echogenic-walled hepatic portal veins at the porta hepatis; HV, hepatic veins; L, normal liver parenchyma, appearing hypoechoic and coarsely granular.

b. Fibrosis (irrespective of primary cause).

c. Any lesion near the surface of the liver.

2. Focal hepatic lesions on ultrasonography (single or multiple).

There is wide variation in the ultrasonographic appearance of focal liver lesions, and the sonographic features are not usually specific for a particular disease process. The lists below therefore give the most probable differentials for a given ultrasonographic appearance.

a. Anechoic.

 – Biliary cyst, pseudocyst or cystadenoma.

 – Parenchymal cyst (may be associated with polycystic kidney disease in cats).

 – Peliosis hepatis – randomly distributed, multiple, blood-filled cavities.

 – Alveolar echinococcosis*.

b. Hypoechoic (Fig. 9.11).

 – Primary hepatic or metastatic neoplasia.

 – Lymphoma.

 – Mast cell disease.

 – Histiocytic neoplasms.

 – Nodular hyperplasia.

 – Abscess.

 – Granuloma.

 – Necrosis or acute infarction.

 – Hepatocutaneous syndrome.

c. Isoechoic or hyperechoic.

 – Primary hepatic or metastatic neoplasia.

 – Histiocytic neoplasms.

 – Nodular hyperplasia.

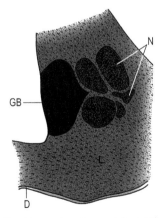

Figure 9.11 Focal hypoechoic liver nodules on ultrasonography. D, diaphragm; GB, gall bladder deformed by adjacent nodules; L, normal liver parenchyma; N, hypoechoic liver nodules.

 – Abscess.

 – Granuloma.

 – Organized infarct.

 – Acute parenchymal haemorrhage.

d. Target lesions – have a hypoechoic rim and a hyperechoic or isoechoic centre.

 – Multiple lesions are more likely to be malignant than benign.

 – Benign target lesions include nodular hyperplasia, pyogranulomatous hepatitis, cirrhosis and chronic active hepatitis.

e. Complex.

 – Haemorrhagic or infected cyst.

 – Primary hepatic or metastatic neoplasia.

 – Histiocytic neoplasm.

 – Abscess.

 – Organizing haematoma.

 – Alveolar echinococcosis* – large cavitary masses, with or without wall mineralization.

 – Telangiectasis.

 – Liver lobe torsion – can result in a large mass of mixed echogenicity with multiple cyst-like areas, which is continuous with the liver.

3. Diffuse hepatic changes on ultrasonography – in order to appreciate diffuse changes in echogenicity, the echogenicity of the liver should be compared with that of the renal cortex and the spleen at the same tissue depth and with the same machine settings. The normal liver is the same echogenicity or slightly more echoic than the normal renal cortex, and slightly less echoic than the normal spleen.

a. Increased echogenicity, normal architecture (portal vein margins tend to become obscured, sound attenuation may be increased).

 – Fatty infiltration.

 – Steroid hepatopathy.

 – Fibrosis (irrespective of primary cause).

 – Lymphoma.

 – Mast cell infiltration in dogs.

b. Decreased echogenicity, normal architecture (portal vein margins tend to be enhanced).

 – Acute hepatitis.

 – Diffuse infiltrative disease (e.g. lymphoma).

- Amyloidosis.
- Passive congestion (usually see distended hepatic veins).
c. Normal echogenicity, normal architecture.
- Normal.
- Acute hepatitis.
- Toxic hepatopathy.
- Diffuse infiltrative disease.
d. Disordered architecture.
- Primary hepatic or widespread metastatic neoplasia.
- Fibrosis with regenerative nodules.
- Amyloidosis in cats.
- Hepatocutaneous syndrome – Swiss cheese or lacy appearance.

9.23 ULTRASONOGRAPHIC ABNORMALITIES OF THE BILIARY TRACT

1. Thickened gall bladder wall on ultrasonography – the normal thickness of the gall bladder wall in dogs is up to 3 mm. In cats, a wall thickness of > 1 mm is accurate in predicting gall bladder disease, although a thickness of < 1 mm cannot rule out mild or chronic inflammation.
   a. Smooth.
   - Contracted gall bladder.
   - Oedema due to congestive cardiac failure or hypoalbuminaemia.
   - Cholecystitis.
   b. Irregular.
   - Mucosal hyperplasia (incidental in middle-aged or older dogs).
   - Neoplasia.
2. Echoes within the lumen of the gall bladder on ultrasonography.
   a. Slice thickness artefact (see Appendix).
   b. Sludge (in the dependent part of the gall bladder).
   - Often seen in normal dogs.
   - Fasting.
   - Cholestasis.
   - Cholecystitis.
   c. Choleliths (in the dependent part of the gall bladder; variable acoustic shadowing depending on mineral content).
   d. Mucosal hyperplasia.

e. Mucocele – typical kiwi fruit appearance.
   f. Neoplasia.
3. Dilation of the biliary tract on ultrasonography – the first sign of obstruction is dilation of the gall bladder and cystic duct, then the common bile duct dilates and finally the extra- and intrahepatic ducts dilate. The common bile duct may remain distended even after an obstruction is removed. In cats, a common bile duct diameter of > 5 mm is strongly suggestive of obstruction. Obstruction may lead to gall bladder rupture.
   a. Gall bladder alone.
   - Fasted or anorexic.
   - Early extrahepatic biliary obstruction.
   - Mucocele.
   b. Gall bladder and other parts of the biliary tract.
   - Extrahepatic biliary obstruction (e.g. due to pancreatitis, pancreatic neoplasia, choleliths, lymphadenopathy, bile duct atresia).
4. Duplex gall bladder – cats; usually incidental.
5. Hepatic cysts secondary to congenital biliary atresia – one feline case report.
6. Gall bladder agenesis – one canine case report.

9.24 ULTRASONOGRAPHIC ABNORMALITIES OF THE HEPATIC VASCULAR SYSTEM

1. Distension of hepatic veins and CdVC on ultrasonography (often with ascites).
   a. Congestive heart failure.
   b. Obstruction of the CdVC between the heart and the liver.
   - Thrombus.
   - Neoplasm.
   - Adhesions.
   c. Large fraction portocaval shunt; turbulence may be seen in the CdVC at the point of termination of the shunting vessel.
2. Distension of the hepatic portal vein on ultrasonography.
   a. Portal hypertension secondary to liver disease (may see secondary shunting vessels and ascites; decreased or reversed portal flow may be seen on Doppler studies).

b. Obstruction of the portal vein near the porta hepatis.
  – Thrombus.
  – Neoplasm.
  – Adhesions.
  c. Hepatic arteriovenous fistula.
3. Small hepatic portal vein – it can be useful to measure portal vein:aorta diameters. Dogs with a portal vein:aorta of ≤ 0.65 are likely to have an extrahepatic portosystemic shunt or idiopathic noncirrhotic portal hypertension, whereas a portal vein:aorta ≥ 0.8 suggests that these conditions are unlikely.
  a. Congenital extrahepatic portosystemic shunt.
  b. Idiopathic noncirrhotic portal hypertension.
  c. Obstruction of portal vein distant from porta hepatis.
4. Anomalous blood vessel(s) on ultrasonography.
  a. Within the liver parenchyma.
    – Congenital intrahepatic portosystemic shunt.
    – Hepatic arteriovenous fistula.
  b. Outside the liver parenchyma.
    – Congenital extrahepatic portosystemic shunt.
    – Acquired portosystemic shunt (usually multiple vessels).
    – Arteriovenous fistula.

SPLEEN

The spleen is a strap-shaped organ that is roughly triangular in cross-section. It is proportionately larger in dogs than in cats. The head of the spleen lies in the left cranial abdomen between the fundus of the stomach cranially and the left kidney caudally (if the liver is small and the stomach is empty, it may abut the diaphragm). It is visible on a VD radiograph in both dogs and cats as a triangular structure adjacent to the left body wall and is also often seen on the lateral view, cranial to the left kidney. The body and tail of the spleen form its ventral part and are more variable in location. In dogs, they are usually seen in cross-section in the ventral abdomen on the lateral radiograph as a triangular or ovoid structure lying caudal to the liver, especially on an RLR radiograph. In some cases, it may be difficult to differentiate the spleen from the liver if the two organs are in contact. The body and tail of the spleen are often not seen on the lateral view in cats, unless enlarged.

The borders of the spleen should be smooth and well defined. Splenic size is very variable radiographically, and so evaluation of size is highly subjective; splenic size also increases with certain anaesthetic agents. Splenic disease is less common in cats than in dogs.

9.25 ABSENCE OF THE SPLENIC SHADOW

1. Normal variation on the lateral view (the head of the spleen is reliably seen on VD views in both dogs and cats).
  a. The splenic body and tail are not usually seen on the lateral view in cats.
  b. The splenic body and tail are less likely to be seen in an LLR radiograph in dogs than in an RLR radiograph.
2. Previous splenectomy.
3. Small spleen (e.g. hypovolaemia), when the ventral part of the spleen may not be visible in dogs on the lateral view.
4. Splenic mass or torsion, not identified as spleen.
5. Displacement through a diaphragmatic or body wall rupture or hernia.
6. Situs inversus of abdominal organs, with right-sided spleen overlooked.

9.26 VARIATIONS IN LOCATION OF THE SPLEEN

The head of the spleen is attached to the stomach by the gastrosplenic ligament and will not be displaced unless rupture of the ligament or gastric enlargement or displacement has occurred. The body and tail of the spleen create the triangular or ovoid splenic shadow seen on lateral radiographs and are more mobile.

1. Cranial displacement of the ventral part of the spleen.
  a. Normal cranial location in deep-chested breeds of dog.
  b. Displacement by caudal abdominal organomegaly.
  c. Small liver, allowing spleen to slide cranially.
  d. Diaphragmatic rupture.

e. Pericardioperitoneal diaphragmatic hernia.
2. Caudal displacement of the spleen.
   a. Gastric distension (see 10.3.4 and 10.3.5).
   b. Hepatomegaly.
   c. Gastric mass.
3. Ventral displacement of the spleen.
   a. Ventral body wall rupture.
   b. Gastric dilation and volvulus.
4. Dorsal or contralateral displacement of the spleen.
   a. Splenic torsion.
      – Isolated.
      – With GDV.

9.27 VARIATIONS IN SPLENIC SIZE AND SHAPE

Due to the normal wide anatomical and physiological variation in splenic size, substantial change must be present before it may be considered abnormal. Apparent variation in size may also be due to altered orientation, as the splenic body and tail are mobile. An occasional variant is the development of ectopic splenic tissue giving a segmented appearance to the splenic shadow.

1. Generalized splenic enlargement with a normal shape and smooth outline.
   a. Normal variant; especially in the German Shepherd dog and Greyhound.
   b. Passive splenic congestion (spleen may be obscured by ascites).
      – Right heart failure.
      – Portal hypertension.
      – Sedative, tranquilizing and anaesthetic agents, especially barbiturates and phenothiazines.
      – Gastric dilation and volvulus involving the spleen (spleen also in an abnormal location).
      – Isolated splenic torsion (spleen C-shaped or in abnormal location); mainly large, deep-chested dogs such as German Shepherd dog and Great Dane; acute or chronic signs.
      – Splenic thrombosis.
   c. Neoplasia.
      – Lymphoma (liver ± lymph nodes also often enlarged – see 9.16.1 and Fig. 9.6).

      – Malignant histiocytosis; especially Bernese Mountain Dog, Golden and Flat-coated Retrievers and Rottweilers, ± pulmonary and hepatic masses and lymphadenopathy.
      – Acute and chronic leukaemias.
      – Systemic mastocytosis.
      – Myeloproliferative disease.
      – Haemangioma, haemangiosarcoma or metastatic neoplasia more often results in an irregular splenic outline.
   d. Inflammatory splenomegaly – many causes, including:
      – Penetrating wounds.
      – Migrating foreign bodies.
      – Septicaemia and bacteraemia.
      – Toxoplasmosis*.
      – Salmonellosis.
      – Mycobacteriosis.
      – Brucellosis.
      – Leishmaniasis*.
      – Fungal infections*.
      – Ehrlichiosis*.
      – Babesiosis*.
      – Haemobartonellosis.
      – Infectious canine hepatitis.
      – Cats – feline infectious peritonitis.
   e. Chronic anaemia or haemolysis – splenic hyperplasia.
   f. Chronic infection – splenic hyperplasia.
   g. Severe nodular lymphoid hyperplasia (liver margins may be smooth or irregular).
   h. Extramedullary haemopoiesis.
   i. Toxaemia.
   j. Amyloidosis.
   k. Systemic lupus erythematosus.
   l. Cats – hypereosinophilic syndrome.
   m. Cats – feline hypertrophic muscular dystrophy.
2. Diffusely enlarged, C-shaped spleen.
   a. Splenic torsion – ascites may obscure the spleen and splenic emphysema may also be present.
3. Focal or irregular splenic enlargement or splenic mass (see 9.39.2 and Fig. 9.17).
   a. Neoplasia.
      – Haemangiosarcoma (especially German Shepherd dog); spleen may be obscured by abdominal fluid due to splenic

haemorrhage; highly metastatic (e.g. to liver, mesentery, lungs, right atrium and pericardial sac).
- Haemangioma – as above.
- Malignant histiocytosis; especially Bernese Mountain Dog, Golden and Flat-coated Retrievers and Rottweilers; concurrent pulmonary and hepatic masses and lymphadenopathy too.
- Leiomyosarcoma.
- Fibrosarcoma.
- Other primary and metastatic tumours.
   b. Nodular lymphoid hyperplasia.
   c. Splenic haematoma.
   - Spontaneous.
   - Traumatic.
   - Secondary to splenic neoplasia.
   d. Splenic abscess.
   e. Splenic hamartoma.
   f. Inflammatory pseudotumour – benign, tumour-like inflammatory–reparative lesion of unknown aetiology; rare.
   g. Pedunculated liver mass or liver lobe torsion may mimic a splenic mass.
4. Reduction in splenic size.
   a. Severe dehydration.
   b. Severe shock.
5. Miscellaneous.
   a. Accessory spleen – heterotopic splenic tissue growing into visible nodules; developmental or following splenic trauma (splenosis). Differential diagnosis is metastases, especially of haemangiosarcoma.

9.28 VARIATIONS IN SPLENIC RADIOPACITY

Variations in splenic opacity are rare.
1. Mineralization of the spleen.
   a. Mineralization of chronic haematoma or abscess – may be shell-like marginal mineralization.
   b. Histoplasmosis*.
   c. Extraskeletal osteosarcoma.
2. Gas lucency in the spleen.
   a. Emphysema due to gas-forming organisms, secondary to splenic torsion.
   b. Splenic abscess or splenitis.

c. Post-mortem change, occurring within 12 h of death.

9.29 ULTRASONOGRAPHIC TECHNIQUE FOR THE SPLEEN

The spleen lies superficially within the abdomen, so a high-frequency transducer (≥ 7.5 MHz) may be used. The head of the spleen lies close to the gastric fundus in the left cranial abdomen. The body and tail of the spleen can be followed along the left flank or running obliquely across the floor of the abdomen.

Contrast ultrasound techniques can be used to enhance the visibility and improve differentiation of benign and malignant lesions. For the underlying principles of contrast ultrasound techniques, see 9.20. Focal malignant lesions in the spleen are hypoechoic to surrounding spleen 30 s after starting contrast injection. Tortuous feeding vessels may also be seen associated with malignancy. Benign lesions tend to have the same perfusion pattern as surrounding spleen.

9.30 NORMAL ULTRASONOGRAPHIC APPEARANCE OF THE SPLEEN

The spleen should be smooth in outline with a dense, even echotexture. The echogenicity of the spleen is usually greater that that of the liver at the same depth and machine settings. Splenic veins may be seen leaving the spleen at the hilus.

9.31 ULTRASONOGRAPHIC ABNORMALITIES OF THE SPLEEN

1. Focal splenic parenchymal lesions on ultrasonography (Fig. 9.12) – focal lesions may be single or multiple and often distort the normal smooth outline of the spleen. They have a very variable ultrasonographic appearance, which is rarely specific for a particular disease process. The lists given below therefore give only the most probable differential diagnoses.
   a. Focal anechoic, hypoechoic or isoechoic lesions.
   - Primary splenic neoplasia.
   - Metastatic neoplasia.
   - Lymphoma.

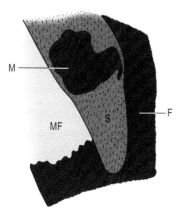

Figure 9.12 Splenic mass and ascites on ultrasonography: the splenic outline would be obscured radiographically by the abdominal effusion, but this enhances the ultrasonographic examination. F, free abdominal fluid; M, focal splenic mass, deforming the outline of the spleen slightly; MF, mesenteric fat; S, tail of spleen.

- Mast cell disease.
- Histiocytic neoplasms.
- Nodular lymphoid hyperplasia.
- Extramedullary haematopoiesis, especially following anaemic episodes such as autoimmune haemolytic anaemia and babesiosis.
- Small splenic haematoma.
- Necrosis or acute infarct – sharply demarcated with decreased or absent flow on Doppler examination.
- Splenic abscess.
- Granuloma (e.g. histoplasmosis*).
- Splenic cyst (uncommon).

b. Focal hyperechoic lesions.
- Normal fat around hilar splenic veins.
- Primary splenic neoplasia.
- Mast cell tumours (uncommon).
- Metastatic neoplasia.
- Myelolipomata – peripheral or adjacent to blood vessels.
- Splenic abscess containing gas.
- Granuloma containing mineralization.
- Organized infarct.
- Acute intraparenchymal haemorrhage.
- Triangular hyperechoic area at the hilus of the spleen between the splenic parenchyma and the splenic veins,

continuous with hyperechoic mesentery – associated with acute splenic torsion but also seen with diffuse neoplastic infiltration.
- Gas bubbles, with emphysema secondary to splenic torsion.

c. Complex lesions.
- Primary splenic neoplasia.
- Metastatic neoplasia.
- Lymphoma (less common).
- Splenic haematoma.
- Splenic abscess.
- Telangiectasia.

d. Target lesions – target lesions have a hypoechoic rim and a hyperechoic or an isoechoic centre. Differential diagnoses for target lesions are as for the liver (9.22.2d).

2. Diffuse splenic parenchymal changes on ultrasonography.
a. Reduced or normal echogenicity, normal architecture.
- Passive splenic congestion (for differential diagnoses, see 9.27.1).
- Acute systemic inflammatory diseases.
- Diffuse neoplastic infiltration (e.g. lymphoma, mast cell infiltration, histiocytic neoplasms).
- Arterial thrombosis.

b. Increased echogenicity, normal architecture.
- Chronic congestion.
- Chronic inflammatory diseases.
- Chronic granulomatous diseases (e.g. histoplasmosis*).
- Mast cell tumours in cats (uncommon).

c. Disturbed architecture – hypoechoic.
- Lymphoma – multiple tiny hypoechoic nodules, resulting in a Swiss cheese appearance.
- Mast cell disease – diffuse mottling described in cats.
- Splenic torsion – initially see progressive enlargement of the spleen with decreased blood flow; later see a hypoechoic parenchyma with short, linear echogenicities forming a lacy appearance, the so-called starry sky appearance; may also see thrombi in splenic vessels.
- Arterial thombosis.

- Nodular hyperplasia.
- Extramedullary haematopoiesis.

PANCREAS

9.32 PANCREATIC RADIOLOGY

The normal pancreas is not visible radiographically due to its small size, although it can be imaged using ultrasound by experienced ultrasonographers. Radiography is poorly sensitive for pancreatic disease and false negative findings are common, but radiography is helpful to rule out other causes of an acutely painful abdomen.

Severe inflammatory or neoplastic pancreatic disease may produce the radiographic appearance of focal peritonitis, with or without a mild mass effect, in the right cranial quadrant of the abdomen. The adjacent descending duodenum may be displaced laterally and show focal, gas-dilated ileus, sometimes assuming a C-shaped course with thickened and corrugated walls (Fig. 9.13). The stomach and colon may also be displaced, but barium should not be used to demonstrate this, as it may exacerbate the clinical signs by provoking pancreatic enzyme release. Secondary abdominal effusion may arise.

1. Localized loss of serosal detail, right cranial abdominal quadrant (due to inflammation of surrounding mesentery).
   a. Pancreatitis.
   b. Pancreatic neoplasia, usually (adeno) carcinoma.
      - Secondary pancreatitis.
      - Local metastasis.
2. Localized mass effect.
   a. Pancreatitis.

b. Sequelae to pancreatitis.
   - Pancreatic pseudocyst.
   - Pancreatic necrosis.
   - Pancreatic abscess.
c. Pancreatic neoplasia.
d. Pancreatic pseudocyst.
e. Pancreatic nodular hyperplasia – usually too small to be seen radiographically.
3. Pancreatic mineralization – rare.
   a. Chronic pancreatitis.
   b. Pancreatic neoplasia.
   c. Fat necrosis.

9.33 ULTRASONOGRAPHIC TECHNIQUE FOR THE PANCREAS

The patient should ideally be starved overnight to ensure that the stomach is empty but may be allowed access to water. Acute cases usually involve vomiting, so the stomach is often already empty. Ultrasonography of the pancreas should be scheduled before barium contrast studies, as barium will interfere with passage of the sound beam.

In order to image the pancreas, a high-frequency ($\geq$ 7.5 MHz) transducer is essential. The animal may be placed on its right side to encourage gas to rise away from the area of interest in the right cranial abdomen; some operators prefer to perform the examination with the dog in dorsal recumbency. The stomach, descending duodenum and right kidney should be located as landmarks. The right limb of the pancreas lies dorsomedial to the descending duodenum and ventral to the right kidney, while the left limb of the pancreas lies caudal to the stomach and cranial to the transverse colon. The portal vein lies just dorsal and to the left of the body of the pancreas. The left lobe is often larger and easier to image than the right lobe in the cat. Conversely, the right lobe of the pancreas is often easier to image in the dog, as the left lobe may be obscured by gas in the adjacent stomach or transverse colon.

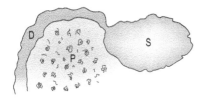

Figure 9.13 Pancreatic disease: ventrodorsal view (detail). The duodenum is dilated and spastic and follows a curved, C-shaped course. There is a mottled radiopacity suggestive of peritonitis in the region of the pancreas. D, duodenum; P, pancreas; S, stomach.

9.34 NORMAL ULTRASONOGRAPHIC APPEARANCE OF THE PANCREAS

The pancreas is an ill-defined organ that may not be recognized if imaging conditions are not optimal. It is moderately echoic, usually intermediate in echogenicity between the liver and spleen, and of even echotexture. The pancreaticoduodenal vein running through the length of the right limb of the pancreas may aid in identification.

A study in normal cats showed the mean thickness of the right lobe of the pancreas to be 4.5 mm; that of the body, 6.6 mm; and that of the left lobe, 5.4 mm. The pancreatic duct is consistently seen within the left lobe of the pancreas in cats but not in dogs. The width of the normal pancreatic duct varies between 0.8 and 2.4 mm; it tends to be wider in older cats, but no association has been found between pancreatic disease and pancreatic duct width.

9.35 ULTRASONOGRAPHIC ABNORMALITIES OF THE PANCREAS

1. Pancreas not seen on ultrasonography.
   a. Low-resolution imaging system.
   b. Operator inexperience.
   c. Patient factors such as obesity, gastrointestinal gas, panting, abdominal rigidity or pain (e.g. if pancreatitis is present).
   d. Pancreatic atrophy.
   e. Pneumoperitoneum (e.g. post laparotomy).
2. Focal pancreatic lesions on ultrasonography.
   a. Inflammatory pseudocysts – anechoic or hypoechoic with acoustic enhancement.
   b. Congenital cysts or retention cysts – similar appearance to pseudocysts.
   c. Pancreatic abscess – may have anechoic or hypoechoic contents and thus resemble cysts, or echoic contents and thus resemble a solid mass.
   d. Small neoplasm (e.g. insulinoma).
   e. Nodular changes secondary to chronic pancreatitis.
   f. Nodular hyperplasia – occasional finding in older dogs and cats; well-defined hypoechoic to isoechoic nodules.
3. Diffuse pancreatic disturbance on ultrasonography – usually includes enlargement of the pancreas, which is of a heterogeneous echogenicity and texture. Surrounding fat may be hyperechoic due to saponification. May be associated abdominal fluid, thickening and reduced motility of adjacent stomach and descending duodenum, corrugation of the duodenum (see 10.34) and/or evidence of

biliary obstruction. Inflammatory and neoplastic disease cannot be differentiated on ultrasonographic criteria alone.
   a. Pancreatitis.
      – Acute necrotizing pancreatitis – irregular hypoechoic foci due to haemorrhage and necrosis of the pancreas and surrounding tissues.
      – Subacute to chronic active pancreatitis – well-defined hypoechoic organ surrounded by hyperechoic mesentery; may see irregular margins and foci of mineralization.
   b. Pancreatic neoplasia.
      – Adenocarcinoma – poorly echogenic nodules or mass; as these develop, they may compress the common bile duct, invade adjacent stomach and duodenum, and spread to liver and draining lymph nodes.
      – Insulinoma – solitary or multiple nodules, or an ill-defined area of abnormal echogenicity; nodules usually ≤ 2.5 cm in diameter.
   c. Pancreatic oedema – pancreas enlarged, with hypoechoic lines demarcating pancreatic lobules; may be associated with pancreatitis, hypoalbuminaemia or hypotension.

ADRENAL GLANDS

9.36 ADRENAL GLAND RADIOLOGY

The adrenal glands lie in the retroperitoneal space medial or craniomedial to the ipsilateral kidney. The normal adrenal gland is too small to be visible radiographically; radiography is usually unrewarding for imaging adrenal disease, and ultrasonography, CT and MRI are usually more helpful. Large adrenal masses may sometimes be recognized cranial to the ipsilateral kidney, which may be displaced caudally or laterally (see 9.38.4 and Fig. 9.16), and intravenous urography may be helpful to differentiate the adrenal gland and kidney. Diffuse retroperitoneal changes may also be present (see 9.9 and 9.10). Adrenal hyperplasia secondary to a pituitary tumour is not usually visible radiographically, although non-specific secondary signs of hyperadrenocorticism may be seen (pendulous abdomen, hepatomegaly, bronchial and pulmonary mineralization, calcinosis cutis, abdominal soft tissue mineralization, osteopenia). In the case of suspected pituitary or adrenal neoplasia, an imaging search for metastasis should also be made. Animals with hyperadrenocorticism are predisposed to pulmonary thromboembolism (see 6.23.6). Functional imaging of the adrenal gland may be performed with scintigraphy.

1. Adrenal mass – adrenal tumours may invade local blood vessels and provoke thrombus formation; venography of the CdVC or other imaging techniques are useful in surgical planning. Rupture of an adrenal tumour may cause retroperitoneal or intraperitoneal haemorrhage.
   a. Adeno(carcin)oma – cortex.
   b. Phaeochromocytoma – medulla; often locally invasive.
   c. Metastasis.
   d. Neuroblastoma, ganglioblastoma, myelolipoma – medulla.
   e. Haemorrhage.
   f. Hyperplasia.
   g. Inflammation or infection.
   h. Cyst.
2. Adrenal mineralization.
   a. Common incidental finding in old cats, usually bilateral.
   b. Neoplasia – the usual cause of adrenal mineralization in dogs.

9.37 ULTRASONOGRAPHY OF THE ADRENAL GLANDS

If the adrenal glands are to be identified ultrasonographically, it is essential that a high-frequency transducer is used (≥ 7.5 MHz) and that the operator has a clear understanding of the vascular anatomy of the retroperitoneal space. A ventral abdominal or flank approach may be used.

In the dog, the left adrenal gland is a bilobed or elongated oval shape lying ventrolateral to the aorta, between the origins of the cranial mesenteric artery and the left renal artery. The right adrenal gland often has a triangular shape and lies dorsolateral to the CdVC, near the hilus of the right kidney. In the cat, both adrenal glands are a flattened oval shape. The adrenal glands are usually hypoechoic, but occasionally a hypoechoic cortex and a slightly more echoic medulla may be seen. The size of the adrenal glands in normal dogs has

been found to be variable and not proportional to body weight. In dogs, the maximum diameter of the adrenal at its caudal pole seems to be the most reliable indicator of adrenal size, and a maximum normal diameter of 7.4 mm gives reasonable sensitivity and specificity. In cats, the normal adrenals are 10–11 mm long and up to 4.3 ± 0.3 mm in diameter.

1. Adrenal glands not seen on ultrasonography.
   a. Low-resolution imaging system.
   b. Poor image quality (e.g. bowel gas, obesity, panting).
   c. Inexperienced operator.
   d. Adrenal atrophy (e.g. functional contralateral adrenal tumour).
   e. Previous adrenalectomy.
   f. Exogenous steroid administration.
   g. Hypoadrenocorticism (Addison's disease).
2. Adrenal glands enlarged on ultrasonography – it is not possible to distinguish adrenal-dependent and pituitary-dependent hyperadrenocorticism by the appearance of the adrenal glands alone. Primary adrenal tumours may be uni- or bilateral and of varying echogenicity. It is important to check ultrasonographically for invasion of adjacent blood vessels; right adrenal masses in particular may invade the CdVC. If a nodule in the adrenal exceeds 2 cm in diameter, it is more likely to be neoplastic than hyperplastic; if it exceeds 4 cm, then a malignant lesion is more likely than a benign one.
   a. Retention of normal basic shape.
      – Adrenal hyperplasia secondary to pituitary disease; bilateral and often more hypoechoic.
      – Small adrenal tumours.
      – Trilostane administration.
   b. Loss of normal basic shape.
      – Severe adrenal hyperplasia secondary to pituitary tumour.
      – Trilostane administration.
      – Adrenal tumour (adenoma, adenocarcinoma, phaeochromocytoma, metastasis).
3. Hyperechoic specks $\pm$ acoustic shadowing.
   a. Incidental, particularly in the cat.
   b. Mineralization of an adrenal tumour.

4. Adrenal glands small on ultrasonography.
    a. Unilateral – functional contralateral adrenal tumour.
    b. Bilateral – hypoadrenocorticism (Addison's disease).

ABDOMINAL MASSES

Radiographic identification of the organ of origin of an abdominal mass is based on location of the mass, displacement or compression of adjacent organs, and absence of identification of normal organs. Further information may be obtained radiographically using special radiographic views such as horizontal beam projections, abdominal compression and radiographic contrast techniques, but ultrasonography is usually the next diagnostic step. Ultrasonographic diagnosis is easiest if some normal organ tissue remains attached to the mass; if the entire organ is abnormal, then diagnosis may be based on failure to identify a given organ. If neoplasia is suspected, thoracic radiographs should also be obtained.

Abdominal masses may be associated with peritoneal effusion. This may mask the mass radiographically, although displacement of other structures may allow the presence of a mass to be inferred. Ultrasonographic examination is enhanced by the presence of free abdominal fluid.

The stomach, bladder and uterus are capable of considerable physiological enlargement, which should be differentiated from disease processes. The following sections are intended as a guide to the likely organ of origin of masses in various parts of the abdomen; having identified the likely organ(s), the relevant section of Chapters 9, 10 or 11 should be consulted for possible causes.

9.38 CRANIAL ABDOMINAL MASSES (LARGELY WITHIN THE COSTAL ARCH)

1. Liver – the most cranial abdominal organ, lying immediately caudal to the diaphragm. The administration of barium may be helpful in showing the precise location of the stomach and by inference the caudal margin of the liver.
    a. Generalized liver enlargement (see 9.16.1 and Fig. 9.6).

Lateral view
    – Caudodorsal displacement of the pylorus: tilting of the gastric axis nearer to the horizontal plane.
    – Caudodorsal displacement of the cranial duodenal flexure.
    – Caudal displacement of spleen and small intestine.
    – Abdominal distension giving pot-bellied appearance.
Ventrodorsal view
    – Caudal and medial (left) displacement of the pylorus.
    – Caudal displacement of small intestine.
    b. Right lateral or middle lobe enlargement (Fig. 9.14).
Lateral view
    – Caudodorsal displacement of the pylorus, small intestine and ascending colon.
    – If large and pedunculated, the mass may lie caudal to the stomach, mimicking a splenic mass.
Ventrodorsal view
    – Caudal and medial (left) displacement of the pylorus, small intestine and ascending colon.
    – ± caudal displacement of the right kidney.
    c. Left lateral or middle lobe enlargement (Fig. 9.15).
Lateral view
    – Dorsal displacement of the fundus of the stomach.
    – Caudodorsal displacement of small intestine.
    – May appear very similar to right-sided enlargement on this view, but differs on the VD view.
Ventrodorsal view
    – Caudal and medial (right) displacement of the fundus and small intestine.
    – Caudal displacement of the head of the spleen.
    – ± caudal displacement of the left kidney.
    d. Central lobe enlargement.
Lateral view
    – Caudodorsal displacement and indentation of the body of the stomach.
Ventrodorsal view
    – As for the lateral view.

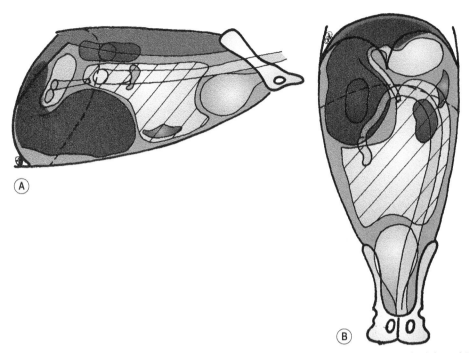

Figure 9.14 Right-sided liver enlargement: (A) lateral and (B) ventrodorsal view. *(From Thrall, D.E. (ed.) (1998)* Textbook of Veterinary Diagnostic Radiology, *4th edition. Philadelphia: Saunders, with permission.)*

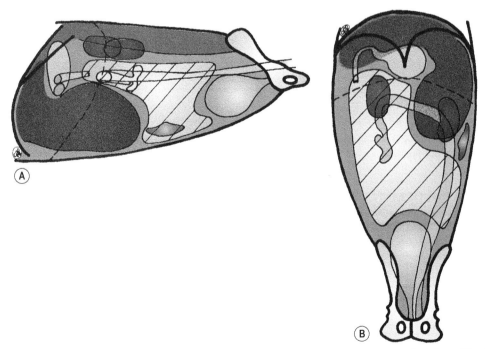

Figure 9.15 Left-sided liver enlargement: (A) lateral and (B) ventrodorsal view. *(From Thrall, D.E. (ed.) (1998)* Textbook of Veterinary Diagnostic Radiology, *4th edition. Philadelphia: Saunders, with permission.)*

2. Stomach – lies immediately caudal to, and
supported on, the liver.
Lateral view
   – Caudal displacement of the small intestine,
     transverse colon and spleen.
   – Increased distance between gastric
     lumen and transverse colon, if the cause
     is thickening of the caudal stomach wall.
   – If the stomach is torsed, the spleen may
     also be displaced in other directions.
Ventrodorsal view
   – As for the lateral view.

3. Pancreas – pancreatic masses are rarely
seen as discrete soft tissue structures, but
enlargement of the pancreas may be inferred by
displacement of adjacent organs and localized
loss of abdominal detail (Fig. 9.13).
a. Right limb of pancreas.
Lateral view
   – Ventral displacement of the duodenum.
Ventrodorsal view
   – Lateral (right) displacement of the
     duodenum.
   – Cranial and medial (left) displacement of
     the pylorus.
   – The pylorus and duodenum may form a
     wide, fixed C shape.
b. Left limb or body of pancreas.
Lateral view
   – Ventral displacement of the duodenum.
Ventrodorsal view
   – Indentation of the caudal stomach wall.
   – Caudal displacement of the small intestine
     and transverse colon.

4. Adrenal glands – lie in the retroperitoneal
space craniomedial to the ipsilateral kidney.
Adrenal masses that are visible radiographically
are likely to be neoplastic and are often
mineralized.
Lateral view
   – Caudal displacement of the ipsilateral
     kidney, with ventral displacement of its
     cranial pole.
   – Ventral displacement of the small and
     large intestines.
Ventrodorsal view
   – Caudolateral displacement of the cranial
     pole of the ipsilateral kidney, so that the
     left kidney appears rotated clockwise and
     the right kidney anticlockwise, depending
     on which adrenal is enlarged (Fig. 9.16).

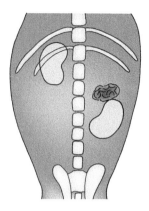

Figure 9.16 Adrenal mass on the ventrodorsal view: the
ipsilateral kidney is displaced caudally and its cranial pole
is rotated outwards.

9.39 MID–ABDOMINAL MASSES

1. Liver – focal ventral liver masses may
occasionally extend into the mid-ventral
abdomen, displacing the stomach cranially and
mimicking other mid-abdominal masses such as
splenic lesions.

2. Spleen.
a. Head of spleen (proximal) – relatively
   immobile due to the gastrosplenic ligament.
Lateral view
   – Cranial displacement of the fundus of the
     stomach.
   – Caudal displacement of the left kidney.
   – Depending on the exact location of the
     mass within the spleen, small intestine
     may be displaced ventrally or dorsally.
Ventrodorsal view
   – Cranial displacement of the fundus of the
     stomach.
   – Caudal displacement of the left kidney.
   – Caudal and medial (right) displacement of
     the small intestine and adjacent parts of
     transverse and descending colon.
b. Body and tail (distal) – these portions of the
   spleen are highly mobile, and masses can be
   seen in a variety of mid-abdominal locations
   (Fig. 9.17).
Lateral view
   – Dorsal and cranial and/or caudal
     displacement of small intestines, which
     may appear draped over a ventral
     abdominal mass.

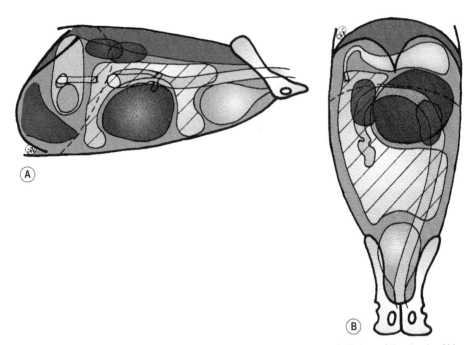

Figure 9.17 Splenic mass: (A) lateral and (B) ventrodorsal view. *(From Thrall, D.E. (ed.) (1998)* Textbook of Veterinary Diagnostic Radiology, *4th edition. Philadelphia: Saunders, with permission.)*

  – Dorsal displacement of the large
   intestine.
  – Cranial displacement of the stomach if the
   mass is large.
 Ventrodorsal view
  – Small intestine most likely to be displaced
   to the right by a left-sided mass, but it may
   also be displaced to the left, cranially,
   caudally or peripherally.
  – Cranial displacement of the stomach if the
   mass is large.
3. Kidneys – the kidneys lie in the retroperitoneal
 space and so remain dorsally located in the
 abdomen, even when markedly enlarged.
 a. Right kidney.
 Lateral view
  – Ventral displacement of the small intestine
   and ascending and transverse colon.
 Ventrodorsal view
  – Medial (left) displacement of the small
   intestine and ascending and transverse colon.
 b. Left kidney (Figs 9.18 and 11.1).
 Lateral view
  – Ventral displacement of the small intestine
   and descending colon.

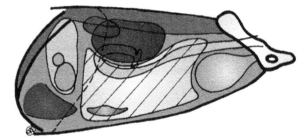

Figure 9.18 Left renal mass on the lateral view (see Fig. 11.1 for ventrodorsal view). *(From Thrall, D.E. (ed.) (1998)* Textbook of Veterinary Diagnostic Radiology, *4th edition. Philadelphia: Saunders, with permission.)*

 Ventrodorsal view
  – Medial (right) displacement of the small
   intestine and descending colon.
4. Small intestine – small intestinal masses are usually
 also associated with radiographic signs of intestinal
 obstruction (e.g. dilated loops and gravel sign).
 Lateral view
  – Displacement of other structures
   depending on size and location of mass.
 Ventrodorsal view
  – As for the lateral view.

5. Large intestine (including caecum) – the wide normal diameter of the large intestine means that without contrast studies, smaller masses may be overlooked.
   Lateral view
   – Ventral displacement of small intestine.
   Ventrodorsal view
   – Left, right or caudal displacement of small intestine, depending on the part of the large intestine that is affected.
6. Omentum and mesentery – variable effects depending on the location of the mass.
   a. Root of mesentery.
   Lateral view
   – Mid-dorsal mass with ventral and cranial or caudal displacement of small intestine.
   Ventrodorsal view
   – Mid-abdominal mass displacing small intestines peripherally, which is unusual for a splenic mass.
   b. Mesenteric lymph nodes.
   Lateral view
   – Peripheral displacement of small intestines.
   Ventrodorsal view
   – As for the lateral view.
   c. Colic lymph nodes.
   Lateral view
   – Ventral displacement of the ascending colon, especially on the LLR view.
   Ventrodorsal view
   – Lateral (right) displacement of the ascending colon.
7. Ovaries – ovaries are intraperitoneal, therefore, unlike the kidneys, they may lie more ventrally in the abdomen when markedly enlarged. They arise caudal to the ipsilateral kidney.
   a. Right ovary.
   Lateral view
   – Variable ventral displacement of small intestine.
   – If large, cranial displacement of the right kidney ± ventral deviation of its caudal pole.
   Ventrodorsal view
   – Medial (left) displacement of the small intestine and ascending colon.
   b. Left ovary.

Lateral view
   – Variable ventral displacement of small intestine.
   – If large, cranial displacement of the left kidney ± ventral deviation of its caudal pole.
   Ventrodorsal view
   – Medial (right) displacement of the small intestine and descending colon.
8. Retained testicle (more often right) – variable location between the caudal pole of the ipsilateral kidney and the inguinal region; displacement of other structures accordingly. May torse or develop neoplasia, abscess or haematoma.
9. Retroperitoneal masses.
   Lateral view
   – Ventral displacement of the kidneys and small intestine.
   Ventrodorsal view
   – Less helpful, but there may be lateral (right or left) displacement of the kidneys or small intestine if the mass is lateralized.

9.40 CAUDAL ABDOMINAL MASSES

1. Urinary bladder – bladder masses are rarely visible on plain radiographs and require cystography for demonstration. The mass effect caused by distension of the bladder is described below; such distension may be physiological, or pathological due to inability to urinate.
   Lateral view
   ● Cranial displacement of small intestine.
   ● Dorsal displacement of the descending colon.
   Ventrodorsal view
   ● Cranial displacement of small intestine.
   ● Lateral (left or right) displacement of the descending colon.
2. Uterus – mild uterine enlargement may not be detected, because uterine horns mimic the appearance of small intestinal loops. Most types of uterine enlargement affect the whole organ and are described below; focal masses will create effects depending on their location (see 11.40.1 and Fig. 11.16). A vaginal or uterine stump mass creates a more localized swelling between the descending colon and bladder neck,

which may displace and/or compress the bladder.

Lateral view

- Cranial or craniodorsal displacement of small intestine.
- Dorsal displacement of the descending colon.
- ± separation of the descending colon and bladder by a soft tissue structure.

Ventrodorsal view

- Cranial ± medial displacement of small intestine.

3. Prostate – the location of the prostate gland varies depending on the degree of filling of the bladder; it lies more cranially when the bladder is full (see 11.48 and Fig. 11.18).

Lateral view

- Cranial displacement of the bladder.
- Asymmetric prostatic diseases may also cause dorsal or ventral displacement of bladder; paraprostatic cysts may even lie cranial to the bladder, and contrast studies or ultrasonography are required to locate the bladder (see 11.49.1 and Fig. 11.19).
- Dorsal displacement ± compression of the distal descending colon and rectum.

Ventrodorsal view

- Cranial displacement of the bladder.
- Asymmetric prostatic diseases may also cause displacement of the bladder to the right or left.
- Lateral (left) displacement of the distal descending colon and rectum.

4. Large intestine – distal descending colon.

Lateral view

- Ventral displacement of the bladder ± prostate.

Ventrodorsal view

- Little value; possible lateral displacement of the bladder.

5. Sublumbar area (Fig. 9.19).

Lateral view

- Ventral displacement ± compression of the distal descending colon.
- Ventral displacement of the bladder if the mass is large.

Ventrodorsal view

- Little value; possible further lateral (left) displacement of the distal descending colon.

6. Retained testicle – see 9.39.8.

MISCELLANEOUS

9.41 MINERALIZATION ON ABDOMINAL RADIOGRAPHS

The following list of causes of mineralization seen on abdominal radiographs is based on the review paper 'Diagnosis of calcification on abdominal radiographs' (Lamb et al. 1991 *Veterinary Radiology and Ultrasound* 32, 211–220, with permission).

Intestinal tract

- Ingesta (e.g. bones – accumulation may indicate partial obstruction).
- Foreign bodies (e.g. stones).
- Medication (e.g. kaolin).
- Enterolith.
- Uraemic gastritis.

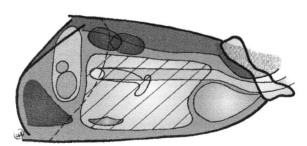

Figure 9.19 Sublumbar mass: lateral view. *(From Thrall, D.E. (ed.) (1998) Textbook of Veterinary Diagnostic Radiology, 4th edition. Philadelphia: Saunders, with permission.)*

Liver (see also 9.18)
- Cholelithiasis (if radiopaque).
- Chronic cholecystitis (gall bladder wall).
- Chronic hepatopathy.
- Cyst (developmental or parasitic, e.g. alveolar echinococcosis*).
- Hepatic nodular hyperplasia.
- Neoplasms (e.g. osteosarcoma).
- Long-standing haematoma, abscess or granuloma.
- Unknown aetiology – especially Yorkshire Terriers.

Spleen (see also 9.28)
- Histoplasmosis*.
- Long-standing haematoma or abscess.
- Extraskeletal osteosarcoma.

Pancreas
- Chronic pancreatitis (including pseudocyst).
- Fat necrosis.
- Neoplasm (e.g. adenocarcinoma).

Kidney (see also 11.3)
- Nephrolithiasis.
- Nephrocalcinosis.
  - Nephrotoxic drugs (e.g. gentamicin).
  - Hypervitaminosis D.
  - Chronic nephritis (e.g. pyelonephritis).
  - Chronic renal insufficiency.
  - Hyperparathyroidism.
  - Hyperadrenocorticism.
  - Renal telangiectasia of Corgis.
- Long-standing haematoma or abscess.
- Parasitic granuloma (e.g. *Toxocara canis*).

Ureter
- Calculus.

Urinary bladder (see also 11.23)
- Calculus.
- Chronic cystitis.
- Transitional cell carcinoma.

Adrenal
- Adrenocortical neoplasm (e.g. adenoma, carcinoma).
- Idiopathic, especially old cats.

Ovary
- Neoplasm (e.g. teratoma).
- Cyst.
- Suture reaction to ovariohysterectomy.

Uterus
- Normal fetus (skeletal calcification is normally visible 35 days after mating in the cat, and approximately 41 days after mating in the dog).
- Mummified fetus.
- Suture reaction to ovariohysterectomy.

Prostate
- Calculus.
- Chronic prostatitis.
- Neoplasm (e.g. adenocarcinoma).
- Cyst (including paraprostatic cyst; may also be intrapelvic).

Vascular
- Chronic renal insufficiency.
- Hypervitaminosis D.
- Idiopathic.

Lymph node
- Chronic inflammation (e.g. fungal* infection).
- Metastatic neoplasm (e.g. osteosarcoma, prostatic adenocarcinoma).

Peritoneal cavity
- Chronic peritonitis.
- Uroliths from ruptured urinary bladder.
- Choleliths from ruptured gall bladder.
- Ectopic pregnancy or rupture of gravid uterus.
- Previous barium extravasation may mimic peritoneal calcification.

Abdominal fat
- Idiopathic nodular fat necrosis – usually cats.
- Pansteatitis in cats.
- Mineralization of lipoma (intra-abdominal or in abdominal wall).
- Chondrolipoma.

Retained intra-abdominal testicle
Penetrating foreign body
Urethra
- Calculus.
- Chronic urethritis.
- Separate centres of ossification of the caudal os penis.

Muscle (see also 12.2)
- Myositis ossificans (e.g. affecting the gluteal muscles).

Skin
- Calcinosis cutis associated with hyperadrenocorticism.

- Calcifying surgical scar.
- Chronic hygroma.

Rib

- Neoplasm (e.g. chondrosarcoma).
- Fracture callus.

Mammary gland

- Neoplasm (e.g. mixed mammary tumour).

Miscellaneous

- Parasitic cyst – may contain motile, mineralized sediment.
- Neoplasm with old haemorrhage.
- Mineralized arteriosclerosis (hypertension, renal secondary hyperparathyroidism).

Further reading

General and miscellaneous

Blackwood, L., Sullivan, M., Lawson, H., 1997. Radiographic abnormalities in canine multicentric lymphoma: a review of 84 cases. J. Small Anim. Pract. 38, 62–69.

Bradbury, C.A., Westropp, J.L., Pollard, E., 2009. Relationship between prostatomegaly, prostatic mineralization, and cytological diagnosis. Vet. Radiol. Ultrasound 50, 167–171.

Cruz-Arambulo, R., Wrigley, R., Powers, B., 2004. Sonographic features of histiocytic neoplasms in the canine abdomen. Vet. Radiol. Ultrasound 45, 554–558.

Haers, H., Saunders, J.H., 2009. Review of clinical characteristics and applications of contrast-enhanced ultrasonography in dogs. J. Am. Vet. Med. Assoc. 234, 460–470.

Hayward, N., 2006. Practical guide to imaging abdominal masses. In Pract. 28, 84–93.

Heeren, V., Edwards, L., Mazzaferro, E.M., 2004. Acute abdomen: diagnosis. Compend. Contin. Educ. Pract. Veterinarian (Small Animal) 26, 350–362.

Heng, H.G., Teoh, W.T., Sheikh-Moar, R., 2008. Postmortem abdominal radiographic findings in feline cadavers. Vet. Radiol. Ultrasound 49, 26–29.

Keppie, N., Nelson, N., Rosenstein, D., 2006. Imaging diagnosis: Mineralization of the aorta, celiac and cranial mesenteric arteries in a cat with chronic renal failure. Vet. Radiol. Ultrasound 47, 69–71.

Lamb, C.R., 1990. Abdominal ultrasonography in small animals: Examination of the liver, spleen and pancreas (review). J. Small Anim. Pract. 31, 6–15.

Lamb, C.R., 1990. Abdominal ultrasonography in small animals: Intestinal tract and mesentery, kidneys, adrenal glands, uterus and prostate (review). J. Small Anim. Pract. 31, 295–304.

Lamb, C.R., Hartzband, L.E., Tidwell, A.S., Pearson, S.H., 1991. Ultrasonographic findings in hepatic and splenic lymphoma in dogs and cats. Vet. Radiol. 32, 117–120.

Lamb, C.R., Kleine, L.J., McMillan, M.C., 1991. Diagnosis of calcification on abdominal radiographs. Vet. Radiol. Ultrasound 32, 211–220.

Lee, R., Leowijuk, C., 1982. Normal parameters in abdominal radiology of the dog and cat. J. Small Anim. Pract. 23, 251–269.

Lefbom, B.K., Adams, W.H., Weddle, D.L., 1996. Mineralized arteriosclerosis in a cat. Vet. Radiol. Ultrasound 37, 420–423.

Llabres Diaz, F., 2006. Practical contrast radiogahy 5. Other techniques. In Pract. 28, 32–40.

Melian, C., Stefanacci, J., Petersen, M.E., Kintzer, P.P., 1999. Radiographic findings in dogs with naturally occurring primary hypoadrenocorticism. J. Am. Anim. Hosp. Assoc. 35, 208–212.

Merlo, M., Lamb, C.R., 2000. Radiographic and ultrasonographic features of retained surgical sponge in eight dogs. Vet. Radiol. Ultrasound 41, 279–283.

Miles, K., 1997. Imaging abdominal masses. Vet. Clin. North Am. Small Anim. Pract. 27, 1403–1431.

Monteiro, C.B., O'Brien, R.T., 2004. A retrospective study on the sonographic findings of abdominal carcinomatosis in 14 cats. Vet. Radiol. Ultrasound 45, 559–564.

Moores, A.P., Bell, A.M.D., Costello, M., 2002. Urinoma (para-ureteral pseudocyst) as a consequence of trauma in a cat. J. Small Anim. Pract. 43, 213–216.

Ramirez, S., Douglass, J.P., Robertson, I.D., 2002. Ultrasonographic features of canine abdominal malignant histiocytosis. Vet. Radiol. Ultrasound 43, 167–170.

Root, C.R., 1998. Abdominal masses. In: Thrall, D.E. (Ed.), Textbook of Veterinary Diagnostic Radiology. 3rd ed. Saunders, Philadelphia, pp. 417–439.

Root, C.R., Lord, P.F., 1971. Peritoneal carcinomatosis in the dog and cat: its radiographic appearance. Vet. Radiol. 12, 54–59.

Sato, A.F., Solano, M., 2004. Ultrasonographic findings in abdominal mast cell disease: a retrospective study of 19 patients. Vet. Radiol. Ultrasound 45, 51–57.

Saunders, H.M., 1998. Ultrasonography of abdominal cavitary parenchymal lesions. Vet. Clin. North Am. Small Anim. Pract. 28, 755–776.

Saunders, H.M., Pugh, C.R., Rhodes, W.H., 1992. Expanding applications of abdominal ultrasonography. J. Am. Anim. Hosp. Assoc. 28, 369–374.

Schwarz, T., Morandi, F., Gnudi, G., Wisner, E., Paterson, C., Sullivan, M., et al., 2000. Nodular fat necrosis in the feline and canine abdomen. Vet. Radiol. Ultrasound 41, 335–339.

Shaiken, L.C., Evans, S.M., Goldschmidt, M.H., 1991. Radiographic findings in canine malignant histiocytosis. Vet. Radiol. 32, 237–242.

Spaulding, K.A., 1993. Ultrasound corner: Sonographic evaluation of peritoneal effusion in small animals. Vet. Radiol. Ultrasound 34, 427–431.

Thrall, D.E., 1992. Radiology corner: Intraperitoneal vs. extraperitoneal fluid. Vet. Radiol. Ultrasound 33, 138–140.

Tidwell, A.S., Ullman, S.L., Schelling, S.H., 1990. Urinoma (para-ureteral pseudocyst) in a dog. Vet. Radiol. Ultrasound 31, 203–206.

Venco, L., Kramer, L., Pagliaro, L., Genchi, C., 2005. Ultrasonographic features of peritoneal cestodiasis caused by mesocestoides sp in a dog and in a cat. Vet. Radiol. Ultrasound 46, 417–422.

Liver

Austin, B., Tillson, D.M., Kuhnt, L.A., 2006. Gallbladder agenesis in a Maltese dog. J. Am. Anim. Hosp. Assoc. 42, 308–311.

Barr, F.J., 1992. Ultrasonographic assessment of liver size in the dog. J. Small Anim. Pract. 33, 359–364.

Barr, F.J., 1992. Normal hepatic measurements in mature dogs. J. Small Anim. Pract. 33, 367–370.

Beatty, J.A., Barrs, V.R., Martin, P.A., Nicoll, R.G., France, M.P., Foster, S.F., et al., 2002. Spontaneous hepatic rupture in

six cats with systemic amyloidosis. J. Small Anim. Pract. 43, 355–363.

Berry, C.R., Ackerman, N., Charach, M., Lawrence, D., 1992. Iatrogenic biloma (biliary pseudocyst) in a cat with hepatic lipidosis. Vet. Radiol. Ultrasound 33, 145–149.

Biller, D.S., Kantrowitz, B., Miyabayashi, T., 1992. Ultrasonography of diffuse liver disease: a review. J. Vet. Intern. Med. 6, 71–76.

Birchard, S.J., Biller, D.S., Johnson, S.E., 1989. Differentiation of intrahepatic versus extrahepatic portosystemic shunts using positive contrast portography. J. Am. Anim. Hosp. Assoc. 25, 13–17.

Blaxter, A.C., Holt, P.E., Pearson, G.R., Gibbs, C., Gruffydd-Jones, T.J., 1988. Congenital portosystemic shunts in the cat: a report of nine cases. J. Small Anim. Pract. 29, 631–645.

Broemel, C., Barthez, P.Y., Leveille, R., Scrivani, P., 1998. Prevalence of gallbladder sludge in dogs as assessed by ultrasonography. Vet. Radiol. Ultrasound 39, 206–210.

Cornejo, L., Webster, C.R.L., 2005. Canine gallbladder mucoceles. Compend. Contin. Euca. Pract. Veterinarian 27, 912–928.

Cuccovillo, A., Lamb, C.R., 2002. Cellular features of sonographic target lesions of the liver and spleen in 21 dogs and a cat. Vet. Radiol. Ultrasound 43, 275–278.

D'Anjou, M.A., Penninck, D.G., Cornejo, L., Pibarot, P., 2004. Ultrasonographic diagnosis of portosystemic shunting in dogs and cats. Vet. Radiol. Ultrasound 45, 424–437.

Evans, S.M., 1987. The radiographic appearance of primary liver neoplasia in dogs. Vet. Radiol. 28, 192–196.

Ferrell, E.A., Graham, J.P., Hanel, R., Randell, S., Farese, J.P., Castleman, W.L., 2003.

Simultaneous congenital and acquired extrahepatic portosystemic shunts in two dogs. Vet. Radiol. Ultrasound 44, 38–42.

Gaillot, H.A., Penninck, D.G., Webster, C.R.L., Crawford, S., 2007. Ultrasonographic features of extrahepatic biliary obstruction in 30 cats. Vet. Radiol. Ultrasound 48, 439–447.

Gaschan, L., 2009. Update on hepatobiliary imaging. Vet. Clin. Small Anim. 39, 349–467.

Hampson, E.C.G.M., Filippich, L.J., Kelly, W.R., Evans, K., 1987. Congenital biliary atresia in a cat: a case report. J. Small Anim. Pract. 28, 39–48.

Hinkle Schwartz, S.G., Mitchell, S.L., Keating, J.H., Chan, D.L., 2006. Liver lobe torsion in dogs: 13 cases (1995–2004). J. Am. Vet. Med. Assoc. 228, 242–247.

Hittmair, K.M., Vielgrader, H.D., Loupal, G., 2001. Ultrasono-graphic evaluation of gall bladder wall thickness in cats. Vet. Radiol. Ultrasound 42, 149–155.

Holt, D.E., Schelling, C.G., Saunders, H.M., Orsher, R.J., 1995. Correlation of ultrasonographic findings with surgical, portographic, and necropsy findings in dogs and cats with portosystemic shunts: 63 cases (1987–1993). J. Am. Vet. Med. Assoc. 207, 1190–1193.

Jacobson, L.S., Kirberger, R.M., Nesbit, J.W., 1995. Hepatic ultrasonography and pathological findings in dogs with hepatocutaneous syndrome: new concepts. J. Vet. Intern. Med. 9, 399–404.

Lamb, C.R., 1996. Ultrasonographic diagnosis of congenital portosystemic shunts in dogs: results of a prospective study. Vet. Radiol. Ultrasound 37, 281–288.

Lamb, C.R., 1998. Ultrasonography of portosystemic shunts in dogs and cats. Vet. Clin. North Am. Small Anim. Pract. 28, 725–754.

Lamb, C.R., Daniel, G.B., 2002. Diagnostic imaging of dogs with suspected portosystemic shunting. Compend. Contin. Educ. Pract. Veterinarian (Small Animal) 24, 626–635.

Lamb, C.R., Forster-van Hyfte, M.A., White, R.N., McEvoy, F.J., Rutgers, H.C., 1996. Ultrasonographic diagnosis of congenital portosystemic shunts in 14 cats. J. Small Anim. Pract. 37, 205–209.

Lamb, C.R., Wrigley, R.H., Simpson, K.W., Forster-van Hyfte, M., Garden, O.A., Smyth, B.A., et al., 1996. Ultrasonographic diagnosis of portal vein thrombosis in 4 dogs. Vet. Radiol. Ultrasound 37, 121–129.

Lee, K.C.L., Lipscomb, V.J., Lamb, C.R., Gregory, S.P., Guitian, J., Brockman, D.J., 2006. Association of portovenographic findings with outcome in dogs receiving surgical treatment for single congenital portosystemic shunts: 45 cases (2000–2004). J. Am. Vet. Med. Assoc. 229, 1122–1129.

Leveille, R., Biller, D.S., Shiroma, J.T., 1996. Sonographic evaluation of the common bile duct in cats. J. Vet. Intern. Med. 10, 296–299.

Moores, A.L., Gregory, S.P., 2007. Duplex gall bladder associated with choledocholithiasis, cholecystitis, gall bladder rupture and peritonitis in a cat. J. Small Anim. Pract. 48, 404–409.

Newell, S.M., Selcer, B.A., Girard, E., Roberts, G.D., Thompson, J.P., Harrison, J.M., 1998. Correlations between ultrasonographic findings and specific hepatic diseases in cats: 72 cases (1985–1997). J. Am. Vet. Med. Assoc. 213, 94–98.

Nyland, T.G., Barthez, P.Y., Ortega, T.M., Davis, C.R., 1996. Hepatic ultrasonographic and pathologic findings in dogs with canine superficial necrolytic dermatitis. Vet. Radiol. Ultrasound 37, 200–205.

Nyland, T.G., Koblik, P.D., Tellyer, S.E., 1999. Ultrasonographic features of splenic lymphoma in dogs – 12 cases. J. Am. Vet. Med. Assoc. 12, 1565–1568.

O'Brien, R.T., Iani, M., Matheson, J., Delaney, F., Young, K., 2004. Contrast harmonic ultrasound of spontaneous liver nodules in 32 dogs. Vet. Radiol. Ultrasound 45, 547–553.

Partington, B.P., Biller, D.S., 1995. Hepatic imaging with radiology and ultrasound. Vet. Clin. North Am. Small Anim. Pract. 25, 305–335.

Reed, A.L., 1995. Ultrasonographic findings of diseases of the gallbladder and biliary tract. Vet. Med. 190, 950–957.

Sato, A.F., Solano, M., 1998. Radiographic diagnosis: liver lobe entrapment and associated emphysematous hepatitis. Vet. Radiol. Ultrasound 39, 123–124.

Scharf, G., Kaser-Hotz, B., Borer, L., Hasler, A., Haller, M., Fluckiger, M., Radiographic, ultrasonographic, and computed tomographic appearance of alveolar echinococcosis in dogs. Vet. Radiol. Ultrasound 45, 411–418.

Schwarz, L.A., Penninck, D.G., Leveille-Webster, C., 1998. Hepatic abscesses in 13 dogs: a review of the ultrasonographic findings, clinical data and therapeutic options. Vet. Radiol. Ultrasound 39, 357–365.

Scrivani, P.V., Yeager, A.E., Dykes, N.L., Scarlett, J.M., 2001. Influence of patient positioning on sensitivity of mesenteric portography for detecting an anomalous portosystemic blood vessel in dogs: 34 cases (1997–2000). J. Am. Vet. Med. Assoc. 219, 1251–1253.

Smith, S.A., Biller, D.S., Goggin, J.M., Kraft, S.L., Hoskinson, J.J., 1998. Diagnostic imaging of biliary obstruction. Compend. Contin. Educ. Pract. Veterinarian (Small Animal) 20, 1225–1234.

Sonnenfield, J.M., Armbrust, L.J., Radlinsky, M.A., Chun, R., Hoskinson, J.J., Kennedy, G.A., 2001. Radiographic and ultrasonographic findings of liver lobe torsion in a dog. Vet. Radiol. Ultrasound 42, 344–346.

Suter, P.F., 1982. Radiographic diagnosis of liver disease in dogs and cats. Vet. Clin. North Am. Small Anim. Pract. 12, 153–173.

White, R.N., Burton, C.A., McEvoy, F.J., 1998. Surgical treatment of intrahepatic portosystemic shunts in 45 dogs. Vet. Rec. 142, 358–365.

Wrigley, R.H., Konde, L.J., Park, R.D., Lebel, J.L., 1987. Ultrasonographic diagnosis of portacaval shunts in young dogs. J. Am. Vet. Med. Assoc. 191, 421–424.

Spleen

Gärtner, F., Santos, M., Gillette, D., Schmitt, F., 2002. Inflammatory pseudotumour of the spleen in a dog. Vet. Rec. 150, 697–698.

Gaschen, L., Kircher, P., Venziri, C., Hurter, K., Lang, J., 2003. Imaging diagnosis: the abdominal air-vasculogram in a dog with splenic torsion and clostridial infection. Vet. Radiol. Ultrasound 44, 553–555.

Hanson, J.A., Papageorges, M., Girard, E., Menard, M., Hebert, P., 2001. Ultrasonographic appearance of splenic disease in 101 cats. Vet. Radiol. Ultrasound 42, 441–445.

Konde, L.J., Wrigley, R.H., Lebel, J.L., Park, R.D., Pugh, C., Finn, S., 1989. Sonographic and radiographic changes associated with splenic torsion in the dog. Vet. Radiol. 30, 41–45.

Mai, W., 2006. The hilar perivenous hyperechoic triangle as a sign of acute splenic torsion in dogs. Vet. Radiol. Ultrasound 47, 487–491.

Neath, P.J., Brockman, D.J., Saunders, H.M., 1997. Retrospective analysis of 19 cases of isolated torsion of the splenic pedicle in dogs. J. Small Anim. Pract. 38, 387–392.

O'Brien, R.T., Waller, K.R., Osgood, T.L., 2004. Sonographic features of drug-induced splenic congestion. Vet. Radiol. Ultrasound 45, 225–227.

Patnaik, A.K., Lieberman, P.H., Macewen, E.G., 1985. Splenosis in a dog. J. Small Anim. Pract. 26, 23–31.

Rossi, F., Leone, V.F., Vignoli, M., Laddaga, E., Terragni, R., 2008. Use of contrast-enhanced ultrasound for characterization of focal splenic lesions. Vet. Radiol. Ultrasound 49, 154–164.

Saunders, H.M., Neath, P.J., Brockman, D.J., 1998. B-mode and Doppler ultrasound imaging of the spleen with canine splenic torsion: a retrospective evaluation. Vet. Radiol. Ultrasound 39, 349–353.

Schwarz, L.A., Penninck, D.G., Gliatto, J., 2001. Ultrasound corner: Canine splenic myelolipomas. Vet. Radiol. Ultrasound 42, 347–348.

Stickle, R.L., 1989. Radiographic signs of isolated splenic torsion in dogs: eight cases (1980–1987). J. Am. Vet. Med. Assoc. 194, 103–106.

Wrigley, R.H., Konde, L.J., Park, R.D., Lebel, J.L., 1988. Ultrasonographic features of splenic lymphoma in dogs – 12 cases. J. Am. Vet. Med. Assoc. 192, 1565–1568.

Wrigley, R.H., Park, R.D., Konde, L.J., Lebel, J.L., 1988. Ultrasonographic features of splenic haemangio-sarcoma in dogs: 18 cases. J. Am. Vet. Med. Assoc. 192, 1113–1117.

Pancreas

Etue, S.M., Penninck, D.G., Labato, M.A., Pearson, S., Tidwell, A., 2001. Ultrasono-graphy of the normal feline pancreas and associated anatomic landmarks: a pros-pective study of 20 cats. Vet. Radiol. Ultrasound 42, 330–336.

Hecht, S., Henry, G., 2007. Sonographic evaluation of the normal and abnormal pancreas. Clin. Tech. Small Anim. Pract. 22, 115–121.

Hecht, S., Penninck, D.G., Mahoney, O.M., King, R., Rand, W.M., 2006. Relationship of pancreatic duct dilation to age and clinical findings in cats. Vet. Radiol. Ultrasound 47, 287–294.

Hecht, S., Penninck, D.G., Keating, J.H., 2007. Imaging findings in pancreatic neoplasia and nodular hyperplasia in 19 cats. Vet. Radiol. Ultrasound 48, 45–50.

Hess, R.S., Saunders, H.M., Van Winkle, T.J., Shofer, F.S., Washabau, R.J., 1998. Clinical, clinicopathologic, radiographic, and ultrasonographic abnormalities in dogs with fatal acute pancreatitis: 70 cases (1986–1995). J. Am. Vet. Med. Assoc. 213, 665–670.

Lamb, C.R., Simpson, K.W., Boswood, A., Matthewman, L.A., 1995. Ultrasonography of pancreatic neoplasia in the dog: a retrospective review of 16 cases. Vet. Rec. 137, 65–68.

Adrenal glands

Barthez, P.Y., Nyland, T.G., Feldman, E.C., 1995. Ultrasonographic evaluation of the adrenal glands in the dog. J. Am. Vet. Med. Assoc. 207, 1180–1183.

Besso, J.G., Penninck, D.G., Gliatto, J.M., 1997. Retrospective ultrasonographic evaluation of adrenal gland lesions in 26 dogs. Vet. Radiol. Ultrasound 38, 448–455.

Douglass, J.P., Berry, C.R., James, S., 1997. Ultrasonographic adrenal gland measurements in dogs without evidence of adrenal gland disease. Vet. Radiol. Ultrasound 38, 124–130.

Grooters, A.M., Biller, D.S., Miyabayashi, T., Leveille, R., 1994. Evaluation of routine abdominal ultrasonography as a technique for imaging the canine adrenal glands. J. Am. Anim. Hosp. Assoc. 30, 457–462.

Grooters, A.M., Biller, D.S., Merryman, J., 1995. Ultrasonographic parameters of normal canine adrenal glands: comparison to necropsy findings. Vet. Radiol. Ultrasound 36, 126–130.

Grooters, A.M., Biller, D.S., Theisen, S.K., Miyabayashi, T., 1996. Ultrasonographic characteristics of adrenal glands in dogs with pituitary-dependent hyperadrenocorticism: comparison with normal dogs. J. Vet. Intern. Med. 10, 110–115.

Mantis, P., Lamb, C.R., Witt, A.L., Neiger, R., 2003. Changes in ultrasonographic appearance of adrenal glands in dogs with pituitary-dependent hyperadrenocorticism treated with Trilostane. Vet. Radiol. Ultrasound 44, 682–685.

Rosenstein, D.S., 2000. Diagnostic imaging in canine pheochromocytoma. Vet. Radiol. Ultrasound 41, 499–506.

Schelling, C.G., 1991. Ultrasonogra-phy of the adrenal gland. Probl. Vet. Med. 3, 604–617.

Tidwell, A.S., Penninck, D.G., Besso, J.G., 1997. Imaging of adrenal gland disorders. Vet. Clin. North Am. Small Anim. Pract. 27, 237–254.

Whittemore, J.C., Preston, C.A., Kyles, A.E., Hardie, E.M., Feldman, E.C., 2001. Nontraumatic rupture of an adrenal gland tumor causing intra-abdominal or retroperito-neal hemorrhage in four dogs. J. Am. Vet. Med. Assoc. 219, 329–333.

Abdominal blood vessels

Finn-Bodner, S.T., Hudson, J.A., 1998. Abdominal vascular sonography. Vet. Clin. North Am. Small Anim. Pract. 28, 887–942.

Spaulding, K.A., 1992. Ultrasound corner: Helpful hints in identifying the caudal abdominal aorta and caudal vena cava. Vet. Radiol. Ultrasound 33, 90–92.

Spaulding, K.A., 1997. A review of sonographic identification of abdominal vessels and juxtavascular organs. Vet. Radiol. Ultrasound 38, 4–23.

Abdominal lymph nodes

Kinns, J., Mai, W., 2007. Association between malignancy and sonographic heterogeneity in canine and feline abdominal lymph nodes. Vet. Radiol. Ultrasound 48, 565–569.

Pugh, C.R., 1994. Ultrasonographic examination of abdominal lymph nodes in the dog. Vet. Radiol. Ultrasound 35, 110–115.

Chapter 10

Gastrointestinal tract

CHAPTER CONTENTS

Oesophagus (see 8.14–8.20)

Stomach 268
10.1 Normal radiographic appearance of the stomach 268
10.2 Displacement of the stomach 269
10.3 Variations in stomach size 269
10.4 Variations in stomach contents 270
10.5 Variations in the stomach wall 271
10.6 Gastric contrast studies: technique and normal appearance 272
10.7 Technical errors on the gastrogram 273
10.8 Gastric luminal filling defects on contrast studies 273
10.9 Abnormal gastric mucosal pattern on contrast studies 274
10.10 Variations in gastric emptying time 274
10.11 Ultrasonographic technique for the stomach 275
10.12 Normal ultrasonographic appearance of the stomach 276
10.13 Variations in gastric contents on ultrasonography 276
10.14 Lack of visualization of the normal gastric wall layered architecture on ultrasonography 277
10.15 Focal thickening of the gastric wall on ultrasonography 277
10.16 Diffuse thickening of the gastric wall on ultrasonography 277

Small intestine 277
10.17 Normal radiographic appearance of the small intestine 277
10.18 Variations in the number of small intestinal loops visible 278
10.19 Displacement of the small intestine 278
10.20 Bunching of small intestinal loops 278
10.21 Increased width of small intestinal loops 279
10.22 Variations in small intestinal contents 280
10.23 Small intestinal contrast studies: technique and normal appearance 282
10.24 Technical errors with small intestinal contrast studies 282
10.25 Variations in small intestinal luminal diameter on contrast studies 283
10.26 Small intestinal luminal filling defects on contrast studies 283
10.27 Variations in the small intestinal wall on contrast studies 283
10.28 Variations in small intestinal transit time on contrast studies 284
10.29 Ultrasonographic technique for the small intestine 285
10.30 Normal ultrasonographic appearance of the small intestine 285
10.31 Variations in small intestinal contents on ultrasonography 285
10.32 Dilation of the small intestinal lumen on ultrasonography 285
10.33 Lack of visualization of the normal small intestinal wall layered architecture on ultrasonography 285

10.34 Abnormal arrangement of the small intestine on ultrasonography 286

10.35 Focal thickening of the small intestinal wall on ultrasonography 286

10.36 Diffuse thickening of the small intestinal wall on ultrasonography 287

10.37 Mucosal layer alterations of the small intestine 287

Large intestine 287

10.38 Normal radiographic appearance of the large intestine 287

10.39 Displacement of the large intestine 288

10.40 Large intestinal dilation 289

10.41 Variations in large intestinal contents 289

10.42 Variations in large intestinal wall opacity 290

10.43 Large intestinal contrast studies: technique and normal appearance 290

10.44 Technical errors with large intestinal contrast studies 291

10.45 Large intestinal luminal filling defects on contrast studies 291

10.46 Increased large intestinal wall thickness on contrast studies 291

10.47 Abnormal large intestinal mucosal pattern on contrast studies 291

10.48 Ultrasonographic technique for the large intestine 292

10.49 Normal ultrasonographic appearance of the large intestine 292

10.50 Ultrasonographic changes in large intestinal disease 292

STOMACH

10.1 NORMAL RADIOGRAPHIC APPEARANCE OF THE STOMACH

The stomach consists of a fundus (dome-like out-pouching dorsally on the left), cardia (junction with the oesophagus), body (middle portion) and pyloric portion (pyloric antrum and canal ventrally on the right). An imaginary line joining the fundus, body and pylorus is known as the gastric axis. The position of the stomach differs between dogs and cats and between conformational types of dog. In cats and in most breeds of dog, the gastric axis lies parallel to the caudal ribs on the lateral view, against the liver, and so displacement of the

stomach axis reflects a change in liver size or position (Fig. 10.1A and B). In deep-chested dog breeds, the gastric axis is perpendicular to the spine, and this may mimic reduced liver size. The pylorus may lie slightly cranial to the rest of the stomach, and its position and appearance vary slightly between right and left lateral recumbency. In right lateral recumbency, the pylorus is likely to be fluid-filled and appears as a round soft tissue mass; in left lateral recumbency it may contain gas, which may extend into the descending duodenum. Gas rises to the uppermost portion of the stomach and fluid pools in the dependent part, so positional radiography may be used to highlight certain areas with gas, for example left lateral recumbency to assess pyloric and proximal duodenal pathology such as mural masses and foreign bodies. In deep-chested dog breeds, on the ventrodorsal (VD) view the gastric axis lies transversely approximately at the level of the tenth intercostal space, with the fundus to the left and the pylorus to the right of the midline (Fig. 10.1C). In barrel-chested breeds, the stomach is more curved, with the fundus lying more cranially and the pylorus

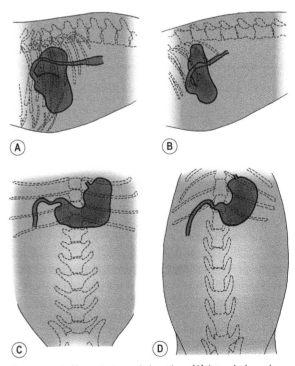

Figure 10.1 Normal stomach location: (A) lateral view, dog; (B) lateral view, cat; (C) ventrodorsal (VD) view, dog; (D) VD view, cat.

closer to the midline. In cats, on the VD view an empty stomach is located with the pylorus in the midline and the remainder of the stomach to the left side (Fig. 10.1D). Distension of the feline stomach results in displacement of the pylorus to the right side. The amount of air or ingesta present combined with normal gastric contractions will affect the size and shape of the stomach, and opacity depends on the nature of the gastric contents.

10.2 DISPLACEMENT OF THE STOMACH

1. Cranial displacement of the gastric axis.
   a. Reduced liver size (see 9.16.3 and Fig. 9.7).
   b. Diaphragmatic hernia or rupture.
   c. Peritoneopericardial diaphragmatic hernia (see 7.6.3).
   d. Gastro-oesophageal intussusception (see 8.19.2).
   e. Hiatal hernia (see 8.19.3 and 8.19.7).
2. Caudal indentation or distortion of the stomach.
   a. Distension or mass of the transverse colon.
   b. Pancreatic mass, left limb (see 9.38.3).
   c. Mesenteric mass (see 9.39.6).
   d. Other large abdominal masses, including late pregnancy.
3. Caudal displacement of the gastric axis.
   a. Enlarged liver (see 9.16.1 and Fig. 9.6).
   b. Thoracic expansion.
4. Stomach displaced towards the right.
   a. Enlarged spleen.
   b. Left-sided liver enlargement.
5. Stomach displaced towards the left.
   a. Enlarged pancreas, particularly body.
   b. Right-sided liver enlargement.

The stomach may also be variably displaced in cases of gastric dilation and volvulus (GDV); chronic gastric volvulus without dilation is also seen, in which the stomach is in an abnormal location but is not markedly distended.

10.3 VARIATIONS IN STOMACH SIZE

A small amount of gas and/or fluid is normally observed in the stomach after an 8 h fast.

1. Stomach not visible.
   a. Completely empty.
   b. Absence of abdominal fat.
   – Young animals.
   – Emaciation.
   c. Peritoneal effusion.
2. Stomach visible but empty.
   a. Fasted or anorexic (NB: this does not rule out obstruction if the animal has vomited recently).
3. Stomach normal shape and size; gas and/or fluid contents.
   a. Normal, with some aerophagia.
   b. Recent drink.
   c. Acute gastritis.
4. Stomach distended but normal in shape. The fundus and body tend to enlarge more than the pylorus and do so mainly on the left side of the abdomen.
   a. Endotracheal tube in oesophagus not trachea – dilation with gas.
   b. Excessive ingestion of food.
   c. Acute dilation by air and/or fluid.
   – Aerophagia due to dyspnoea.
   – Aerophagia secondary to any painful condition such as pancreatitis or blunt trauma.
   – Acute gastritis.
   – Outflow obstructed by a foreign body.
   – After abdominal surgery.
   – Anticholinergic drugs.
   – After endoscopy.
   d. Chronic dilation – may show a *gravel sign* (see 10.4.2 and Fig. 10.3).
   – Chronic obstruction by foreign bodies in the stomach or duodenum.
   – Pyloric outflow problem (see 10.10.3).
   e. Pancreatitis.
   f. Dysautonomia – may also see small intestinal, oesophageal and urinary bladder dilation.
5. Stomach distended with an abnormal shape.
   a. Gastric dilation and volvulus (Fig. 10.2) – especially in large, deep-chested dogs. The stomach will be abnormally distended by food, liquid and gas, with the stomach lumen apparently divided into two by a soft tissue band, giving a double-gas bubble appearance, also known as *compartmentalization* or a *boxing glove sign*. This is due to the soft tissue of the lesser curvature and proximal duodenum coursing caudally from their abnormal position in the

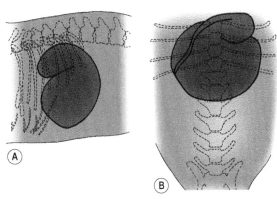

Figure 10.2 Gastric dilation and volvulus: (A) lateral view and (B) ventrodorsal (VD) view. The stomach is markedly distended with gas ± ingesta and shows compartmentalization. It may be difficult to identify which is the pylorus and which the fundus unless gas is present in the duodenum (seen here on the VD view).

craniodorsal quadrant of the abdomen. Frequently, the pylorus will be displaced dorsally and towards the left side; the fundus will be displaced ventrally and towards the right side unless the degree of rotation approaches 360 °. It is helpful to perform both right and left lateral recumbent radiographs, as gas will move around in the stomach and may help to identify the position of the pylorus. Other signs of GDV include splenic displacement, ileus, pneumatosis (intramural gas), pneumoperitoneum and megaoesophagus. GDV is rare in cats and is usually associated with diaphragmatic rupture.

b. Acute dilatation with gas or food in a dog that previously had a gastropexy – the stomach will fold on itself, resulting in an abnormal, boxing glove appearance.

Radiography is not necessary to diagnose severe gastric dilation but is invaluable in detecting volvulus, because easy passage of a stomach tube does not rule out rotation.

10.4 VARIATIONS IN STOMACH CONTENTS

The animal should ideally be fasted for 12 h prior to elective abdominal radiography. Retention of food in the stomach after 12 h is usually abnormal; however, sometimes the animal eats unknown to

the owner during the fast, so the radiographs should be repeated under a more controlled fasting situation. Obtaining radiographs with the animal in different positions may be helpful in outlining abnormal stomach contents, as gas rises to the highest part of the stomach.

1. Small amount of gas and/or fluid – normal.
2. Mineral opacity material.
   a. Foreign bodies (sometimes incidental findings in dogs).
      – Metallic materials such as fish hooks, needles and staples.
      – Stones, pebbles, etc.
      – Bones or bone fragments; differential diagnosis is mineralization of rugal folds secondary to chronic renal failure.
      – Dense rubber or glass.
   b. Gravel sign – accumulation of small mineralized fragments of ingesta that may develop proximal to chronic partial obstructions, in this case secondary to a pyloric outflow problem (see 10.10.3 and Fig. 10.3). Not reliably seen, as material may be vomited up.
   c. Barium from a previous contrast study.
   d. Medications containing bismuth and kaolin.
   e. Mimicked by mineralization of the stomach wall (see 10.5.3).
3. Soft tissue radiopacity with interspersed small gas bubbles.
   a. Food – normal if not fasted.
   b. Abnormal retention of food if fasted for more than 12 h (e.g. due to outflow obstruction to

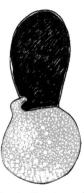

Figure 10.3 Gravel sign in the stomach due to a chronic, partial outflow obstruction. Small, radiopaque fragments of ingesta accumulate in a distended pylorus. A gravel sign is not always seen, as the material may be vomited up.

the pylorus and/or duodenum, or nervous pylorospasm if hospitalized).

  c. Foreign bodies.

- Plastic or cellophane.
- Fabrics, carpet or string.
- Phytobezoar (e.g. grass).
- Trichobezoar (e.g. hairball).

4. Uniform soft tissue radiopacity.

  a. Recently ingested liquid.

  b. Retained liquids.

- Acute gastric dilation.
- Outflow obstruction of the pylorus and duodenum.

  c. Foreign bodies.

  d. Large gastric tumour or polyp.

  e. Blood clot.

  f. Pylorogastric (gastrogastric) or duodenogastric intussusception – rare, as intussusceptions are more often in the aboral than the oral direction.

5. Gas.

  a. Aerophagia.

  b. Gastric dilation and volvulus (see 10.3.5 and Fig. 10.2).

6. Homogeneous, grey-appearing stomach content is usually due to equal amounts of water and fluid content superimposed.

10.5 VARIATIONS IN THE STOMACH WALL

The gastric wall thickness can be evaluated accurately only when the stomach is moderately distended by gas or radiopaque contrast medium (see 10.6). Rugal folds are predominantly located in the fundus and are smaller and more numerous in dogs than in cats. Few rugal folds are observed in the pyloric antral region.

1. Focally thickened stomach wall.

  a. Pseudomass.

- Transient wall contraction of an empty stomach.
- Fluid accumulation in pylorus in right lateral recumbency.

  b. Neoplasia (Fig. 10.4), often associated with localized poor distension and lack of peristalsis.

- Adenocarcinoma – usually lesser curvature and pylorus; Staffordshire Bull Terrier, Rough Collie and Belgian Shepherd dog predisposed.

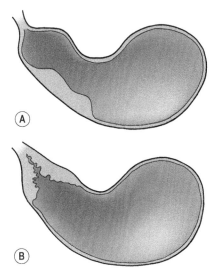

Figure 10.4 Gastric tumours (best seen on contrast radiography): (A) not affecting the pylorus; often seen as a smooth thickening of the stomach wall with raised edges; (B) around the pyloric canal; often ragged and circumferential with poor distension producing an apple core appearance.

- Leiomyoma or leiomyosarcoma.
- Lymphoma (especially cats).

  c. Pyloric muscular or mucosal hypertrophy.

  d. Polyp.

  e. Focal chronic hyperplastic gastropathy (syn. giant hypertrophic gastritis, Ménétrier's disease); unlike neoplasia, the stomach wall remains mobile.

  f. Focal infiltrative gastritis.

- Eosinophilic.
- Granulomatous.
- Fungal infections, especially *Pythium insidiosum**.

  g. Aberrant *Spirocerca lupi** granuloma.

2. Diffusely thickened stomach wall.

  a. Secondary to persistent vomiting.

  b. Chronic gastritis.

  c. Eosinophilic gastritis.

  d. Lymphoma (especially cats).

  e. Non-beta tumour of pancreas (gastrinoma or APUDoma) due to trophic effect on gastric mucosa causing rugal fold hypertrophy.

  f. Chronic hyperplastic gastropathy.

  g. Fungal infections, especially *Pythium insidiosum**.

3. Mineralization of the stomach wall.
   a. Mimicked by mineralized stomach contents (see 10.4.2).
   b. Artefactual due to the presence of linear gastric foreign bodies.
   c. Rugal fold mineralization.
      – Uraemic gastropathy, due to renal secondary hyperparathyroidism.
      – Other causes of severe hypercalcaemia, especially toxicity with vitamin D and analogues (e.g. cholecalficerol rodenticide, calcipotriol in antipsoriasis cream).
   d. Dystrophic mineralization in masses.
      – Neoplasm.
      – Granuloma (e.g. *Pythium insidiosum**, aberrant *Spirocerca lupi** granuloma, which may also undergo neoplastic transformation).
4. Gas in the stomach wall (gastric pneumatosis).
   a. Gastric ulceration.
   b. Partial gastric wall perforation.
   c. Necrosis secondary to GDV.
   d. Secondary to pancreatitis.
5. Fat layer in the stomach wall.
   a. May be seen in normal cats.

10.6 GASTRIC CONTRAST STUDIES: TECHNIQUE AND NORMAL APPEARANCE

Indications for contrast studies of the stomach include the following:

- Position of the stomach, including assessment of liver size and investigation of an unidentified abdominal mass.
- Orientation of the stomach (e.g. chronic torsion).
- Presence and location of suspected gastric foreign bodies.
- Vomiting, especially haematemesis.
- Melaena.
- Weight loss with possible gastric cause.
- Assessment of stomach wall thickness and mucosal pattern.
- Assessment of gastric emptying.

Pneumogastrography is a useful, simple and safe technique that is helpful for space-occupying diseases but gives no information about the mucosal surface, for which positive and double-contrast studies are required. If rupture of the stomach is suspected, low-osmolarity iodinated contrast medium rather than barium should be used. Following administration of contrast medium, fluoroscopy may be helpful to identify areas of poor gastric wall motility associated with neoplasia.

If the procedure is elective, preparation should involve a fast of at least 12 h and appropriate chemical restraint. Radiographs should be taken in right lateral, left lateral, sternal and dorsal recumbency. The exposure factors used should be reduced following administration of air and increased with positive contrast media.

Pneumogastrogram

Pass a stomach tube and inflate the stomach with room air. Shows:

- Stomach location.
- Radiolucent foreign bodies and intraluminal masses.
- Stomach wall thickness.
- Little or no information about the mucosal surface.

Positive contrast gastrogram

a. Small-volume barium sulphate or iodinated contrast medium: shows stomach location.
b. Barium-impregnated polyethylene spheres (BIPS): gives some information about stomach emptying.
c. Large-volume (7–12 mL/kg) 30% w/v barium sulphate using a stomach tube or 2–3 mL/kg isotonic iodinated contrast medium. Shows:
   – Stomach size.
   – Stomach shape.
   – Contractility.
   – Contents (as filling defects).
   – Liquid phase of stomach emptying.
d. Large-volume food studies (barium or BIPS mixed in food). Shows the solid phase of stomach emptying.

Double–contrast gastrogram

First, 1 mL/kg barium 100% w/v is given by stomach tube, then the stomach is distended with air. Shows:

- Excellent mucosal detail.
- Stomach wall thickness.
- Radiolucent foreign bodies.

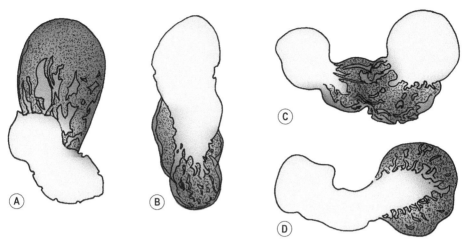

Figure 10.5 Normal double-contrast gastrogram: (A) right lateral recumbency, with barium in the pylorus and gas in the fundus; (B) left lateral recumbency, with barium in the fundus and gas in the pylorus (± the duodenum); (C) dorsal recumbency for the ventrodorsal view, with barium in the fundus and pylorus and gas in the body of the stomach; (D) sternal recumbency for the dorsoventral view, with barium in the body of the stomach and gas in the fundus ± pylorus.

The normal gastrogram (Fig. 10.5) shows positive contrast medium pooling in dependent areas and luminal gas uppermost. Positive contrast medium in the inter-rugal clefts creates gently curving lines when seen *en face* and a serrated margin to the stomach when seen tangentially. On a correctly exposed radiograph of a patient in reasonable body condition, the thickness of the stomach wall can be assessed. Peristaltic waves create symmetrical, smooth indentations to the shape of the stomach, varying from image to image. The stomach should distend appropriately for the amount of filling, and poor distension suggests neoplasia or severe gastritis.

10.7 TECHNICAL ERRORS ON THE GASTROGRAM

1. Lack of plain (survey) radiographs.
   a. Radiopaque foreign bodies overlooked.
   b. Incorrect exposure factors used for the contrast study.
   c. Patient not adequately fasted.
2. Inappropriate exposure factors – add 5–10 kVp to settings used to obtain plain radiographs for positive contrast studies.
   a. Underexposed positive contrast studies will hinder detection of smaller radiolucent foreign bodies.
   b. Overexposed pneumogastrogram will hinder detection of smaller radiopaque foreign bodies.
3. Inadequate distension of the stomach.
   a. Precludes accurate evaluation of wall thickness and of masses.
   b. Results in a longer gastric emptying time, as inadequate distension fails to stimulate emptying reflexes.
4. Too much positive contrast used – small foreign bodies will be 'drowned'; later radiographs should be taken to look for residual contrast adhering to foreign material.
5. Inadequate number of images (in absence of fluoroscopic examination) – may preclude the detection of gastric wall stiffness, foreign bodies, soft tissue masses and ulceration.
6. Over-diagnosis based on single or few images – mural lesions must be confirmed on multiple radiographs, as peristaltic waves lead to transient gastric wall thickening, which may give rise to false positive diagnoses.

10.8 GASTRIC LUMINAL FILLING DEFECTS ON CONTRAST STUDIES

Smaller foreign bodies may be hidden by large-volume positive gastrograms. See also 10.4, *Variations in stomach contents*.

1. Retained food.
2. Phytobezoar (e.g. grass) or trichobezoar (e.g. hairball).
3. Foreign bodies.
4. Stomach wall masses projecting into the lumen.
   a. Neoplasm.
   b. Polyp.
   c. Granuloma.
   d. Abscess.
   e. Haematoma.
   f. Pylorogastric (gastrogastric) or duodenogastric intussusception.
   g. Chronic hyperplastic gastropathy (syn. giant hypertrophic gastritis, Ménétrier's disease).
5. Blood clots and mucus.

10.9 ABNORMAL GASTRIC MUCOSAL PATTERN ON CONTRAST STUDIES

Mild ulcerative gastritis and shallow ulcers may be difficult to detect; consider using endoscopy instead, because normal radiographs do not rule out disease. The mucosal pattern is normally of parallel bands of barium in the inter-rugal clefts, with rugae seen as parallel-sided, band-like filling defects. Rugae are sparse near the pylorus and are less obvious in cats than in dogs.

1. Normal variant – the presence of ingesta or mucus creates an irregular, patchy rugal fold pattern mimicking pathology (flocculation).
2. Gastritis – irregular, patchy rugal fold pattern (Fig. 10.6); barium persists after the stomach has

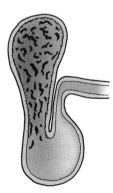

Figure 10.6 Severe gastritis on a barium or double-contrast gastrogram: poorly distensible stomach with an irregular mucosal surface and a broken-up rugal fold pattern.

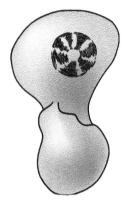

Figure 10.7 Gastric ulcer on a barium or double-contrast gastrogram with the animal in right lateral recumbency: barium collects in the centre of the ulcer and rugal folds are 'gathered' towards it.

largely emptied, as it adheres to inflamed or ulcerated areas.

3. Ulceration – crater-like in profile and circular when seen *en face* (Fig. 10.7). Barium persists in the ulcer crater long after stomach has emptied (12 to 24 h films are therefore useful) and rugal folds may be gathered towards the ulcer.
   a. Drugs.
      – Non-steroidal anti-inflammatory drugs (e.g. aspirin and ibuprofen).
   b. Neoplasia.
      – Primary gastric (e.g. adenocarcinoma and lymphoma).
      – Pancreatic gastrinoma.
   c. Secondary to mast cell tumours elsewhere.
   d. Stress.
   e. Inflammatory bowel disease.
   f. Secondary to chronic hepatic and renal disease.
   g. Due to the presence of abrasive foreign material.
4. Chronic hyperplastic gastropathy – greatly enlarged rugal folds; may cause secondary pyloric stenosis.

10.10 VARIATIONS IN GASTRIC EMPTYING TIME

Scintigraphy is considered the method of choice for assessment of gastric emptying, because radiography is less likely to represent normal physiological conditions. The use of ultrasonography has also been described. Factors affecting the passage of radiographic contrast media through the gut include the following:

- period of prior fasting
- use and nature of chemical restraint
- degree of relaxation of the patient
- type of contrast medium used
- quantity of contrast medium administered.

If the stomach was empty prior to administration of the contrast medium, barium suspensions should begin to exit within 30 min in the dog and 15 min in the cat (provided an adequate quantity was given), and the stomach should be completely empty by 4 h in the dog and 2 h in the cat. Hypertonic iodine solutions empty faster, as they induce hyperperistalsis. Barium mixed with food (or food alone) empties more slowly, taking up to 12 h to empty completely. When food and BIPS are fed together, half the BIPS should have left the stomach by 6 h ($\pm$ 3 h) and three-quarters by 8.5 h ($\pm$ 2.75 h). Radiographs made 12–24 h after barium administration may show a barium-outlined or impregnated ulcerative lesion or foreign body causing partial obstruction.

Fluoroscopy with image intensification is an invaluable method of assessing gut motility. In the absence of fluoroscopy, it may also be possible to detect presence or absence of peristalsis on serial radiographs.

1. Rapid gastric emptying.
   a. Normal variant – liquid contrast medium given on an empty stomach.
   b. Gastric emptying time is shorter in puppies than in adult dogs.
   c. Gastroenteritis.
2. Delayed gastric emptying with decreased gastric motility (seen with fluoroscopy or on serial radiographs).
   a. Sedation or general anaesthesia, or use of spasmolytics.
   b. Gastric or duodenal ulceration.
   c. Gastritis.
      - Parvovirus.
      - Cats – panleucopenia.
   d. Small intestinal obstruction.
   e. Pancreatitis.
   f. Peritonitis.
   g. Hypokalaemia due to vomiting.
   h. Dysautonomia – may also see small intestinal, oesophageal and urinary bladder dilation.

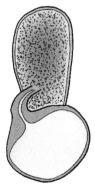

Figure 10.8 Pyloric stenosis on a barium gastrogram with the animal in right lateral recumbency: the pyloric antrum is distended and little barium enters the duodenum. In the case of malignant neoplasia, the pylorus may be poorly distended and irregularly marginated (see also Fig. 10.4B).

3. Delayed gastric emptying with normal or increased gastric motility.
   a. Diet – fatty food takes longer to exit stomach.
   b. Pyloric obstructions and stenoses (Fig. 10.8).
      - Foreign bodies.
      - Pyloric muscular or mucosal hypertrophy.
      - Pyloric, duodenal, pancreatic or gall bladder neoplasia.
      - Pyloric or duodenal scar tissue.
      - Pyloric or duodenal ulceration.
      - Pyloric or duodenal granuloma.
      - Pyloric or duodenal polyp.
      - Chronic hyperplastic gastropathy; large rugal folds.
      - Idiopathic – especially Siamese cats, and may be associated with megaoesophagus.
   c. Pylorospasm.
      - Nervous pylorospasm.
      - Small intestinal obstruction.

10.11 ULTRASONOGRAPHIC TECHNIQUE FOR THE STOMACH

The patient should ideally be fasted for 12 h prior to ultrasonographic examination of the stomach but allowed free access to water. The presence of food or gas in the stomach will result in artefacts preventing complete examination of the gastric lumen and wall. Water administered by stomach tube at 10–15 mL/kg will enhance visibility of mural pathology.

The hair should be clipped from the cranial ventral abdomen, between the xiphisternum and the umbilicus, the skin cleaned with surgical spirit and liberal quantities of acoustic gel applied. The transducer should be placed just behind the xiphisternum and the sound beam angled craniodorsally to image the stomach. The entire stomach should be imaged in both longitudinal and transverse planes relative to the luminal axis. It may be helpful to vary the position of the animal in order to allow fluid to pool in different regions of the stomach.

A sector or curvilinear transducer of as high a frequency as possible compatible with adequate tissue penetration should be used (7.5 MHz in cats or small or medium dogs; 5 MHz in large or obese dogs). Endoscopic ultrasonography is especially useful but is still not widely available in veterinary medicine.

10.12 NORMAL ULTRASONOGRAPHIC APPEARANCE OF THE STOMACH

The gastric wall has a characteristic layered appearance when imaged with a high-resolution system. The ultrasonographic layers are generally considered to correspond to histological regions (Fig. 10.9).

The gastric wall is arranged to form rugal folds but should otherwise be smooth and of uniform thickness. If the stomach is empty and contracted, the wall will appear thicker than if the stomach is distended. Peristaltic and segmental contractions are normally seen, at a rate of 4–5 contractions per minute in the normal dog. Normal wall thickness is given in Table 10.1.

10.13 VARIATIONS IN GASTRIC CONTENTS ON ULTRASONOGRAPHY

1. Anechoic with hyperechoic specks – indicates fluid content with air bubbles, debris or mucus.

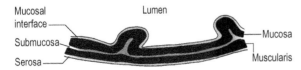

Mucosal interface
Lumen
Submucosa
Serosa
Mucosa
Muscularis

Figure 10.9 Gastric (or small intestinal) wall layers identified on ultrasonography.

Table 10.1 Wall thickness of various parts of the gastrointestinal tract

REGION AND WEIGHT OF ANIMAL	WALL THICKNESS (MM)	
	Dog[b]	Cat
Stomach: inter-rugal	3–5	3–5
Duodenum[a]	3–6	2–3[c]
< 20 kg	< 5.1	
20–30kg	< 5.3	
> 30 kg	< 6	
Jejunum[a]	2–5	2–2.5
< 20 kg	< 4.1	
20–30 kg	< 4.4	
> 30 kg	< 4.7	
Colon	2–3	1.5–2

[a]Delaney, F., O'Brien, R.T. and Waller, K. (2003) Ultrasound evaluation of small bowel thickness compared to weight in normal dogs. *Veterinary Radiology and Ultrasound* **44**, 577–580.
[b]Puppy values will be at the lower limits.
[c]May be thicker in sedated cats.

a. Normal – recent ingestion of fluid.
b. Retained fluid secondary to gastric outflow obstruction or proximal small intestinal obstruction (peristalsis may be increased or diminished).
c. Retained fluid secondary to functional ileus (peristalsis diminished or absent).
   – After abdominal surgery.
   – Peritonitis or pancreatitis.
   – Electrolyte disturbances.
   – Renal failure.
d. Gastrointestinal perforation.
e. Gastric ulcers.

2. Solid material of variable echogenicity outlined by fluid.
   a. Food remnants.
   b. Foreign material.
   c. Pedunculated gastric mass.

3. Heterogeneous material filling the stomach, with or without acoustic shadowing.
   a. Recent ingestion of food.
   b. Retained food secondary to gastric outflow obstruction.
   c. Foreign material.
   d. Blood clot.

4. Extensive acoustic shadowing preventing visualization of contents.
   a. Gastric gas.
   b. Pneumoperitoneum.

10.14 LACK OF VISUALIZATION OF THE NORMAL GASTRIC WALL LAYERED ARCHITECTURE ON ULTRASONOGRAPHY

1. Gas or food contents.
2. Use of a low-frequency transducer (5 MHz or lower).
3. Generally poor image quality.
   a. Poor skin preparation.
   b. Poor skin–transducer contact.
   c. Obese patient.
4. Gastric disease (see 10.15 and 10.16).

10.15 FOCAL THICKENING OF THE GASTRIC WALL ON ULTRASONOGRAPHY

1. Retention of the normal layered architecture.
   a. Normal rugal folds.
   b. Localized hyperplastic gastropathy.
   c. Pyloric hypertrophy – circumferential thickening of the pylorus (in the dog, wall thickness ≥ 9 mm, with the muscular layer ≥ 4 mm).
   d. Neoplasia.
      – Leiomyoma.
      – Malignant histiocytosis.
   e. Polyp – may be sessile or pedunculated; usually echogenic and confined to mucosa.
   f. Increased number of layers – pylorogastric intussusception.
2. Loss of the normal layered architecture.
   a. Neoplasia.
      – Adenocarcinoma (typically asymmetrical, heteroechoic thickening).
      – Leiomyoma or leiomyosarcoma.
      – Lymphoma (typically symmetrical, hypoechoic thickening) – especially cats.
      – Malignant histiocytosis.
   b. Gastric ulcer – may contain hyperechoic gas speckles.
   c. Necrotizing gastritis – may contain hyperechoic gas speckles.
   d. Pyogranulomatous disease, especially *Pythium insidiosum**.

10.16 DIFFUSE THICKENING OF THE GASTRIC WALL ON ULTRASONOGRAPHY

1. Retention of the normal layered architecture.
   a. Contracted, empty stomach.
   b. Severe gastritis.
   c. Chronic hyperplastic gastropathy.
   d. Wall oedema.
      – Right heart failure.
      – Hypoproteinaemia.
      – Acute gastritis.
   e. Uraemic gastropathy.
2. Loss of the normal layered architecture.
   a. Diffuse neoplasia (see 10.15; although neoplasia is more often focal).
   b. Necrotizing gastritis.
   c. Uraemic gastritis.
   d. Severe haemorrhage (e.g. coagulopathy).
   e. Pyogranulomatous disease, especially *Pythium insidiosum**.
3. Abnormal layering.
   a. Hyperechoic line at mucosal luminal interface due to mineralization.
      – Uraemic gastropathy, due to renal secondary hyperparathyroidism.
      – Other causes of severe hypercalcaemia, especially toxicity with vitamin D and analogues (e.g. cholecalciferol rodenticide, calcipotriol in antipsoriasis cream).

SMALL INTESTINE

10.17 NORMAL RADIOGRAPHIC APPEARANCE OF THE SMALL INTESTINE

The animal should ideally be fasted for 12 h before the radiographic examination. When much faecal material is present in the colon, an enema may also be necessary, with radiography repeated some hours later. Evaluation of the stomach contents should be made, as radiopaque stomach contents and gas from aerophagia will also pass through to the small intestine. In left lateral recumbency, gas from the stomach often passes into the proximal duodenum, and this is helpful if duodenal pathology such as neoplasia or foreign body is suspected.

The descending duodenum runs along the right abdominal wall and is slightly larger in diameter than the remaining small intestine. The jejunum and ileum cannot be differentiated except at the ileocaecocolic junction. The small intestine fills much of the abdominal cavity, lying caudal to the stomach and cranial to the urinary bladder and filling the space not taken by other organs. In obese animals, the small intestine lies more centrally.

10.18 VARIATIONS IN THE NUMBER OF SMALL INTESTINAL LOOPS VISIBLE

1. Increased number of small intestinal loops visible.
   a. Artefactual – a false impression of increased number is given if the intestine is distended by gas, food or fluid (see 10.21); evaluate the stomach, which may contain similar material.
      – Mechanical obstruction.
      – Functional obstruction (paralytic ileus).
2. Decreased number of small intestinal loops visible.
   a. Artefactual.
      – Small intestine empty and collapsed.
      – Obesity, making the intestines lie more centrally.
      – Poor abdominal detail in very thin or young animals.
   b. Abnormal.
      – Abdominal effusion masking serosal detail.
      – Displacement through hernias or body wall ruptures.
      – Plication along a linear foreign body.
      – Intussusception.
      – Previous enterectomy.

10.19 DISPLACEMENT OF THE SMALL INTESTINE

1. Small intestine displaced into the thoracic cavity.
   a. Ruptured diaphragm.
   b. Peritoneopericardial diaphragmatic hernia.
   c. Congenital diaphragmatic hernia (incomplete formation of the diaphragm).
2. Cranial displacement of the small intestine.
   a. Against the dorsal part of the diaphragm, sometimes seen in normal deep-chested dogs when the stomach is empty.
   b. Small liver.

   c. Ruptured diaphragm with displacement of the liver into the thorax allowing small intestines to lie more cranially.
   d. Distended urinary bladder.
   e. Uterine enlargement.
      – Pregnancy.
      – Pyometra.
   f. Ruptured attachment of abdominal muscles to ribs.
3. Caudal displacement of the small intestine.
   a. Liver enlargement.
   b. Stomach distension.
   c. Empty urinary bladder.
   d. Inguinal hernia.
   e. Large perineal hernia.
   f. Ruptured caudal abdominal muscles.
4. Displacement of the small intestine to the right or left.
   a. Previous prolonged lateral recumbency.
   b. Asymmetrical enlargement of liver.
   c. Enlargement of the spleen.
   d. Severe enlargement of a kidney.
   e. Rupture of right or left abdominal muscles.
5. Fixed location of distended small intestinal loops on serial radiographs.
   a. Previous surgery.
   b. Adhesions.
   c. Peritonitis.
6. Central bunching of the small intestine (see 10.20).
7. Peripheral displacement of the small intestine.
   a. Mid-abdominal mass.
      – Mesenteric lymph nodes.
      – Mesenteric mass.
      – Certain parts of spleen.

10.20 BUNCHING OF SMALL INTESTINAL LOOPS

1. Obesity causing intestines to lie centrally, especially in cats.
2. Severe ascites – gas-filled small intestines float to the highest area and appear bunched.
3. Plication along a linear foreign body – usually see teardrop-shaped gas bubbles (see 10.22.1 and 10.25.4 and Figs 10.11 and 10.13). May be associated with focal peritonitis if bowel is lacerated.

4. Adhesions.
5. Sclerosing encapsulating peritonitis.
   a. Secondary to abdominal neoplasia with involvement of omentum or mesentery.
   b. Mesothelioma.
   c. Previous perforating foreign body or surgery.
   d. Infectious agents.

10.21 INCREASED WIDTH OF SMALL INTESTINAL LOOPS

Sufficient abdominal fat is necessary to provide contrast to see the serosal surface of intestinal loops. On lateral radiographs, the small intestine usually has a diameter less than the height of lumbar vertebral bodies or two rib widths in dogs and less than 12 mm in cats. Generally, no loop should be more than twice the diameter of the other loops. In dogs, a ratio of > 1.6 between the diameter of the small intestine and the mid-vertebral body height of L5 is highly suggestive of obstruction. Increased width of small intestinal loops may be due to dilation of the lumen, thickening of the wall or a combination of both processes. Fluid-filled dilation can be differentiated from wall thickening only using contrast studies or ultrasonography. Multiple dilated loops of intestine tend to appear to stack up against one another and to curve abnormally like a hairpin or paperclip (Fig. 10.10).

The number of dilated loops should be assessed, as complete obstructions located in distal jejunum or ileum and generalized paralytic ileus will cause many loops to be dilated, while higher obstructions and segmental paralytic ileus will affect fewer loops. The degree of dilation depends on the aetiology and the duration of the problem. Acute obstructions or chronic, partial obstructions that have become total tend to result in marked dilation, whereas partial obstructions tend to result in milder dilation. Distal to the obstruction, the loops may be smaller than normal. Chronic, partial obstructions also often show a gravel sign. Normal intestinal diameter does not rule out obstruction, especially when the obstruction is in the duodenum.

Causes of small intestinal obstruction are shown in Boxes 10.1 and 10.2.

Ultrasonographic assessment of peristalsis is helpful in differentiating functional ileus from

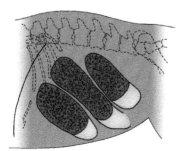

Figure 10.10 Dilated, gas- and fluid-filled small intestinal loops.

> **BOX 10.1   Causes of mechanical small intestinal obstruction (intraluminal, extraluminal or mural)**
>
> - Foreign body, tricho- or phytobezoar or enterolith – may be radiolucent.
> - Neoplasia – mainly lymphoma (especially cats), adenocarcinoma, leiomyoma or leiomyosarcoma.
> - Polyp.
> - Granuloma.
> - Abscess.
> - Stricture.
> - Intussusception – most common in young dogs, often with parvovirus, or soon after surgery.
> - Adhesions (e.g. from previous surgery).
> - Intestinal diverticulum (intestinal duplication).
> - Strangulation in a hernia or omental or mesenteric tear.
> - Intestinal volvulus (partly a functional obstruction as well).

> **BOX 10.2   Causes of functional small intestinal obstruction (paralytic ileus)**
>
> - Secondary to chronic mechanical obstruction.
> - Recent abdominal surgery.
> - Severe dehydration.
> - Electrolyte imbalances.
> - Certain drugs (e.g. parasympatholytics, analgesics, general anaesthetics and sedatives).
> - Gastric dilation and volvulus.
> - Severe gastroenteritis (e.g. parvovirus).
> - Peritonitis (generalized or localized, e.g. pancreatitis).
> - Gastrointestinal perforation.
> - Ischaemia (e.g. due to intestinal volvulus).
> - Blunt abdominal trauma.
> - Dysautonomia (may also see gastric, oesophageal and urinary bladder dilation).
> - Spinal trauma with neurological injury.

low mechanical obstruction; in both cases many small intestinal loops will be dilated.

1. Single dilated or thickened small intestinal loop.
   a. Mass due to:
      - Neoplasia.
      - Foreign body.
      - Granuloma.
      - Abscess.
      - Intussusception.
   b. Obstruction with local effect only (e.g. intestinal entrapment in torn mesentery).
   c. Partial functional obstruction (paralytic ileus) – sentinel loop (e.g. due to localized peritonitis).
2. Few dilated small intestinal loops.
   a. Colon or enlarged uterus mistaken for small intestine.
   b. Proximal mechanical small intestinal obstruction (see Box 10.1 for causes); often accompanied by a gravel sign if a chronic, partial obstruction (see 10.4.2. and Fig. 10.3).
   c. Localized functional small intestinal obstruction (paralytic ileus; see Box 10.2 for causes) – descending duodenum if due to pancreatitis.
   d. Vascular compromise.
      - Jejunal artery thrombosis.
      - Segmental small intestinal volvulus not involving the root of the mesentery (also partly a mechanical obstruction).
      - Strangulation of a few loops in a hernia or mesenteric tear (also partly a mechanical obstruction).
3. Many dilated small intestinal loops.
   a. Distal small intestinal obstruction (see Box 10.1 for causes).
      - Also caecal impaction (faecolithiasis).
   b. Generalized functional small intestinal obstruction (paralytic ileus; see Box 10.2 for causes).
   c. Vascular compromise.
      - Small intestinal volvulus at the root of the mesentery; occlusion of the cranial mesenteric artery causes ischaemia, leading to functional as well as mechanical obstruction. Often Great Danes and German Shepherd dogs; the latter also often suffer from exocrine pancreatic insufficiency.
      - Strangulation of many loops in a hernia or mesenteric tear (also partly a mechanical obstruction).
   d. Diffuse neoplasia – mainly alimentary lymphoma.
   e. Intestinal pseudo-obstruction secondary to tunica muscularis atrophy or fibrosis (tends to be marked dilation).

10.22 VARIATIONS IN SMALL INTESTINAL CONTENTS

In a fasted animal with an empty stomach, the small intestine should be of homogeneous fluid opacity with some gas-filled segments. There is normally less gas seen in the small intestine of the cat than the dog.

1. Gas-filled small intestine.
   a. Normal diameter small intestine with normal luminal shape.
      - Normal.
      - In descending duodenum in left lateral recumbent radiograph.
      - Aerophagia (e.g. due to dyspnoea – evaluate stomach contents).
      - Following pneumogastrogram.
      - Following anaesthesia using nitrous oxide.
      - Recent enema.
      - Enteritis.
      - Incomplete obstruction.
      - Debilitated, recumbent animal.
   b. Non-dilated, but gas accumulation of abnormal shape.
      - Transient, due to peristalsis (repeat the radiograph).
      - Intussusception (crescentic gas shadow, lying between intussuscipiens and intussusceptum).
      - Plication along a linear foreign body (gas bubbles small and triangular or teardrop-shaped, or forming a corkscrew pattern) (Figs 10.11 and 10.13D); look also for signs of peritonitis that would suggest perforation (see 9.6.2).
      - Small gas bubbles trapped in a radiolucent foreign body; some have a characteristic pattern (e.g. corn cob).
      - Adhesions from previous surgery or peritonitis.
   c. Increased diameter small intestine.

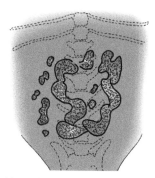

Figure 10.11 Linear foreign body seen on plain radiography; irregular accumulations of small intestinal gas, often in corkscrew or teardrop shapes (see also 10.25.4 and Fig. 10.13D).

- Colon or caecum mistaken for small intestine.
- Following anaesthesia using nitrous oxide.
- Mechanical obstruction (see Box 10.1 for causes); look also for signs of peritonitis that would suggest perforation (see 9.6.2).
- Functional obstruction (paralytic ileus; see Box 10.2 for causes).
- Intestinal pseudo-obstruction secondary to tunica muscularis atrophy or fibrosis.
- Free abdominal gas mimicking intestinal gas (see 9.7.2).
- Emphysematous pyometritis mistaken for small intestine.

2. Fluid radiopacity of the small intestine.
   a. Normal diameter small intestine.
      - Normal.
      - Intestinal disease without dilation of lumen or marked mural thickening.
   b. Small intestine of increased diameter.
      - Colon or enlarged uterus mistaken for small intestine.
      - Mechanical obstruction (see Box 10.1 for causes).
      - Functional obstruction (paralytic ileus) (see Box 10.2 for causes).
      - Severe gastroenteritis.
      - Diffuse neoplasia – mainly lymphoma.
      - Other infiltrative bowel wall disease.

When dilated intestine is filled with both gas and fluid, standing lateral abdominal radiographs made using a horizontal X-ray beam can be useful. Mechanical obstructions tend to cause different levels between the gas-capped fluid lines in the same intestinal loop (look for inverted, U-shaped loops and compare the gas cap level on each vertical side; Fig. 10.12A). Functional obstructions (paralytic ileus) tend to have gas-capped fluid lines at the same level in a given U-shaped section of intestine (Fig. 10.12B).

3. Radiopaque contents in the small intestine (evaluate stomach contents as well).
   a. Small intestine of normal diameter.
      - Radiopaque food.
      - Barium or iodine contrast media.
      - Radiopaque medications.
      - Incidental foreign material.
      - Faeces mistaken for small intestinal contents.
      - Enterolith.
   b. Small intestine of increased diameter.
      - Radiopaque foreign bodies (fluid- or gas-dilated loops too).
      - Enterolith.

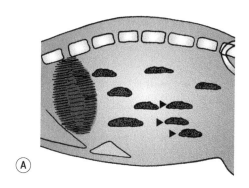

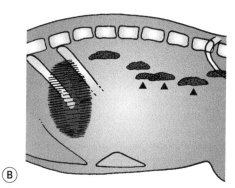

Figure 10.12 Standing horizontal beam abdominal radiograph: (A) dog with total mechanical bowel obstruction, with gas-capped fluid lines at different levels in the abdomen; (B) dog with paralytic ileus with gas-capped fluid lines roughly at the same level in the dorsal abdomen.

- Food debris lodged proximal to an obstruction.
- Dense, focal accumulation of mineral debris (gravel sign) – proximal to a chronic, partial obstruction.
- Sand impaction.
- Caecal impaction (faecolithiasis) mistaken for an area of small intestine.

10.23 SMALL INTESTINAL CONTRAST STUDIES: TECHNIQUE AND NORMAL APPEARANCE

Indications for contrast studies of the small intestine include the following:

- Position of the intestines (e.g. rupture or hernia, or abdominal mass).
- Presence and location of suspected intestinal foreign bodies.
- Vomiting, especially if a structural cause is suspected.
- Melaena.
- Chronic diarrhoea.
- Weight loss with possible intestinal cause.
- Assessment of small intestinal wall thickness and mucosal surface.
- Assessment of small intestinal transit time.

If rupture of the small intestine is suspected, low-osmolarity iodinated contrast medium rather than barium should be used. If the procedure is elective, preparation should involve a fast of at least 12 h and enemas to remove superimposed colonic faecal material, followed by appropriate chemical restraint (mild sedation of a type that does not significantly affect transit time). 30% w/v barium sulphate is given by stomach tube or oral syringing at a dose rate of 5–12 mL/kg depending on body weight (larger doses per kg for smaller breeds). An alternative technique is to use BIPS and to observe the passage of the radiopaque spheres through the gastrointestinal tract. The small BIPS show transit rate of ingesta and the large BIPS are used to demonstrate obstructions. Radiographs should be taken in lateral and dorsal recumbency at regular intervals to follow the passage of contrast medium along the gut (e.g. 15, 30, 60 min after dosing and then hourly until most of the contrast is in the colon).

The normal appearance of the small intestine on a barium study is of a mass of sinuous tubes, with slight variations in radiopacity as barium mixes

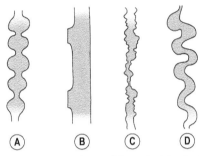

Figure 10.13 Variations in small intestinal luminal diameter: (A) string of pearls appearance in cat duodenum; (B) pseudoulcers in dog duodenum; (C) diffuse neoplasia; (D) linear foreign body.

with luminal gas. The diameter of the loops varies slightly due to peristalsis. A hazy, spiculated or brush border appearance seen in some animals is normal and is due to barium extending between clumps of intestinal villi, so-called fimbriation. Normal variants in the duodenum are duodenal beading (cats), pseudoulcers (dogs) (see 10.25.1, 10.25.4 and Fig. 10.13A and B) and flocculation, when barium mixes with intestinal mucus. With iodine studies, progressive dilution of the contrast medium as it passes along the gut creates a less radiopaque and hazier appearance.

10.24 TECHNICAL ERRORS WITH SMALL INTESTINAL CONTRAST STUDIES

1. Lack of plain (survey) radiographs.
   a. Radiopaque foreign bodies overlooked.
   b. Incorrect exposure factors used for contrast study.
   c. Animal not adequately fasted.
   d. Much faecal material present – inadequate enema.
2. Inappropriate exposure factors – add 5–10 kVp to settings used to obtain plain radiographs.
3. Inadequate amount of contrast medium.
   a. Under-dosing.
   b. Vomiting after administration.
4. Inadequate number of images (in absence of fluoroscopic evaluation) may preclude thorough evaluation; accurate diagnosis can be improved by taking sufficient radiographs and viewing them together for consistency of findings.
5. Over-diagnosis based on single or few images because peristaltic waves may mimic lesions.

10.25 VARIATIONS IN SMALL INTESTINAL LUMINAL DIAMETER ON CONTRAST STUDIES

Normal intestinal diameter is approximately the same as the depth of a lumbar vertebra or twice the width of a rib in the dog and 12 mm in the cat. In dogs, a ratio of > 1.6 between the diameter of the small intestine and the mid-vertebral body height of L5 is highly suggestive of obstruction. The jejunum and ileum are similar in size; the duodenum is slightly wider.

1. Segmental narrowing of diameter.
   a. Normal peristaltic waves – will be transient and symmetrical.
   b. Cats – a bead-like string of pearls appearance to the duodenum is normal (duodenal segmentation – Fig. 10.13A).
   c. Intestinal neoplasia – may have circumferential, ragged, apple core appearance.
   d. Contrast medium dissecting past an impacted foreign body.
   e. Intestinal scarring following foreign body impaction or previous surgery.
2. Generalized narrowing of small intestinal diameter.
   a. Inadequate contrast medium given.
   b. Contrast medium mixing with ingesta already present in the stomach and emptying at the slower rate of solid material.
   c. Thickening of the intestinal wall (see 10.27.1).
3. Dilation of the small intestine (see 10.21).
4. Irregular luminal diameter.
   a. Normal pseudoulcers in young dogs are outpouchings of the duodenal lumen along the antimesenteric border, due to mucosal thinning over submucosal lymphoid follicles (Fig. 10.13B).
   b. Intestinal neoplasia (e.g. alimentary lymphoma – Fig. 10.13C).
   c. Peritonitis.
   d. Linear foreign body – intestines bunched and plicated (Fig. 10.13D).
   e. Ulceration – focal outpouching of lumen.
      – Benign.
      – Malignant (ulcerated neoplasm).

10.26 SMALL INTESTINAL LUMINAL FILLING DEFECTS ON CONTRAST STUDIES

1. Ingesta – usually multiple, small filling defects.
2. Foreign bodies – variable in shape.

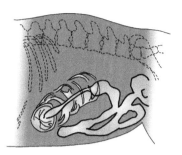

Figure 10.14 Intussusception at the ileocaecocolic junction. The intussusceptum is seen as a thin band of barium entering the intussusception, which produces a corrugated watch spring appearance due to barium leaking back into the space between the two outer layers of intestinal wall.

3. Worms – linear (transverse lines may be seen with tapeworms).
4. Polyps – oriental cats may be predisposed to duodenal polyps.
5. Intestinal neoplasia.
6. Intussusception (especially at ileocaecocolic junction) – luminal mass ± watch spring appearance as the barium dissects between the intussusceptum and intussuscipiens (Fig. 10.14).

Where obstruction has occurred, the shape of the leading edge of the barium column may give a clue as to the cause of the obstruction (Fig. 10.15).

10.27 VARIATIONS IN THE SMALL INTESTINAL WALL ON CONTRAST STUDIES

1. Increased wall thickness – small intestinal wall thickness can only be adequately assessed using contrast studies or ultrasonography. On plain recumbent radiographs, a linear gas bubble lying along the top of a partially filled intestinal loop will mimic intestinal wall thickening (Fig. 10.16).
   a. Severe chronic enteritis.
   b. Ulcerative enteritis.
   c. Inflammatory or infiltrative bowel wall disease.
   d. Neoplasia.
      – Lymphoma (especially in cats).
      – Adenocarcinoma – focal thickening.
      – Leiomyoma or leiomyosarcoma – focal thickening.
   e. Fungal infections, especially *Pythium insidiosum*.
   f. Muscular hypertrophy.
   g. Lymphangiectasia.

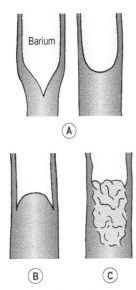

Figure 10.15 In cases of obstruction, assessment of the shape of the leading edge of barium may be helpful in suggesting the cause of the obstruction: (A) single point or convex shape suggests mural or extramural lesion (e.g. neoplasia, granuloma, stricture); (B) double point or concave shape suggests luminal mass or foreign body; (C) irregular contour suggests foreign body.

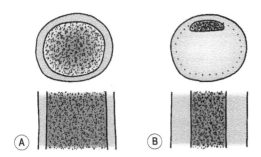

Figure 10.16 Formation of artefactual intestinal wall 'thickening' on plain radiographs: (A) a gas-filled loop in which only the intestinal wall is of soft tissue radiopacity; (B) a gas- and fluid-filled loop in which the soft tissue radiopacity of the fluid lying beneath the gas summates with the intestinal wall, producing the appearance of wall thickening.

2. Increased wall opacity – rare.
   a. Severe hypercalcaemia.
     – Renal secondary hyperparathyroidism.
     – Toxicity with vitamin D and analogues (e.g. cholecalciferol rodenticide, calcipotriol in antipsoriasis cream).

3. Decreased wall opacity – pneumatosis intestinalis due to wall necrosis; rare.

10.28 VARIATIONS IN SMALL INTESTINAL TRANSIT TIME ON CONTRAST STUDIES

In dogs, barium sulphate should begin to reach the colon within 90–120 min; in cats the normal transit time is 30–60 min. Hypertonic iodinated media induce hyperperistalsis and reduce the transit time. Persistent accumulation of BIPS in a loop of small intestine is highly suggestive of physical obstruction, whereas scattered distribution of BIPS through the small intestine suggests increased transit time. Radiographs made 12–24 h after barium administration may show a barium outlined or impregnated ulcerative lesion or foreign body causing partial obstruction.

See also 10.10 for factors that may affect intestinal transit time.

1. Reduced small intestinal transit time (rapid transit).
   a. Iodinated contrast medium, especially if hypertonic but also with low-osmolarity, water-soluble contrast medium (e.g. iohexol).
   b. Hypermotility due to enteritis.
   c. Prior surgical resection of significant lengths of intestine.
2. Increased small intestinal transit time (delayed transit).
   a. Sedation, general anaesthesia or use of spasmolytics.
   b. Partial obstruction (see Box 10.1 for causes), but most commonly:
     – Foreign body.
     – Intestinal neoplasia.
     – Polyp.
     – Intussusception.
   c. Inflammatory or infiltrative bowel wall disease.
   d. Pancreatitis.
   e. Hypomotility due to enteritis.
     – Parvovirus infection.
     – Cats – panleucopenia.
   f. Functional obstruction (paralytic ileus – see Box 10.2 for causes).
   g. Intestinal pseudo-obstruction secondary to tunica muscularis atrophy or fibrosis.
   h. Dysautonomia.
   i. Peritonitis.

10.29 ULTRASONOGRAPHIC TECHNIQUE FOR THE SMALL INTESTINE

For elective studies, the patient should be fasted for 12 h while allowing free access to water and given an opportunity to defecate before carrying out the examination. Because barium sulphate interferes with image quality, the ultrasonographic examination should be performed before any barium contrast studies.

A ventral abdominal approach should be used, and a high-frequency ($\geq$ 7.5 MHz) sector or curvilinear transducer chosen. The spleen may be used as an acoustic window to examine underlying intestinal loops. To avoid interference from intraluminal gas, the position of the patient may be varied so that fluid drops into, and gas rises away from, the area of interest.

The descending loop of the duodenum may be identified in the right cranial abdomen as a superficially located, straight segment of small intestine. It is not usually possible to differentiate other specific intestinal regions, except the terminal ileum as it approaches the ileocaecocolic junction.

10.30 NORMAL ULTRASONOGRAPHIC APPEARANCE OF THE SMALL INTESTINE

In high-quality images, layering of the small intestinal wall will be apparent as in the stomach (see 10.12 and Fig. 10.9). The mucosa is the thickest layer, and both dogs and particularly cats have a very prominent echogenic submucosal layer in the ileum. Normal wall thicknesses are given in Table 10.1; thickness increases with increasing weight, and sedation in the cat may increase mean duodenal wall thickness to 2.7 mm. The normal proximal duodenum shows peristaltic waves at four or five contractions per minute, whereas small intestinal contractions in the mid-abdomen are generally seen one to three times per minute.

10.31 VARIATIONS IN SMALL INTESTINAL CONTENTS ON ULTRASONOGRAPHY

1. Echogenic small intestinal contents without acoustic shadowing.
   a. Mucus.
   b. Food material.
   c. Some types of foreign material.
2. Echogenic small intestinal contents with significant acoustic shadowing.
   a. Gas.
   b. Bone fragments.
   c. Linear foreign body, often with bowel plication.
   d. Other foreign bodies, such as stones, palm seeds and corn cob pieces.
3. Anechoic or hypoechoic small intestinal contents.
   a. Fluid.

10.32 DILATION OF THE SMALL INTESTINAL LUMEN ON ULTRASONOGRAPHY

Motility is generally decreased if the small intestine is dilated, but may be normal to increased in cases of acute mechanical obstruction.

1. Few dilated small intestinal loops – localized dilation.
   a. Normal peristalsis.
   b. Proximal small intestinal mechanical obstruction (see Box 10.1 for causes).
   c. Partial functional obstruction (see Box 10.2 for causes).
   d. Adhesions.
2. Many dilated small intestinal loops – generalized dilation.
   a. Acute distal small intestinal mechanical obstruction (see Box 10.1 for causes).
   b. Chronic distal partial obstruction (may become total).
   c. Functional obstruction (paralytic ileus; see Box 10.2 for causes).
   d. Diffuse neoplasia – mainly lymphoma.

10.33 LACK OF VISUALIZATION OF THE NORMAL SMALL INTESTINAL WALL LAYERED ARCHITECTURE ON ULTRASONOGRAPHY

As for the stomach (see 10.14). Loss of intestinal wall layering is more likely to occur with neoplasia than with inflammatory disease. Adenocarcinoma is likely to be asymmetrical with irregular margins and heterogeneous echogenicity, whereas lymphoma more often produces symmetrical, hypoechoic thickening that may be focal, multifocal or diffuse. Lymphoma often does not produce complete obstruction, whereas other tumours may. Abdominal lymphadenopathy may also be seen but is a non-specific finding.

10.34 ABNORMAL ARRANGEMENT OF THE SMALL INTESTINE ON ULTRASONOGRAPHY

1. Corrugated small intestine.
   a. Secondary to peritonitis.
   b. Duodenum, secondary to pancreatitis.
   c. Enteritis.
      – Parvovirus enteritis.
      – Inflammatory bowel disease.
      – Lymphocytic or plasmacytic enteritis.
   d. Neoplasia.
      – Pancreatic.
      – Intestinal lymphoma.
      – Diffuse abdominal neoplasia (usually carcinomatosis).
   e. Protein-losing enteropathy.
   f. Lymphangiectasia.
   g. Linear foreign body.
   h. Entrapment in omental or mesenteric tear or by adhesion.
   i. Infarction (e.g. secondary to hypertrophic cardiomyopathy thromboembolism in cats).
2. Plicated or bunched small intestine.
   a. Linear foreign body (see 10.22.1 and 10.25.4 and Figs 10.11 and 10.13D).
   b. Sclerosing encapsulating peritonitis (see 10.20.5).
3. Increased number of layers – intussusception (see 10.35.3 and Fig. 10.17).

10.35 FOCAL THICKENING OF THE SMALL INTESTINAL WALL ON ULTRASONOGRAPHY

The small intestinal wall in the dog is generally considered to be abnormally thick if it is > 5 mm or > 6 mm for the duodenum. The duodenal papilla may be seen in cats and cause a slight focal thickening. Generally, neoplasia is likely to cause greater increase in thickening and more wall disruption than inflammatory disease and is more likely to be focal. Marked regional lymphadenopathy occurs most often with neoplasia.

1. Retention of the normal layered architecture – bowel may be slightly thickened; thickness > 10 mm may occur but is rare.
   a. Enteritis.
   b. Ulceration or perforation.

   c. Duodenitis secondary to pancreatitis.
   d. Smooth muscle hypertrophy.
      – Idiopathic; especially cats.
      – Chronic enteritis.
      – Proximal to stenosis or foreign body.
      – Lymphoma.
   e. Cats – feline infectious peritonitis; pyogranulomatous mass that may be up to 30 mm thick, mainly at ileocaecocolic junction and colon, rarely small bowel.
2. Loss of the normal layered architecture.
   a. Intestinal neoplasia – may have associated regional lymphadenopathy.
      – Adenocarcinoma (usually asymmetrical thickening of wall).
      – Lymphoma (especially cats; usually symmetrical, hypoechoic thickening).
      – Leiomyoma or leiomyosarcoma – may be complex, cystic or solid masses.
      – Mast cell tumour in cats.
   b. Severe duodenitis secondary to pancreatitis.
   c. Fungal infections, especially *Pythium insidiosum**.
   d. Other chronic inflammatory lesion or granuloma.
   e. Indolent ulcer.
   f. Ischaemic change.
   g. Focal lymphangiectasia.
   h. Vascular malformation.
   i. Cats – feline infectious peritonitis (see 10.35.1).
3. Increased number of layers – intussusception (Fig. 10.17), usually occurring in aboral

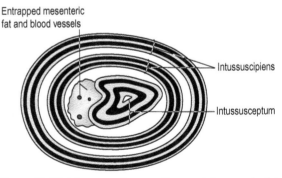

Entrapped mesenteric fat and blood vessels

Intussuscipiens

Intussusceptum

Figure 10.17 Intussusception on ultrasound: increase in the number of concentric tissue layers visible.

direction; may be predisposed to by pedunculated luminal masses (polyps or benign or low-grade tumours), so a careful search should be made for other pathology. Colour Doppler to assess blood flow in entrapped mesentery has been found to be useful for predicting reducibility.

4. Intestinal duplication (intestinal diverticulum) – cystic structure intimately associated with bowel wall – may have common muscular layer.

10.36 DIFFUSE THICKENING OF THE SMALL INTESTINAL WALL ON ULTRASONOGRAPHY

See 10.35 for normal wall thickness measurements.

1. Retention of the normal layered architecture – bowel may be slightly thickened but normal layering and thickness does not rule out disease.
   a. Enteritis.
   b. Inflammatory bowel disease.
   c. Bacterial infection and overgrowth.
   d. Food allergy.
   e. Protein-losing enteropathy.
   f. Lymphangiectasia.
   g. Oedema secondary to portal hypertension.
   h. Smooth muscle hypertrophy – especially cats.
   i. Involuting uterus *post partum* mimicking small intestine.
2. Loss of normal layered architecture, or decreased definition.
   a. Severe necrotizing enteritis.
   b. Lymphocytic or plasmacytic enteritis.
   c. Diffuse lymphoma.
   d. Fungal infections, especially *Pythium insidiosum**.
   e. Infarction (e.g. secondary to hypertrophic cardiomyopathy thromboembolism in cats).

10.37 MUCOSAL LAYER ALTERATIONS OF THE SMALL INTESTINE

1. Artefact – extended mucosal interface on transverse images.
2. Parvovirus infection – thinner mucosa due to sloughing.

3. Hyperechoic mucosal striations or speckles.
   a. Lymphangiectasia with protein-losing enteropathy and often with ascites.
   b. Primary inflammatory bowel disease (e.g. lymphocytic or plasmacytic enteritis).
   c. Neoplasia – histiocytic sarcoma.
   d. Mural gas with ulceration.

LARGE INTESTINE

10.38 NORMAL RADIOGRAPHIC APPEARANCE OF THE LARGE INTESTINE

The caecum is located in the right side of the mid abdomen at the level of L3 and is often gas-filled and corkscrew-shaped in dogs (Fig. 10.18). In cats,

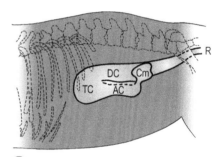

(A)

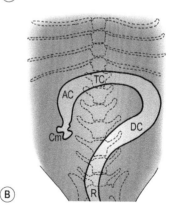

(B)

Figure 10.18 Normal large intestine in the dog: (A) lateral view and (B) ventrodorsal view. The appearance is similar in the cat, but the caecum is not usually visible. AC, ascending colon; Cm, caecum; DC, descending colon; R, rectum; TC, transverse colon.

it is very small and not usually detectable. The ascending colon runs cranially and to the right of the spine, adjacent to the duodenum and pancreas. The transverse colon crosses the cranial abdomen caudal to the stomach. The descending colon runs caudally to the pelvic inlet, to the left of the spine. In large-breed dogs, the terminal descending colon may be observed to the right of the spine, especially if the dog lay in right lateral recumbency before the VD radiograph was obtained. Extra bends in the descending colon are termed *redundant colon* and also occur more frequently in large-breed dogs; this is normal unless there is simultaneous dilation. Through the pelvis, the large intestine is called the rectum. The colon and rectum will be filled to a variable degree by gas and faeces; the radiopacity of the faeces depends on diet and on faecal consistency.

10.39 DISPLACEMENT OF THE LARGE INTESTINE

1. Displacement of the ascending colon.
   a. Further to the right.
      - Enlarged right kidney.
      - Enlarged right colic lymph nodes.
      - Right adrenal mass.
   b. Towards the midline.
      - Dilation of the duodenum.
      - Enlargement of the right limb of the pancreas.
      - Enlargement of the right side of the liver.
2. Displacement of the transverse colon.
   a. Caudally.
      - Dilation of the stomach.
      - Enlarged liver.
      - Enlargement of the left limb of the pancreas.
   b. Cranially.
      - Reduced liver size.
      - Ruptured diaphragm.
      - Gross urinary retention.
      - Uterine enlargement.
      - Enlargement of the middle colic lymph nodes.
      - Other mid-abdominal mass.
3. Displacement of the proximal descending colon.
   a. Further to the left.
      - Enlarged left kidney.

   - Left adrenal mass.
   b. Towards the midline or to the right side.
      - Enlargement of the left side of the liver.
      - Enlarged spleen.
   c. Ventrally.
      - Enlarged left kidney.
      - Retroperitoneal pathology (see 9.9).
4. Displacement of the distal descending colon.
   a. Medially or laterally.
      - Normal variant, especially in large-breed dogs and following previous right lateral recumbency.
      - Full bladder.
      - Enlarged prostate.
   b. Ventrally.
      - Enlarged sublumbar (mainly medial iliac) lymph nodes.
      - Dorsal soft tissue mass (e.g. lipoma, leiomyoma).
      - Severe spondylosis.
      - Retroperitoneal pathology (see 9.9).
   c. Dorsally.
      - Full bladder.
      - Enlarged uterus.
      - Enlarged prostate or paraprostatic cyst.
5. Abnormally short colon.
   a. Developmental anomaly that may predispose to soft, unformed faeces.
   b. Severe colitis.
   c. Previous surgical resection.
6. Kinked or tortuous descending colon.
   a. Normal variant – redundancy.
7. Displacement of the rectum.
   a. Dorsally.
      - Enlarged prostate.
      - Intrapelvic paraprostatic cyst.
      - Full, intrapelvic bladder.
      - Retroflexed bladder (e.g. perineal hernia).
      - Vaginal mass.
      - Urethral mass.
      - Pelvic bone mass.
      - Other ventral intrapelvic soft tissue masses.
   b. Ventrally.
      - Dorsal intrapelvic soft tissue mass or cellulitis secondary to lumbosacral discospondylitis.
      - Sacral or caudal vertebral mass.

10.40 LARGE INTESTINAL DILATION

The colonic diameter should be less than 1.5 times the length of L7. A dilated colon is usually filled with faeces of increased radiopacity.

1. Congenital conditions leading to large intestinal dilation.
   a. Atresia ani or coli – radiography is useful for assessing the degree of deformity, which may vary from anal stenosis to segmental aplasia of parts of the distal large intestine, ± rectogenital or rectourethral fistula; rectal or oral contrast medium or insertion of a radiopaque probe into the anus may be useful in assessing the extent of the deformity.
   b. Colonic duplication.
   c. Short, straight colon with caecum in left abdomen.
   d. Myelodysplasia in Manx cats.
   e. Spina bifida manifesta.
2. Acquired causes of large intestinal dilation with faeces due to mechanical obstruction (obstipation).
   a. Prostatomegaly or paraprostatic cyst (may be intrapelvic).
   b. Sublumbar swelling – usually due to lymphadenopathy.
   c. Intrapelvic soft tissue mass.
   d. Pelvic canal deformity.
      – Traumatic fracture with malunion.
      – Nutritional secondary hyperparathyroidism with folding fractures of the pelvis in puppies and kittens or obstructive effects seen in later life.
      – Pelvic bone neoplasia.
   e. Perineal hernia – usually a localized rectal distension that may be outlined caudally by a crescentic gas shadow; usually associated with prostatomegaly.
   f. Distal large intestinal stricture.
      – Colonic or rectal adenocarcinoma.
      – Adhesions following ovariohysterectomy.
3. Acquired causes of large intestinal dilation with faeces due to functional obstruction (constipation).
   a. Neurological.
      – Spinal cord pathology.
      – Cauda equina pathology.
      – Lumbar nerve pathology.

   b. Colonic neuropathy – megacolon.
   c. Hypertrophic megacolon – predisposed to by predominantly bony diet and inactivity.
   d. Certain drugs (e.g. opioids).
   e. Cats – idiopathic megacolon.
   f. Psychological – unwillingness to defecate due to pain or to behavioural or environmental reasons.
4. Gas-dilation of the large intestine (see 10.41.1).

10.41 VARIATIONS IN LARGE INTESTINAL CONTENTS

Diarrhoea is often associated with a hypermotile colon, which results in the colon being empty of faeces although it may be gas-filled to a variable degree. Colonic impaction can be diagnosed by observing a dilated colon filled with radiopaque faecal material. Surprisingly, faecal impaction can also lead to diarrhoea.

1. Empty or gas-filled large intestine.
   a. Normal – recent defecation.
   b. Following enema.
   c. Colitis.
      – Infectious.
      – Parasitic.
      – Abrasive dietary materials.
      – Ulcerative.
      – Lymphocytic, plasmacytic or eosinophilic.
   d. Diarrhoea.
   e. Caecal inversion.
   f. Intussusception.
   g. Neoplasia.
   h. Typhlitis (caecal inflammation).
   i. Volvulus of the colon (may be hard to identify as large intestine).
2. Soft tissue mass in the large intestine – outlined by air or seen on a contrast study.
   a. Ileocolic intussusception.
   b. Neoplasia (e.g. leiomyoma).
   c. Polyp.
   d. Foreign body of soft tissue opacity.
   e. Caecal inversion.
3. Increased radiopacity of the large intestine, normal diameter.
   a. Bones in diet.
   b. Constipation.
      – Lack of opportunity to defecate.

– Psychogenic.

– Old age.

– Dietary.

– Chronic abdominal pain or pain on defecation.

4. Increased radiopacity of the large intestine, dilated.

a. Megacolon.

b. Obstipation.

– Bony or soft tissue pelvic narrowing.

– Colonic or rectal masses.

c. Caecal impaction due to foreign body, neoplasia, spontaneous inversion or faecolithiasis – focal area of soft tissue, faecal or mineralized radiopacity in the region of the caecum; may cause obstruction.

10.42 VARIATIONS IN LARGE INTESTINAL WALL OPACITY

1. Reduced opacity – air (pneumatosis coli); leads to a reduced radiopacity of the colonic wall in a linear or scattered pattern.

a. Ulcerative colitis.

b. Ulceration due to neoplasia.

c. Iatrogenic mucosal perforation.

2. Increased radiopacity.

a. Artefactual due to adherent faeces.

b. Metastatic calcification.

c. Dystrophic calcification of colonic or rectal wall lesions.

10.43 LARGE INTESTINAL CONTRAST STUDIES: TECHNIQUE AND NORMAL APPEARANCE

Indications for contrast studies of the large intestine include the following:

● position of the colon and rectum, especially in relation to abdominal or pelvic masses

● obstipation

● tenesmus

● fresh blood in the faeces

● suspected intussusception.

If colonic rupture is suspected, a contrast study should not be performed, as it will encourage passage of faecal material into the peritoneal cavity, resulting in peritonitis. Colonic filling after an oral contrast study is usually inadequate and misleading, as the residual contrast medium is mixed with faeces. Thorough radiographic examination requires a large volume of contrast medium administered per rectum. The normal appearance of the large intestine is of a wide, gently curving tube with little variation in diameter and smooth, featureless walls and mucosal pattern.

Pneumocolon

A quick and useful study. A flexible catheter (e.g. Foley or urinary catheter) is passed into the rectum and approximately 10 mL/kg room air administered to fill the colon.

● Differentiates colon from gas-filled small intestine.

● Shows colonic or rectal strictures.

● Shows colonic masses and ileocaecocolic intussusceptions.

● Gives little or no information about the mucosal surface.

Barium enema

The animal should be fasted for 24 h and the colon cleansed with warm water and saline enemas at least 6 h prior to the study. The animal should be heavily sedated or anaesthetized. A balloon-tipped enema tube or Foley catheter is inserted into the rectum and 7–14 mL/kg of 10–20% w/v warmed barium sulphate suspension is run in under gravity. If the animal is anaesthetized and the anal sphincter relaxed, an anal purse-string suture may be required to prevent leakage. Radiographs are taken in lateral and dorsal recumbency.

● Differentiates colon from gas-filled small intestine.

● Shows colonic or rectal strictures.

● Shows large colonic or rectal masses and ileocaecocolic intussusceptions (small masses may be obscured).

● Gives more information about the mucosal surface than pneumocolon.

Double-contrast enema

Following the above radiographs, barium is allowed to drain out of the anus (e.g. by placing the enema bag on the floor) and the large intestine is then distended with room air. Radiographs are repeated.

- Shows colonic or rectal masses and strictures.
- Gives detailed visualization of the mucosal surface.

10.44 TECHNICAL ERRORS WITH LARGE INTESTINAL CONTRAST STUDIES

1. Lack of plain (survey) radiographs.
   a. Incorrect exposure factors used for contrast study.
   b. Animal not adequately cleansed of faeces, the retained faeces giving rise to filling defects in the contrast medium.
2. Inappropriate exposure factors – add 5–10 kVp to settings used to obtain plain radiographs for a positive contrast study and reduce by 5–10 kVp for pneumocolon.
3. Small lesions masked by overlying barium – double-contrast studies overcome this problem.
4. Perforation and peritonitis.
5. Colonic spasm.
   a. Cold contrast medium.
   b. Catheter irritation.

10.45 LARGE INTESTINAL LUMINAL FILLING DEFECTS ON CONTRAST STUDIES

1. Retained faeces.
2. Foreign bodies.
3. Masses.
   a. Pedunculated (e.g. polyp, leiomyoma).
   b. Sessile (e.g. neoplasia of large intestinal wall; Fig. 10.19) – often circumferential.

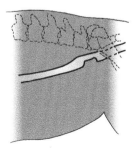

Figure 10.19 Large intestinal tumour shown on contrast enema – focal thickening of the colonic wall.

4. Ileocaecocolic intussusception.
5. Caecal inversion.

10.46 INCREASED LARGE INTESTINAL WALL THICKNESS ON CONTRAST STUDIES

1. Diffuse thickening of the large intestinal wall.
   a. Severe colitis.
      - Infectious.
      - Parasitic.
      - Abrasive dietary materials.
      - Ulcerative.
      - Lymphocytic, plasmacytic or eosinophilic.
   b. Diffuse neoplasia.
   c. Hypertrophic megacolon – predisposed to by predominantly bony diet and inactivity.
2. Focal thickening of the large intestinal wall.
   a. Neoplasia – usually asymmetric wall thickening, lumen narrowing ± proximal obstipation.
      - Adenocarcinoma.
      - Lymphoma.
      - Leiomyoma or leiomyosarcoma.
      - Mast cell tumour in cats.
   b. Focal colitis.
      - Histiocytic.
      - Granulomatous.
      - Fungal infections*, especially phycomycoses such as pythiosis.
   c. Scar tissue from a previous lesion or surgery (narrow lumen ± wall thickening).

10.47 ABNORMAL LARGE INTESTINAL MUCOSAL PATTERN ON CONTRAST STUDIES

1. Artefactual – incomplete removal of faeces.
2. Colitis.
   a. Mild colitis may not be detected – consider using proctoscopy or colonoscopy; suggested by observing thickened mucosal folds and fine spiculation of the contrast–mucosal interface.
   b. Severe, ulcerative colitis – deeper spiculation and ulceration at the contrast–mucosal interface; the colon may be rigid and shortened with a thickened wall and/or a corrugated mucosal pattern (Fig. 10.20).

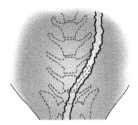

Figure 10.20 Severe colitis on a double-contrast enema: poor distension of the colon with an irregular mucosal pattern.

Tends not to be focal although may not involve the entire colon.

10.48 ULTRASONOGRAPHIC TECHNIQUE FOR THE LARGE INTESTINE

As for the small intestine (see 10.29). A water enema may be used to aid imaging, but this may necessitate sedation or even general anaesthesia. Transrectal ultrasound can be used to image the wall of the rectum and descending colon.

10.49 NORMAL ULTRASONOGRAPHIC APPEARANCE OF THE LARGE INTESTINE

The large intestine of the cat and dog does not have sacculations or bands as are seen in other species. Accordingly, the appearance of the large intestine is similar to that of the small intestine (see 10.30), although the diameter of large intestine tends to be greater than that of small intestine. The descending colon can be identified by its relationship to the bladder and often by the presence of hyperechoic gas shadows. The layers of the large intestinal wall are often not clearly seen due to the presence of gas and faecal material, causing acoustic shadowing and reverberation artefacts. Peristaltic contractions are not usually seen. Normal colonic wall thickness is given in Table 10.1.

10.50 ULTRASONOGRAPHIC CHANGES IN LARGE INTESTINAL DISEASE

Similar to those described for the small intestine (see 10.31–37).

Further reading

General

Agut, A., Sanchez-Valverde, M.A., Lasaosa, J.M., Murciano, J., Molina, F., 1993. Use of iohexol as a gastrointestinal contrast medium in the dog. Vet. Radiol. Ultrasound 34, 171–177.

Borgarelli, M., Biller, D.S., Goggin, J.M., Bussadori, C., 1996. Ultrasonographic examination of the gastrointestinal system. Part 1. Ultrasonographic anatomy and normal findings. Part 2. Ultrasonographic identification of gastrointestinal disease. Veterinaria 10, 37–47.

Boysen, S.R., Tidwell, A.S., Penninck, D.G., 2003. Ultrasonographic findings in dogs and cats with gastrointestinal perforation. Vet. Radiol. Ultrasound 44, 556–564.

Bradley, K., 2005. Practical contrast radiography 2. Gastrointestinal studies. In Pract. 27, 412–417.

Dennis, R., 1992. Barium meal techniques in dogs and cats. In Pract. 14, 237–248.

Detweiler, D.A., Biller, D.S., Hoskinson, J.J., Harkin, K.R., 2001. Radiographic findings in canine dysautonomia in twenty-four dogs. Vet. Radiol. Ultrasound 42, 108–112.

Gaschen, L., 2005. The role of imaging in dogs and cats with vomiting and chronic diarrhoea. Eur. J. Compan. Anim. Pract. 15, 197–203.

Gibbs, C., Pearson, H., 1973. The radiological diagnosis of gastrointestinal obstruction in the dog. J. Small Anim. Pract. 14, 61–82.

Goggin, J.M., Biller, D.S., Debey, B.M., Pickar, J.G., Mason, D., 2000. Ultrasonographic measurement of gastrointestinal wall thickness and the ultrasonographic appearance of the ileocolic region in healthy cats.

J. Am. Anim. Hosp. Assoc. 36, 224–228.

Graham, J.P., Newell, S.M., Roberts, G.D., Lester, N.V., 2000. Ultrasonographic features of canine gastrointestinal pythiosis. Vet. Radiol. Ultrasound 41, 273–277.

Grooters, A.M., Biller, D.S., Ward, H., Miyabayashi, C., Couto, C., 1994. Ultrasonographic appearance of feline alimentary lymphoma. Vet. Radiol. Ultrasound 35, 468–472.

Hunt, G.B., Worth, A., Marchevsky, A., 2004. Migration of wooden skewer foreign bodies form the gastrointestinal tract in eight dogs. J. Small Anim. Pract. 45, 362–367.

Kleine, L.J., Lamb, C.R., 1989. Comparative organ imaging: the gastrointestinal tract. Vet. Radiol. 30, 133–141.

Lamb, C.R., 1990. Abdominal ultrasonography in small animals: intestinal tract and mesentery, kidneys, adrenal glands, uterus and prostate. J. Small Anim. Pract. 31, 295–304.

Lamb, C.R., 1999. Recent developments in diagnostic imaging of the gastrointestinal tract of the dog and cat. Vet. Clin. North Am. Small Anim. Pract. 29, 307–342.

Miyabayashi, T., Morgan, J.P., 1991. Upper gastrointestinal examinations: a radiographic study of clinically normal beagle puppies. J. Small Anim. Pract. 32, 83–88.

Myers, N., Penninck, D.G., 1994. Ultrasonographic diagnosis of gastrointestinal smooth muscle tumors in the dog. Vet. Radiol. Ultrasound 35, 391–397.

Newell, S.M., Graham, J.P., Roberts, G.D., Ginn, P.E., Harrison, J.M., 1999. Sonography of the normal feline gastrointestinal tract. Vet. Radiol. Ultrasound 40, 40–43.

Penninck, D.G., 1998. Characterization of gastrointestinal tumors. Vet. Clin. North Am. Small Anim. Pract. 28, 777–798.

Penninck, D.G., Nyland, T.G., Fisher, P.E., Kerr, L.Y., 1989. Ultrasonography of the normal canine gastrointestinal tract. Vet. Radiol. 30, 272–276.

Penninck, D.G., Nyland, T.G., Kerr, L.Y., Fisher, P.E., 1990. Ultrasonographic evaluation of gastrointestinal diseases in small animals. Vet. Radiol. Ultrasound 31, 134–141.

Penninck, D.G., Moore, A.S., Tidwell, A.S., Matz, M.E., Freden, G.O., 1994. Ultrasonography of alimentary lymphosarcoma in the cat. Vet. Radiol. Ultrasound 35, 299–304.

Robertson, I.D., Burbidge, H.M., 2000. Pros and cons of barium-impregnated polyethylene spheres in gastrointestinal disease. Vet. Clin. North Am. Small Anim. Pract. 30, 449–465.

Sato, A.F., Solano, M., 2004. Ultrasonographic findings in abdominal mast cell disease: a retrospective study of 19 patients. Vet. Radiol. Ultrasound 45, 51–57.

Sparkes, A.H., Papasouliotis, K., Barr, F.J., Gruffydd-Jones, T.J., 1997. Reference ranges for gastrointestinal transit of barium-impregnated polyethylene spheres in healthy cats. J. Small Anim. Pract. 38, 340–343.

Tidwell, A.S., Penninck, D.G., 1992. Ultrasonography of gastrointestinal foreign bodies. Vet. Radiol. Ultrasound 33, 160–169.

Stomach

Allan, F.J., Guilford, W.G., Robertson, I.D., Jones, B.R., 1996. Gastric emptying time of solid radio-opaque markers in healthy dogs. Vet. Radiol. Ultrasound 37, 336–344.

Applewhite, A.A., Cornell, K.K., Selcer, B.A., 2001. Pylorogastric intussusception in the dog: a case report and literature review. J. Am. Anim. Hosp. Assoc. 37, 238–243.

Barber, D.L., 1982. Radiographic aspects of gastric ulcers in dogs: a comparative review and report of 5 case histories. Vet. Radiol. 23, 109–116.

Biller, D.S., Partington, B.P., Miyabayashi, R., Leveille, R., 1994. Ultrasonographic appearance of chronic hypertrophic pyloric gastropathy in the dog. Vet. Radiol. Ultrasound 35, 30–33.

Bowlus, R.A., Biller, D.S., Armbrust, L.J., Henrikson, T.D., 2005. Clinical utility of pneumogastrography in dogs. J. Am. Anim. Hosp. Assoc. 41, 171–178.

Dennis, R., Herrtage, M.E., Jefferies, A.R., Matic, S.E., White, R.A.S., 1987. A case of

hyperplastic gastropathy in a cat. J. Small Anim. Pract. 28, 491–504.

Diana, A., Penninck, D.G., Keating, J.H., 2009. Ultrasonographic appearance of canine gastric polyps. Vet. Radiol. Ultrasound 50, 201–204.

Evans, S.M., 1983. Double versus single contrast gastrography in the dog and cat. Vet. Radiol. 24, 6–10.

Evans, S.M., Biery, D.N., 1983. Double contrast gastrography in the cat: technique and normal radiographic appearance. Vet. Radiol. 24, 3–5.

Funkquist, B., 1979. Gastric torsion in the dog. I. Radiological picture during nonsurgical treatment related to the pathological anatomy and to the further clinical course. J. Small Anim. Pract. 20, 73–91.

Grooters, A.M., Miyabayashi, T., Biller, D.S., Merryman, J., 1994. Sonographic appearance of uremic gastropathy in four dogs. Vet. Radiol. Ultrasound 35, 35–40.

Heng, H.G., Wrigley, R.H., Kraft, S.L., Powers, B.E., 2005. Fat is responsible for an intramural radiolucent band in the feline stomach wall. Vet. Radiol. Ultrasound 46, 54–56.

Hittmair, K., Krebitz-Gressl, E., Kübber-Heiss, A., Möstl, K., 2000. Feline alimentary lymphosarcoma: radiographical, ultrasonographical, histological and virological findings. Wien. Tierärztl. Monatsschr. 87, 174–183 reprinted in the Eur. J.Compan. Anim. Prac. (2001) 11, 119–128.

Jakovljevic, S., 1988. Gastric radiology and gastroscopy in the dog. Vet. Annu. 28, 172–182.

Jakovljevic, S., Gibbs, C., 1993. Radiographic assessment of gastric mucosal fold thickness in dogs. Am. J. Vet. Res. 54, 1827–1830.

Kaser-Hotz, B., Hauser, B., Arnold, P., 1996. Ultrasonographic findings in canine gastric neoplasia in 13 patients. Vet. Radiol. Ultrasound 37, 51–56.

Lamb, C.R., Grierson, J., 1999. Ultrasonographic appearance of primary gastric neoplasia in 21 dogs. J. Small Anim. Pract. 40, 211–215.

Lee, H., Yeon, S., Chang, D., Eom, K., Yoon, H., Choi, H., et al., 2005. Ultrasonographic diagnosis – Pylorogastric intussusception in a dog. Vet. Radiol. Ultrasound 46, 317–318.

Love, N.E., 1993. Radiology corner: The appearance of the canine pyloric region in right versus left lateral recumbent radiographs. Vet. Radiol. Ultrasound 34, 169–170.

Pearson, H., Gaskell, C.J., Gibbs, C., Waterman, A., 1974. Pyloric and oesophageal dysfunction in the cat. J. Small Anim. Pract. 15, 487–504.

Penninck, D.G., Moore, A.S., Gliatto, J., 1998. Ultrasonography of canine gastric epithelial neoplasia. Vet. Radiol. Ultrasound 39, 342–348.

Rallis, T.S., Patsikas, M.N., Mylonakis, M.E., Day, M.J., Petanides, T.A., Papazoglou, L.G., et al., 2007. Giant hypertrophic gastritis (Ménétrier's-like disease) in an Old English sheepdog. J. Am. Anim. Hosp. Assoc. 43, 122–127.

Sullivan, M., Lee, R., Fisher, E.W., Nash, A.S., McCandlish, I.A.P., 1987. A study of 31 cases of gastric carcinoma in dogs. Vet. Rec. 120, 79–83.

Wyse, C.A., McLellan, J., Dickie, A.M., Sutton, D.G.M., Preston, T., Yam, P.S., 2003. A review of methods for assessment of the rate of gastric emptying in the dog and cat: 1898–2002. J. Vet. Intern. Med. 17, 609–621.

Intestines

Ablin, L.W., Moore, F.M., Shields Henney, L.H., Berg, J., 1991. Intestinal diverticular malformation in dogs and cats. Compend. Contin. Educ. Pract.

Veterinarian (Small Animal) 13, 426–430.

Baez, J.L., Hendrick, M.J., Walker, L.M., Washabau, R.J., 1999. Radiographic, ultrasonographic, and endoscopic findings in cats with inflammatory bowel disease of the stomach and small intestine: 33 cases (1990–1997). J. Am. Vet. Med. Assoc. 215, 349–354.

Bruce, S.J., Guilford, W.G., Hedderley, D.L., McCauley, M., 1999. Development of reference intervals for the large intestinal transit of radio-opaque markers in dogs. Vet. Radiol. Ultrasound 40, 472–476.

Cairo, J., Font, J., Gorraiz, J., Martin, C., Pons, C., 1999. Intestinal volvulus in dogs: a study of four clinical cases. J. Small Anim. Pract. 40, 136–140.

Couraud, L., Jermyn, K., Yam, P.S., Ramsey, I.K., Philbey, A.W., 2006. Intestinal pseudo-obstruction, lymphocytic leiomyositis and atrophy of the muscularis externa in a dog. Vet. Rec. 159, 86–87.

Delaney, F., O'Brien, R.T., Waller, K., 2003. Ultrasound evaluation of small bowel thickness compared to weight in normal dogs. Vet. Radiol. Ultrasound 44, 577–580.

Diana, A., Pietra, M., Guglielmini, C., Boari, G., Bettini, G., Cipone, M., 2003. Ultrasonography and pathological features of intestinal smooth muscle hypertrophy in four cats. Vet. Radiol. Ultrasound 44, 566–569.

Dvir, E., Leisewitz, A.L., Van der Lugt, J.J., 2001. Chronic idiopathic intestinal pseudo-obstruction in an English bulldog. J. Small Anim. Pract. 42, 243–247.

Gibbs, C., Pearson, H., 1986. Localized tumours of the canine small intestine: a report of twenty cases. J. Small Anim. Pract. 27, 507–519.

Graham, J.P., Lord, P.F., Harrison, J.M., 1998. Quantitative estimation of

intestinal dilation as a predictor of obstruction in the dog. J. Small Anim. Pract. 39, 521–524.

Harvey, C.J., Lopez, J.W., Hendrick, M.J., 1996. An uncommon intestinal manifestation of feline infectious peritonitis: 26 cases (1986–1993). J. Am. Vet. Med. Assoc. 209, 1117–1120.

Hoffmann, K.L., 2003. Sonographic signs of gastroduodenal linear foreign body in 3 dogs. Vet. Radiol. Ultrasound 44, 466–469.

Junius, A.M., Appeldoorn, A.M., Schrauwen, E., 2004. Mesenteric volvulus in the dog: a retrospective study of 12 cases. J. Small Anim. Pract. 45, 104–107.

Kinns, J., Sears, K., Seiler, G., 2008. Imaging diagnosis – Jejunal vascular malformation in a dog. Vet. Radiol. Ultrasound 40, 179–181.

Lamb, C.R., Hansson, K., 1994. Radiology corner: Radiological identification of nonopaque intestinal foreign bodies. Vet. Radiol. Ultrasound 35, 87–88.

Lamb, C.R., Mantis, P., 1998. Ultrasonographic features of intestinal intussusception in 10 dogs. J. Small Anim. Pract. 39, 437–441.

Louvet, A., Denis, B., 2004. Ultrasonographic diagnosis – Small bowel lymphangiectasia in a dog. Vet. Radiol. Ultrasound 45, 565–567.

Moon, M.M., Biller, D.S., Armbrust, L.J., 2003. Ulrasonographic appearance and etiology of corrugated small intestine. Vet. Radiol. Ultrasound 44, 199–203.

Newell, S.M., Graham, J.P., Roberts, G.D., Ginn, P.E., Harrison, J.M., 1999. Sonography of the normal feline gastrointestinal tract. Vet. Radiol. Ultrasound 40, 40–43.

Patsikas, M., Papazoglou, L.G., Papaioannou, N.G., Dessiris, A.K.,

2004. Normal and abnormal ultrasonographic findings that mimic small intestinal intussusception in the dog. J. Am. Anim. Hosp. Assoc. 40, 147–151.

Patsikas, M., Papazoglou, L.G., Jakovlevic, A.K., Dessiris, A.K., 2005. Color Doppler ultrasonography in prediction of the reducibility of intussuscepted bowel in 15 young dogs. Vet. Radiol. Ultrasound 46, 313–316.

Patsikas, M., Papazoglou, L.G., Papaioannou, N.G., Savvas, I., Kazakos, G.M., Dessiris, A.K., 2009. Ultrasonographic findings of intestinal intussusception in seven cats. J. Feline Med. Surg. 5, 335–343.

Penninck, D., Seyers, B.S., Webster, C.R.L., Rand, W.,

Moore, A.S., 2003. Diagnostic value of ultrasonography in differentiating enteritis from intestinal neoplasia in dogs. Vet. Radiol. Ultrasound 44, 570–575.

Rault, D.N., Besso, J.G., Boulouha, L., Begon, Y., Ruel, Y., 2004. Significance of a common extended mucosal interface observed in transverse small intestine sonogram. Vet. Radiol. Ultrasound 45, 177–179.

Russell, N.J., Tyrrell, D., Irwin, P.J., Beck, C., 2008. Pneumatosis coli in a dog. J. Am. Anim. Hosp. Assoc. 44, 32–35.

Standler, N., Wagner, W.M., Goddard, A., Kirberger, R.M., 2010. Normal canine pediatric gastrointestinal ultrasonography.

Vet. Radiol. Ultrasound 51, in press.

Standler, N., Wagner, W.M., Goddard, A., Kirberger, R.M., 2010. Ultrasonographic appearance of canine porvoviral enteritis in puppies. Vet. Radiol. Ultrasound 51, in press.

Sutherland-Smith, J., Penninck, D.G., Keating, J.H., Webster, C.R.L., 2007. Ultrasonographic intestinal hyperechoic mucosal striations in dogs are associated with lacteal dilation. Vet. Radiol. Ultrasound 48, 51–57.

Swift, I., 2009. Ultrasonographic features of intestinal entrapment in dogs. Vet. Radiol. Ultrasound 50, 205–207.

Chapter 11

Urogenital tract

CHAPTER CONTENTS

Urinary tract   298

Kidneys   298
11.1 Non-visualization of the kidneys   299
11.2 Variations in kidney size and
      shape   299
11.3 Variations in kidney radiopacity   300
11.4 Variations in kidney location   301
11.5 Upper urinary tract contrast studies:
      technique and normal
      appearance   301
11.6 Absent nephrogram   303
11.7 Abnormal timing of the nephrogram   303
11.8 Uneven radiopacity of the
      nephrogram   303
11.9 Abnormalities of the pyelogram   304
11.10 Ultrasonographic examination of the
       kidneys   305
11.11 Normal ultrasonographic appearance of the
       kidneys   305
11.12 Abnormalities of the renal pelvis on
       ultrasonography   306
11.13 Focal parenchymal abnormalities of
       the kidney on ultrasonography   306
11.14 Diffuse parenchymal abnormalities of
       the kidney on ultrasonography   307
11.15 Perirenal abnormalities on
       ultrasonography   307

Ureters   308
11.16 Dilated ureter   309
11.17 Normal ultrasonographic appearance of the
       ureters   309

11.18 Dilation of the ureter on ultrasonography   310

Urinary bladder   310
11.19 Non-visualization of the urinary
       bladder   310
11.20 Displacement of the urinary
       bladder   310
11.21 Variations in urinary bladder size   311
11.22 Variations in urinary bladder shape   311
11.23 Variations in urinary bladder
       radiopacity   311
11.24 Urinary bladder contrast studies: technique
       and normal appearance   312
11.25 Reflux of contrast medium up a ureter
       following cystography   313
11.26 Abnormal bladder lumen on
       cystography   313
11.27 Thickening of the urinary bladder wall on
       cystography   314
11.28 Ultrasonographic examination of the
       bladder   315
11.29 Normal ultrasonographic appearance of the
       bladder   315
11.30 Thickening of the bladder wall on
       ultrasonography   315
11.31 Changes in echogenicity of the bladder
       wall   316
11.32 Cystic structures within or near the bladder
       wall on ultrasonography   316
11.33 Changes in urinary bladder contents on
       ultrasonography   316

Urethra and vagina   317
11.34 Urethral and vaginal contrast studies:
       technique and normal appearance   317

11.35 Abnormalities of the
       (vagino)urethrogram 318
11.36 Ultrasonography of the urethra and vagina
       319

Female genital tract 319

Ovaries 319
11.37 Ovarian enlargement 320
11.38 Ultrasonographic examination of the ovaries
       320
11.39 Normal ultrasonographic appearance
       of the ovary 320
11.40 Ovarian abnormalities on
       ultrasonography 320

Uterus 320
11.41 Uterine enlargement 320
11.42 Variations in uterine radiopacity 321
11.43 Radiographic signs of dystocia
       and fetal death 321
11.44 Ultrasonographic examination of the
       uterus 322
11.45 Normal ultrasonographic appearance of the
       uterus 322
11.46 Variation in uterine contents on
       ultrasonography 322
11.47 Thickening of the uterine wall on
       ultrasonography 322

Male genital tract 322

Prostate 322
11.48 Variations in location of the
       prostate 323
11.49 Variations in prostatic size 323
11.50 Variations in prostatic shape and
       outline 324
11.51 Variations in prostatic radiopacity 324
11.52 Ultrasonographic examination of the prostate
       324
11.53 Normal ultrasonographic appearance of the
       prostate 324
11.54 Focal parenchymal changes of the prostate on
       ultrasonography 325
11.55 Diffuse parenchymal changes of the prostate
       on ultrasonography 325
11.56 Paraprostatic lesions on
       ultrasonography 325

Testes 325
11.57 Ultrasonographic examination of
       the testes 325

11.58 Normal ultrasonographic appearance of the
       testes 326
11.59 Testicular abnormalities on ultrasonography
       326
11.60 Paratesticular abnormalities on
       ultrasonography 326

URINARY TRACT

KIDNEYS

The kidneys lie in the retroperitoneal space, and visualization of the renal outline depends on the presence of sufficient surrounding fat. In the dog, the cranial pole of the right kidney lies in the renal fossa of the caudate lobe of the liver at the level of T13–L1 and may be difficult to discern, especially in thin or deep-chested dogs or if the gastrointestinal tract contains much ingesta. The left kidney usually lies approximately half a kidney length more caudally, and more ventrally, and is more mobile. The kidneys are best seen on a right lateral recumbent expiratory film, in which the dependent right kidney slides cranially and there is least superimposition. They are bean-shaped, with a hilar notch where the vessels and ureters enter; depending on their orientation relative to the X-ray beam, they may be seen as either ovoid or bean-shaped structures. In lateral recumbency, the dependent kidney usually appears ovoid, whereas the uppermost kidney droops so that the hilus is profiled and the kidney appears bean-shaped.

In cats, the kidneys tend to be more easily visible, as the right kidney is usually separated from the liver by fat and both kidneys are mobile. The kidneys appear smaller, rounder and more variable in location than in the dog. On a lateral view, partial superimposition of the kidneys may mimic a smaller mass in both cats and dogs.

Kidney size is best assessed on a ventrodorsal (VD) radiograph to avoid a difference between the two kidneys due to magnification of the uppermost one, which may occur in lateral recumbency (Fig. 11.1). Measurements should be made on plain films, as the kidneys swell slightly during an intravenous urogram (IVU), the increase in size being dose- and time-dependent. The size range of the

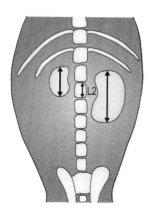

Figure 11.1 Decreased and increased kidney size in the dog, as assessed on the ventrodorsal radiograph (normal size range, 2.5–3.5 times L2).

canine kidney is usually quoted as 2.5–3.5 times the length of L2, although 2.75–3.25 may be more realistic; the normal feline kidney size range is 1.9–2.6 times the length of L2 in neutered cats and 2.1–3.2 in entire cats. The two kidneys should be the same size in a given patient.

11.1 NON-VISUALIZATION OF THE KIDNEYS

1. Normal variant (especially for the right kidney on a VD view).
   a. Inappropriate exposure setting or processing (especially underexposure).
   b. Little abdominal fat.
      – Young animals.
      – Very thin animals.
   c. Deep-chested conformation, kidneys therefore lying more cranially.
   d. Food, gas or faeces in the gastrointestinal tract, obscuring a kidney.
2. Kidney in abnormal location (see 11.4).
3. Nephrectomy.
4. Very small kidney (see 11.2.5).
5. Renal agenesis.
   a. Unilateral (either right or left may be absent), with compensatory hypertrophy of the remaining kidney; the ureter may still be present.
   b. Bilateral – rare; animal dies soon after birth.
6. Severe peritoneal effusion.
7. Retroperitoneal disease.
   a. Urine leakage.

b. Haemorrhage.
c. Inflammation.
d. Diffuse neoplasia.

11.2 VARIATIONS IN KIDNEY SIZE AND SHAPE

1. Normal size kidney, smooth outline.
   a. Normal.
   b. Acute nephritis.
   c. Acute renal toxicity.
      – Ethylene glycol (antifreeze) poisoning.
      – Other toxins.
      – Certain drugs (e.g. gentamicin, cisplatin).
   d. Amyloidosis.
   e. Early stages of other disease processes.
2. Normal size kidney, irregular outline.
   a. Disease processes listed below that have not produced a detectable size change.
   b. Renal infarct.
   c. Trauma.
3. Mildly enlarged kidney, smooth outline.
   a. Nephrogram phase of IVU – bilateral.
   b. Acute renal failure – bilateral; numerous causes.
   c. Acute glomerulo- or interstitial nephritis – often bilateral.
   d. Acute pyelonephritis – often bilateral.
   e. Hydronephrosis – unilateral or bilateral, depending on the cause.
   f. Congenital portosystemic shunts – dogs often show bilateral kidney hypertrophy ± urinary tract calculi and haematogenous osteomyelitis.
   g. Compensatory renal hypertrophy – unilateral; opposite kidney small or absent.
   h. Renal neoplasia – usually unilateral; more often irregular than smooth (other than lymphoma); in cats, lymphoma is the commonest renal tumour and is usually bilateral.
   i. Subcapsular abscess, haematoma or urine – unilateral or bilateral depending on the cause.
   j. Perirenal fluid associated with acute renal failure.
   k. Amyloidosis – often bilateral.
   l. Acromegaly – bilateral.
   m. Parasitic – *Dioctophyma renale** infection.
   n. Hypertrophic feline muscular dystrophy – bilateral.

4. Markedly enlarged kidney, smooth outline.
   a. Hydronephrosis – unilateral or bilateral, depending on the cause (see 11.9.1 and Fig. 11.3).
   b. Renal neoplasia – usually unilateral; more often irregular than smooth.
   c. Subcapsular abscess, haematoma or urine – unilateral or bilateral.
   d. Renal lymphoma – common in cats; less common in dogs.
   e. Perirenal (perinephric) pseudocysts; usually elderly male cats; often grossly enlarged 'kidney' outline – usually bilateral.
   f. Cats – feline infectious peritonitis (FIP) causing pyogranulomatous nephritis, although the kidneys are more likely to be irregular in outline.
5. Enlarged kidney, irregular outline.
   a. Primary renal neoplasia – usually unilateral but may be bilateral; benign and malignant neoplasms cannot be differentiated on radiographic appearance alone.
      - Renal cell carcinoma.
      - Transitional cell carcinoma.
      - Nephroblastoma; usually young dogs.
      - Hereditary multifocal renal cystadenoma or cystadenocarcinoma (see p. 306) – usually German Shepherd dogs, together with nodular dermatofibrosis lesions and uterine leiomyomas.
      - Renal lymphoma – especially cats, bilateral; often other organs are affected too, and there is an association with nasal lymphoma.
      - Others: adenoma, haemangioma, haemangiosarcoma, papilloma, anaplastic sarcoma, extraskeletal osteosarcoma, etc.
   b. Metastatic neoplasia – unilateral or bilateral.
      - Metastasis from a primary in the opposite kidney.
      - Many other primary tumours metastasize to the kidneys.
   c. Renal abscess – usually unilateral.
   d. Renal haematoma – usually unilateral.
   e. Renal granuloma – unilateral or bilateral.
   f. Renal cyst(s).
   g. Renal hamartoma – a benign, focal malformation that may cause renal haemorrhage.
   h. Polycystic kidney disease (PKD) – heritable condition in long-haired cats, especially Persians and Persian crosses, and also in Cairn and Bull Terriers; usually bilateral.
   i. Cats – FIP, causing pyogranulomatous nephritis.
6. Small kidney, smooth or irregular in outline.
   a. Chronic renal disease.
      - Chronic glomerulonephritis.
      - Chronic pyelonephritis.
      - Chronic interstitial nephritis.
      - Chronic renal calculi.
   b. Developmental renal hypoplasia or dysplasia – younger dogs, with a familial tendency in some breeds, including Cocker Spaniel, Lhasa Apso, Shih Tzu, Norwegian Elkhound, Samoyed, Boxer and Dobermann.
   With both (a) and (b), metastatic soft tissue mineralization (e.g. gastric rugae, blood vessels) and renal secondary hyperparathyroidism (rubber jaw; see 4.9.5 and Fig. 4.5) may also be present.
   c. Chronic hydronephrosis.
   d. Parenchymal atrophy secondary to renal infarcts.
   e. Amyloidosis, especially in cats.

11.3 VARIATIONS IN KIDNEY RADIOPACITY

The radiopacity of the kidneys is normally the same as for other soft tissue structures. On VD radiographs, a slight radiolucency may be observed in the central medial area of each kidney due to fat within the pelvic region. Incidental adrenal gland mineralization in older cats should not be mistaken for renal changes.

1. Focal increased radiopacity of the kidney – mineralization of parenchyma may be differentiated from renal pelvic calculi by means of IVU, as the latter will be obscured by the pyelogram.
   a. Artefactual due to superimposition of the other kidney (lateral view), nipple (VD view) or ingesta (either view).
   b. Mineralized nephroliths in the renal pelvis – large ones can become staghorn in shape; ureteric calculi may also be seen.
   c. Mineralized nephroliths in the renal diverticula – often multiple (especially in cats).
   d. Dystrophic mineralization of parenchyma.
      - Neoplasia.
      - Chronic haematoma, granuloma, cyst or abscess.

e. Parasitic granuloma (e.g. *Toxocara canis*).

f. Osseous metaplasia.

2. Diffuse or multifocal increased radiopacity of the kidney – nephrocalcinosis.

   a. Chronic renal disease.

   b. Ethylene glycol (antifreeze) poisoning.

   c. Hyperparathyroidism – primary or secondary.

   d. Hyperadrenocorticism.

   e. Hypercalcaemia syndromes.

   f. Nephrotoxic drugs (e.g. gentamicin).

   g. Hypervitaminosis D.

   h. Renal telangiectasia – Corgi.

3. Reduced radiopacity of the renal pelvis.

   a. Pelvic fat, especially in obese cats.

   b. Reflux of air from the urinary bladder under high pressure during pneumocystography; gas lucency may also be seen in the ureters.
      – Overinflation of a normal bladder.
      – Inflation of a poorly distensible bladder.

   c. Inadvertent catheterization of an ectopic ureter followed by air injection.

   d. Infection with gas-producing bacteria.

11.4 VARIATIONS IN KIDNEY LOCATION

Both congenital and acquired causes of abnormal location occur. The majority are acquired, due to displacement by masses or through ruptures. Congenital malposition constitutes renal ectopia and is unusual.

1. Cranial displacement.

   a. Intrathoracic; right kidney herniation following diaphragmatic rupture is reported in cats.

   b. By large mid- or caudal abdominal mass.

2. Caudal displacement.

   a. Due to intrathoracic expansion.

   b. By distended stomach.

   c. Left kidney by mass in head of spleen.

   d. Right kidney by hepatomegaly.

   e. Ectopic kidney (e.g. sublumbar).

   f. Situs inversus of abdominal organs – right kidney caudal to left kidney.

3. Ventral displacement.

   a. By retroperitoneal fat in obese animal.

   b. By pathological retroperitoneal swelling or effusion (see 9.9).

c. By ipsilateral adrenal mass (cranial pole usually displaced more than caudal pole).

d. Large renal masses may lie more ventrally than normal due to gravity.

e. Ectopic kidney in peritoneal cavity.

4. Dorsal displacement.

   a. By ventral abdominal mass.

5. Lateral displacement.

   a. By ipsilateral adrenal mass (cranial pole usually displaced more than caudal pole).

6. Medial displacement.

   a. Simple renal ectopia – kidney, ureter and vesicoureteral junction are on the same side of the abdomen.

   b. Crossed renal ectopia – kidney lies on the opposite side to normal, but the ureter crosses the midline; may be fused to contralateral kidney.

   c. Horseshoe kidney – both kidneys medially displaced and fused together.

11.5 UPPER URINARY TRACT CONTRAST STUDIES: TECHNIQUE AND NORMAL APPEARANCE

Indications for contrast studies of the kidneys and ureters include the following:

- Identification of number, location, size and shape of the kidneys; some information is given about kidney function and internal architecture, especially of the renal pelvis.
- Investigation of abdominal masses.
- Investigation of haematuria or pyuria not arising from the lower urogenital tract.
- Investigation of the location of possible urinary tract calculi, and differentiation from gastrointestinal material.
- Investigation of urinary incontinence.
- After trauma with suspected urinary tract damage.

Intravenous urography or *IVU (excretion urography)* is especially useful for evaluation of the renal pelvis and ureters. Lesions of the renal parenchyma are more difficult to diagnose, and generally such diseases are more readily detected by ultrasonography. Selective renal angiography is not often performed; contrast medium deposited near the renal artery via a femoral arterial catheter will outline the renal blood supply and demonstrate features of kidneys that are failing and therefore not likely to opacify well following an IVU.

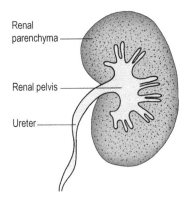

Figure 11.2 Nephrogram and pyelogram phase of intravenous urogram.

Labels in figure:
Renal parenchyma
Renal pelvis
Ureter

During and for a few seconds immediately after the contrast medium injection, the vascular supply to the kidney is outlined, forming the *angiogram* phase. This is quickly followed by a diffuse increase in radiopacity of the kidney parenchyma, the *nephrogram* phase. Occasionally, the cortex transiently appears more radiopaque than the medulla; the medulla is approximately twice the thickness of the cortex. The nephrogram persists for about 1–3 h. Within 1–2 min of the injection in normal kidneys, the renal pelvis and ureters are filled by contrast medium, which is being concentrated in the urine; this is the *pyelogram* phase (Fig. 11.2). The radiographic appearance of the renal pelvis is very variable in dogs, and the renal diverticula are not consistently seen.

Preparation

- Blood tests: blood urea nitrogen level > 17 mmol/L (> 100 mg%) and/or blood creatinine levels > 350 μmol/L (> 4 mg%) indicate severe renal compromise, which is likely to preclude opacification of the upper urinary tract and is a contraindication for the study (if the urea and creatinine are only moderately increased, consideration should be given to increasing the dose of iodine up to two-fold to improve visualization of the urinary system).
- Assessment of circulation and hydration status: injection of hypertonic contrast medium should not be made in patients that are dehydrated or in hypotensive shock in case of induction of acute renal shut-down. Non-ionic (low-osmolar) iodinated contrast media are safer for such patients and for cats.

- Twelve-hour fast and colonic enema.
- Placement of an intravenous catheter, because extravasation of contrast medium outside the vein is irritant.
- Sedation or anaesthesia of the patient, as appropriate.
- Plain (survey) lateral and VD radiographs to check patient preparation and exposure factors.

Side effects

- Induction of dehydration.
- Acute renal failure due to precipitation of proteins in renal tubules (more likely if the urine protein is elevated).
- Rare anaphylactic shock (severe reaction or death).

Bolus intravenous urogram (low volume, high concentration)

Inject up to 850 mg I/kg of body weight of 300–400 mg I/mL contrast medium rapidly with the patient in dorsal recumbency; take an immediate VD radiograph (the kidneys are seen separately, as they are not superimposed) followed by laterals and VDs as necessary. Identify the angiogram, nephrogram and pyelogram phases of opacification. Caudal abdominal compression to occlude the ureters and increase pelvic filling has been described, although this can produce the artefactual appearance of mild hydronephrosis.

Infusion intravenous urogram (large volume, low concentration): an alternative technique for the ureters

Inject approximately 1200 mg I/kg of body weight of 150 mg I/mL contrast medium slowly as a drip infusion; this creates more osmotic diuresis and better visualization of the ureters. Rapid radiographic exposure is not necessary. Only the nephrogram and pyelogram phases are seen. It is particularly important to ensure that the colon is empty of faeces, and performing a pneumocystogram first will increase bladder pressure and improve opacification of the ureters as well as providing a radiolucent background against which ureter endings are easier to see. Both right and left lateral recumbent and oblique views as well as VDs are helpful for identification of ureter terminations, and fluoroscopy may also be useful.

Selective renal angiography

Catheterize the femoral artery and advance the catheter up the aorta until the tip is at the level of the renal arteries; inject a few millilitres of high-concentration contrast medium as a bolus and make an immediate VD radiograph. An angiogram phase is seen (unless the vascular supply is disrupted), and a nephrogram and pyelogram are seen in functioning kidneys.

Ultrasound-guided antegrade pyelography

This technique permits assessment of the pelvis and ureters in animals with obstructive uropathy, which are anuric or oliguric and in which an IVU is likely to be non-diagnostic. Under ultrasound guidance, a small amount of positive contrast medium is injected into the renal pelvis and opacifies the ureters as far distally as any obstruction. Nephropyelocentesis is also possible, of value in the diagnosis of pyelonephritis.

11.6 ABSENT NEPHROGRAM

1. Inadequate dose of contrast medium.
2. Severe renal disease with marked azotaemia.
3. Prior nephrectomy.
4. Very small kidney overlooked.
5. Renal aplasia.
6. Obstructed or avulsed renal artery.
7. Absence of functional renal tissue.
   a. Extensive neoplasia.
   b. Extreme hydronephrosis.
   c. Large abscess.

11.7 ABNORMAL TIMING OF THE NEPHROGRAM

The normal appearance is of uniformly increased kidney radiopacity and improved visualization of kidney outline, which occurs due to the presence of contrast medium in the renal vasculature and tubules. The opacity should be greatest initially, followed by a gradual decrease. Abnormalities in timing are shown in Table 11.1.

11.8 UNEVEN RADIOPACITY OF THE NEPHROGRAM

Areas of poor vascularity show initial absent or poor opacification, but there may be variable increase with time.

1. Well-defined areas of non-opacification.
   a. Renal cyst – solitary cysts are an occasional incidental finding.
   b. Renal abscess, granuloma or haematoma.
   c. Renal infarct – single or multiple; wedge-shaped area with the apex directed towards the hilus.
   d. Polycystic kidney disease – heritable condition in long-haired cats, especially Persians and Persian crosses, and also in Cairn and Bull Terriers; usually bilateral.
   e. Hereditary multifocal renal cystadenoma or carcinoma – usually German Shepherd dogs, together with nodular dermatofibrosis lesions and uterine leiomyomas.
2. Poorly defined areas of non-opacification.
   a. Renal neoplasia (may also see areas of increased opacity due to contrast medium extravasation and pooling).
      – Renal cell carcinoma.
      – Transitional cell carcinoma.
      – Nephroblastoma.
      – Renal adenoma, haemangioma or papilloma.
      – Anaplastic sarcoma.
      – Hereditary multifocal renal cystadenoma or cystadenocarcinoma – German Shepherd dog.
      – Renal lymphoma – especially cats, bilateral; often wedge-shaped areas of reduced opacification.
   b. Renal infarct – may be ill defined.
   c. Severe nephritis.
   d. Cats – FIP.
3. Peripheral rim of opacification only – severe hydronephrosis (Fig. 11.3B).
4. Peripheral rim of non-opacification.
   a. Subcapsular fluid accumulation (e.g. perirenal pseudocysts, acute renal failure, urinoma).
   b. Cats – subcapsular lymphoma.
5. Areas of increased opacity due to accumulation of contrast medium.
   a. Neoplasia.
   b. Hamartoma.
   c. Leaking blood vessel (often the cause of 'idiopathic' renal haemorrhage).
   d. Trauma.
6. Extravasation of contrast medium outside the kidney shadow.
   a. Trauma.

Table 11.1	Differential diagnoses for changes in renal opacification during intravenous urogram			
INITIAL OPACIFICATION	**SUBSEQUENT OPACIFICATION**			
Good	Progressive decrease	Normal		
Fair to good	Progressive increase	Systemic hypotension induced by the contrast medium	Contrast medium-induced renal failure	Acute renal obstruction
Fair to good	Persistent	Systemic hypotension induced by the contrast medium	Contrast medium-induced renal failure	Acute tubular necrosis
Poor	Progressive decrease	Insufficient contrast medium dose	Primary polyuric renal failure	Intravenous fluids given during the procedure
Poor	Progressive increase	Systemic hypotension prior to contrast medium administration	Renal ischaemia	Acute extrarenal obstruction
Poor	Persistent	Primary glomerular dysfunction	Severe acute or chronic renal disease	
Slow opacification of abnormal and poorly vascularized tissue		● Neoplasia ● Abscess ● Granuloma ● Haematoma ● Cyst		
None	None	Insufficient contrast medium dose	Prior nephrectomy or non-functional kidney	Renal aplasia Arterial obstruction or traumatic avulsion of renal artery

(After Feeney, D.A., Barber, D.L. and Osborne, C.A., 1982, Functional aspects of the nephrogram in excretion urography: a review. *Veterinary Radiology* 23, 42–45, with permission.)

11.9 ABNORMALITIES OF THE PYELOGRAM

The pyelogram (demonstrating renal diverticula, pelvis and ureters) should be visible approximately 1 min after the injection and persists for up to several hours. In the dog, the pelvis is usually ≤ 2 mm wide and diverticula ≤ 1 mm wide; figures are not available for cats.

1. Dilation of the renal pelvis ± diverticula.
   a. Caudal abdominal compression used.
   b. Physiological due to polyuria and polydipsia or intravenous fluid therapy.
   c. Diuresis due to hyperosomolar contrast medium, fluid therapy or drugs – bilaterally symmetrical and usually mild.
   d. Hydronephrosis – pelvic dilation may become very gross, with only a thin rim of surrounding parenchymal tissue (Fig. 11.3).
      – Idiopathic.

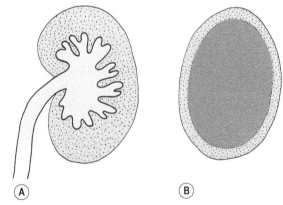

Figure 11.3 Hydronephrosis on intravenous urogram. (A) Mild hydronephrosis: slight distension and rounding of the renal pelvis and diverticula with dilation of the ureter. (B) Severe hydronephrosis: only a thin rim of parenchyma remains, opacified by its blood supply rather than by filtering urine. The ureter may not be visible if the kidney is non-functional. The radiographic signs depend on the degree of urine outflow obstruction and the duration of the condition.

- Secondary to ureteric obstruction (see 11.16.3).
e. Renal calculus (radiopaque calculi may be obscured by the similar radiopacity of the contrast medium).
f. Chronic pyelonephritis or pyonephrosis – filling defects may also be seen due to debris, and mild hydroureter may be present; often pelvis dilated only, not diverticula; ± irregular pelvic outline.
g. Renal neoplasia.
  - Secondary dilation of the pelvis and proximal ureter is often seen.
  - Mechanical obstruction of the pelvis.
h. Ectopic ureter – due to stenosis of the ureter ending and/or ascending infection (see 11.16.1 and Fig. 11.8).
i. Renal pelvic blood clot.
  - Coagulopathy.
  - Bleeding neoplasm.
  - Trauma.
  - After renal biopsy or antegrade pyelography.
  - Idiopathic renal haemorrhage.
j. *Dioctophyma renale** (giant kidney worm).
2. Distortion of the renal pelvis.
  a. Renal neoplasia (Fig. 11.4).
  b. Other renal parenchymal mass lesions (cyst, abscess, haematoma, granuloma).
  c. Large renal calculus.
  d. Chronic pyelonephritis.
  e. Blood clot.
    - Coagulopathy.

- Bleeding neoplasm.
- Trauma.
- After renal biopsy or antegrade pyelography.
- Idiopathic renal haemorrhage.
f. Polycystic kidney disease – heritable condition in long-haired cats, especially Persians and Persian crosses, and also in Cairn and Bull Terriers; usually bilateral.
3. Filling defects in the pyelogram.
  a. Normal interlobar blood vessels – linear radiolucencies within the diverticula.
  b. Air bubbles refluxed from overdistended pneumocystogram.
  c. Calculi.
  d. Debris due to pyelonephritis.
  e. Neoplasia.
  f. Blood clot.
  g. *Dioctophyma renale** (giant kidney worm).

11.10 ULTRASONOGRAPHIC EXAMINATION OF THE KIDNEYS

The kidneys may be examined from either a ventral abdominal or a flank approach. The advantages of the latter approach include the superficial location of the kidneys and the absence of intervening bowel. The main disadvantage is that the clipped areas of flank may be less acceptable to the owner.

A high-frequency (7.5 MHz) transducer should be used. Each kidney should be imaged in the transverse and either sagittal or dorsal (coronal) section, ensuring that the entire renal volume is examined. Where possible, the renal artery and vein entering and leaving the hilus should be identified.

11.11 NORMAL ULTRASONOGRAPHIC APPEARANCE OF THE KIDNEYS

The normal kidney is smooth and bean-shaped. A thin, echogenic capsule may be visible except at the poles, where the tissue interfaces are parallel to the ultrasound beam. The renal cortex is hypoechoic and finely granular in texture (Fig. 11.5). It is usually isoechoic or slightly hypoechoic relative to the liver if a 5 MHz transducer is used, but may appear mildly hyperechoic relative to the liver with a 7.5 MHz transducer or higher. The renal cortex should normally be less echogenic than the spleen. The renal medulla is usually virtually

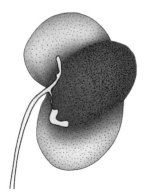

Figure 11.4 Renal tumour on intravenous urogram: normal cranial and caudal poles of the kidney, but a central bulging and poorly opacifying area with distortion of the renal pelvis.

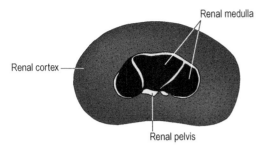

Figure 11.5 Normal ultrasonographic appearance of the kidney in the dorsal plane; the medulla is almost anechoic, the cortex is hypoechoic and fat in the renal pelvis is hyperechoic.

anechoic and divided into segments by the echogenic diverticula and interlobar vessels. A linear hyperechoic zone has been described, lying parallel to the corticomedullary junction in the medulla of some normal cats (medullary rim sign). Echogenic specks at the corticomedullary junction represent arcuate arteries. Fat in the renal sinus forms an intensely hyperechoic region at the hilus, which may cast a faint acoustic shadow.

The kidney size may be measured ultrasonographically, and normal size ranges are given for cats, being 37–44 mm long (the right kidney may be slightly larger than the left). In dogs, kidney size varies with body weight. The ratio of kidney length to aortic diameter may be calculated: renal size is considered to be reduced if kidney:aorta is < 5.5 and to be increased if kidney:aorta is > 9.1.

An increase in renal cross-sectional area is a sensitive indicator of acute renal allograft rejection in dogs and cats.

11.12 ABNORMALITIES OF THE RENAL PELVIS ON ULTRASONOGRAPHY

Causes of renal pelvic abnormalities are listed in Section 11.9, *Abnormalities of the pyelogram*, and the same principles apply to ultrasonography.

1. Pelvic dilation, leading to hydronephrosis – an anechoic accumulation of fluid is seen in the renal pelvis; as the severity of the dilation increases, there is progressive compression of the surrounding renal parenchyma (Fig. 11.6) and there may be associated ureteral dilation.
2. Distortion of the renal pelvis – less easy to recognize on ultrasonography than with an IVU.
3. Material within the pelvis, such as inflammatory debris, blood clots, neoplasm or calculi, result

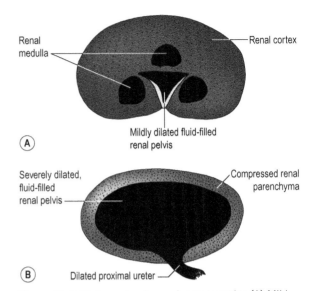

Figure 11.6 Hydronephrosis on ultrasonography. (A) Mild hydronephrosis: anechoic fluid is visible in the renal pelvis. (B) Severe hydronephrosis: a thin rim of parenchyma surrounds a large collection of fluid.

in masses of variable size and echogenicity; in the case of renal calculi, there is a strongly reflective surface with distal acoustic shadowing, irrespective of mineral composition. Multiple ring-like structures, 5–10 mm in diameter, have been described in the renal pelvis in *Dioctophyma renale** infection in the dog.

11.13 FOCAL PARENCHYMAL ABNORMALITIES OF THE KIDNEY ON ULTRASONOGRAPHY

1. Well-circumscribed, anechoic parenchymal lesion; simple or complex.
   a. Thin, smooth wall.
      – Cyst – single or multiple. PKD is heritable in long-haired cats, mainly Persians and Persian crosses, and also in Cairn and Bull Terriers, and may be associated with foci of mineralization and an indistinct corticomedullary junction. Cysts are also seen in familial nephropathy of Shih Tzus and Lhasa Apsos; solitary cysts may be seen in other breeds as incidental findings.
      – Hereditary multifocal renal cystadenoma or cystadenocarcinoma – complex, cystic structures; usually German Shepherd dogs, together with nodular dermatofibrosis lesions and uterine leiomyomas.

b. Thick or irregular wall.
  - Cyst.
  - Haematoma.
  - Abscess.
  - Neoplasia (e.g. renal cystadenoma or cystadenocarcinoma in the German Shepherd dog).

2. Hypoechoic parenchymal lesion.
  a. Neoplasia.
    - Lymphoma (nodular or wedge-shaped).
    - Malignant histiocytosis (although more commonly there is involvement of the liver, spleen and lymph nodes).
    - Mast cell infiltration.
    - Others (see 11.2.4).

3. Hyperechoic parenchymal lesion.
  a. Neoplasia.
    - Primary tumour containing blood or mineralization (e.g. haemangioma, chondrosarcoma).
    - Lymphoma.
    - Metastatic (e.g. haemangiosarcoma, thyroid adenocarcinoma).
  b. Chronic infarct (wedge-shaped).
  c. Parenchymal calcification or calculus.
  d. Parenchymal gas.
  e. A large number of very small cysts (Polycystic disease, PKD) – especially Persian and Persian cross cats; also reported in Cairn and Bull Terriers.
  f. Cats – FIP.

4. Heterogeneous or complex parenchymal lesion.
  a. Neoplasia.
    - Primary renal carcinoma.
    - Others (see 11.2.4).
  b. Abscess.
  c. Haematoma.
  d. Granuloma.
  e. Acute infarct.
  f. A large number of very small cysts (PKD) – especially Persian and Persian cross cats; also reported in Cairn and Bull Terriers.

5. Medullary rim sign – an echogenic line in the outer zone of the renal medulla that parallels the corticomedullary junction.
  a. Normal variant.
  b. Nephrocalcinosis, hypercalcaemic nephropathy.
  c. Ethylene glycol (antifreeze) toxicity.
  d. Chronic interstitial nephritis.
  e. Lymphoma.

f. Acute tubular necrosis.
g. Portosystemic shunt.
h. Leptospirosis.
i. Mineral deposit in tubule lumen.
j. Cats – FIP.

6. Acoustic shadowing.
  a. Deep to pelvic fat.
  b. Renal calculus – strongly reflective surface.
  c. Nephrolithiasis – reflective surface.
  d. Dystrophic mineralization of a chronic abscess or neoplasm.
  e. Gas.

11.14 DIFFUSE PARENCHYMAL ABNORMALITIES OF THE KIDNEY ON ULTRASONOGRAPHY

Corticomedullary definition may be increased or decreased, depending on whether only the cortex or both cortex and medulla are affected.

1. Increased cortical echogenicity, with retained or enhanced corticomedullary definition.
  a. Normal variant in cats (fat deposition in the tubules).
  b. Inflammatory disease.
    - Glomerulonephritis.
    - Interstitial nephritis.
    - Cats – FIP.
  c. End-stage renal disease – kidney also small and irregular.
  d. Acute tubular necrosis or nephrosis due to toxins, for example ethylene glycol (antifreeze) toxicity.
  e. Renal dysplasia – kidney also small and irregular.
  f. Nephrocalcinosis, hypercalcaemic nephropathy.
  g. Neoplasia.
    - Diffuse lymphoma (especially cats).
    - Metastatic squamous cell carcinoma.
  h. Amyloidosis.

2. Reduced corticomedullary definition.
  a. Chronic renal disease (end-stage kidneys).
  b. Renal dysplasia.
  c. Multiple small cysts.

11.15 PERIRENAL ABNORMALITIES ON ULTRASONOGRAPHY

Abnormal perirenal material may be identified on ultrasonography or IVU. On ultrasonography, the material is usually anechoic to hypoechoic but in

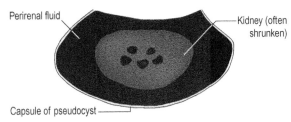

Figure 11.7 Perirenal fluid on ultrasonography: anechoic fluid outlines the kidney, which is often shrunken and hyperechoic with loss of corticomedullary definition.

some cases contains debris or is complex in echogenicity. Sonographically, subcapsular fluid may be difficult to distinguish from perirenal retroperitoneal fluid (Fig. 11.7), and both types of abnormality are considered in this section.

1. Perirenal or perinephric pseudocyst – especially elderly cats, usually unknown aetiology, although in one cat transitional cell carcinoma affecting the capsule was identified. Usually large amounts of unilateral or bilateral anechoic, subcapsular transudate. The kidneys are also often abnormal.
2. Perirenal abscess – affects cats more often than dogs; usually associated with pyelonephritis. Anechoic to hypoechoic perirenal fluid containing small specks of echogenic debris; usually unilateral.
3. Perirenal haemorrhage – unilateral or bilateral, depending on cause.
   a. Trauma.
   b. After renal biopsy.
   c. Coagulopathy.
   d. Neoplastic erosion of a blood vessel.
   e. Chronic expanding haematoma (rare) – complex sonographic appearance.
4. Neoplasia.
   a. Renal lymphoma in cats – a subcapsular hypoechoic rim is due to lymphoma infiltrate rather than free fluid; usually bilateral.
   b. Transitional cell carcinoma has been reported as producing unilateral subcapsular transudate in a cat.
5. Urinoma – anechoic fluid, secondary to rupture of the kidney or proximal ureter; usually unilateral.
6. Acute renal failure – anechoic fluid, ± renal abnormalities depending on the cause; usually bilateral.
7. Retroperitoneal fluid secondary to trauma or urethral obstruction with very full bladder.

URETERS

The ureters lie in the retroperitoneal space until they approach the bladder, where they enter the peritoneal cavity. They are not normally visible on plain radiographs unless they are markedly dilated, although occasionally they may be seen as fine, radiopaque lines in obese animals. An IVU or ultrasound-guided antegrade pyelography is required for the assessment of ureteric location, diameter, patency and integrity (see 11.5). Retrograde (vagino)urethrography is also helpful in demonstration of ectopic ureter endings. Normal ureters move urine to the bladder in peristaltic waves, so their diameter is variable and the entire ureter may not be visible on a single IVU radiograph. The normal termination of the ureter within the bladder wall is characteristically hook-shaped, the right normally lying slightly more cranially than the left (Fig. 11.8). IVU with CT is an excellent imaging modality for evaluation of the ureters.

Dislodged nephroliths may lead to ureteral obstruction and dilation but are easily mistaken for radiopaque bowel contents on plain radiographs. They may be obscured by contrast medium on IVU (confirming their location) or seen as filling defects. The osmotic diuresis caused by an IVU may also flush the calculi into the bladder.

Traumatic rupture of a ureter will result in uroretroperitoneum and/or uroabdomen with loss of visualization of retroperitoneal and/or abdominal detail. IVU shows contrast medium leakage; the

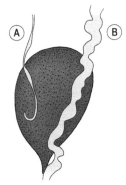

Figure 11.8 Normal and ectopic ureters shown by combined intravenous urogram and pneumocystogram. The normal ureter (A) is narrow and ends in a terminal hook in the trigone area of the bladder. The ectopic ureter (B) is dilated and tortuous, and extends caudal to the bladder neck.

site of leakage may be hard to identify, but the proximal ureter is likely to be dilated and hydronephrosis may ensue. Perirenal or paraureteral urinoma (uriniferous pseudocyst) is an occasional sequel, being a retroperitoneal accumulation of extravasated urine in a thick, fibrous sac. It is usually associated with ipsilateral hydronephrosis.

11.16 DILATED URETER

Not seen on plain radiographs unless the dilation is gross; otherwise requires an IVU or ultrasound-guided antegrade pyelography for demonstration (see 11.5). The normal canine ureter seen on an IVU is ≤ 3 mm in diameter, depending on the dog's size; ureters are very fine in the cat. Dilation of a ureter with urine due to obstruction is known as hydroureter.

1. Ectopic ureter – dilation due to stenosis at the ectopic ending and/or ascending infection (Fig. 11.8); unilateral or bilateral. The ureter usually opens into the urethra, occasionally vagina or rectum; the precise location may be shown using concomitant pneumocystogram and/or retrograde (vagino)urethrogram. In dogs, the ureter usually tunnels through the bladder wall to its ending, whereas in cats the ectopic ureters usually bypass the bladder. Absence of bladder opacification suggests that both ureters are ectopic, but the converse does not apply because urine from an ectopic ureter ending may seep cranially into the bladder. The ipsilateral kidney may be small and/or irregular, with hydronephrosis and associated pyelonephritis.
   a. Congenital – females usually show incontinence from a young age, although males may remain continent due to the longer urethra; females are affected more often than males, dogs more often than cats (especially Golden and Labrador Retrievers).
   b. Acquired (e.g. accidental ligation of the ureters with the uterine stump at ovariohysterectomy, leading to ureterovaginal fistula).
2. Ascending infection (the ureters may also be narrow and/or lacking peristalsis) – pyelonephritis may also be present, causing pelvic dilation and filling defects ± irregularity of the kidney outline.

3. Proximal to an acquired ureteric obstruction.
   a. Calculus dislodged from kidney.
   b. Ureteric stricture or obstruction.
      – Following calculus impaction.
      – Following trauma.
      – Blood clot in animals with renal haemorrhage or coagulopathy.
      – Uterine stump granuloma and adhesions.
      – Severe inflammation of the ureter.
      – Ureteric neoplasm or polyp.
      – Iatrogenic due to inadvertent ligation (e.g. during ovariohysterectomy).
   c. Any retroperitoneal or abdominal lesion causing extrinsic ureteric compression (e.g. bladder neck lesions, uterine stump granuloma, prostatic disease, retroperitoneal pathology).
4. Ureterocele – focal, cystic dilation of ureter at or near its entry into the bladder, often projecting into the bladder lumen; may cause hydroureter by obstruction. May also be at the termination of an ectopic ureter.
5. Ureteral diverticulum – small sacculation protruding from the lumen secondary to chronic, partial ureteral obstruction. Multiple, small diverticula of ≤ 1 mm diameter have also been reported.
6. Proximal to a congenital ureteric obstruction.
   a. Torsion, kinking, stenosis, stricture or atresia.
   b. Aberrant blood vessels encircling the ureter.
   c. Circumcaval (retrocaval) ureter.
7. Ureteral duplication has been described in two dogs (one complete, one incomplete); in the dog with complete duplication, one of the ureters ended blindly at the bladder and was markedly dilated and urine-filled.

11.17 NORMAL ULTRASONOGRAPHIC APPEARANCE OF THE URETERS

The normal ureters are not generally visible ultrasonographically, although their terminations in the trigone may be seen as small mounds. Periodic flow of urine from the ureters into the bladder (ureteric jets) can be demonstrated using colour flow techniques (or occasionally without colour if the specific gravity of the urine entering from the ureters differs significantly from that in the bladder) or after administration of furosemide.

11.18 DILATION OF THE URETER ON ULTRASONOGRAPHY

This is most clearly seen proximally, as the ureter leaves the kidney, or distally as it passes dorsal to the bladder. For differential diagnoses, see 11.16. Ureteric ectopia may be diagnosed in some cases by absence of the normal ureteric jet or urine or the ability to trace a dilated ureter to the urethra. Ureteroceles may also be seen on ultrasonography.

URINARY BLADDER

The urinary bladder is most easily seen on the lateral radiograph, outlined by fat. The neck of the bladder is located in the retroperitoneum and is more difficult to see than the more cranial portions, especially if overlain by hind limb musculature. In bitches, the bladder neck is located at or near the pelvic inlet; in entire male dogs, it is displaced cranially to a variable degree depending on the size of the prostate. In fat cats, the bladder may lie far cranially, with a long, thin soft tissue band extending to the pubis, representing the urethra.

11.19 NON-VISUALIZATION OF THE URINARY BLADDER

1. Technical factors.
   a. Obscured by hind limb musculature (lateral view), faeces (VD view) or the prepuce in male dogs (VD view).
   b. Underexposure.
2. Poor serosal detail (emaciation or ascites).
3. Small bladder.
   a. Normal – recent urination; may be partly intrapelvic.
   b. Severe cystitis.
   c. Bilateral ectopic ureters.
   d. Hypoplastic bladder.
4. Displacement through a hernia or rupture.
   a. Perineal.
   b. Inguinal.
   c. Body wall.
5. Urinary bladder rupture – free abdominal fluid with loss of serosal detail; more likely to rupture following trauma or obstruction in males than in females, due to the longer, narrower urethra.

Note that visualization of a bladder shadow does not rule out a small tear. Skeletal and thoracic injuries may also be present.

11.20 DISPLACEMENT OF THE URINARY BLADDER

Displacement of the bladder may result in urethral occlusion, diagnosed using retrograde urethrography.

1. Caudal displacement.
   a. Perineal hernia (usually male dogs); may retroflex.
   b. Short urethra syndrome or sphincter mechanism incompetence (usually bitches).
   c. Large abdominal mass.
2. Ventral displacement.
   a. Ventral abdominal wall weakness (e.g. hyperadrenocorticism), rupture or surgical dehiscence.
   b. Colonic distension.
      – Constipation or megacolon.
      – Colonic masses.
   c. Severe sublumbar lymphadenopathy or other swelling.
   d. Uterine or uterine stump enlargement.
   e. Paraprostatic cyst or asymmetrical prostatomegaly.
   f. Prepubic tendon rupture.
   g. Inguinal hernia.
3. Cranial displacement.
   a. Normal appearance in many cats, due to the long and sometimes poorly visible intra-abdominal urethra.
   b. Very full bladder, especially in animals with abdominal wall weakness.
   c. Prostatomegaly or paraprostatic cyst.
   d. Ruptured or avulsed urethra.
   e. Obesity – cats.
4. Dorsal displacement.
   a. Distended descending colon falling ventral to the bladder under gravity.
   b. Paraprostatic cyst or asymmetrical prostatomegaly.
   c. Retained testicle.
5. Lateral displacement.
   a. Normal on VD view.
   b. Distended descending colon.
   c. Paraprostatic cyst or asymmetrical prostatomegaly.
   d. Inguinal hernia.

11.21 VARIATIONS IN URINARY BLADDER SIZE

The bladder size is very variable, as it depends on the rate of urine production, time elapsed since last urination and degree of dysuria. House-trained animals may be reluctant to urinate in the confines of a veterinary hospital, and so large bladders are often seen on radiographs.

1. Large urinary bladder.
    a. Normal lack of urination, especially if polyuric.
    b. Non-obstructive urinary retention.
        – Psychogenic urinary retention.
        – Neurological dysfunction (e.g. cauda equina syndrome, dysautonomia; sacrocaudal luxation, especially in cats).
        – Orthopaedic disease or injury leading to reluctance or inability to adopt posture for urination.
        – Atonic following chronic distension.
    c. Outflow obstruction.
        – Bladder neck neoplasm (usually transitional cell carcinoma).
        – Large calculus lodged in the bladder neck.
        – Urethral calculus.
        – Urethral tumour.
        – Urethral stricture.
        – Mucosal slough.
        – Prostatic disease.
        – Neurological dysfunction (e.g. urethral spasm).
        – Penile urethral plug – male cats.
2. Small urinary bladder.
    a. Recent urination.
    b. Oliguria or anuria.
    c. Large tear in the bladder wall (free abdominal fluid present).
    d. Ureteric rupture (retroperitoneal and/or abdominal fluid present).
    e. Ectopic ureter(s).
    f. Non-distensible bladder due to disease or spasm.
        – Severe cystitis (see 11.27.2 and Fig. 11.12).
        – Diffuse bladder wall neoplasia.
    g. Hypoplastic bladder.

11.22 VARIATIONS IN URINARY BLADDER SHAPE

1. Artefactual due to superimposition of a paraprostatic cyst, or cyst mistaken for bladder.

2. Compression by adjacent structures.
3. Inadequate distension during contrast cystography.
4. Part-filled, atonic bladder.
5. Sphincter mechanism incompetence – bladder often elongated, rectangular or bilobed.
6. Recent bladder surgery.
7. Extensive bladder neoplasia.
8. Bladder rupture.
9. Diverticulum.
    a Congenital – usually apical and often associated with cystitis.
    b. Acquired due to trauma, outflow obstruction or previous surgery.
10. Spasticity due to trauma.
11. Persistent urachus – pointed bladder apex that may be patent; rare in small animals.

11.23 VARIATIONS IN URINARY BLADDER RADIOPACITY

Overlying objects (e.g. radiopacities in the small and large intestine, nipples and dirt in the hair coat) can be mistaken for bladder calculi. Additional radiographs made after urination, other views or simultaneous compression with a radiolucent paddle should help to differentiate opacities within the bladder from overlying structures.

1. Increased bladder radiopacity.
    a. Superimposed radiopaque objects.
    b. Radiopaque calculi – usually larger in females, as smaller ones are voided; may be associated with cystitis; central in bladder shadow.
    c. Dystrophic mineralization in a tumour – any location.
    d. Dystrophic mineralization secondary to severe cystitis – mainly cranioventral.
    e. Ballistics.
    f. Cats – crystalline debris (standing lateral radiographs may help to show abnormal sediment), although most bladder debris in cats is radiolucent.
2. Gas lucency associated with the bladder.
    a. Iatrogenic from catheterization or cystocentesis – most likely to be central in location on a recumbent lateral radiograph, as it rises to the highest level.
    b. Emphysematous cystitis – infection with gas-producing bacteria, predisposed to by diabetes mellitus; streaks of gas lucency

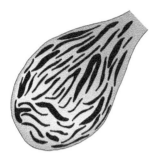

Figure 11.9 Emphysematous cystitis: streaks of gas lucency are seen in the region of the bladder.

associated with the bladder wall and ligaments (Fig. 11.9); ultrasound is more sensitive than radiography for the detection of small amounts of gas in the bladder wall.

11.24 URINARY BLADDER CONTRAST STUDIES: TECHNIQUE AND NORMAL APPEARANCE

Indications for contrast studies of the bladder include the following:

- Identification of location and integrity of the bladder.
- Investigation of caudal abdominal masses.
- Dysuria, stranguria, urinary tenesmus or pollakiuria.
- Haematuria or pyuria.
- Urinary retention.
- Urinary incontinence.

Cystography is used to demonstrate the location, integrity, wall thickness, luminal filling defects and mucosal detail of the urinary bladder. Different techniques can be used depending on the requirement of the examination (e.g. pneumocystography is used for bladder location, positive cystography for small ruptures and double-contrast cystography for mucosal detail and radiolucent calculi). Following contrast medium administration, VD, right and left lateral recumbent views and oblique radiographs should be obtained to demonstrate different areas of the bladder wall and lumen.

Bladder wall thickness is best assessed on a pneumocystogram or double-contrast study. The normal bladder wall is about 1–2 mm thick when the bladder is reasonably well distended. With a double-contrast study, the mucosal surface will be highlighted by a fine margin of contrast medium,

residual contrast pooling centrally (in the dependent area) as a 'contrast puddle', within which free luminal structures will be seen as filling defects. Note that the bladder may appear normal in acute cystitis.

Preparation

- Fasting to remove intestinal ingesta that may overlie the bladder.
- Enema, so that faeces do not indent or obscure the bladder.
- Sedation or anaesthesia of the patient, as appropriate.
- Plain lateral and VD radiographs.
- Bladder catheterization and urine drainage, noting the quantity removed (aids in establishing how much contrast can safely be instilled).

Pneumocystogram

Good for location and shape of the bladder. Shows large luminal filling defects, mural masses and marked increase in wall thickness. Poor for mucosal detail, small filling defects and minor changes in wall thickness; small tears may be overlooked, as escaping gas mimics intestinal gas.

The patient is laid in left lateral recumbency, as this reduces the risk of significant air embolism to the lungs. Fatal air emboli have been reported when the bladder was overinflated with air, especially in cats. The bladder is inflated slowly with room air until it feels turgid by abdominal palpation (cats, 10–40 mL; dogs, usually 50–300 mL depending on patient size and observation of the amount of urine removed). Oxygen, nitrous oxide or carbon dioxide can also be used. Both underdistension and overdistension must be avoided, as both can produce false diagnoses. To avoid overexposure, the mAs should be reduced by 30%.

Positive contrast cystography

Good for location and shape of the bladder and for detecting contrast leakage from the bladder or proximal urethra, although post-evacuation films may be required for detection of small leaks that are otherwise obscured. Adequate for assessment of wall thickness and large filling defects. Poor for small filling defects, which may be 'drowned' by contrast medium; poor for mucosal detail.

The bladder is inflated slowly using iodinated positive contrast medium, best diluted to approximately 100–150 mg I/mL to avoid irritation of bladder wall due to high osmolarity; alternatively, a non-ionic (low-osmolarity) contrast medium may be preferred. Positive cystography may be combined with a retrograde urethrogram as retrograde urethrocystography. To avoid underexposure, the mAs should be increased by 30%.

Double–contrast cystography

Good for all requirements; excellent for mucosal detail, because contrast medium will adhere to inflamed and ulcerated areas, and for detection of small filling defects, because free bodies will be seen within the central contrast puddle.

Between 2 and 20 mL of positive contrast medium is instilled depending on patient size, the patient rolled or the bladder area massaged to encourage coating of the bladder wall, and then the bladder is inflated with air. Alternatively, a positive contrast study can be performed first, excess contrast drained and then the bladder inflated with air.

Cystogram following intravenous urogram

Undertaken if bladder catheterization is impossible.

Following an IVU, positive contrast will enter the bladder and mix with urine. There is no control over the degree of bladder distension.

11.25 REFLUX OF CONTRAST MEDIUM UP A URETER FOLLOWING CYSTOGRAPHY

1. Normal in immature animals and occasionally observed in normal adults.
2. Contrast medium under high pressure.
   a. Overinflation of a normal bladder.
   b. Inflation of a poorly distensible bladder.
3. Cystitis (likely to predispose to pyelonephritis).
4. Neoplasia of the trigone of the bladder.
5. Previous ureteral transplant surgery.
6. Following accidental catheterization of an ectopic ureter followed by injection of contrast medium.

11.26 ABNORMAL BLADDER LUMEN ON CYSTOGRAPHY

1. Luminal opacities seen on pneumocystography.
   a. Calculi – usually lie in the centre of the bladder shadow in lateral recumbency.

Variable opacity and may easily be overexposed (use a bright light or adjust greyscale).
   b. Blood clot – irregular in outline; any location (may be attached to the bladder wall); soft tissue opacity. Differential diagnosis is mural masses – try flushing bladder with saline and repeating the cystogram.
   c. Bladder tumour – attached to the wall, usually near the dorsal aspect of the bladder neck (trigone); soft tissue opacity (Fig. 11.13).
   d. Polyp – smooth, pedunculated, soft tissue opacity.
2. Filling defects (relative lucencies) seen on double-contrast cystography (Fig. 11.10); with positive contrast studies, smaller structures are obscured by the contrast medium.
   a. Artefactual from overlying gas-filled bowel or incomplete bladder distension.
   b. Air bubbles – coalesce to produce a soap bubble appearance, lying in the centre of the bladder shadow on a positive contrast cystogram (rise to the highest point) and around the periphery of the contrast puddle on a double-contrast cystogram.
   c. Calculi – usually lie in the centre of the bladder shadow in lateral and dorsal recumbency. Radiolucent compared with contrast medium; may be obscured by large amounts of contrast medium so best seen with a double-contrast cystogram, in which they lie in the central contrast puddle.

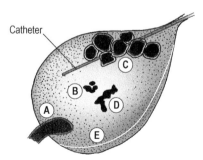

Figure 11.10 Various filling defects seen on double-contrast cystography. (A) Overlying gas-filled bowel. (B) Calculi in the centre of the contrast puddle. (C) Air bubbles around the periphery of the contrast puddle. (D) Blood clots: variable in location. (E) Mucosal slough. Air bubbles are the most distinctly marginated filling defects, calculi are semidistinct and blood clots are the least clearly outlined.

d. Blood clots.
 – Small, free clots may simulate the appearance of calculi.
 – Large, free clots produce irregular filling defects.
 – Clots attached to the bladder wall mimic tumours; may be dislodged on bladder flushing.
e. Mucosal slough – fine, linear filling defects or masses.
 – Severe cystitis, especially in cats.
 – Iatrogenic from poor catheterization technique.
f. Bladder wall neoplasm or polyp whose attachment to the wall is not seen in profile.

3. Altered luminal shape.
a. Small and/or irregular – incomplete distension.
b. Bladder wall lesions (see 11.27).
c. Diverticula (see 11.22.9); small vesicourachal diverticula at the bladder apex may be seen only on cystography; sometimes seen with cystitis but may also be incidental findings (Fig. 11.11).
d. Leakage of contrast medium into the bladder wall and peritoneal space.
 – Trauma.
 – Severe cystitis, especially in cats.
 – Post cystocentesis (occasional).

11.27 THICKENING OF THE URINARY BLADDER WALL ON CYSTOGRAPHY

Best seen on a double-contrast cystogram with the bladder distended to a normal size. However, chronic cystitis and neoplasia can result in a reduction in bladder capacity, so proceed with caution when trying to distend the bladder, especially when only a small volume of urine has been obtained on catheterization.

1. Diffuse bladder wall thickening with a smooth mucosal surface.
a. Normal, inadequately distended bladder.
b. Artefact – incomplete urine drainage prior to pneumocystography, resulting in a large gas bubble lying centrally above a pool of urine.
c. Chronic cystitis (mainly cranioventral).
d. Muscular hypertrophy due to chronic urinary outflow obstruction.
e. Diffuse mesenchymal neoplasia – unusual.

2. Diffuse bladder wall thickening with an irregular mucosal surface; abnormal contrast medium adherence may be present.
a. Chronic cystitis (mainly cranioventral) (Fig. 11.12) – more common in females than in males.
 – Idiopathic cystitis; common in cats and may lead to contrast leakage into the peritoneal cavity in the absence of bladder rupture.
 – Infectious.
 – Mechanical due to bladder calculi.
 – Chemical.
 – Traumatic.
 – Emphysematous – gas streaks seen too; usually diabetic animals.
b. Diffuse neoplasia – unusual.

3. Diffuse bladder wall thickening with a nodular mucosal surface.

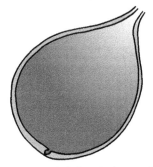

Figure 11.11 Vesicourachal diverticulum at the bladder apex, seen on cystography. The adjacent bladder wall is thickened as a result of chronic cystitis.

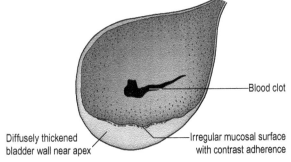

Blood clot

Diffusely thickened bladder wall near apex

Irregular mucosal surface with contrast adherence

Figure 11.12 Chronic cystitis on double-contrast cystography.

a. Ulcerative cystitis with adherent blood clots (usually cranioventral).
b. Polypoid cystitis (cranioventral or widespread).
c. Diffuse neoplasia – unusual.

4. Diffuse bladder wall thickening with contrast medium passing into or through the bladder wall.
   a. Small bladder tear.
   b. Urachal diverticulum (cranioventral; may be associated with chronic cystitis).
   c. Severe, ulcerative cystitis.
   d. Mucosal slough.

5. Focal bladder wall thickening.
   a. Neoplasia (usually but not always near the dorsal aspect of the bladder neck; Fig. 11.13); may cause hydroureter and hydronephrosis if the ureters are involved. Sublumbar lymphadenopathy, lumbosacral bony changes, pulmonary metastases and hypertrophic osteopathy may also be sequelae.
      – Epithelial types are more common (e.g. transitional cell carcinoma, squamous cell carcinoma, adenocarcinoma, papilloma); often a roughened surface with contrast adherence.
      – Mesenchymal types are less common (e.g. leiomyoma, leiomyosarcoma, rhabdomyosarcoma, fibrosarcoma, lymphoma, metastatic tumours); usually a smoother mucosal surface – rhabdomyosarcoma may occur in young dogs.
   b. Polyp or polypoid cystitis.
   c. Granuloma.
   d. Ureterocele – focal dilation of the ureter adjacent to or within the bladder wall at the trigone.

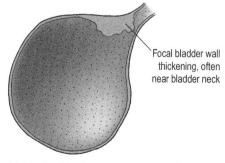

Focal bladder wall thickening, often near bladder neck

Figure 11.13 Bladder tumour on cystography.

11.28 ULTRASONOGRAPHIC EXAMINATION OF THE BLADDER

Ideally, urine should be present in the bladder, so avoid giving the patient the opportunity to urinate before carrying out the ultrasonographic examination.

The bladder is imaged from the caudal ventral abdominal wall, adopting a parapreputial approach in the male dog. A high-frequency (7.5 MHz) transducer should be used and placed just cranial to the pubic brim, moving cranially until the bladder is identified. A stand-off may be necessary to image the near wall. The bladder is imaged in both sagittal and transverse planes of section. If necessary, the position of the animal can be altered and/or imaging performed from the flank to ensure that all parts of the bladder wall and lumen are adequately evaluated.

The introduction of microbubbled saline into the bladder has been described as a technique for diagnosis of bladder rupture. The immediate presence of microbubbles in the fluid around the bladder is diagnostic of rupture.

11.29 NORMAL ULTRASONOGRAPHIC APPEARANCE OF THE BLADDER

The bladder should be oval or ellipsoid in shape with thin, smooth walls. The normal wall thickness is 1–2 mm when fully distended but may be up to 5 mm thick when empty. If a high-frequency transducer is used and the bladder is not full, three distinct wall layers may be seen – hyperechoic serosa, hypoechoic muscular layer and hyperechoic mucosa – producing a double reflective line. However, these layers are not usually clear in the distended bladder. The dorsal bladder wall may be hard to assess due to adjacent colonic gas and faeces. Indentation of the dorsal bladder wall by a full colon may mimic pathology, but reorientation of the scan plane from transverse to longitudinal will show change in shape of the structure from circular to linear, confirming its origin as colon.

11.30 THICKENING OF THE BLADDER WALL ON ULTRASONOGRAPHY

1. Focal bladder wall thickening – ultrasound-guided suction or brush biopsy may be possible.
   a. Neoplasm – the histological type cannot be determined by the ultrasonographic

appearance alone, but the following ultrasonographic features may give an indication of the most likely tumour type.

– Transitional cell carcinoma – single or multiple masses of complex echogenicity, usually irregular in shape and broad-based, most commonly located at the bladder neck, usually dorsally; usually highly vascular.

– Leiomyoma or leiomyosarcoma – most commonly single, smoothly marginated masses of reduced or mixed echogenicity that can involve any part of the bladder; no blood flow seen within the mass on Doppler examination.

– Lymphoma – homogeneous or heterogeneous, smoothly marginated masses that can involve any part of the bladder.

b. Polyp – may be single or multiple; usually well defined with a narrow point of attachment.

c. Granuloma.

d. Scarring and adhesions by mesentery at site of rupture or previous bladder surgery.

e. Artefact due to indentation of the dorsal bladder wall by the colon.

2. Diffuse bladder wall thickening – for differential diagnoses, see 11.27.

11.31 CHANGES IN ECHOGENICITY OF THE BLADDER WALL

1. Artefactual.
   a. Gas and faeces in the colon adjacent to the dorsal bladder wall.
   b. Calculi or sediment lying adjacent to the bladder wall.
2. Gas within the bladder wall produces bright echoes with reverberation; the location of the echoes within the bladder wall does not alter when the animal changes position.
3. Dystrophic mineralization also produces fixed, bright echoes within the bladder wall but tends to produce acoustic shadowing rather than reverberation.
   a. Neoplasm.
   b. Granuloma or abscess.
   c. Cyclophosphamide toxicity – if the dog does not urinate, mural necrosis occurs.

4. Suture material post cystotomy may create focal echogenicities within the bladder wall.

11.32 CYSTIC STRUCTURES WITHIN OR NEAR THE BLADDER WALL ON ULTRASONOGRAPHY

1. Distinct from the bladder lumen.
   a. Hydroureter (dorsal to bladder).
   b. Ureterocele (in the region of the trigone).
   c. Urachal cyst (cranial to bladder).
   d. Prostatic or paraprostatic lesions (see 11.54–11.56 and Fig. 11.20).
   e. Uterine or vaginal lesions (see 11.46 and Fig. 11.17).
2. Extending from the bladder lumen – diverticulum.
   a. Urachal (cranioventral bladder).
   b. Congenital (apical or trigone).
   c. Traumatic (any location).
   d. Stomatized ureterocele.

11.33 CHANGES IN URINARY BLADDER CONTENTS ON ULTRASONOGRAPHY

To distinguish dependent free luminal content from a mural mass, the bladder can be balloted, the animal can be scanned standing up or a cystocentesis can be performed and some of the urine withdrawn squirted back into the bladder.

1. Small, scattered echoes within the anechoic urine.
   a. Artefact – slice thickness or reverberation artefact.
   b. Sediment.
      – Blood or cellular debris.
      – Crystalline material (may be normal).
   c. Air bubbles (usually secondary to cystocentesis).
2. Hypo- or hyperechoic mass, non-shadowing.
   a. Blood clot (may be free in the lumen or adherent to the wall).
   b. Polyp or neoplasm (can usually be shown to be attached to wall).
   c. Mucosal slough (linear or mass-like).
3. Hyperechoic mass, shadowing.
   a. Artefact – full colon impinging on the bladder.
   b. Calculus (in the dependent part of the bladder).
   c. Calcified mural mass.

URETHRA AND VAGINA

The male and female urethra are not visible on plain radiographs. Radiopaque calculi may be seen in the region of the urethra, and mineralized structures in the distal urethral area may be due to a vestigial os penis in an intersex (hermaphrodite or pseudohermaphrodite) animal. In male dogs, the os penis is seen; its base may appear roughened or fragmented due to the presence of separate centres of ossification, mimicking urethral calculi. Large, intrapelvic masses associated with the urethra may be seen to displace the rectum, but further evaluation of the urethra requires examination with contrast medium.

11.34 URETHRAL AND VAGINAL CONTRAST STUDIES: TECHNIQUE AND NORMAL APPEARANCE

Indications for urethral contrast studies include the following:

- Urinary incontinence (for ectopic ureters and urethral length).
- Urinary retention.
- Stranguria, dysuria, urinary tenesmus, haematuria or vulval or penile bleeding.
- Investigation of suspected prostatic disease.
- Investigation of intrapelvic and caudal abdominal masses.
- Investigation of suspected vestibular and vaginal lesions.
- Investigation of intersex animals.
- After pelvic trauma.

Retrograde urethrography (males) and retrograde vaginourethrography (females) are used to examine the urethra, and with larger quantities of contrast medium the bladder will also be demonstrated (retrograde urethrocystography).

In the male animal, the urethra is seen as a smoothly bordered tube with occasional symmetrical narrowing due to peristalsis (Fig. 11.14A). In male dogs, the prostatic urethra is often of wider diameter than the rest and lies slightly dorsal to the centre of the gland. In the bitch, the urethra appears very narrow and the vestibule and vagina are spindle-shaped, terminating in a spoon-shaped cervix (in both intact and neutered animals) (Fig. 11.14B). The vagina may be shorter in neutered bitches than in entire animals. Voiding urethrography during manual compression of the bladder is possible but creates radiation hazard for the operator.

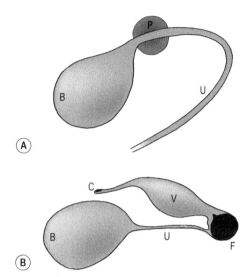

Figure 11.14 (A) Normal retrograde urethrogram: male dog (B, bladder; P, prostate; U, urethra). (B) Normal retrograde vaginourethrogram: bitch (B, bladder; C, cervix; F, bulb of Foley catheter; U, urethra; V, vagina).

Preparation

- Enema to empty the rectum and distal colon of faeces.
- The urinary bladder should be reasonably full of urine or contrast medium to create a little backflow resistance and encourage urethral distension (in cats with feline lower urinary tract disease, the retrograde study should be performed before catheterizing the bladder).
- Sedation or anaesthesia of the patient, as appropriate.
- Tilting the table to elevate the animal's head will increase the abdominal pressure on the urethra and may improve filling.
- Plain lateral and VD radiographs: care must be taken not to misidentify the pelvic floor as the urethra on the lateral view, so comparison of the urethrogram with precontrast films is important.
- Prefill the catheter with contrast medium to avoid the introduction of air bubbles during the injection.

Retrograde urethrography (males)

The urethra is catheterized with the catheter tip lying distal to the area of interest. The external urethral orifice is occluded by a soft clamp during injection or by the use of a balloon catheter.

Iodinated contrast medium (used alone or mixed with an equal quantity of K-Y Jelly) is injected at a dose rate of about 1 mL/kg of body weight. Air should not be used, as it can occasionally enter the corpus cavernosum of the penis. The exposure is made as soon as possible after injection consistent with radiation safety of the operator.

In the male dog, different positions, centring points and exposures may be needed to show different areas of the urethra in lateral recumbency. Oblique VD views are used to avoid superimposition of the penile and prostatic urethra.

Retrograde vaginourethrography (females)

In bitches, a standard or Foley catheter is inserted between the lips of the vulva and held in place with a soft clamp. If using a Foley, the tip of the catheter distal to the bulb is cut off to prevent it entering the vagina and occluding the urethra, and the bulb is inflated. In cats, it may not be possible to use a Foley catheter. An alternative procedure is to inject contrast medium as the catheter is withdrawn from the bladder.

Then, 1 mL/kg of body weight of iodinated contrast medium is injected carefully (vaginal rupture has been reported in Rough Collies and Shetland Sheepdogs). Larger volumes may be required in bitches in season and those with pyometra. Lateral and oblique VD radiographs are obtained.

For vaginal masses and strictures, air alone may be adequate (pneumovaginography).

11.35 ABNORMALITIES OF THE (VAGINO)URETHROGRAM

1. Short or absent urethra with caudally displaced bladder neck.
   a. Sphincter mechanism incompetence, although radiographs may also be normal, and this is a functional disease and not a radiographic diagnosis: radiography is mainly used to rule out ectopic ureters in incontinent animals, although in most continent bitches the bladder neck is at or cranial to the pubic brim, and with sphincter mechanism incompetence it lies more caudally.
   b. Urethral hypoplasia.
   c. Intersexuality (e.g. common vagina and urethra).

2. Urethral filling defects.
   a. Air bubbles accidentally injected into the urethra (will not distend its lumen and will move freely up the urethra into the bladder).
   b. Calculi (may distend the urethra) – more common in males; often at the ischial arch or caudal os penis (in the latter site, mimicked by multiple centres of ossification).
   c. Blood clots.
   d. Urethral plugs in male cats.
   e. Urethral neoplasia – more common in bitches and rare in cats; usually transitional cell carcinoma, although a number of other types are reported. May also involve the bladder neck. The rectum may be elevated if a significant mass arises in the intrapelvic urethra.

3. Urethral stricture – may be associated with urinary retention.
   a. Simulated by a peristaltic wave or inadequate distension – repeat the radiograph to see whether it is consistent.
   b. Previous calculus impaction.
   c. Previous surgery or trauma.
   d. Prostatic disease, especially neoplasia.
   e. Urethral or periurethral neoplasia.
   f. Severe urethritis.

4. Urethral mucosal surface irregularity.
   a. Urethral or prostatic neoplasia (Fig. 11.15).
   b. Severe urethritis.

5. Urethral displacement.
   a. Adjacent or encircling mass.
   b. Perineal or inguinal hernia and bladder displacement.
   c. Asymmetric prostatic disease.
      – Prostatic retention cyst(s).
      – Prostatic abscess.
      – Prostatic neoplasia.

6. Contrast medium extravasation or extension outside the urethra.
   a. Normal – small amount of extravasation into prostatic ductules in male dogs.
   b. Artefact – leakage of contrast medium on to the hair coat.
   c. Contrast medium may occasionally enter uterine horns, especially during oestrus; Differential diagnosis is ectopic ureter.
   d. Urethrotomy or urethrostomy.
   e. Urethral rupture.

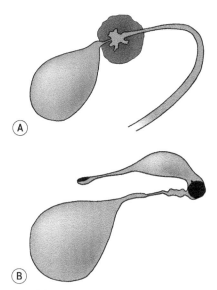

Figure 11.15 (A) Prostatic neoplasia seen on retrograde urethrography: extravasation of contrast medium, urethral stricture and irregular prostatic outline (cf. Fig. 11.14A). (B) Urethral neoplasia seen on retrograde vaginourethrography: narrow and irregular urethra (cf. Fig. 11.14B).

   – Trauma.
   – Iatrogenic from poor catheterization technique.
f. Urethral fistula, usually to rectum or vagina.
   – Congenital.
   – Acquired.
g. Prostatic disease.
   – Cystic hyperplasia.
   – Cystic prostatitis.
   – Prostatic neoplasia.
   – Prostatic abscess.
h. Urethral duplication ± cyst formation.
i. Into cavities representing Müllerian duct remnants in intersex dogs.
7. Vaginal abnormalities.
   a. Congenital.
      – Vestibulovaginal stenosis.
      – Stricture.
      – Partial or complete aplasia.
      – Persistent hymen.
      – Secondary vaginal pouch (vaginal diverticulum, double vagina).
      – Vaginal cyst.
      – Conformational abnormalities in intersex animals.

   b. Filling defects.
      – Cyst.
      – Polyp.
      – Neoplasia – various types, benign or malignant; leiomyoma most common.
   c. Ectopic ureters entering the vagina.
   d. Poor distensibility or mucosal irregularity.
      – Vaginitis.
      – Vaginal neoplasia.
   e. Vaginal enlargement – may produce an intrapelvic or caudal abdominal soft tissue mass.
      – Hyperplasia.
      – Oestrogen treatment.
      – Neoplasia.
      – Hydrocolpos – accumulation of uterine and vaginal secretions due to a congenital vaginal obstruction.
      – Secondary vaginal pouch.
   f. Contrast leakage.
      – Vaginal rupture – can be iatrogenic during retrograde vaginourethrography.
      – Vaginoperitoneal fistula after ovariohysterectomy – may be an incidental finding.

11.36 ULTRASONOGRAPHY OF THE URETHRA AND VAGINA

There is limited ultrasonographic visualization of the pelvic urethra unless a high-frequency rectal or vaginal transducer is available. From a ventral abdominal approach, the prostatic urethra may be visible in the male dog. The male urethra distal to the ischial arch can be imaged percutaneously.

Similarly, the vagina is not normally seen ultrasonographically. A large vaginal mass may be seen in the caudal abdomen dorsal to the bladder.

FEMALE GENITAL TRACT

OVARIES

Normal ovaries are not visible radiographically. Ovarian masses are usually located caudal to the ipsilateral kidney but are intraperitoneal and may migrate ventrally if large.

11.37 OVARIAN ENLARGEMENT

For the radiographic appearance of ovarian masses, see 9.39.7.

1. Mimicked by other mid-abdominal masses – use contrast techniques or ultrasonography to investigate further.
   a. Composite shadow – take orthogonal view.
   b. Enlarged kidney.
   c. Enlarged lymph node.
   d. Small intestinal mass.
2. Ovarian neoplasia – abdominal effusion may also be present.
   a. Granulosa cell tumour.
   b. Teratoma – may contain mineralized material.
   c. Dysgerminoma.
   d. Adenoma or adenocarcinoma.
   e. Metastasis.
   f. Others.
3. Ovarian cyst or cystadenoma – may develop a calcified rim.
4. Ovarian bursal abscess – may be associated with peritonitis.

11.38 ULTRASONOGRAPHIC EXAMINATION OF THE OVARIES

Ultrasonographic examination may be carried out with the animal in dorsal or lateral recumbency. A high-frequency (7.5 MHz) transducer is used and each kidney identified. The region caudal and ventral to the caudal pole of each kidney is then searched. The ovaries may be particularly difficult to identify during anoestrus.

11.39 NORMAL ULTRASONOGRAPHIC APPEARANCE OF THE OVARY

In anoestrus, the ovary is smoothly rounded and uniformly hypoechoic relative to the surrounding fat. Multiple follicles develop during pro-oestrus; these are thin-walled and anechoic. During oestrus and dioestrus, the follicles regress and corpora lutea develop, but immature corpora lutea and follicles have a very similar ultrasonographic appearance. Mature corpora lutea appear oval and hypoechoic.

11.40 OVARIAN ABNORMALITIES ON ULTRASONOGRAPHY

1. Rounded foci, anechoic contents, thin walls – benign cysts. May be single or multiple, uni- or bilateral.
   a. Non-functional.
   b. Functional.
2. Rounded foci, hypoechoic contents, thick irregular walls.
   a. Neoplasia with a cystic component.
   b. Haemorrhagic cyst.
   c. Abscess.
3. Hyperechoic foci (± shadowing).
   a. Teratoma containing fat, bone or tooth.
   b. Dystrophic mineralization (other tumours).
4. Solid mass, variable echogenicity.
   a. Neoplasia.

UTERUS

A normal, non-gravid uterus is not seen radiographically except in very obese dogs, in which it may be outlined by fat. Mild uterine enlargement is best seen as a tubular soft tissue structure ventral to the descending colon and dorsal to the bladder neck; more cranially, the uterine horns mimic fluid-filled small intestine. When enlargement of the uterine horns exceeds the diameter of small intestine, they may be seen as convoluted soft tissue structures cranial to the bladder. On the VD view, an enlarged uterus can give rise to kidney-shaped radiopacities (the 'extra kidney' sign).

11.41 UTERINE ENLARGEMENT

1. Generalized uterine enlargement (Fig. 11.16).
   a. Fluid-filled small intestine mistaken for uterus.
   b. Normal, gravid uterus prior to detection of fetal mineralization (cats < 35 days' gestation, dogs < 41 days' gestation). A lobular shape may be noted by mid-pregnancy.
   c. Normal *post-partum* uterus – the involuting uterus will remain visible for at least a week after parturition.

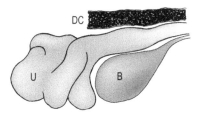

Figure 11.16 Uterine enlargement: the descending colon and bladder are separated by a soft tissue viscus, which continues cranial to the bladder. B, bladder; DC, descending colon; U, uterus.

   d. Pyometra – the commonest cause of pathological generalized enlargement.
   e. Haematometra.
   f. Hydrometra or mucometra.
     – Secondary to uterine neoplasia or endometrial hyperplasia.
     – Obstructive – absence of internal cervical os.
   g. Uterine torsion – gravid uterus or other uterine distension (e.g. haematometra).
2. Focal uterine enlargement.
   a. Small litter size.
   b. Mid-pregnancy, before fetal ossification.
   c. Pyometra localized to one uterine horn or entrapped in inguinal hernia (metrocele).
   d. Stump pyometra or granuloma – mass lesion dorsal or craniodorsal to the bladder neck.
   e. Uterine neoplasia.
     – Leiomyo(sarco)mas, especially in German Shepherd dogs with renal hereditary multifocal cystadenoma or cystadenocarcinoma and nodular dermatofibrosis.
     – Adenocarcinoma.
     – Fibroadenoma.
     – Lipoma.
     – Others.
   f. Adenomyosis – enlarged, ectopic uterine glands.
   g. Uterine torsion – single horn.

11.42 VARIATIONS IN UTERINE RADIOPACITY

Fetal mineralization will be detected from about 35 days' gestation in the cat and 41 days in dogs. It is easier to detect on lateral radiographs, because the spine is partly superimposed over the abdomen on the VD view. Increasing bone opacity develops during the last trimester – the skull, vertebrae and long bones are the most apparent. Just before parturition, mineralization of the bones of the paws will become visible. Assessment of fetal numbers is best achieved by counting the number of skulls.

1. Increased uterine radiopacity – mineralization.
   a. Mimicked by gastrointestinal mineralization from an ingested bird, rodent, fetus or other foreign object.
   b. Third trimester pregnancy.
   c. Fetal mummification, especially if ectopic – coiled and dense fetal skeletal remnants.
2. Decreased uterine radiopacity – gas.
   a. Mimicked by overlying gastrointestinal gas.
   b. Fetal death – gas in fetal heart cavities or cranial cavity.
   c. Emphysematous pyometra (physometra) – gas in the uterus due to metritis and/or fetal death; differential diagnosis is intestinal ileus – rule out using gastrointestinal contrast study.

11.43 RADIOGRAPHIC SIGNS OF DYSTOCIA AND FETAL DEATH

Radiographs are useful to evaluate the number of fetuses, their size relative to the pelvic diameter, their presentation to the pelvic canal and the size and shape of the pelvic canal. Live fetuses normally lie in a neutral or semiflexed position. Ultrasonography is needed to check for fetal distress or recent death, because radiographs will be normal.

1. Fetal oversize – pregnancy with single or few fetuses tends to result in larger fetuses, which are more likely to lead to dystocia.
2. Fetal malpresentation (e.g. lying at the pelvic inlet but with head or limb back).
3. Maternal dystocia.
   a. Uterine inertia – fetuses normal but none close to pelvic inlet.
   b. Physical obstruction (e.g. small pelvic canal or pelvic fracture malunion).
4. Fetal death.
   a. Fetal or uterine gas.
   b. Abnormal position of the fetus (e.g. hyperextension).
   c. Disintegration of the fetus.

d. Overlapping of cranial bones – Spalding's sign.

e. Demineralization of fetal bones.

f. Mummification – dense, compacted fetuses.

11.44 ULTRASONOGRAPHIC EXAMINATION OF THE UTERUS

The cervix and body of the uterus are located dorsal to the bladder and ventral to the descending colon. The uterine horns cranial to the bladder are not usually recognized unless distended; they are typically less than 1 cm in diameter and are hidden among the small intestine and mesenteric fat.

11.45 NORMAL ULTRASONOGRAPHIC APPEARANCE OF THE UTERUS

The normal non-gravid uterus is a hypoechoic tubular structure with a focal thickening at the cervix. A central linear echo may be apparent during pro-oestrus, oestrus and dioestrus.

During pregnancy, the uterus begins to enlarge within days. This is, however, a non-specific effect due to hormonal changes. Pregnancy can be positively confirmed only when gestational sacs (comprising the fetus surrounded by fetal fluids and membranes) become visible – at around 20–25 days after the last mating and sometimes earlier. Fetal cardiac activity and generalized fetal movements indicate viability. As pregnancy progresses, the fetus grows and differentiation of fetal organs and mineralization of the fetal skeleton become apparent. Following parturition, the involuting uterus remains detectable for 3–4 weeks.

11.46 VARIATION IN UTERINE CONTENTS ON ULTRASONOGRAPHY

1. Anechoic uterine contents (fluid).
   a. Early pregnancy (10–20 days post mating, before the fetus is visible).
   b. Pyometra.
   c. Haematometra.
   d. Hydrometra or mucometra.
2. Hypoechoic uterine contents (fluid containing variable quantities of swirling echoes).
   a. Pyometra (Fig. 11.17).
   b. Haematometra.
   c. Mucometra.

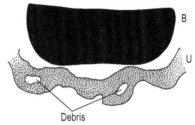

Figure 11.17 Pyometra on ultrasonography: a hypoechoic tubular structure deep to the anechoic bladder. B, bladder; U, uterus.

3. Mixed echogenicity uterine contents.
   a. Normal pregnancy (defined fetal structures surrounded by fluid, with fetal cardiac activity).
   b. Dead fetuses (fetal structure becomes progressively less well defined as decomposition or mummification occurs, no fetal cardiac activity).
   c. Pyometra (fluid with unstructured debris).
   d. Post-partum uterus (fluid with unstructured debris).

11.47 THICKENING OF THE UTERINE WALL ON ULTRASONOGRAPHY

1. Diffuse thickening of the uterine wall.
   a. Early pregnancy.
   b. Post partum.
   c. Endometritis or cystic endometrial hyperplasia (may be heterogeneous; may see multiple, small cysts).
2. Focal thickening of the uterine wall – may be isoechoic with the surrounding uterine wall or of complex echogenicity; may have a cystic component.
   a. Uterine neoplasia.
   b. Uterine granuloma or abscess.

MALE GENITAL TRACT

PROSTATE

Radiographic examination of the male reproductive organs is limited to the prostate gland and testes in male dogs. In cats, the prostate is very small and prostatic disease is rare. The prostate lies in the caudal retroperitoneum caudal to the bladder neck and ventral to the descending colon. It is normally smooth, rounded and bilobed, and encircles the urethra symmetrically. As it enlarges, it displaces the bladder cranially, and a larger proportion will be seen cranial to the pelvic brim. Prostate size is variable and related to age, breed, presence of disease and benign hyperplasia, which occurs from middle age. The prostate is less well seen on VD radiographs and is therefore best assessed on lateral views. Radiography is insensitive for precise diagnosis of prostatic disease, because different conditions can produce similar changes (e.g. increase in size) or may coexist. Prostatic disease can be investigated further using retrograde urethrography to assess the location, diameter and integrity of the prostatic urethra (see 11.33, 11.34 and Figs 11.1 and 11.14). Ultrasonographic examination of the prostate often yields further information and allows guided aspiration or biopsy.

11.48 VARIATIONS IN LOCATION OF THE PROSTATE

1. Cranial displacement of the cranial margin of the prostate.
   a. Full bladder.
   b. Ventral abdominal wall weakness (e.g. hyperadrenocorticism), rupture or surgical dehiscence.
   c. Prostatomegaly (see 11.49.2).
2. Caudal displacement of the prostate.
   a. Small and often intrapelvic in castrated dogs (not usually visible).
   b. Perineal hernia.

11.49 VARIATIONS IN PROSTATIC SIZE

Prostatic size can be assessed on a lateral radiograph by comparing the craniocaudal prostate dimension to the pelvic inlet dimension (the distance between the cranioventral border of the sacrum and the cranial tip, or promontory, of the pubis). In normal entire males, the craniocaudal prostate dimension should not exceed 70% of the pelvic inlet dimension (Fig. 11.18). Prostatic size increases until middle age and then decreases again. Severe prostatomegaly may compress the descending colon, leading to faecal tenesmus and

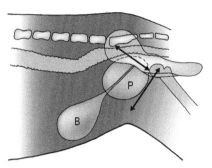

Figure 11.18 Measurement of prostatic size. The craniocaudal prostatic dimension should not exceed 70% of the pelvic inlet dimension. This figure shows prostatomegaly, with cranial displacement of the bladder and dorsal displacement of the colon. B, bladder; P, prostate.

obstipation, and may also cause chronic dysuria and urinary retention.

1. Normal size.
   a. Normal prostate.
   b. Enlargement due to disease in a dog previously castrated.
   c. Neoplasia – may be present without obvious enlargement.
   d. Prostatitis.
2. Enlarged prostate.
   a. Normal size but cranial displacement due to a full bladder or abdominal wall weakness.
   b. Benign prostatic hyperplasia – smooth, symmetrical about the urethra, remains bilobed; common in entire, middle-aged male dogs.
   c. Squamous metaplasia – smooth and symmetrical; associated with oestrogen-producing testicular neoplasia or administration of oestrogens.
   d. Prostatitis – irregular, ill-defined ± caudal abdominal peritonitis.
   e. Large intraprostatic cyst(s) – may be asymmetric about the urethra.
   f. Prostatic abscess(es) – may be asymmetric about the urethra.
   g. Prostatic neoplasia – older entire or neutered dogs; may be asymmetric about the urethra and spread to bladder; the commonest cause of prostatic urethral stricture; may see periosteal new bone on caudal lumbar spine, sacrum, tail base and pelvis (see 5.4.3 and Fig. 5.7), lung and skeletal metastases.
      – Adenocarcinoma.

- Extension of bladder transitional cell carcinoma.
- Other types are unusual.
3. Small or non-visible prostate.
   a. Poor radiographic technique (e.g. hind legs not pulled far enough caudally).
   b. Normal.
      - Young dog – prostate small and intrapelvic.
      - Castrated dog.
      - Aged entire dog – atrophy.
      - Emaciation – lack of fat to outline prostate.
   c. Caudal displacement.
      - Perineal hernia.
   d. Chronic prostatitis.

11.50 VARIATIONS IN PROSTATIC SHAPE AND OUTLINE

Benign hyperplasia and squamous metaplasia remain symmetrical and smooth in outline.

1. Asymmetry of the prostate about the urethra.
   a. Prostatic abscess.
   b. Prostatic neoplasia.
   c. Large intraprostatic cyst.
   d. Paraprostatic cyst – cystic vestiges of the Müllerian duct (uterus masculinus) or may arise from prostatic retention cysts or neoplasia; single or multiple, may calcify. Large paraprostatic cysts may be hard to differentiate from the bladder without cystography or ultrasonography (Fig. 11.19).
2. Irregularity or loss of clarity of the prostatic margins; loss of clarity arises due to surrounding inflammation.
   a. Prostatitis.
   b. Prostatic abscess (may rupture).
   c. Large intraprostatic cyst(s).
   d. Prostatic neoplasia.

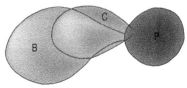

Figure 11.19 Paraprostatic cyst: 'extra bladder' shadow. B, bladder; C, paraprostatic cyst; P, prostate.

11.51 VARIATIONS IN PROSTATIC RADIOPACITY

1. Increased prostatic radiopacity – mineralization.
   a. Eggshell-like rim radiopacity.
      - Paraprostatic cyst (may be intra-abdominal, intrapelvic or perineal).
      - Resolving abscess.
   b. Irregular patches or nodules of mineralization.
      - Dystrophic mineralization due to neoplasia; neutered dogs with prostatic mineralization are very likely to have prostatic neoplasia.
      - Parts of paraprostatic cysts, including mineralized stalk.
      - Severe, chronic prostatitis.
      - Prostatic calculi – may be incidental.
2. Decreased prostatic radiopacity – gas.
   a. Normal – iatrogenic reflux of air into prostatic ductules during pneumocystography.
   b. Cystic prostatitis.
   c. Abscessation.
   d. Prostatic neoplasia with pneumocystogram performed.

11.52 ULTRASONOGRAPHIC EXAMINATION OF THE PROSTATE

No special patient preparation is required, although it can be useful to allow defecation before the examination. A high-frequency (7.5 MHz, or in large dogs, 5 MHz) transducer is placed on one side of the prepuce, cranial to the pubic brim, to locate the bladder. Having found the bladder neck, the transducer is moved caudally to identify the prostate. If the prostate is small or intrapelvic, it may be helpful to push it forwards gently using a gloved finger per rectum. The prostate is imaged in both the sagittal and the transverse planes of section, ensuring that the entire volume of the gland is imaged.

A transrectal approach can be used to image the prostate if an appropriate transducer is available.

11.53 NORMAL ULTRASONOGRAPHIC APPEARANCE OF THE PROSTATE

The normal canine prostate is smooth in outline and oval or bilobed in shape. The parenchyma is moderately echoic with an evenly granular texture. A central linear echo, the hilar echo, may be evident. The open prostatic urethra is usually seen only in sedated or anaesthetized animals or if there is urethral obstruction further distally.

For differential diagnoses related to changes in size of the prostate, see 11.49.

11.54 FOCAL PARENCHYMAL CHANGES OF THE PROSTATE ON ULTRASONOGRAPHY

1. Anechoic contents, smooth thin walls.
   a. Intraprostatic cyst.
      – < 1 cm diameter considered normal and may be seen with benign hyperplasia.
      – Prostatic retention cysts.
      – Cysts associated with squamous metaplasia.
   b. Haematocyst.
   c. Abscess.
2. Anechoic or hypoechoic contents, thick irregular walls.
   a. Abscess.
   b. Neoplasm with necrotic centre or cystic component.
3. Hypoechoic nodules.
   a. Neoplasia – more commonly involves most or all of the prostate by the time of presentation.
4. Hyperechoic foci.
   a. Prostatic calculus.
   b. Focal calcification (see 11.51.1).
   c. Gas within cavitating lesion.
      – Abscess.
      – Necrotic neoplasm.
      – Cyst.

11.55 DIFFUSE PARENCHYMAL CHANGES OF THE PROSTATE ON ULTRASONOGRAPHY

1. Normal echogenicity and echotexture.
   a. Normal prostate.
   b. Benign prostatic hyperplasia.
   c. Squamous metaplasia.
2. Increased echogenicity, uniform echotexture.
   a. Benign prostatic hyperplasia.
   b. Squamous metaplasia.
3. Increased echogenicity, heterogeneous echotexture.

a. Chronic bacterial prostatitis.
   b. Granulomatous prostatitis (blastomycosis*, cryptococcosis*).
   c. Neoplasia (may contain focal mineralization, leading to acoustic shadowing).
4. Decreased echogenicity, heterogeneous echotexture.
   a. Acute inflammation or abscessation.
   b. Neoplasia (less common); prostatic lymphoma is rare, but multiple ill-defined hypoechoic nodules have been described.

11.56 PARAPROSTATIC LESIONS ON ULTRASONOGRAPHY

1. Paraprostatic cysts – vary in appearance from simple cysts to complex septated structures (Fig. 11.20). May be multiple and can be difficult to distinguish from the urine-filled bladder. Variable mineralization of the cyst wall may produce acoustic shadowing. Concurrent benign or malignant prostatic disease may be present.
2. Retained testicle (may become neoplastic or torse).
3. Other caudal abdominal masses (see 9.40).

TESTES

11.57 ULTRASONOGRAPHIC EXAMINATION OF THE TESTES

The testicles normally lie in the scrotum and so may be imaged by placing a high-frequency transducer directly on the scrotal skin. If a testicle is not fully descended, then a search may be made, starting in the inguinal region and progressing to the abdominal cavity. Within the abdomen, the testicle most commonly lies near the bladder but

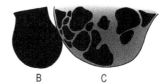

Figure 11.20 Paraprostatic cyst on ultrasonography. Internal septation is often seen, with variable amounts of solid tissue. B, bladder; C, paraprostatic cyst.

may lie anywhere between the kidneys and the bladder.

11.58 NORMAL ULTRASONOGRAPHIC APPEARANCE OF THE TESTES

The normal canine testis is smoothly rounded and moderately echoic with an even, granular echotexture. A central linear echo may be seen, representing the mediastinum testis. The epididymis, found at the head and tail of the testis, is less echoic and more coarsely textured.

11.59 TESTICULAR ABNORMALITIES ON ULTRASONOGRAPHY

1. Focal parenchymal abnormalities.
   a. Neoplasia (interstitial cell, Sertoli cell, seminoma) – may be single or multiple, and of variable echogenicity. Very large lesions tend to have a complex appearance. Intra-abdominal testes are more likely to become neoplastic.
   b. Abscess – anechoic or hypoechoic contents, irregular wall.
   c. Infarct – hyperechoic, wedge-shaped.
2. Diffuse parenchymal abnormalities.

a. Orchitis – patchy hypoechoic appearance, often associated with epididymitis.
b. Torsion – diffusely hypoechoic, concurrent enlargement of epididymis; decreased blood flow seen with Doppler.
c. Atrophy – hypoechoic or isoechoic.
   – Senile.
   – Neoplasm in contralateral testis.

11.60 PARATESTICULAR ABNORMALITIES ON ULTRASONOGRAPHY

1. Enlargement of epididymis.
   a. Epididymitis.
   b. Torsion.
2. Abnormal scrotal contents.
   a. Scrotal hernia (mixed echogenicity, often with shadowing or reverberation due to gas).
   b. Haemorrhage (usually anechoic).
      – Trauma.
      – Extension from abdominal or retroperitoneal haemorrhage (see 9.6.1 and 9.9.2).

Further reading

General

Baines, E., 2005. Practical contrast radiography 3. Urogenital studies. In Pract. 27, 466–473.

Hotston Moore, A., 2001. Urinary incontinence in adult bitches 1. Investigation. In Pract. 23, 534–540.

Hotston Moore, A., 2001. Urinary incontinence in adult bitches 2. Differential diagnosis and treatment. In Pract. 23, 588–595.

Johnston, G.R., Walter, P.S., Feeney, D.A., 1986. Radiographic and ultrasonographic features of uroliths and other urinary tract fillings defects. Vet. Clin. North Am. Small Anim. Pract. 16, 261–292.

Lamb, C.R., 1990. Abdominal ultrasonography in small animals: intestinal tract and mesentery, kidneys, adrenal glands, uterus and prostate (review). J. Small Anim. Pract. 31, 295–304.

Pugh, C.R., Rhodes, W.H., Biery, D. N., 1993. Contrast studies of the urogenital system. Vet. Clin. North Am. Small Anim. Pract. 23, 281–306.

Silverman, S., Long, C.D., 2000. The diagnosis of urinary incontinence and abnormal urination in dogs and cats. Vet. Clin. North Am. Small Anim. Pract. 30, 427–448.

Webster, N., 2009. Ultrasonography of the urogenital tract in dogs and cats. In Pract. 31, 210–217.

Kidneys

Allworth, M.S., Hoffmann, K.L., 1999. Crossed renal ectopia with fusion in a cat. Vet. Radiol. Ultrasound 40, 357–360.

Barr, F.J., 1990. Evaluation of ultrasound as a method of assessing renal size in the dog. J. Small Anim. Pract. 31, 174–179.

Barr, F.J., Holt, P.E., Gibbs, C., 1990. Ultrasonographic measurement of normal renal parameters. J. Small Anim. Pract. 31, 180–184.

Beraud, R., Carozzo, C., 2007. Perirenal expanding haematoma in a cat. J. Small Anim. Pract. 48, 43–45.

Biller, D.S., Schenkman, D.I., Bortnoski, H., 1991. Ultrasonographic appearance of renal infarcts in a dog. J. Am. Anim. Hosp. Assoc. 27, 370–372.

Biller, D.S., Bradley, G.A., Partington, B.P., 1992. Renal medullary rim sign: ultrasonographic evidence of renal disease. Vet. Radiol. 33, 286–290.

Castellano, M.C., Idiart, J.R., 2005. Multifocal renal

cystadenocarcinoma and nodular dermatofibrosis in dogs. Compendium on Continuing Education for the Practicing Veterinarian (Small Animal) 27, 846–853.

Felkai, C.S., Voros, K., Vrabely, T., Karsai, F., 1992. Ultrasonographic determination of renal volume in the dog. Vet. Radiol. Ultrasound 33, 292–296.

Forrest, L.J., O'Brien, R.T., Tremelling, M.S., Steinberg, H., Cooley, A.J., Kerlin, R.L., 1998. Sonographic renal findings in 20 dogs with leptospirosis. Vet. Radiol. Ultrasound 39, 337–340.

Grandage, J., 1975. Some effects of posture on the radiographic appearance of the kidneys of the dog. J. Am. Vet. Med. Assoc. 166, 165–166.

Grooters, A.M., Cuypers, M.D., Partington, B.P., Williams, J., Pechman, R.D., 1997. Renomegaly in dogs and cats. Part II. Diagnostic approach. Compendium on Continuing Education for the Practicing Veterinarian (Small Animal) 19, 1213–1229.

Holloway, A., O'Brien, R., 2007. Perirenal effusion in dogs and cats with acute renal failure. Vet. Radiol. Ultrasound 48, 574–579.

Katic, N., Bartolomaeus, E., Böhler, A., Dupré, G., 2997. Traumatic diaphragmatic rupture in a cat with partial kidney displacement into the thorax. J. Small Anim. Pract. 48, 705–708.

Konde, L.J., Wrigley, R.H., Park, R.D., Lebel, J.L., 1984. Ultrasonographic anatomy of the normal canine kidney. Vet. Radiol. 25, 173–178.

Mareschal, A., d'Anjou, M.A., Moreau, K., Alexander, K., Beauregard, G., 2007. Ultrasonographic measurement of kidney-to-aorta ratio as a method of estimating renal size in dogs. Vet. Radiol. Ultrasound 48, 434–438.

Marolf, A., Kraft, S., Lowry, J., Pelsue, J., Veir, J., 2002. Radiographic diagnosis – right kidney herniation in a cat. Vet. Radiol. Ultrasound 43, 237–240.

Moe, L., Lium, B., 1997. Hereditary multifocal renal cystadenocarcinomas and nodular dermatofibrosis in 51 German shepherd dogs. J. Small Anim. Pract. 38, 498–505.

Mosenco, A.S., Culp, W.T.N., Johnson, A., French, A., Mehler, S.J., 2008. Renal cystadenoma in a domestic shorthair. J. Feline. Med. Surg. 10, 102–105.

Nyland, T.G., Kantrowitz, B.M., Fisher, H.J., Olander, H.J., Hornof, W.J., 1989. Ultrasonic determination of kidney volume in the dog. Vet. Radiol. 30, 174–180.

Ochoa, V.B., DiBartola, S.P., Chew, D.J., Westropp, J., Carothers, D.S., Biller, D.S., 1999. Perinephric pseudocysts in the cat: a retrospective study and review of the literature. J. Vet. Intern. Med. 13, 47–55.

Raffan, E., Kipar, A., Barber, P.J., Freeman, A.I., 2008. Transitional cell carcinoma forming a perirenal cyst in a cat. J. Small Anim. Pract. 49, 144–147.

Reichle, J.K., DiBartola, S.P., Leveille, R., 2002. Renal ultrasonographic and computed tomographic appearance, volume and function of cats with autosomal dominant polycystic kidney disease. Vet. Radiol. Ultrasound 43, 368–373.

Rivers, B.J., Johnston, G.R., 1996. Diagnostic imaging strategies in small animal nephrology. Vet. Clin. North Am. Small Anim. Pract. 26, 1505–1517.

Shiroma, J.T., Gabriel, J.K., Carter, R.L., Scruggs, S.L., Stubbs, P.W., 1999. Effect of reproductive status on feline renal size. Vet. Radiol. Ultrasound 40, 242–245.

Soler, M., Teixeira, M., Agut, A., 2008. Imaging diagnosis –

Dioctophyma renale in a dog. Vet. Radiol. Ultrasound 49, 307–308.

Triolo, A.J., Miles, K.G., 1995. Renal imaging techniques in dogs and cats. Vet. Med. 13, 959–966.

Valdés-Martínez, A., Cianciolo, R., Mai, W., 2007. Association between renal hypoechoic subcapsular thickening and lymphosarcoma in cats. Vet. Radiol. Ultrasound 48, 357–360.

Zatelli, A., D'Ippolito, P., 2004. Bilateral perirenal abscesses in a domestic neuter shorthair cat. J. Vet. Intern. Med. 18, 902–903.

Ureters

Adin, C.A., Herrgesell, E.J., Nyland, T.J., Hughes, J.M., Gregory, C.R., Kyles, A.E., et al., 2003. Antegrade pyelography for suspected ureteral obstruction in cats: 11 cases (1995–2001). J. Am. Vet. Med. Assoc. 222, 1576–1581.

Dean, P.W., Bojrab, M.J., Constantinescu, G.M., 1988. Canine ectopic ureter. Compendium on Continuing Education for the Practicing Veterinarian (Small Animal) 10, 146–157.

Doust, R.T., Clarke, S.P., Hammond, C., Paterson, C., King, A., 2006. Circumcaval ureter associated with an intrahepatic portosystemic shunt in a dog. J. Am. Vet. Med. Assoc. 228, 389–391.

Eisele, J.G., Jackson, J., Hager, D., 2005. Ectopic ureterocele in a cat. J. Am. Anim. Hosp. Assoc. 41, 332–335.

Esterline, M.L., Biller, D.S., Sicard, G.K., 2005. Ureteral duplication in a dog. Vet. Radiol. Ultrasound 46, 485–489.

Ewers, R.S., Holt, P.E., 1992. Urological complications following ovariohysterectomy in a bitch. J. Small Anim. Pract. 33, 236–238.

Holt, P.E., Gibbs, C., 1992. Congenital urinary incontinence in cats: a review of 19 cases. Vet. Radiol. 130, 437–442.

Holt, P.E., Gibbs, C., Pearson, H., 1982. Canine ectopic ureter – a review of twenty-nine cases. J. Small Anim. Pract. 23, 195–208.

Jakovljevic, S., Van Alstine, W.G., Adams, L.G., 1998. Ureteral diverticula in two dogs. Vet. Radiol. Ultrasound 39, 425–429.

Lamb, C.R., 1994. Acquired ureterovaginal fistula secondary to ovariohysterectomy in a dog: diagnosis using ultrasound-guided nephropyelocentesis and antegrade pyelography. Vet. Radiol. Ultrasound 35, 201–203.

Lamb, C.R., 1998. Ultrasonography of the ureters. Vet. Clin. North Am. Small Anim. Pract. 28, 823–848.

Lamb, C.R., Gregory, S.P., 1994. Ultrasonography of the ureterovesicular junction in the dog: a preliminary report. Vet. Rec. 134, 36–38.

Lamb, C.R., Gregory, S.P., 1998. Ultrasonographic findings in 14 dogs with ectopic ureter. Vet. Radiol. Ultrasound 39, 218–223.

Lautzenhiser, S.J., Bjorling, D.E., 2002. Urinary incontinence in a dog with an ectopic ureterocele. J. Am. Anim. Hosp. Assoc. 38, 29–32.

Reichle, J.K., Peterson, R.A., Mahaffey, M.B., Schelling, C.G., Barthez, P.Y., 2003. Ureteral fibroepithelial polyps in four dogs. Vet. Radiol. Ultrasound 44, 433–437.

Rivers, B.J., Walter, P.A., Polzin, D.J., 1997. Ultrasonographic-guided, percutaneous antegrade pyelography: technique and clinical application in the dog and cat. J. Am. Anim. Hosp. Assoc. 33, 61–68.

Stiffler, K.S., Stevenson, M.A.M., Mahaffey, M.B., Howerth, E.W., Barsanti, J.A., 2002. Intravesical ureterocele with concurrent renal dysfunction in a dog: a case report and proposed classification system. J. Am. Anim. Hosp. Assoc. 38, 33–39.

Sutherland-Smith, J., Jerram, J.M., Walker, A.M., Warman, C.G.A., 2004. Ectopic ureters and ureteroceles in dogs: presentation, cause, and diagnosis. Compendium on Continuing Education for the Practicing Veterinarian (Small Animal) 26, 303–310.

Tattersall, J., Welsh, E., 2006. Ectopic ureterocele in a male dog: a case report and review of surgical management. J. Am. Anim. Hosp. Assoc. 42, 395–400.

Bladder

Atalan, G., Barr, F.J., Holt, P.E., 1998. Estimation of bladder volume using ultrasonographic determination of cross-sectional areas and linear measurements. Vet. Radiol. Ultrasound 39, 446–450.

Benigni, L., Lamb, C.R., Corzo-Menendez, N., Holloway, A., Eastwood, J.M., 2006. Lymphoma affecting the urinary bladder in three dogs and a cat. Vet. Radiol. Ultrasound 47, 592–596.

Cote, E., Carroll, M.C., Beck, K.A., Good, K., Gannon, K., 2002. Diagnosis of urinary bladder rupture using ultrasound contrast cystography: in vitro model and two case history reports. Vet. Radiol. Ultrasound 43, 281–286.

Feeney, D.A., Weichselbaum, R.C., Jessen, C.R., Osborne, C.A., 1999. Imaging canine urocystoliths. Vet. Clin. North Am. Small Anim. Pract. 29, 59–72.

Geisse, A.L., Lowry, J.E., Schaeffer, D.J., Smith, C.W., 1997. Sonographic evaluation of urinary bladder wall thickness in normal dogs. Vet. Radiol. Ultrasound 38, 132–137.

Groesslinger, K., Tham, T., Egerbacher, D., Lorinson, D., 2005. Prevalence and radiologic and histologic appearance of vesicourachal diverticula in dogs without clinical signs of urinary tract disease. J. Am. Vet. Med. Assoc. 226, 383–386.

Gunn-Moore, D., 2000. Feline lower urinary tract disease: an update. In Pract. 22, 534–542.

Hanson, J.A., Tidwell, A.S., 1996. Ultrasonographic appearance of urethral transitional cell carcinoma in ten dogs. Vet. Radiol. Ultrasound 37, 293–299.

Heng, H.G., Lowry, J.E., Boston, S., Gabel, N., Ehrhart, N., Gulden, S.M. S., 2006. Smooth muscle neoplasia of the urinary bladder wall in three dogs. Vet. Radiol. Ultrasound 47, 83–86.

Johnston, G.R., Feeney, D.A., Rivers, W.J., Weichselbaum, R., 1996. Diagnostic imaging of the feline lower urinary tract. Vet. Clin. North Am. Small Anim. Pract. 26, 401–415.

Lamb, C.R., Trower, N.D., Gregory, S.P., 1996. Ultrasound-guided catheter biopsy of the lower urinary tract: technique and results in 12 dogs. J. Small Anim. Pract. 37, 413–416.

Leveille, R., 1998. Ultrasonography of urinary bladder disorders. Vet. Clin. North Am. Small Anim. Pract. 28, 799–822.

Leveille, R., Biller, D.S., Partington, B. P., Miyabayashi, T., 1992. Sonographic investigation of transitional cell carcinoma of the urinary bladder in small animals. Vet. Radiol. Ultrasound 33, 103–107.

Mahaffey, M.B., Barsanti, J.A., Crowell, W.A., Shotts, E., Barber, D.L., 1989. Cystography: effect of technique on diagnosis of cystitis in dogs. Vet. Radiol. Ultrasound 30, 261–267.

Petite, A., Busoni, V., Heinen, M.P., Billen, F., Snaps, F., 2006. Radiographic and ultrasonographic findings of emphysematous cystitis in four nondiabetic dogs. Vet. Radiol. Ultrasound 47, 90–93.

Scheepens, E.T.F., L'Eplattenier, H., 2005. Acquired urinary bladder diverticulum in a dog. J. Small Anim. Pract. 46, 578–581.

Scrivani, P.V., Léveillé, R., Collins, R.L., 1997. The effect of patient positioning on mural filling defects during double contrast cystography. Vet. Radiol. Ultrasound 38, 355–359.

Scrivani, P.V., Chew, D.J., Buffington, C.A.T., Kendall, M., 1998. Results of double-contrast cystography in cats with idiopathic cystitis: 45 cases (1993–1995). J. Am. Vet. Med. Assoc. 212, 1907–1909.

White, R.A.S., Herrtage, M.E., 1986. Bladder retroflexion in the dog. J. Small Anim. Pract. 27, 735–746.

Urethra

Duffey, M.H., Barnhart, M.D., Barthez, P.Y., Smeak, D.D., 1998. Incomplete urethral duplication with cyst formation in a dog. J. Am. Vet. Med. Assoc. 213, 1287–1289.

Holt, P.E., Gibbs, C., Latham, J., 1984. An evaluation of positive contrast vaginourethrography as a diagnostic aid in the bitch. J. Small Anim. Pract. 25, 531–549.

Scrivani, P.V., Chew, D.J., Buffington, C.A.T., Kendall, M., Leveille, D.M., 1997. Results of retrograde urethrography in cats with idiopathic non obstructive lower urinary tract disease and their association with pathogenesis in 53 cases (1993–1995). J. Am. Vet. Med. Assoc. 211, 741–748.

Silverstone, A.M., Adams, W.M., 2001. Radiographic diagnosis of a rectourethral fistula in a dog. J. Am. Anim. Hosp. Assoc. 37, 573–576.

Ticer, J.W., Spencer, C.P., Ackerman, N., 1980. Positive contrast retrograde urethrography: a useful procedure for evaluating urethral disorders in the dog. Vet. Radiol. 21, 2–11.

Genital system: general

Holt, P.E., Long, S.E., Gibbs, C., 1983. Disorders of urination associated with canine intersexuality. J. Small Anim. Pract. 24, 475–487.

Kneller, S.K., 1986. Radiologic examination. In: Burke, T.J (Ed.), Small Animal Reproduction and Infertility. Lea & Febiger, Philadelphia, pp. 158–185.

Root, C.R., Spaulding, K.A., 1994. Diagnostic imaging in companion animal theriogenology. Semin. Vet. Med. Surg. (Small Anim.) 9, 7–27.

Female genital system

Diez-Bru, N., Garcia-Real, I., Martinez, E.M., Rollan, E., Mayenco, P., Llorens, P., 1998. Ultrasonographic appearance of ovarian tumors in 10 dogs. Vet. Radiol. Ultrasound 39, 226–233.

England, G.C.W., 1998. Ultrasonographic assessment of abnormal pregnancy. Vet. Clin. North Am. Small Anim. Pract. 28, 849–868.

England, G.C.W., Allen, W.E., 1989. Ultrasonographic and histological appearance of the canine ovary. Vet. Rec. 125, 555–556.

England, G.C.W., Yeager, A.E., 1993. Ultrasonographic appearance of the ovary and uterus of the bitch during oestrus, ovulation and early pregnancy. J. Reprod. Fertil. Suppl. 47, 107–117.

Fayrer-Hosken, R.A., Mahaffey, M., Miller-Liebl, D., Caudle, A.B., 1991. Early diagnosis of canine pyometra using ultrasonography. Vet. Radiol. Ultrasound 32, 287–289.

Ferretti, L.M., Newell, S.M., Graham, J.P., Roberts, G.D., 2000. Radiographic and ultrasonographic evaluation of the normal feline postpartum uterus. Vet. Radiol. Ultrasound 41, 287–291.

Holt, P.E., Bohannon, J., Day, M.J., 2006. Vaginoperitoneal fistula after ovariohysterectomy in three bitches. J. Small Anim. Pract. 47, 744–746.

Kydd, D.M., Burnie, A.G., 1986. Vaginal neoplasia in the bitch: a review of forty clinical cases. J. Small Anim. Pract. 27, 255–263.

Mayenco-Aguirre, A.M., Garcia-Real, R., Cediel-Algovia, R., Llorens-Pena, P., Sánchez-Muela, M., 2002. Secondary vaginal pouch in a bitch. Vet. Rec. 150, 152–153.

Miles, K., 1995. Imaging pregnant dogs and cats. Compendium on Continuing Education for the Practicing Veterinarian (Small Animal) 17, 1217–1226.

Misumi, K., Fujiki, M., Miura, N., Sakamoto, H., 2000. Uterine horn torsion in two non-gravid bitches. J. Small Anim. Pract. 41, 468–471.

Pharr, J.W., Post, K., 1992. Ultrasonography and radiography of the canine post partum uterus. Vet. Radiol. Ultrasound 33, 35–40.

Stöcklin-Gautschi, N.M., Guscetti, F., Reichler, I.M., Geissbühler, U., Braun, S.A., Arnold, S., 2001. Identification of focal adenomyosis as a uterine lesion in two dogs. J. Small Anim. Pract. 42, 413–416.

Viehoff, F.W., Sjollema, B.E., 2003. Hydrocolpos in dogs: surgical treatment in two cases. J. Small Anim. Pract. 44, 404–407.

Male genital system

Atalan, G., Holt, P.E., Barr, F.J., 1999. Ultrasonographic estimation of prostate size in normal dogs, and relationship to bodyweight and age. J. Small Anim. Pract. 40, 119–122.

Atalan, G., Barr, F.J., Holt, P.E., 1999. Comparison of ultrasonographic and radiographic measurements of canine prostatic dimensions. Vet. Radiol. Ultrasound 40, 408–412.

Bradbury, C.A., Westropp, J.L., Pollard, R.E., 2009. Relationship between prostatomegaly, prostatic mineralization and cytologic diagnosis. Vet. Radiol. Ultrasound 50, 167–171.

Caney, S.M.A., Holt, P.E., Day, M.J., Rudorf, T.J., Gruffydd-Jones, T.J., 1998. Prostatic carcinoma in two cats. J. Small Anim. Pract. 39, 140–143.

Dorfman, M., Barsanti, J., 1995. Diseases of the canine prostate gland. Compendium on Continuing Education for the Practicing Veterinarian (Small Animal) 17, 791–810.

Feeney, D.A., Johnston, G.R., Klausner, J.S., Perman, V., Leininger, J.R., Tomlinson, M.J., 1987. Canine prostatic disease – comparison of ultrasonographic appearance with morphologic and microbiologic findings: 30 cases (1981–1985). J. Am. Vet. Med. Assoc. 190, 1027–1034.

Feeney, D.A., Johnston, G.R., Klausner, J.S., Bell, F.W., 1989. Canine prostatic ultrasonography. Semin. Vet. Med. Surg. (Small Anim.) 4, 44–57.

Gumbsch, P., Gabler, C., Holzmann, A., 2002. Colour-coded duplex sonography of the testes of dogs. Vet. Rec. 151, 140–144.

Hecht, S., King, R., Tidwell, A.S., Gorman, S.C., 2004. Ultrasound diagnosis: intra-abdominal torsion of a non-neoplastic testicle in a cryptorchid dog. Vet. Radiol. Ultrasound 45, 58–61.

Johnston, G.R., Feeney, D.A., Johnston, S.D., O'Brien, T.D., 1991. Ultrasonographic features of testicular neoplasia in dogs: 16 cases (1989–1988). J. Am. Vet. Med. Assoc. 198, 1779–1784.

Newell, S.M., Mahaffey, M.B., Binhazim, C.E., Greene, C.E., 1992. Paraprostatic cyst in a cat. J. Small Anim. Pract. 33, 399–401.

Pugh, C.R., Konde, L.J., 1991. Sonographic evaluation of canine testicular and scrotal abnormalities: a review of 26 case histories. Vet. Radiol. 32, 243–250.

Pugh, C.R., Konde, L.J., Park, R.D., 1990. Testicular ultrasound in the normal dog. Vet. Radiol. 31, 195–199.

Ruel, Y., Barthez, P.Y., Mailles, A., Begon, D., 1998. Ultrasonographic evaluation of the prostate in healthy intact dogs. Vet. Radiol. Ultrasound 39, 212–216.

Stowater, J.L., Lamb, C.R., 1989. Ultrasonographic features of paraprostatic cysts in nine dogs. Vet. Radiol. 30, 232–239.

White, R.A.S., Herrtage, M.E., Dennis, R., 1987. The diagnosis and management of paraprostatic and prostatic retention cysts in the dog. J. Small Anim. Pract. 28, 551–574.

Williams, J., Niles, J., 1999. Prostatic disease in the dog. In Pract. 21, 558–575.

Winter, M.D., Locke, J.E., Penninck, D.G., 2006. Imaging diagnosis: urinary obstruction secondary to prostatic lymphoma in a young dog. Vet. Radiol. Ultrasound 47, 597–601.

Chapter 12

Soft tissues

CHAPTER CONTENTS

12.1 Variations in thickness of soft tissues 331
12.2 Variations in radiopacity of soft tissues 332
12.3 Contrast studies of sinus tracts and fistulae
(sinography, fistulography) 334
12.4 Contrast studies of the lymphatic system
(lymphography, lymphangiography) 334
12.5 Contrast studies of peripheral arteries
and veins (angiography, arteriography,
venography) 335
12.6 Ultrasonography of soft tissues 336
12.7 Ultrasonography of muscles, tendons
and nerves 337
12.8 Ultrasonography of superficial lymph
nodes 338

Soft tissues and fluid have a similar radiopacity, which is less than that of bone and other mineralized material and greater than that of gas. Fat is slightly less radiopaque than fluid and other soft tissues and can usually be distinguished from them. It is not usually possible, therefore, to distinguish different components of fluid or soft tissue structures within a region unless they are outlined by fat, gas or mineralized material, or unless contrast techniques are used. Fat in areas such as the abdominal cavity, pericardial sac, fascial planes and joints provides helpful contrast with other soft tissues and often aids interpretation. Magnetic resonance imaging (and to a lesser extent, CT) is the preferred technique when detailed soft tissue information is required. The use of ultrasonography for the

musculoskeletal system is described briefly in Chapter 3. In the case of the limbs, evaluation of imaging abnormalities may be easier if the presumed normal contralateral body part is also evaluated for comparison.

12.1 VARIATIONS IN THICKNESS OF SOFT TISSUES

1. Diffuse increase in thickness of soft tissue.
   a. Fat deposition – obesity; distinguished by fat radiopacity that is less than that of other soft tissues (seen subcutaneously, within fascial planes, and in the thoracic and abdominal cavities).
   b. Muscular hypertrophy.
      – In response to activity.
      – Cats – feline hypertrophic muscular dystrophy; uncommon, leads to progressive muscular hypertrophy.
   c. Oedema.
      – Obstruction to venous drainage.
      – Congestive heart failure.
      – Hypoproteinaemia (secondary to renal, hepatic or intestinal disease).
   d. Lymphoedema.
      – Developmental anomaly of lymphatic drainage.
      – Acquired obstruction to lymphatic drainage.
      – Lymphangiosarcoma.
   e. Cellulitis.
   f. Diffuse or extensive neoplasia.

g. Subcutaneous administration of fluids.

h. Emphysema (gas bubbles and streaks visible).

2. Focal increase in thickness of soft tissues.

a. Subcutaneous administration of fluids.

b. Skin folds – especially certain breeds, such as the English Bulldog and Shar Pei.

c. Seroma (e.g. following surgery).

d. Neoplasia – benign or malignant.

e. Cellulitis or abscess.

f. Haematoma.

g. Granuloma (e.g. lick granuloma, or soft tissue callus over a pressure point).

h. Hygroma.

i. Cyst.

j. Hamartoma.

k. Vascular malformation.

l. Compartment syndrome – elevation of interstitial pressure in a closed osseofascial compartment, usually due to vascular injury or trauma ± fracture; most commonly in a limb.

3. Decrease in thickness of soft tissues.

a. Emaciation – primarily loss of fat layer.

b. Muscular atrophy.
   – Disuse (e.g. chronic lameness).
   – Neurogenic.
   – As a consequence of myositis.

12.2 VARIATIONS IN RADIOPACITY OF SOFT TISSUES

1. Increased radiopacity – but remaining of soft tissue opacity.

a. Increased thickness of soft tissues (e.g. given the same exposure, the soft tissues of the thigh will appear more radiopaque than those of the distal limb, due to their increased bulk).

b. Superimposition of skin or subcutaneous masses.

c. Superimposition of nipples.

d. Superimposition of engorged ticks.

e. Skin folds.

f. Positioning aids (e.g. foam wedges).

g. Wet or dirty hair or fur, or ultrasound gel – usually gives a streaky appearance.

2. Increased radiopacity – unstructured mineral opacity due to deposition of calcium salts or other minerals.

a. Artefactual, due to dirty intensifying screens or cassettes.

b. Surface application of some lotions or ointments.

c. Foreign material (e.g. dirt, glass).

d. Secondary to injection of corticosteroids.

e. Hyperadrenocorticism (Cushing's disease) – calcinosis cutis (see below) and also mineralization of bronchopulmonary structures, kidney and sometimes other soft tissues; other features include hepatomegaly, osteopenia and adrenal masses.

f. Dystrophic calcification, i.e. deposition of calcium salts in damaged or diseased tissue.
   – Secondary to trauma (e.g. calcifying tendinopathy).
   – Chronic haematoma.
   – Chronic abscess, granuloma or granulation tissue.
   – Chronic necrosis (e.g. abdominal fat necrosis).
   – Within a neoplasm.
   – Cyst wall.

g. Metastatic calcification – calcification of soft tissues secondary to disorders of calcium and phosphorus homeostasis (e.g. kidneys, major blood vessels, gut wall).
   – Chronic renal failure and renal secondary hyperparathyroidism (see 1.16.4 and 4.9.5 and Fig. 4.5); paw calcification also seen in cats.
   – Pseudohyperparathyroidism (hypercalcaemia of malignancy), usually secondary to anal sac adenocarcinoma or lymphoma.
   – Primary hyperparathyroidism – uncommon; usually older dogs, particularly Keeshond.
   – Vitamin D toxicosis – cats are more sensitive than dogs; may die from renal failure prior to visible soft tissue mineralization.

h. Calcinosis cutis – granular deposits of calcium in the skin and/or linear streaks of calcium in fascial planes; usually secondary to hyperadrenocorticism (Cushing's disease) but may also be seen secondary to hyperparathyroidism.

i. Calcinosis circumscripta (tumoral calcinosis) (Fig. 12.1) – young, larger-breed dogs, especially German Shepherd dogs, and rare in cats; amorphous calcium deposits

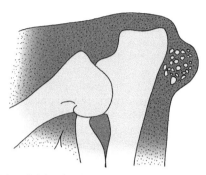

Figure 12.1 Calcinosis circumscripta near the elbow of a dog; a cluster of stippled mineral opacities within an area of focal soft tissue swelling.

within soft tissues, often attached to tendons, joint capsules or periosteum. Possibly associated with trauma, such as pressure points and at sites of previous surgery. Commonly recognized sites include the extremities or prominences of the limbs, the neck and the tongue, and it has also been reported in the spine, causing neurological deficits.

j. Chondrocalcinosis (pseudogout, calcium pyrophosphate deposition disease) – rare; unknown aetiology and mainly older animals; articular or periarticular deposition of calcium pyrophosphate crystals.

k. Idiopathic vascular calcification.

l. Iatrogenic – percutaneous injection of calcium-containing drug or long-acting corticosteroid.

3. Increased radiopacity – more structured mineral opacity that in some cases has trabecular detail suggestive of bone formation.

a. Normal anatomical structures or variants (e.g. sesamoids, clavicle, hyoid apparatus, separate centres of ossification).

b. Fragments of bone displaced from their normal position due to avulsion or other fractures.

c. Chronic tendinopathy.

d. Neoplasia.
   - Extraskeletal osteosarcoma – described in a wide range of sites in both dogs and cats; variable degrees of mineralization, and some appear as soft tissue masses only.
   - Multilobular tumour of bone – usually attached to adjacent bone but has been reported in axillary soft tissues.
   - Other neoplasms may occasionally contain mineralization.

e. Heterotopic osteochondrofibrosis in association with von Willebrand's disease – Dobermann, hip area (see 3.9.12).

f. Myositis ossificans – formation of non-neoplastic bone within striated muscle; termed *heterotopic* because it is in an abnormal position.
   - Idiopathic.
   - Secondary to trauma or chronic disease.

g. Cats – hypervitaminosis A; there may be extensive periarticular mineralization as well as periarticular and vertebral osteophytes (see 5.4.8).

h. Cats – osteochondromatosis: may have widespread soft tissue mineralization unconnected to adjacent bone.

i. Fibrodysplasia ossificans (Fig. 12.2) – rare, progressive disorder, especially cats; similar to myositis ossificans but differs in that the bone may displace muscle but does not involve it. Typically multiple, symmetrical lesions unrelated to trauma.

4. Increased radiopacity – metallic opacity.

a. Artefactual due to dirty intensifying screens or cassettes.

b. Surface application of lotions or ointments containing metallic salts.

c. Surface contamination with contrast medium.

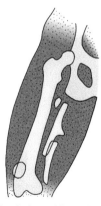

Figure 12.2 Fibrodysplasia ossificans in the pelvic limb of a cat: well-organized deposits of bone in the soft tissues of the medial thigh. Myositis ossificans has a similar radiographic appearance, and the two conditions may be differentiated only if fascial planes can also be seen, because fibrodysplasia ossificans lies within fascial planes, whereas myositis ossificans is within muscle bellies.

d. Contrast medium within a sinus tract or fistula.

e. Foreign material (e.g. bullets, air gun pellets, needles).

f. Migration of metallic implants originally in skeletal structures.

g. Surgical staples or wire sutures.

h. Microchip.

5. Decreased radiopacity of soft tissues.

a. Artefactual – overexposure or overdevelopment.

b. Decreased thickness of soft tissues.

c. Presence of fat.

   – Normal or obese; linear fat deposits in a subcutaneous site and along fascial planes.

   – Localized fatty mass (lipoma, liposarcoma, e.g. intermuscular lipomas in the thigh region of dogs).

d. Presence of gas (Fig. 12.3).

   – Puncture, laceration or incision of skin.

   – Secondary to subcutaneous or intramuscular injection.

   – Penetration of the pharynx, oesophagus or trachea.

   – Extension of pneumomediastinum.

   – Within intestinal loops in a hernia or rupture.

   – Infection with gas-forming organisms (uncommon).

   – Sinus tract or fistula (for dermoid sinus see 5.7.4).

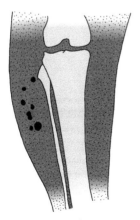

Figure 12.3 Subcutaneous emphysema secondary to a cat bite: multiple small gas bubbles seen within the soft tissues lateral to the fibula.

12.3 CONTRAST STUDIES OF SINUS TRACTS AND FISTULAE (SINOGRAPHY, FISTULOGRAPHY)

A sinus tract is defined as a tract leading from a focus of infection to the body surface or to the lumen of a hollow organ. Sinus tracts are often the result of foreign bodies, such as plant or suture material. A fistula runs from the lumen of a hollow organ or body cavity to another hollow organ or body cavity or to the body surface.

Contrast studies may be used in either case to determine the route of the tract. In the case of a sinus tract, contrast material may, in addition, outline a foreign body at the site of the focus of infection. However, care must be taken with interpretation, as the contrast medium does not always fill the tract(s) completely and so may underestimate the extent of the lesion. In addition, it may be difficult to discriminate between foreign material and filling defects due to gas bubbles, purulent debris and fibrous tissue.

In order to perform a contrast study, a catheter prefilled with contrast medium is placed into the end of the tract opening at the body surface. The catheter is secured in place either by a purse-string suture or atraumatic forceps or by use of a balloon catheter. A water-soluble iodinated contrast medium is then injected slowly and a radiograph of the region taken towards the end of, or after completion of, the injection. The quantity of contrast medium used will depend on the suspected extent of the lesion.

12.4 CONTRAST STUDIES OF THE LYMPHATIC SYSTEM (LYMPHOGRAPHY, LYMPHANGIOGRAPHY)

This contrast technique is not commonly used in veterinary medicine but may be used to investigate causes of lymphoedema. Note that such clinical signs may be due to venous obstruction rather than, or as well as, lymphatic obstruction, and venography may also be required. Lymphography may also be used to assess the conformation of the thoracic duct prior to ligation in cases of chylothorax.

The original technique described involved injecting methylene blue subcutaneously distal to the site of interest; this is taken up by the lymphatic vessels, which can then be identified, surgically exposed and cannulated. A water-soluble iodinated contrast medium may then be injected,

and radiographs of the region taken after completion of the injection, demonstrating draining
lymphatics and lymph nodes.

An alternative method is to inject low-osmolar,
water-soluble contrast medium intradermally distal
to the site of the expected lesion, and this will also
demonstrate lymphatics and lymph nodes. Oily iodinated contrast media may also be used but are difficult to source. More recently, a technique of direct
injection into a popliteal lymph node has been
described as a method of opacifying the thoracic duct
prior to surgical ligation in animals with chylothorax,
and injection may be made into any lymph node distal to the site of interest. If necessary, this may be performed under ultrasound guidance.

Primary congenital lymphoedema has been
described in puppies and is considered to be due
to a dysplasia of lymph vessels and/or nodes. In
the more common localized form, one or both of
the distal pelvic limbs are usually affected; in the
less common generalized form, the nose, pinnae
and vulva may also be affected. Tortuosity and
dilation of local lymphatics is usually seen,
although occasionally the initial dermal lymph vessels are aplastic or hypoplastic. Draining lymph
nodes are usually absent or small.

Lymphoedema may also be due to lymphangio-
sarcoma; lymphographic abnormalities would be
expected to occur but have not yet been reported
in small animals.

12.5 CONTRAST STUDIES OF PERIPHERAL ARTERIES AND VEINS (ANGIOGRAPHY, ARTERIOGRAPHY, VENOGRAPHY)

Contrast studies of peripheral blood vessels may be
indicated when it is important to define the arterial
supply or the venous drainage of a mass or extrem-
ity. If information regarding the arterial supply is
required, then it is usually necessary to surgically
expose and cannulate the feeder artery to the
region. If information only about venous drainage
is required, then it is sufficient to inject the contrast
medium into a peripheral vein distal to the region of
interest. Water-soluble iodinated contrast medium
should be used in both cases, and radiographs of
the region taken towards the end of injection or
immediately on completion of injection.

1. Poor opacification of vessel(s).
   a. Insufficient contrast medium used.
   b. Leakage of contrast around the catheter.

c. Time delay between the completion of
   injection and the radiographic exposure too
   great.
d. Vessel occluded:
   – By a mass within or outside it.
   – By a ligature.
   – By a thrombus or embolus.
e. Vessel disrupted.

2. Filling defects.
   a. Thromboembolism – most often in the aorta
      and external iliac arteries, causing pelvic limb
      weakness, pain and collapse.
      – Secondary to cardiomyopathy, especially
        in cats.
      – Endocarditis.
      – Trauma.
      – Neoplasia.
      – Renal amyloidosis.
      – Hyperadrenocorticism (Cushing's disease).
      – Secondary to thoracic aortic thrombus
        formation in *Spirocerca lupi** infection.
      – For pulmonary thromboembolism see 6.23.6.
   b. Neoplastic invasion.
   c. Heartworms (pulmonary arteries,
      caudal vena cava or aberrant in other
      locations).
   d. Foreign bodies.
   e. Thoracic aortic thrombus formation in *S. lupi**
      infection.

3. Dilation.
   a. Aorta – see 7.10.1.
   b. Pulmonary artery – post-stenotic dilation.
   c. Aneurysm.
      – True aneurysm (saccular or fusiform),
        due to weakening of the arterial
        media with intact, stretched intima
        and adventitia; common in *S. lupi**
        infection.
      – Pseudoaneurysm – rupture of an artery or
        aneurysm with haemorrhage confined to
        periarticular structures.

4. Contrast medium extravasation.
   a. Trauma involving blood vessel – in the
      limbs may lead to compartment syndrome –
      see 12.1.2.
   b. Ruptured aneurysm, especially in *S. lupi**
      infection.
   c. Neoplastic erosion of blood vessel.

5. Additional abnormal vessels seen.

a. Developmental anomaly of arterial supply and/or venous drainage.
  – Developmental angiomatosis (benign vascular anomaly).
  – Hamartoma.
b. Acquired anomaly of arterial supply and/or venous drainage.
  – Development of collateral circulation in response to disruption or occlusion of normal vessels.
  – Development of abnormal vessels supplying and draining a neoplasm.
  – Acquired angiomatosis.
c. Arteriovenous malformation.
  – Congenital.
  – Acquired (e.g. secondary to trauma, biopsy, surgery, neoplasia).

12.6 ULTRASONOGRAPHY OF SOFT TISSUES

Changes in thickness of soft tissues (see 12.1) may be appreciated ultrasonographically, and in addition, it may be possible to determine which soft tissue component is responsible for the change in thickness. Changes in echogenicity may give added information, and vascularity can be assessed using colour flow or power Doppler. Ultrasound-guided fine needle aspiration or biopsy of abnormal tissues may be performed.

1. Increased echogenicity of soft tissues, ± acoustic shadowing.
   a. Diffuse.
      – Inappropriate control settings.
      – Obesity.
      – Subcutaneous emphysema.
   b. Localized.
      – Foreign material (e.g. grass awns, thorns, wooden splinters and porcupine quills).
      – Localized subcutaneous emphysema.
      – Gas within herniated intestinal loops.
      – Localized mineralization or ossification (see 12.2.2 and 12.2.3).
      – Localized fibrosis.
      – Neoplasm.
      – Granuloma.
      – Abscess.
2. Decreased echogenicity of soft tissues.

   a. Diffuse.
      – Inappropriate control settings.
      – Oedema.
      – Lymphoedema.
      – Obesity.
   b. Localized.
      – Recently injected fluids.
      – Seroma following surgery.
      – Cyst.
      – Haematoma.
      – Severe oedema.
      – Abscess.
      – Neoplasm.
      – Granuloma.
3. Mixed echogenicity of soft tissues.
   a. Abscess (Fig. 12.4).
   b. Foreign body, usually with surrounding reaction or abscess ± draining tract – foreign bodies often produce acoustic shadowing, and in the case of grass awns a characteristic spindle-shaped structure consisting of two or three echogenic lines may be seen (Fig. 12.5).
   c. Haematoma.
   d. Neoplasm.
      – Lipoma – typically well-defined, encapsulated and striated in appearance; most are hypoechoic or isoechoic to surrounding soft tissues and have virtually no blood flow on Doppler ultrasonography.
      – Others.

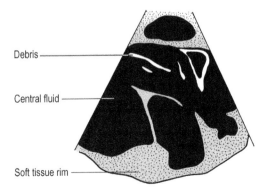

Figure 12.4 Ultrasonographic image of an abscess, showing a soft tissue rim and central fluid containing some debris.

Debris

Central fluid

Soft tissue rim

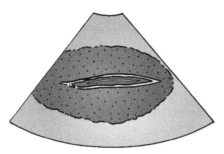

Figure 12.5 Ultrasonographic image of a grass awn in the flank of a dog. A spindle-shaped echogenic structure consisting of three parallel lines is visible, surrounded by a zone of hypoechogenicity representing a surrounding abscess and tissue reaction.

12.7 ULTRASONOGRAPHY OF MUSCLES, TENDONS AND NERVES

Ultrasonography of peripheral muscles is straightforward. Once the scanning site has been prepared by clipping and cleaning, a high-frequency (7.5 MHz or greater) transducer is placed directly over the muscle of interest. Normal muscle appears hypoechoic, with a characteristic striated appearance in longitudinal section and a stippled appearance in transverse section. The hyperechoic striations and stipples represent fibrous tissue around muscle fibre bundles. The boundaries between different muscle bellies are hyperechoic.

The tendons are relatively hyperechoic, with densely packed parallel fibres apparent in longitudinal section. A little fluid around a tendon, within the tendon sheath, may be normal.

Ultrasonography of the normal canine brachial plexus, major nerves of the thoracic limb and sciatic nerve has been described. The nerves appear as hypoechoic, tubular structures with an internal echotexture of discontinuous, hyperechoic bands, surrounded by a thin rim of highly echogenic tissue.

1. Hypoechoic focus within muscle, with consequent disruption of fibre pattern.
   a. Haematoma.
      – Trauma.
      – Coagulopathy.
   b. Abscess.
      – Puncture wound.
      – Haematogenous infection.
   c. Neoplasm.
      – Primary muscle tumour (rhabdomyoma, rhabdomyosarcoma).

   – Metastatic tumour.
2. Hyperechoic focus within muscle, with consequent disruption of fibre pattern: acoustic shadowing may or may not be present.
   a. Fibrosis.
   b. Calcification or ossification (see 12.2.2 and 12.2.3).
   c. Fracture fragments.
   d. Metallic surgical implants.
   e. Gas (see 12.2.5).
   f. Foreign body.
   g. Neoplasm.
      – Primary muscle tumour (rhabdomyoma, rhabdomyosarcoma).
      – Metastatic tumour.
3. Mixed echogenicity within muscle, with disruption of the fibre pattern.
   a. Haematoma ± muscle tearing.
   b. Abscess.
   c. Neoplasm.
4. Change in echogenicity of tendons (Fig. 12.6) – damage to tendons is indicated by disruption of the normally tightly packed, hyperechoic fibres. Anechoic or hypoechoic lesions within the substance of the tendon represent haemorrhage or inflammatory exudate, progressing to granulation tissue. The lesions become more hyperechoic as fibrous tissue replaces granulation tissue, but the fibre alignment remains disrupted until the later stages of healing. See also 3.13.9 and Figure 3.37.
5. Abnormality of nerves – neoplasia of nerves (e.g. in the brachial plexus) produces hypoechoic, tubular masses that lack blood flow and that may separate the artery from its corresponding vein.

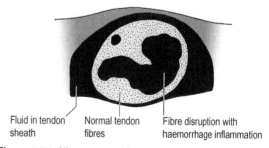

Fluid in tendon sheath   Normal tendon fibres   Fibre disruption with haemorrhage inflammation

Figure 12.6 Ultrasonographic appearance of a damaged Achilles tendon (transverse section). The normal stippled pattern of the tendon fibres is replaced by a hypoechoic region representing fibre disruption and haemorrhage or inflammation. Fluid may be seen in the tendon sheath.

12.8 ULTRASONOGRAPHY OF SUPERFICIAL LYMPH NODES

Normal lymph nodes are typically small oval structures that are isoechoic with surrounding fat or tissue. Where vascularity can be detected using power Doppler or contrast harmonic ultrasound, this is usually hilar. Because ultrasonographic features are usually not specific for a given disease, ultrasound-guided fine needle aspiration is a useful means of obtaining a cytological diagnosis.

1. Enlargement of lymph node.
   a. Reactive.
   b. Lymphoproliferative disease.
   c. Metastatic disease.
   While it is not possible to determine the enlargement of an individual lymph node definitively using ultrasound, the features shown below may be helpful.
2. Change in shape.
   a. Reactive lymph nodes tend to remain oval.
   b. Lymphomatous lymph nodes tend to become more rounded.
   c. Lymph nodes containing metastatic neoplasia vary in shape, with smaller nodes tending to remain oval while larger ones tend to become rounded.
3. Change in echogenicity.
   a. Most lymphomatous and metastatic lymph nodes become hypoechoic to surrounding fat and tissue.
   b. Metastatic lymph nodes may become heterogeneous in echogenicity.
4. Changes in vascularity.
   a. Vascular features that may indicate malignancy include displacement of the central hilar vessel, visibility of pericapsular and subcapsular vessels, and the development of aberrant vessels.
   b. Resistive index (RI) is generally > 0.68 and pulsatility index (PI) > 1.49 in metastatic lymph nodes, with lower values in normal, reactive and lymphomatous lymph nodes.

Further reading

Radiology

Cizinauskas, S., Lang, J., Botteron, C., Tomsa, K., Fatzer, K., Laissue, J., et al., 2002. Idiopathic vascular calcifications in a Labrador retriever puppy. J. Vet. Intern. Med. 16, 192–196.

Clayton Jones, D.G., Allen, W.E., Webbon, P.M., 1981. Arteriovenous fistula in the metatarsal pad of a dog: a case report. J. Small Anim. Pract. 22, 635–639.

Davidson, E.B., Schulz, K.S., Wisner, E., Schwartz, E., 1998. Calcinosis circumscripta of the thoracic wall in a German shepherd dog. J. Am. Anim. Hosp. Assoc. 34, 153–156.

Dueland, R.T., Wagner, S.D., Parker, R.B., 1990. von Willebrand heterotopic osteochondrofibrosis in Doberman Pinschers: five cases (1980–1987). J. Am. Vet. Med. Assoc. 197, 383–388.

Guilliard, M., 2001. Fibrodysplasia ossificans in a German shepherd dog. J. Small Anim. Pract. 42, 550–553.

Hay, C.W., Roberts, R., Latimer, K., 1994. Multilobular tumour of bone at an unusual location in the axilla of a dog. J. Small Anim. Pract. 35, 633–636.

Huntley, K., Frazer, J., Gibbs, C., Gaskell, C.J., 1982. The radiological features of canine Cushing's syndrome: a review of forty-eight cases. J. Small Anim. Pract. 23, 369–380.

Kirberger, R.M., Zambelli, A., 2008. Imaging diagnosis – Aortic thromboembolism associated with spirocercosis in a dog. Vet. Radiol. Ultrasound 48, 418–420.

Kuntz, C.A., Dernell, W.S., Powers, B.E., Withrow, S., 1998. Extraskeletal osteosarcomas in dogs: 14 cases. J. Am. Anim. Hosp. Assoc. 34, 26–30.

Lamb, C.R., White, R.N., McEvoy, F.J., 1994. Sinography in the investigation of draining tracts in small animals: retrospective review of 25 cases. Vet. Surg. 132, 183–185.

Levitin, B., Aroch, A., Aizenberg, I., Foreman, O., Shamir, M., 2003. Linear osteochondromatosis in a cat. Vet. Radiol. Ultrasound 44, 660–664.

Lewis, D.G., Kelly, D.F., 1990. Calcinosis circumscripta in dogs as a cause of spinal ataxia. J. Small Anim. Pract. 31, 36–38.

Llabres Diaz, F., 2006. Practical contrast radiography 5. Other techniques. In Pract. 28, 32–40.

McEvoy, F.J., Peck, G.J., Hilton, G.S., Webbon, P.M., 1994. Normal venographic appearance of the pelvic limb in the dog. Vet. Rec. 134, 641–643.

Naganobu, K., Ohigashi, Y., Akiyoshi, T., Hagio, M.,

Miyamoto, T., Yamaguchi, R., 2003. Lymphography of the thoracic duct by percutaneous injection of iohexol into the popliteal lymph node of dogs: experimental study and clinical application. Vet. Surg. 35, 377–381.

Neu, H., von Rautenfeld, D.B., 1994. Primary congenital lymphoedema in seven Labrador retriever puppies, one German shepherd puppy and one Canadian wolf puppy. Kleintierpraxis 29, 383–405. Reprinted in the European Journal of Companion Animal Practice 5, 52–64 (1995).

Warren, H.B., Carpenter, J.L., 1984. Fibrodysplasia ossificans in three cats. Vet. Pathol. 21, 485–499.

Ultrasonography

Armbrust, L.J., Biller, D.S., Radlinsky, M.G., Hoskinson, J.J., 2003. Ultrasonographic diagnosis of foreign bodies associated with chronic draining tracts and abscesses in dogs. Vet. Radiol. Ultrasound 44, 66–70.

de Bulnes, A.G., Fernandez, P.G., Aguirre, A.M.M., de la Muela, M.S., 1998. Ultrasonographic imaging of canine mammary tumours. Vet. Rec. 143, 687–689.

Fan, T.M., Simpson, K.W., Trasti, S., Birnbaum, N., Center, S.A., Yeager, A., 1998. Calcipotriol toxicity in a dog. J. Small Anim. Pract. 39, 581–586.

Gnudi, G., Volta, A., Bonazzi, M., Gazzola, M., Bertoni, G., 2005. Ultrasonographic features of grass awn migration in the dog. Vet. Radiol. Ultrasound 46, 423–426.

Guilherme, S., Benigni, L., 2008. Ultrasonographic anatomy of the brachial plexus and major nerves of the canine thoracic limb. Vet. Radiol. Ultrasound 49, 577–583.

Kramer, M., Gerwing, M., Hach, V., Schimke, E., 1997. Sonography of the musculoskeletal system in dogs and cats. Vet. Radiol. Ultrasound 38, 139–149.

Lamb, C.R., Duvemois, A., 2005. Ultrasonographic anatomy of the normal canine calcaneal tendon. Vet. Radiol. Ultrasound 46, 326–330.

Nyman, H.T., Kristensen, A.T., Skovgaard, I.M., McEvoy, F.J., 2005. Characterization of normal and abnormal canine lymph nodes using gray-scale B-mode, color flow mapping and spectral ultrasonography: a multivariate study. Vet. Radiol. Ultrasound 46, 404–410.

Nyman, H.T., Kristensen, A.T., Lee, M.H., Martinussen, T., McEvoy, F.J., 2006. Characterization of canine superficial tumors using gray-scale B-mode, color flow mapping and spectral ultrasonography: a multivariate study. Vet. Radiol. Ultrasound 47, 192–198.

Rose, S., Long, C., Knipe, M., Hornof, B., 2005. Ultrasonographic evaluation of brachial plexus tumors in five dogs. Vet. Radiol. Ultrasound 46, 514–517.

Salwei, R.M., O'Brien, R.T., Matheson, J.S., 2005. Characterization of lymphomatous lymph nodes in dogs using contrast harmonic and power Doppler ultrasound. Vet. Radiol. Ultrasound 46, 411–416.

Shah, Z.R., Crass, J.R., Oravec, D.C., Bellon, E.M., 1992. Ultrasonographic detection of foreign bodies in soft tissues using turkey muscle as a model. Vet. Radiol. Ultrasound 33, 94–100.

Stimson, E.L., Cook, W.T., Smith, M.M., Forrester, S.D., Moon, M.L., Saunders, G.K., 2000. Extraskeletal osteosarcoma in the duodenum of a cat. J. Am. Anim. Hosp. Assoc. 36, 332–336.

Volta, A., Bonazzi, M., Gnudi, G., Gazzola, M., Bertoni, G., 2006. Ultrasonographic features of canine lipomas. Vet. Radiol. Ultrasound 47, 589–591.

Both techniques

Benigni, L., Corr, S., Lamb, C.R., 2007. Ultrasonographic assessment of the canine sciatic nerve. Vet. Radiol. Ultrasound 48, 428–433.

Boswood, A., Lamb, C.R., White, R.N., 2000. Aortic and iliac thrombosis in six dogs. J. Small Anim. Pract. 41, 109–114.

Bulman-Fleming, J.C., Gibson, T.W., Kruth, S.A., 2009. Invasive cutaneous angiomatosis and thrombocytopenia in a cat. J. Am. Vet. Med. Assoc. 234, 381–384.

Williams, J., Bailey, M.Q., Schertel, E.R., Valentine, A., 1993. Compartment syndrome in a Labrador retriever. Vet. Radiol. Ultrasound 34, 244–248.

Pathology

Bertazzolo, W., Toscani, L., Calcaterra, S., Crippa, L., Caniatti, M., Bonfanti, U., 2003. Clinicopathological findings in five cats with paw calcification. J. Feline Med. Surg. 5, 11–17.

Appendix

RADIOGRAPHIC FAULTS

Digital radiography

The now widespread use of digital radiography (both direct digital radiography, DR, and computed radiography, CR) has brought with it a new range of faults and artefacts that may degrade image quality and either mask or mimic pathology. These may arise at one of five stages: pre-exposure, during exposure, post exposure, during computerized reading of the image and at the workstation. Pre-exposure, post-exposure and reading artefacts occur only with CR, whereas exposure and workstation artefacts may also arise with DR. Tables A1–A5 summarize causes and remedies of digital radiography artefacts. (Tables A1–A5 are from 'Artifacts in digital radiography' by D.A. Jiménez, L.J. Armbrust, R.T. O'Brien and D.S. Biller, 2008, *Veterinary Radiology and Ultrasound* 49, 321–332, with permission of Wiley-Blackwell.)

One of the most important artefacts that may have clinical relevance is the Überschwinger (halo) artefact, also known as the rebound effect. This arises from a post-processing manoeuvre known as unsharp masking, which is used to create edge enhancement and to improve apparent contrast by accentuating margins. At interfaces between structures of markedly different attenuation, it creates a dark line of even width, or halo. This occurs especially around metallic implants, mimicking loosening of orthopaedic devices such as screws and pins (Fig. A1). It may also give the erroneous impression of a small pneumothorax or pneumomediastinum. Überschwinger artefact is reduced by using minimal edge enhancement algorithms.

Conventional film–screen radiography

Processing faults are generally more common with manual than with automatic processing, although high-quality manual processing can give extremely good results. However, it should not be assumed that automatic processors are foolproof and always trouble-free, as processing faults may arise due to poor maintenance or careless use of the machine. Radiographic faults may also be caused by incorrect use of intensifying screens, film or grids, or the use of damaged equipment. Table A6 gives possible causes and remedies for a variety of radiographic processing faults. Many can occur with both manual and automatic processing; those confined to one or other technique are indicated by (M) or (A), respectively.

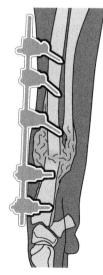

Figure A1 Überschwinger (halo) artefact around metallic implants, seen on a digital radiograph.

Table A1 Pre-exposure artefacts

Artefact	Hardware	Appearance	Cause	Remedy
Storage scatter	CR	• Decreased overall intensity • Decreased image quality • May show pattern of exposure	• Exposure to scatter and background radiation	• Erase imaging plates daily • Protect from scatter radiation
Cracks	CR	• White lines or dots • Often in periphery	• Physical damage to imaging plate • Repeated stress or inappropriate handling	• Handle imaging plates carefully • Perform scheduled maintenance and cleaning • Replace imaging plates as needed
Partial erasure	CR	• Faint superimposition of previous image	• Erasure light failure • Incorrect erasure light intensity	• Replace erasure lights as needed • Incorporate additional ultraviolet light erasure phase
Phantom image	CR	• Faint superimposition of previously erased image	• Prolonged time between erasure and subsequent exposure	• Erase imaging plates daily

CR, computed radiography.

Table A2 Exposure artefacts

Artefact	Hardware	Appearance	Cause	Remedy
Quantum mottle	DR, CR	• Grainy image • Poor overall image quality • Underexposed image	• Insufficient X-ray exposure	• Increase exposure technique as needed
Paradoxical overexposure effect	DR	• Overexposed areas appear lighter	• Severe overexposure	• Reduce exposure technique if possible
Planking	DR	• Rectangular areas of differing intensity	• Variable amplification in separate sections	• Reduce exposure if possible
Upside-down cassette	CR	• Cassette backing superimposed on the image • Severe overall attenuation if cassette has lead backing	• Incorrect cassette placement for exposure	• Check for correct cassette orientation prior to exposure
Grid cut-off	DR, CR	• Regions of increased attenuation	• Incorrect grid placement or alignment	• Check for correct grid location, orientation, and distance from anode
Backscatter	CR	• Fogging and decreased image quality in area underlying scattering structure	• Scatter from object below the cassette • High exposure setting • Gap between scattering object and cassette	• Use cassettes with lead backing
Double exposure	CR, DR	• Images from two exposures superimposed on each other	• Taking multiple radiographs without erasing the cassette • Memory or transfer errors	• Read imaging plates after every exposure • Provide reliable mode of data transfer
Dead pixels	DR	• White dots or lines	• Non-functional detector element(s)	• Use smoothing algorithms for few affected pixels • Replace detector as needed

CR, computed radiography; DR, digital radiography.

Table A3   Post-exposure artefacts

Artefact	Hardware	Appearance	Cause	Remedy
Fading	CR	● More white radiograph ● Decreased overall image quality	● Prolonged time between exposure and reading	● Read imaging plates shortly after exposure
Light leak	CR	● Partial image erasure ● Decreased image quality	● Imaging plate subjected to ambient light	● Read imaging plates shortly after exposure ● Avoid handling imaging plates before reading ● Exercise proper cassette maintenance

CR, computed radiography.

Table A4   Reading artefacts

Artefact	Hardware	Appearance	Cause	Remedy
Debris	CR	● White dots or lines	● Debris blocks emitted light from imaging plate during reading	● Clean imaging plates routinely and as needed
Dirty light guide	CR	● White line in the direction of imaging plate movement during reading	● Dirt on light guide blocks laser from striking the imaging plate	● Perform scheduled reader maintenance ● Clean light guide as needed
Skipped scan lines	CR	● Omission of image information perpendicular to the direction of image plate movement during reading	● Abrupt movement of imaging plate during reading ● Power fluctuation	● Avoid contact with reader during imaging plate reading ● Provide reliable power supply
Unequal phosphors	CR	● Lightened image ● Decreased overall image quality	● Use of imaging plates and image plate reader of differing peak wavelength	● Use imaging plates and readers designed to be used together

CR, computed radiography.

ULTRASOUND TERMINOLOGY AND ARTEFACTS

Terminology

Anechoic – Tissues producing no echoes, appearing black on the image.

Hypoechoic – Tissues producing few echoes, appearing grey on the image.

Hyperechoic – Tissues producing strong echoes, appearing bright on the image.

Most fluids and tissues of homogeneous cellularity produce few or no echoes and therefore appear anechoic or hypoechoic. Gas and mineral interfaces are highly reflective or absorptive and therefore appear hyperechoic. Tissues with a high fibrous tissue or fat content, and tissues containing multiple internal boundaries, tend to produce more echoes and therefore appear brighter than other soft tissues.

Ultrasound artefacts

Some artefacts impair image interpretation and need to be avoided or minimized, while others are incidental features or may even aid interpretation.

Table A5	Workstation artefacts			
Artefact	**Hardware**	**Appearance**	**Cause**	**Remedy**
Diagnostic specifier	DR, CR	● Decreased overall image quality ● Poor image contrast	● Incorrect region of interest designated for post-acquisition processing	● Select correct region of interest for each exposure
Moiré		● Parallel, curved, or wavy lines of increased attenuation	● Interference of grid lines and sampling frequency	● Use oscillating grid ● Use grid with high ratio ● Align grid perpendicular to sampling direction ● Increase exposure time if needed
Border detection	DR, CR	● Image borders placed within the region or interest ● Incorrect image post processing	● Exposure off-centered on cassette ● Highly attenuating objects in area of interest ● Automatic image analysis	● Centre the area of interest ● Use semiautomatic image analysis
Faulty transfer	DR, CR	● Loss or distortion of the image	● Loose cable connection ● Power fluctuation	● Use a reliable transfer method and power supply
Misplacement	DR, CR	● Incorrect localization of sections of the image in the radiograph	● Loose cable connection ● Power fluctuation	● Use a reliable transfer method and power supply
Überschwinger	DR, CR	● Dark zone surrounding highly attenuating objects	● Unsharp masking techniques used to accentuate object borders	● Use moderate settings and kernel size to increase object contrast
Density threshold	DR, CR	● Darkening and decreased contrast of lesser attenuating structures	● Inclusion of high-density objects in histogram analysis and image greyscale	● Create density threshold to exclude metallic objects from histogram analysis

DR, digital radiography; CR, computed radiography.

It is helpful to be able to recognize all common artefacts to prevent their misinterpretation.

Poor transducer contact

Multiple concentric (sector) or straight (linear) lines running across the image, parallel to the scanning surface, obscuring detail. This is usually due to poor preparation of the scanning surface or inadequate use of acoustic gel, but may also occur due to poor congruence between the transducer and body surfaces.

Acoustic shadowing

Seen at highly reflective or absorptive interfaces such as those involving bone or gas. A very strong echo is produced at the interface, but little or no sound passes beyond the interface into deeper tissues. Thus a dark 'shadow' is seen deep to the hyperechoic surface. This may be useful in recognizing small mineral or gas accumulations (e.g. renal calculi) but can also impair visualization of tissues (e.g. rib shadowing may obscure thoracic structures). As far as possible, intervening bone- or gas-containing structures should be avoided when selecting the scanning site (Fig. A2) in order to minimize acoustic shadowing.

Acoustic enhancement

Seen deep to fluid-filled structures as an area of increased echogenicity. As sound passes through tissues, it is scattered and absorbed as well as reflected, but little of this occurs as it passes through fluid. Thus the intensity of sound reaching the far side of a fluid focus is greater than that which has travelled to the same depth through soft tissues. Acoustic enhancement is useful in differentiating fluid foci from tissues that are hypoechoic but solid (Fig. A3).

Table A6   Film faults seen with film–screen radiography

Sign	Causes	Remedies
Radiograph too dark		
Image too dark but area outside primary beam or protected by lead markers normal	Overexposure	Reduce kVp and/or mAs (kVp reduction of 10 is approximately equal to a halving of mAs). Check FFD, and increase it if it is inadvertently too short
Whole film too dark	Overdevelopment	Reduce developer temperature or developing time; ensure starter solution (restrainer) used where necessary
	Fogging (see below)	See below
Radiograph too light		
Image of patient too light, but background black ('soot and whitewash' film)	Underexposure	Increase kVp to increase penetration of patient. Check FFD and reduce if it is inadvertently too long
Image of both patient and background too light, resulting in very low contrast	Underdevelopment	Increase developer temperature or developing time; replenish or replace developer; keep lid on developer tank to delay oxidation (M); check that film is compatible with chemicals used
	Gross underexposure	Increase exposure factors markedly
	Use of incompatible intensifying screens and film (e.g. film not sensitive to light colour emitted by screens)	Check compatibility of intensifying screens and film
Image of patient tolerable (some internal detail), but background is grey not black	Underdevelopment with compensatory overexposure	Correct development and reduce exposure factors
Uneven, marbled appearance to film	Patchy underdevelopment due to uneven developer temperature (M)	Stir developer thoroughly before use to ensure even temperature; use water bath heating method not a direct heater
Fogging (darkening of the film unrelated to the primary beam) – may be generalized or localized	Exposure to white light during storage or processing (exposed area usually black)	Careful storage and use of film; keep lid on developer solution while film in (M)
	Light leakage into darkroom (film diffusely grey and finger shadows may be seen)	Ensure darkroom is light-proof
	Safelight too bright or faulty	Check by laying film on bench with metal object on it for 30 s, then processing it
	Overdevelopment (chemical fog), including lack of starter (restrainer) solution and incompatibility of developer with film	Check developer is correctly made up and that solution is compatible with the film; use at correct temperature and for correct time
	Exposure to scattered radiation	Keep unexposed film away from the radiography area
	Out-of-date film (storage fog)	Use film chronologically and within its use-by date; store at appropriate temperature
Pale patches on the film	Dried splashes of liquid on the intensifying screens; splashes of water or fixer on the unprocessed film (usually M)	Clean intensifying screens regularly; good darkroom design with wet and dry areas (M); handle films with clean, dry hands
Dark or black patches on the film	Splashes of developer on the unprocessed film (usually M)	As above
White specks and lines on the film	Dirt or animal hairs on the intensifying screens; damage to the screens or film emulsion	Clean intensifying screens regularly; handle screens and film carefully; replace screens when damaged
Parallel white or black lines		
Fine lines, close together	Grid faults: damaged grid; grid not perpendicular to primary beam; focused grid used at wrong FFD or upside down; moving grid not activated	Correct use of the grid
Lines of variable width and further apart	Scratches from automatic processor, for example damaged rollers (A)	Regular servicing and cleaning of the automatic processor

Continued

Table A6 Film faults seen with film–screen radiography—Cont'd

Sign	Causes	Remedies
Crescentic black lines	Crimp marks from careless handling of the film before processing	Careful handling of unprocessed film
Branching black lines	Static electricity	Handle film carefully; use antistatic screen cleaner; use a darkroom humidifier
Film background grey and not transparent	Incomplete fixing – fixer exhausted or fixing time too short	Periodically change fixer; correct fixing procedure
Film becomes brown or yellow with time	Incomplete fixing (film background as above) or washing (film surface dirty in reflected light)	Correct fixing and washing
Blurring of the image	Movement of the patient	Restrain patient effectively; use short exposure times; expose during respiratory pause
	Movement of the X-ray tube head	Ensure X-ray stand is stable, especially if exposure cable is attached to tube head
	Poor screen–film contact (test by scattering paper clips on the cassette and making a radiograph)	Replace the cassette
	Large object–film distance	Have part of interest as close to film as possible and largest FFD practicable
	Fogging (see above)	Depending on the cause
	Very rapid film–screen combination used	Use a slower combination consistent with X-ray machine's capabilities
	Movement of the cassette (large-animal radiography)	Use a stable cassette holder on a stand and not held freely

FFD, focus–film distance; A, automatic processing; M, manual processing.

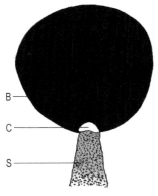

Figure A2 Acoustic shadowing deep to a urinary bladder calculus. B, urinary bladder; C, highly echogenic cystic calculus; S, acoustic shadow.

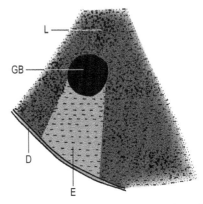

Figure A3 Acoustic enhancement deep to the gall bladder; liver parenchyma in this area appears artefactually hyperechoic compared with adjacent liver. D, diaphragm; E, region of acoustic enhancement deep to the gall bladder; GB, gall bladder; L, liver parenchyma.

Edge shadowing

Shadows seen deep to the edges of rounded, fluid-filled structures such as the gall bladder. Occurs due to refraction and reflection of those parts of the sound beam impinging on the curved edges of the structure (Fig. A4).

Reverberation artefacts

These are produced at highly reflective interfaces such as the surface of air-filled lung or free abdominal gas, due to rapid reverberation of echoes

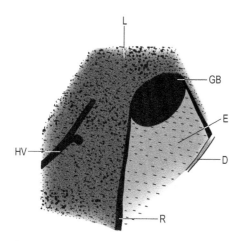

Figure A4   Edge shadowing in the liver, arising from the edge of the gall bladder. D, diaphragm; E, acoustic enhancement; GB, gall bladder; HV, hepatic vein; L, liver parenchyma; R, refractive shadowing.

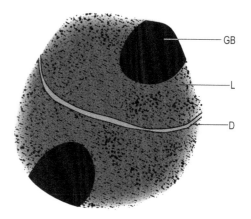

Figure A5   Mirror image artefact arising at the liver–diaphragm–lung interface. D, diaphragm; GB, gall bladder; L, liver parenchyma; M, mirror image – illusion of liver and second gall bladder beyond the diaphragm.

between the interface and the transducer surface. Streams of bright echoes are seen, comprising equidistant parallel lines that eventually trail off.

Comet tail and ring–down artefacts

These appear similar, as closely spaced echoes or solid echogenic streaks distal to the reflector. Their origins are, however, different in that comet tail artefacts usually arise deep to a metallic foreign body whereas ring-down artefacts arise deep to frothy gas accumulations such as those arising in alveolar infiltrates or within a hollow viscus.

Mirror image artefact

This is produced at curved, strongly reflective interfaces and is most commonly seen at the interfaces between liver or diaphragm and lung, and heart and lung. Internal reverberations occur between the interface and the superficial tissues, resulting in spurious reconstructions of superficial tissues at deeper sites. Thus, for example, liver tissue may appear to lie on both sides of the diaphragm, and it is important to recognize that this may be an artefact rather than rupture of the diaphragm (Fig. A5).

Side lobe artefacts

These are spurious echoes that originate from tissue outside the path of the primary sound beam. Minor sound beams travel in a number of

directions, and these are termed *side lobes*. If a side lobe interacts with a highly reflective interface, the returning echoes may be erroneously displayed on the image. Such echoes are much weaker than those originating from the primary beam.

Slice thickness artefact

The ultrasound beam is very thin but still of finite thickness. If part of the thickness of the beam lies within a fluid-filled structure and part lies outside, averaging of the echoes occurs, resulting in the presence of echoes within a fluid-filled structure – pseudosediment. This disappears when the entire thickness of the beam is placed in the fluid-filled structure.

GEOGRAPHIC DISTRIBUTIONS OF DISEASES

Most of the following parasitic and infectious diseases (Table A7) are not found ubiquitously, and their approximate geographic distributions are given. For brevity, these conditions are indicated throughout the text of the preceding 12 chapters with an asterisk (*). However, the increased passage of domestic pets between different countries and the possible effects of climate change should be taken into account, as these may result in 'exotic' diseases arising in non-endemic areas. Fungal diseases are most often encountered in younger animals, usually those less than 4 years old.

Table A7 Geographic distribution of diseases

Disease and organism	Type of organism	Species affected	Main geographic distribution
Actinomycosis (*Actinomyces viscosus, A. hordeovulneris* and other spp.)	Bacterium	● Dogs – sporadic, especially young adult to middle-aged, large-breed hunting dogs or other dogs used or kept in an outdoor environment ● Cats – infrequent ● Infection is usually via aspiration of vegetation or through damaged skin	*A. viscosus* – worldwide; *A. hordeovulneris* – mainly western USA
Aelurostrongylosis – feline lungworm (*Aelurostrongylus abstrusus*)	Helminth: nematode	● Cats, especially hunting cats, as transmitted via gastropods (slugs and snails) ± small rodents, birds, amphibians and reptiles that have eaten the gastropods and are acting as paratenic hosts ● Only causes disease occasionally; usually subclinical	Worldwide; mainly Europe (including UK) and USA
Angiostrongylosis – 'French' heartworm (*Angiostrongylus vasorum*)	Helminth: nematode	● Dogs – usually younger dogs kept in confined groups; also foxes, which may act as a reservoir of infection for dogs. Transmitted via gastropods	Sporadic worldwide, especially Western Europe in focal areas (including southern UK and Ireland). Sporadic in USA in imported dogs. Also Africa, Russia, Asia, South America
Aspergillosis (*Aspergillus* spp.)	Fungus	● Dogs, with systemic form most often in German Shepherd dogs and in immunosuppressed patients ● Cats – rare ● Infection is via inhalation of airborne organism	Worldwide; disseminated form usually in warm, dry climates. Saprophyte in soil and decaying vegetation
Babesiosis (*Babesia canis, B. vogeli, B. rossi* and *B. gibsoni* – dog, and *B. felis* – cat)	Protozoon	● Dogs, transmitted via ticks – *B. canis* by *Dermacentor reticulates* (Europe), *B. vogeli* by *Rhipicephalus sanguineus* (brown dog tick; worldwide), *B. rossi* by *Haemaphysalis elliptica* (sub-Saharan Africa) and *B. gibsoni* by *R. sanguineus* ● Cats – *B. felis*; cycle not known	Worldwide in tropical, subtropical and warm temperate climes (e.g. southern Europe; North, Central and Southern America; Asia; Africa) – increasingly widespread. Feline babesiosis mainly in South Africa
Blastomycosis – North American blastomycosis (*Blastomyces dermatitidis*)	Fungus	● Dogs, especially young, large-breed dogs living close to water ● Cats – rare ● Infection is usually by inhalation	Endemic in North America, mainly close to river valleys and lakes. Sporadic in Central and Africa, Europe and Africa. Soil saprophyte
Borreliosis, Lyme disease (*Borrelia burgdorferi*)	Spirochaete	● Dogs – transmitted by *Ixodes* ticks ● Cats may seroconvert but clinical disease is rare	Worldwide but focal; North America, Europe (including UK), former USSR, Asia, Australia
Capillariasis – fox lungworm (*Capillaria aerophila; syn. Eucoleus aerophila*)	Helminth: nematode	● Dogs and cats are occasionally affected, but the main host is the fox ● Recorded as a zoonosis in some countries ● Infection is via ingestion of eggs from faeces	Mainly North America, Europe, Middle East, Russia, North Africa
Coccidioidomycosis – valley fever or San Joaquin Valley fever (*Coccidioides immitis*)	Fungus	● Dogs, especially young, middle- to large-breed dogs ● Cats – rare ● Infection is usually acquired by inhalation	Endemic in semiarid regions of western and south-western USA, Mexico, Central and South America. Soil saprophyte
Crenosomosis (*Crenosoma vulpis*)	Helminth: nematode	● Dogs are affected occasionally, but the main host is the fox ● Infection is transmitted via gastropods	Worldwide in foxes; occasional in dogs in Europe (including UK), North America and Asia
Cryptococcosis (*Cryptococcus neoformans* and *C. gattii*)	Fungus	● Cats – the most common systemic mycosis of cats; predisposed to by immunosuppression ● Dogs – less common; also predisposed to by immunosuppression ● Infection is acquired from the environment, probably by inhalation, and not from other animals	*C. neoformans* – worldwide; *C. gattii* – tropical and subtropical areas. Soil saprophyte and found in bird excreta, especially that of pigeons

Giant kidney worm (*Dioctyphyma renale*)	Helminth: the largest nematode	● Dogs and cats; definitive host mink ● Infection is via ingestion of annelid worms ± raw fish	Worldwide but sporadic
Dirofilariasis – heartworm (*Dirofilaria immitis*)	Helminth	● Dogs – common ● Cats – occasionally affected but are inherently resistant ● Infection is transmitted by mosquitoes. Humans are occasionally infected, dogs and cats acting as reservoirs	Endemic in tropical, subtropical and warm temperate areas (e.g. southern Europe, North and South America, southern Asia, Africa and Australia)
Alveolar echinococcosis (*Echinococcus multilocularis*)	Helminth: cestode	● Dogs – rare; definitive host fox ● Infection is by ingestion of eggs (e.g. in fox faeces)	Temperate, continental and Arctic zones of northern hemisphere, including Eurasia, North America and Japan
Ehrlichiosis (*Ehrlichia canis*)	Rickettsia	● Dogs – infection is transmitted via the brown dog tick *Rhipicephalus sanguineus*	Most tropical and subtropical regions: reported in the USA, Africa, southern Europe, the Caribbean and parts of Asia; also temperate regions including parts of Europe
Filaroidiasis (*Filaroides hirthi* and *F. milksi*)	Helminth: nematode	● Dogs: *F. hirthi* – sporadic, most often in research colonies or immunosuppressed or stressed dogs; *F. milksi* – a parasite of wildlife of questionable significance in dogs, although morphologically similar to *F. hirthi*. Both have a direct life cycle	Worldwide but sporadic
Tularaemia, rabbit fever (*Francisella* or *Pasteurella tularensis*)	Bacterium	● Dogs and cats are affected occasionally – mainly a disease of rabbits, rodents and other wildlife ● Ticks and other blood-feeding insects are the primary vectors for dogs and cats; infection is also acquired by eating infected rabbits or rodents	Temperate regions of northern hemisphere, mainly between latitudes 30° and 70° N, including much of Eurasia and North America. Type A strains are highly virulent to rabbits and are found only in North America; type B strains are avirulent to rabbits and are also found elsewhere
Hepatozoonosis (*Hepatozoon canis*)	Protozoon	● Dogs, primarily via ingestion of the brown dog tick *Rhipicephalus sanguineus* ● Rarer in cats; causative *Hepatozoon* species and vectors not identified	Worldwide, especially USA, South America, southern Europe, Africa, Middle and Far East
American canine hepatozoooonosis (*Hepatozoon americanum*)	Protozoon	● Dogs, via ingestion of the Gulf Coast tick *Amblyomma maculatum*; much more severe disease than that due to *H. canis*	Southern USA only
Histoplasmosis (*Histoplasma capsulatum*)	Fungus	● Dogs – the most common canine systemic mycosis of North America ● Cats – equally susceptible ● Affected animals are usually less than 4 years old ● Infection is via inhalation	Well-defined warm, humid and moist tropical, subtropical and temperate regions between latitudes 45° N and 30° S; endemic in certain river valleys in USA; also Canada. Sporadic elsewhere. Soil saprophyte, especially in soil rich in bird or bat faeces
Leishmaniasis (*Leishmania donovani* syn. *infantum*)	Protozoon	● Dogs; less common in cats ● Infection is transmitted via sandflies ● Potential zoonosis	Sporadic in tropical, subtropical and temperate climes; mainly between latitudes 50° N and 40° S. Endemic in Central and South America, south-eastern USA, southern Europe, Africa and Asia. Increasingly seen elsewhere due to pet travel
Nocardiosis (*Nocardia asteroides* and other spp.)	Bacterium	● Dogs – sporadic, especially if immunosuppressed ● Cats – less common ● Opportunistic infection ● Male preponderance in both dogs and cats	Worldwide. Soil saprophyte
Oslerus (formerly *Filaroides*) *osleri*	Helminth: nematode	● Dogs ● Direct life cycle	Worldwide

Continued

Table A7   Geographic distribution of diseases—Cont'd

Disease and organism	Type of organism	Species affected	Main geographic distribution
Paragonimiasis, lung fluke (mainly *Paragonimus kellicotti*)	Helminth: trematode	● Dogs and cats ● Infection is transmitted via aquatic or amphibian snails, with crayfish and crab as intermediate host ● Not transmissible directly to humans, but dogs may act as reservoirs of infection	North America, Latin America, Asia, Africa
Canine nasal mite (*Pneumossysus caninum*)	Arthropod	● Dogs – usually non-pathogenic	Worldwide but sporadic
Pneumocystosis (*Pneumocystis carinii*)	Fungus but behaves like a protozoon	● Dogs – sporadic, especially in young Cavalier King Charles Spaniels, Miniature Dachshunds (probably due to immunodeficiency) and immunosuppressed animals ● Otherwise opportunistic and of low virulence ● Acquired by inhalation ● Cats – usually asymptomatic	Worldwide but sporadic in tropical and temperate climates
Pythiosis (*Pythium insidiosum*)	Fungus	● Dogs – especially young, large-breed, male dogs, particularly outdoor working dogs ● Cats – rare ● Mode of infection is not known	Many subtropical countries (e.g. Australasia, South-East Asia, South America, south-eastern USA, Caribbean. Water-borne in fresh water
Rocky Mountain spotted fever (*Rickettsia rickettsii*)	*Rickettsia*	● Dogs – transmitted via dog ticks *Dermacentor variabilis, D. andersoni, Rhipicephalus sanguineus* and *Amblyomma* spp ● Humans may be infected directly or occasionally from dogs	North, Central and South America
Spirocercosis (*Spirocerca lupi*)	Helminth: nematode	● Dogs – very common in some endemic areas ● Cats – seldom reported ● Infection is transmitted via dung beetle or by a variety of small vertebrates that have eaten dung beetles and are acting as paratenic hosts	Most tropical and subtropical countries
Sporotrichosis (*Sporothrix schenckii*)	Fungus	● Cats – especially male cats ● Dogs – less common ● Infection is usually by traumatic inoculation ● The feline disease is zoonotic	Worldwide in warmer areas including USA and Asia; uncommon in Europe. Soil saprophyte, especially if rich in decaying vegetable matter
Toxoplasmosis (*Toxoplasma gondii*)	Protozoon	● Cats – the definitive host, infected via rodents, birds or raw meat ● Dogs – especially if immunosuppressed ● Zoonotic	Worldwide

Further reading

Radiography

Drost, W.T., Reese, D.J., Hornof, W.J., 2008. Digital radiography artifacts. Vet. Radiol. Ultrasound 49 (Suppl. 1), S48–S56.

Ewers, R.S., 1995. Avoiding errors in radiography. Vet. Annu. 35, 47–60.

Jiménez, D.A., Armbrust, L.J., O'Brien, R.T., Biller, D.S., 2008.

Artifacts in digital radiography. Vet. Radiol. Ultrasound 49, 321–332.

Kirberger, R.M., 1999. Radiographic quality evaluation for exposure variables – a review. Vet. Radiol. Ultrasound 40, 220–226.

Kirberger, R.M., Roos, C.J., 1995. Radiographic artefacts. J. S. Afr. Vet. Assoc. 66, 85–94.

Lamb, C.R., 1995. Errors in radiology. Vet. Annu. 35, 33–46.

McLear, R.C., Handmaker, H., Schmidt, C., Walls, C., Gottfried, S., Siegel, E., 2004. "Überschwinger" or "rebound effect" artifact in computed radiographic imaging of metallic implants in veterinary medicine (abstract). Vet. Radiol. Ultrasound 45, 266.

Papageorges, M., 1990. The Mach phenomenon. Vet. Radiol. 31, 274–280.

Papageorges, M., 1998. Visual perception and radiographic interpretation. Compendium on Continuing Education for the Practicing Veterinarian (Small Animal) 20, 1215–1223.

Scrivani, P.V., Bednarski, R.M., Myer, C.W., Dykes, N.L., 1996. Restraint methods for radiography in dogs and cats. Compendium on Continuing Education for the Practicing Veterinarian (Small Animal) 18, 899–916.

Smallwood, J.E., Shively, M.J., Rendano, V.T., Hable, R.E., 1985. A standardized nomenclature for radiographic projections used in veterinary medicine. Vet. Radiol. 26, 2–9.

Ultrasound

Barthez, P.Y., Leveille, R., Scrivani, P. V., 1997. Side lobes and grating lobes artifacts in ultrasound imaging. Vet. Radiol. Ultrasound 38, 387–393.

Kirberger, R.M., 1995. Imaging artefacts in diagnostic ultrasound – a review. Vet. Radiol. Ultrasound 36, 297–306.

Lamb, C.R., Boswood, A., 1995. Ultrasound corner: an artefact resulting from propagation speed error. Vet. Radiol. Ultrasound 36, 549–550.

O'Brien, R.T., Zagzebski, J.A., Delany, F.A., 2001. Ultrasound corner: Range ambiguity artefact.
Vet. Radiol. Ultrasound 42, 542–545.

Penninck, D.G., 2002. Artifacts. In: Nyland, T.G., Mattoon, J.S (Eds.), Small Animal Diagnostic Ultrasound. second ed. Saunders, Philadelphia, pp. 19–29.

Geographic distributions of diseases

Bolt, G., Monrad, J., Koch, J., Jensen, A.L., 1994. Canine angiostrongylosis: a review. Vet. Rec. 135, 447–452.

Clinkenbeard, K.D., Wolf, A.M., Cowell, R.L., Tyler, R.L., 1989. Canine disseminated histoplasmosis. Compendium on Continuing Education for the Practicing Veterinarian (Small Animal) 11, 1347–1360.

Cobb, M.A., Fisher, M.A., 1992. *Crensoma vulpis* infection in a dog. Vet. Rec. 130, 452.

Graupmann-Kuzma, A., Valentine, B. A., Shubitz, L.F., Dial, S.M., Watrous, S.J., Tornquist, S.J., 2008. Coccidioidomycosis in dogs and cats: a review. J. Am. Anim. Hosp. Assoc. 44, 226–235.

Greene, R.T., 1998. Coccidioidomycosis. In: Green, C. E (Ed.), Infectious Diseases of the Dog and Cat. second ed. Saunders, Philadelphia, pp. 391–398.

Hoch, H., Strickland, K., 2008. Canine and feline dirofilariasis: life cycle, pathophysiology and diagnosis. Compendium – Continuing Education for Veterinarians 30, 133–141.

Legendre, A., 1998. Blastomycosis. In: Green, C.E (Ed.), Infectious
Diseases of the Dog and Cat. second ed. Saunders, Philadelphia, pp. 371–377.

Osborne, C.A., Stevens, J.B., Hanlon, G.P., Rosin, E., Bemrick, W.J., 1969. *Dioctyphyma renale* in the dog. J. Am. Vet. Med. Assoc. 155, 605–620.

Quinn, P.J., Donnelly, W.J.C., Carter, M.E., Markey, B.K.J., Torgerson, P.R., Breathnach, R.M. S., 1997. Microbial and Parasitic Diseases of the Dog and Cat. Saunders, London.

Scharf, G., Deplazes, P., Kaser-Hotz, L., Borer, L., Hasler, A., Haller, A., et al., 2004. Radiographic, ultrasonographic, and computed tomographic appearance of alveolar echinococcosis in dogs. Vet. Radiol. Ultrasound 45, 411–418.

Soler, M., Cardoso, L., Teixeira, M., Agut, A., 2008. Imaging diagnosis – *Dioctyphyma renale* in a dog. Vet. Radiol. Ultrasound 49, 307–308.

Torgerson, P.R., McCarthy, G., Donnelly, W.J.C., 1997. *Filaroides hirthi* verminous pneumonia in a West Highland white terrier bred in Ireland. Vet. Rec. 38, 217–219.

Trotz-Williams, L.A., Trees, A.J., 2003. Systematic review of the distribution of the major vector-borne parasitic infections in dogs and cats in Europe. Vet. Rec. 152, 97–105.

Van der Merwe, L.L., Kirberger, R. M., Clift, S., Williams, M., Keller, V., Naidoo, V., 2008. *Spirocerca lupi* infection in the dog. Vet. J. 176, 294–309.

Index

Note: Page numbers in *italics* refer to figures and page numbers in **bold** refer to tables.

A

abdomen
  differences between dogs and
    cats, **231**
  mineralization on radiographs,
    260–2
  radiographic technique and
    positioning, **230**, 230–1
  ultrasonography, 231–2
abdominal masses, 255–60
  caudal abdomen, 259–60
  cranial abdomen, 255–7
  mid-abdomen, 257–9
abdominal wall, *232*, 232–3
abductor pollicis longus
  tenosynovitis, 65
abscess, 337
  abdominal wall, 233
  cavities, 105
  diaphragmatic, 212
  hepatic, 242
  intrahepatic, 241
  laryngeal, 104
  mediastinal, 209–10, 211, 212
  nasopharyngeal, 103
  oesophageal, 211, 215
  ovarian, 320
  paraoesophageal, 218
  paravertebral soft tissues, 130, 131
  perirenal, 308
  peritoneal, 236
  pleural, 204
  prostatic, 323
  pulmonary, 161, 170, 201
  renal, 300, 303
  retrobulbar, 109

  retroperitoneal space, 237
  salivary gland, 109, 110
  soft tissues, 105, 332, 336, *336*
  subcapsular, 299, 300
  testicular, 326
  tooth root, 102, *102*
  tracheal, 151
acanthomatous ameloblastoma, 91
accessory carpal bone fracture, 63, *64*
Achilles tendon lesions, 79, *79*, *337*
achondroplasia, 3
acoustic enhancement, 344, *346*
acoustic shadowing, 343–4, *346*
acromegaly
  calvarium thickening, 89
  frontal bones variation, 101
  mandible, 92
actinomycosis
  geographic distribution, **348**
  lymphadenopathy, 212
  poorly marginated pulmonary
    opacities, 158
  vertebral size and shape variations,
    120
acute idiopathic polyradiculoneuritis,
  141
acute respiratory distress syndrome,
  157
adactyly, 52
adamantinoma, 91
Addison's disease
  see hypoadrenocorticism
adenocarcinoma, 237
  adrenal glands, 254
  ciliary body, 107, 108
  gastric, 271, 277
  large intestine, 291

  ovarian, 320
  pancreatic, 253
  poorly marginated pulmonary
    opacities, 157
  pulmonary, 161
  small intestine, 283, 285
  tracheal, 151
  uterine, 321
adenoma, 237
  ciliary body, 107, 108
  ovarian, 320
  parathyroid gland, 110
  renal, 303
  thyroid gland, 110
adenomyosis, uterine, 321
adrenal glands, 253–5
  mass, 237, 254, 257, *257*
  mineralization on radiographs,
    261
  radiology, 253–4
  ultrasonography, 254–5
aeulurostrongylosis (*Aelurostrongylus
  abstrusus*), 155–6, 158, 162
  geographic distribution, **348**
  interstitial lung pattern, 164, 165
  nodular lung pattern, 163
  vascular lung pattern, 166
ageing, thoracic radiological changes,
  147–8
air embolism, 187
airway obstruction, alveolar lung
  pattern, 156
allergic pulmonary disease
  alveolar lung pattern, 156
  poorly marginated pulmonary
    opacities, 158
alveolar echinococcosis, 242, 246, **349**

alveolar filling, 159
alveolar lung pattern, 154–7, *155*
alveolar nodules, 162
amelia, 52
ameloblastoma, 91
amyloidosis, 299
amyloid-producing odontogenic
    tumour, 91
anaemia, 171
    autoimmune haemolytic, 158,
        167, 251
    chronic, 179, 249
    myelophthistic, 17
    severe, 191, 192
anaphylactic reactions, alveolar lung
        pattern, 156
anconeal process, ununited, 57, *57*
aneurysm
    aortic, 183
    contrast studies, 335
    ventricular, 183, 186
angiography, 188–9, 335–6
    left heart, 188
    non-selective, 189
    renal, 302, 303
    right heart, 189
    selective, 188
angiolipoma, 136
angiomatosis, vertebral, 126
angiostrongylosis (*Angiostrongylus
        vasorum*), 155, 158
    geographic distribution, **348**
    interstitial lung pattern, 165
    mixed lung pattern, 168
    right ventricular enlargement, 185
    vascular lung pattern, 166
ankylosis, temporomandibular
        joint, 94
annulus fibrosus
    dorsally bulging calcified,
        128, *129*
    hypertrophied, 135
anodontia, 101
antebrachium, 60–3
anticoagulant poisoning
    alveolar lung pattern, 156
    interstitial lung pattern, 164
    mediastinal widening, 210
    spinal cord compression, 136
    spinal cord enlargement, 210
anticonvulsant therapy, osteopenia,
        22
anury, 116
aorta
    abdominal, 238–9
    abnormalities, *183*, 183–4, 192
    coarctation of the, 183
aorticopulmonary septal defect, 167,
        182, 183, 185

aortic valve
    abnormalities, 192
    Doppler flow abnormalities, 195
    insufficiency, 182
    stenosis, 182, 183
aplasia, frontal sinuses, 100
aplastic dens, 123
apophysis, 2
APUDoma, 271
arachnoid pseudocyst, spinal, 137–8,
        138
arrhythmias, 176
artefacts, 341, **342**, **343**, **344**, **345–6**
arteriography, 335–6
arteriosclerosis, 179
arteriovenous fistula, 183, 184,
        185, 193
    hepatic, 248
    peripheral, 166
arteriovenous malformation, 110
arthritis *see specific types*
arthrography, 40
arthropathy
    decreased joint space width, 42
    proliferative joint disease, 45
articular cartilage, 1, 2, 42
articular facets
    abnormalities, 129–30
    aplasia, 119, 130
    lesions, spinal cord compression,
        136
ascites, 234, *234*, *236*
aspergillosis (*Aspergillus* spp.)
    geographic distribution, **348**
    mixed osteolytic-osteogenic
        lesions, 27
    poorly marginated pulmonary
        opacities, 158
    rhinitis, 99
    sinusitis, 100
    vertebral endplate irregularities,
        128
    vertebral size and shape variations,
        120
asteroid hyalosis, 107
asthma, feline bronchial, 153, 156,
        168, 207, 224
astrocytoma, 138
ataxia
    hereditary, 140
    hound, 141
atelectasis, 159, 207
    alveolar lung pattern, 156
    consolidated lung lobes, 160
atlantoaxial subluxation, 123,
        123, 129
atresia ani, 289
atresia coli, 289
atrial enlargement, 149, 152, *152*

atrial septal defects, 167, 184, 185,
        193, 194
autoimmune haemolytic anaemia,
        158, 167, 251
avascular necrosis of the femoral
        head, 24, 29, 43, 45, 69, *69*
azygos vein dilation, 210, 212

B

Baastrup's disease, 121
babesiosis
    geographic distribution, **348**
    interstitial lung pattern, 164
barium burger, 214
barium enema, 290
barium-impregnated polyethylene
        spheres (BIPS), 272
barium paste, 214
barrel-chested conformation, 220
basal cell carcinoma, 91
basilar artery, 90
benign prostatic hyperplasia, 323,
        324, 325
biceps brachii tendon rupture, 54
biceps brachii tendon sheath rupture,
        54
biceps femoris calcifying
        tendinopathy, 71
bicipital tenosynovitis, 55
bile peritonitis, 234
biliary tract, 247
biloma, 241
bilothorax, 203
bipartite patella, 72
bladder, urinary, 310–16
    calculi, 311, 313, *313*
    content changes on
        ultrasonography, 316
    contrast studies, 312–15
    displacement, 310
    masses, 259
    mineralization on radiographs, 261
    non-visualization, 310
    normal ultrasonographic
        appearance, 315
    polyps, 313, 314, 315, 316
    radiopacity variations, 311–12
    rupture, 310
    shape variations, 311
    size variations, 311
    ultrasonographic examination, 315
    wall
        cystic structures on
            ultrasonography, 316
        echogenicity changes, 316
        thickening on ultrasonography,
            315–16

blastomycosis, 108
    geographic distribution, **348**
    interstitial lung pattern, 164
    lymphadenopathy, 212
    mixed osteolytic-osteogenic
        lesions, 27
    poorly marginated pulmonary
        opacities, 158
bleb, pulmonary, 169
block vertebrae, 118, 129
blood clot
    bladder, 313, *313*, 314
    ocular, 107
bolus intravenous urogram, 302
bone cysts
    altered shape of bone, 14, 15
    aneurysmal, 25
    metaphyses, 32
    osteolytic areas in diaphyses, 34
    osteolytic lesions, 25, *25*
    radius/ulna, 63
    reduced radiopacity, 28
bone infarcts
    increased radiopacity, 17, 28
    sclerotic areas in diaphyses, 34
bone lesions
    aggressive, 7, **7**, *8*
    non-aggressive, 7, **7**, *7*
bone loss (osteolysis), 3–4
    apparent, 42
    geographic, 4–5, *5*
    mixed pattern, 5, 5–6
    moth-eaten, 5, *5*
    patterns of focal, 4–6
    permeative, 5, *5*
    ribs, 220–1
bone metastases
    increased radiopacity, 28
    mixed osteolytic-osteogenic
        lesions, 26, 34
    mixed radiopacity, 29
    osteolytic areas in diaphyses, 34
    osteolytic lesions, 23, *23*
    reduced radiopacity, 28
    sclerotic areas in diaphyses, 34
bone(s)
    abscess, 25
    altered shape of, 14–15
    anatomy of, 2, *3*
    angulation of, 14–15
    bowing, 14
    cysts *see* bone cysts
    growth plates *see* physis
    increased radiopacity, 16
    infarcts *see* bone infarcts
    lesions *see* bone lesions
    loss *see* bone loss (osteolysis)
    masses *see* bony masses
    metastases *see* bone metastases

ossification *see* ossification
    production, 4
    response to disease or injury, 3–4
    tumours *see* bone tumours
bone tumours
    cranial radiopacity variations, 89
    differentiating from osteomyelitis,
        28
    femur, 71
    humerus, 55
    maxilla/premaxilla, 91
    metaphyses, 31
    mixed osteolytic-osteogenic
        lesions, 25–6, *26*
    radius/ulna, 62–3
    sclerotic areas in diaphyses, 34
    tibia, 77
    see also specific tumours
bony masses, 19–20, *20*
    calvarium thickening, 89–90
    cranial cavity shape variations, 88
    frontal bones variation, 101
    multiple, 29
border effacement, 148, *148*
borreliosis, **348**
boxing glove sign, 269
brachycephalic breeds, 87, *87*, 88, 96
brachycephalic obstructive airway
        syndrome, 103, 104
brachydactyly, 52
brachymelia, 52
brachyury, 116
bradycardia, 178
brain ultrasonography, 90
bronchi
    changes, 152, *152*
    dilation, 154
    occlusion, 160
    perforation, 201
bronchial lumen opacification, 154
bronchial lung pattern, *153*, 153–4
bronchial wall
    calcification, 147
    visibility changes, 153
bronchiectasis, 154, 169
bronchiolitis obliterans, 154, 157
bronchitis, 153
    allergic, 168
    mixed lung pattern, 168
    pulmonary hyperlucency, 168, 169
bronchopneumonia, 155
Brucella canis, 128
Budd-Chiari syndrome, 186–7, 240
bulla
    pulmonary, 169
    tympanic, *96*, 96–7
bursitis, bicipital, 55
butcher's dog disease, 21
butterfly vertebrae, 118, *118*, 140

C

caecal impaction, 290
calcification
    aorta, 184
    bronchial wall, 147, 165
    costochondral junctions, 147
    cranial bone, 89
    external ear canal, 96
    hilar lymph node, 170
    idiopathic vascular, 333
    interstitial, 165
    intra-thoracic, 147
    meniscal, 47, 76
    metastatic, 21, 170, 290, 332
    nipples, 220
    parenchymal, 307
    periarticular, 43
    pulmonary, 170
    soft tissue, 22, 165, 220
    tracheal ring, 147, 170
calcifying tendinopathy
    hip region, 71
    mineralization in or near joints,
        47
    shoulder, *54*, 54–5
    stifle, 76
calcinosis circumscripta, 66, 106,
        332–3, *333*
    bony masses, 29
    intervertebral foramen
        abnormalities, 129
    mineralization in or near joints, 47
    paravertebral soft tissues, 130
    spinal cord compression, 137
calcinosis cutis, 106, 233, 332
calcium phosphate deposition
        disease, 122, 124
calculi
    bladder, 311, 313, *313*
    renal, 305
    salivary gland, 109
    ureteral, 237
    urethra, 318
calicivirus, feline, 46
calvarial hyperostosis, 101
    bony masses, 20
    calvarium thickening, 89
    idiopathic, 88
calvarium, 89, 90
    hyperostosis *see* calvarial
        hyperostosis
    masses, 89–90
    thickening/irregularity, 88, 89–90
    thinning, 89
cancellous bone, 2
canine glycogen storage disease,
        216

canine leucocyte adhesion deficiency, 101
  ear, 96
  frontal sinuses, 100
  mandible, 92
  metaphyses, 33
  mixed osteolytic-osteogenic lesions, 28
  radius/ulna, 62
  temporomandibular joint, 94
canine nasal mite, 98, **350**
capillariasis
  geographic distribution, **348**
  nasal cavity, 98
  poorly marginated pulmonary opacities, 158
carcinoma
  bronchiolar-alveolar, 164, 168
  bronchogenic, 154, 157, 161
  ectopic thyroid, 187
  frontal sinuses, 100
  hepatomegaly, 241
  hereditary multifocal renal, 300, 303, 306
  nasal, 98
  parathyroid gland, 110
  peritoneal, 234, 236
  pulmonary hyperlucency, 170
  salivary gland, 109
  single radiopaque lung lobe, 159
  thyroid gland, 110, 180
cardiac tamponade, 168
cardiogenic pulmonary oedema, 155
cardiomegaly, 148, 176, 181–3, *184*, 184–6
cardiomyopathy, 178–9
  dilated, 186
  hypertrophic, 182, 183
  restrictive, 182
cardiovascular system, 175–96, 225
caries, 102
carotid artery, ultrasonography, 110
carpus, 63–5
cartilaginous cores, retained, 24
  distal ulnar metaphysis, 60, *61*
  metaphyses, 31
cataracts, 108
cauda equina, 115–16
cauda equina syndrome, 135, *136*
caudal circumflex humeral artery, 53
caudal vena cava
  abnormalities, 186–7
  obstruction, 247
  ultrasonography, 238–9
cavitary infarct, 170
cellulitis, 108, 331
  larynx, 104
  mediastinal, 211
  soft tissues, 105, 130, 332

central peripheral neuropathy, 140
cerebral arteries, 90
cervical (cisterna magna) myelography, 131, *133*
cervical spondylopathy (wobbler syndrome), 118, *118*, 121, 122, 123–4, 127
  myelography, 135
  spinal cord compression, 135, 136
chalk bones *see* osteopetrosis
chemodectoma, 183, 187
Chiari syndrome, 88, 140
Chinese Shar Pei fever syndrome, 41, 46, 63, 78
choke chain injuries, 105
cholecystitis, 242
cholecystography, 244
choledocholithiasis, 242
cholelithiasis, 242, 247
cholesteatoma, 96
chondrocalcinosis, 47, 333
chondrodysplasias, 3
  altered shape of long bones, 14
  delayed growth plates closure, 16
  dwarfism, 15
  epiphyses, 30
  metaphyses, 32
  widening of physeal lines, 30
  zinc-responsive, 15
chondroma, 159
chondrometaplasia, 47, *47*, 76
chondrosarcoma
  cardiac, 187
  metastases, 170
  nasal, 98
  ribs, 220
  right ventricular enlargement, 186
  sacroiliac joints, 67
  scapula, 52
  single radiopaque lung lobe, 159
  sternum, 221
  tracheal, 151
  vertebral opacity changes, 125, 126
chordae tendineae, 184, 190
chordoma, 126, 139
chorioretinitis, 107
chronic obstructive pulmonary disease (COPD), 153
chylothorax, 200, 206, 225, 334, 335
chylous effusion, 234
ciliary body enlargement, 108
ciliary dyskinesia, 98
cirrhosis, 241
cisterna magna, 90, 131, *133*
clavicles, 46, 53
coagulopathy
  alveolar lung pattern, 156
  interstitial lung pattern, 164

mediastinal widening, 210
  spinal cord compression, 136–7
  spinal cord enlargement, 139
coarse trabecular pattern, 22
coccidioidomycosis, 108
  geographic distribution, **348**
  interstitial lung pattern, 164
  lymphadenopathy, 212
  mixed osteolytic-osteogenic lesions, 27
  pericardial effusion, 180
  poorly marginated pulmonary opacities, 158
  vertebral size and shape variations, 120
coeliac mesenteric arteriography, 244
coeliography, 244
colitis, 291–2, *292*
collateral ligament
  rupture, 42, *42*, 76
  trauma, 64–5
colon *see* large intestine
comet tail artefacts, 347
common bile duct, 247
common calcaneal tendon lesions, 79
compartmentalization, 269
compartment syndrome, 332
computed tomography (CT), 90, 96, 116, 123, 253, 331
concentric ventricular hypertrophy, 176–7
consolidated lung lobes, *159*, 160
constipation, 289–90
Coonhound paralysis, 141
copper deficiency
  delayed growth plates closure, 16
  osteopenia, 22
  widening of physeal lines, 31
coronary arteries, 185, 186
coronoid disease, *56*, 56–7
corpora lutea, 320
cor pulmonale, 185
cortex, 2, 33
corticosteroid excess, 22
cor triatriatum dexter, 185, 193
cor triatriatum sinister, 182, 185, 190
Corynebacterium, 158
Corynebacterium diphtheria, 128
costal cartilages, 220
costochondral junction, 160
costochondral junction, 160
coxofemoral joint, 68–71
cranial cavity, 88–90
cranial mesenteric arteriography, 244
cranial physes, 116
craniomandibular osteopathy, 92, *92*, 96
  bony masses, 20
  calvarium thickening, 89
  cranial radiopacity variations, 89
  frontal bones, 101

frontal sinuses, 100
metaphyses, 33
periosteal reactions, 19
radius/ulna, 62, *62*
temporomandibular joint, 94
cranium, 88–9
crenosomosis (*Crensoma vulpis*), 155,
    349
cruciate ligament disease, 74–5
cryptococcosis (*Cryptococcus
    neoformans*), 45, 108
geographic distribution, **349**
interstitial lung pattern, 164
lymphadenopathy, 212
mixed osteolytic-osteogenic
    lesions, 28
nasal cavity, 98
poorly marginated pulmonary
    opacities, 158
Cushing's disease *see*
    hyperadrenocorticism
cystadenoma
hereditary multifocal renal, 300,
    303, 306
ovarian, 320
cystic endometrial hyperplasia, 322
cystitis, 311–12, *312*, 314, *314*, 315
cystography, 312–15
abnormal bladder lumen on,
    313–14
double-contrast, 313
following intravenous urogram, 313
positive contrast, 312–13
reflux of contrast media up a ureter
    following, 313
thickening of bladder wall on,
    314–15
cyst(s)
adrenal glands, 254
aneurysmal bone, 121, 125
biliary, 241
bronchogenic, 169
dentigerous, 91, 92, 102–3
dermoid, 111, 139
ganglion, 136
hepatic, 247
intrapericardial, 180, 181
iris, 108
juxta-articular, 136
maxillary bone epithelial, 92
mediastinal, 211, 212
nasal dermoid sinus, 111
nasolacrimal duct, 91
nasopharyngeal, 103
nodular lung pattern, 163
ovarian, 320
paraprostatic, 235, 289, 324, *324*,
    325, *325*
parenchymal, 241

peritoneal, 236
prostatic, 323, 324
prostatomegaly, 289
pulmonary, 161, 169–70, 201
renal, 300, 303, 306
salivary gland, 109
soft tissues, 105, 332
synovial, 136
thyroid, 110
vertebral opacity changes, 125

D

dacryocystorhinography, 106
dactomegaly, 52
Dandy-Walker syndrome, 122
dehydration
microcardia, 178
pulmonary hyperlucency, 168
dens agenesis, 123
dentigerous cysts, 91, 92, 102–3
dentinogenesis imperfecta, 102
dermoid sinus, 119
cyst, 111, 139
vertebral opacity changes, 125
dextrocardia, 177, *177*
diabetes mellitus
hepatomegaly, 240
osteopenia, 22
vertebral opacity changes, 124
diaphragm
rupture, 168, *201*, 201–2, 204, 223,
    224, 225
ultrasonography, 224
variations, 222–4, *223*
diaphragmatic hernia, 159, 160, 180,
    212, 224
diaphysis, 2, 33–4
diarrhoea, 289–90
digital neoplasia, 66
digital radiography faults, 341
dimelia, 52
Dioctophyma renale, 305, 306, **349**
dirofilariasis (*Dirofilaria immitis*), 155,
    158, 162
geographic distribution, **349**
interstitial lung pattern, 165
mixed lung pattern, 168
right ventricular enlargement, 185
vascular lung pattern, 165–6
disc disease, 127
discography, 116, 133
discospondylitis, 121
intervertebral disc space
    abnormalities, 126, 127
paravertebral soft tissue lesions, 131
vertebral endplate irregularities,
    127–8, *128*

vertebral opacity changes, 124, 125
disseminated histiocytic sarcoma, 28
disseminated idiopathic skeletal
    hyperostosis, 45
altered shape of bone, 15
bony masses, 20
paravertebral soft tissues, 130
proliferative joint disease, 44–5
vertebral size and shape variations,
    121
disseminated intravascular
    coagulation, 162
alveolar lung pattern, 156
interstitial lung pattern, 164
nodular lung pattern, 163
distemper, 17
distractio cubiti, 58, 61
distraction index (DI), 69, *69*
diverticulum
bladder, 311, 314, *314*
intestinal, 287
oesophageal, 217, 218
ureteral, 309
dolichocephalic breeds, 87, *87*
Doppler flow abnormalities, 194–6
double-contrast cystography, 313
double-contrast enema, 290–1
double-contrast gastrography, 272–3,
    273
double cortical line, 6
dwarfism, 15, **15**
delayed growth plates closure, 16
pituitary, 30, 31, 119
radius/ulna, 62
widening of physeal lines, 31
dysgerminoma, 320
dyskinesia, primary ciliary, 153, 154
dysmelia, 52
dysostosis enchondralis, 58, 61
dysplasia epiphysealis hemimelica, 29
dystocia, 321

E

ear, *95*, 95–7
Ebstein's anomaly, 184
echinococcosis, alveolar, 242, 246,
    349
echocardiography, 189–96
contrast, 194
Doppler flow abnormalities, 194–6
left heart, 189–92
right heart, 192–4
two-dimensional and M-mode,
    189–94
ectodermal dysplasia, 101
ectopic kidney, 212
ectopic ureters, 305, *308*, 309

ectrodactyly, 52, 66
ectromelia, 52
ehrlichiosis, 46
  geographic distribution, **349**
  joint effusion/soft tissue swelling, 41
Eisenmenger's syndrome, 185–6
elbow, 45, 55–60, *56–60*
emaciation, 332
emphysema, 168–9, 332
  bullous, 201
  lobar, 167, 200
  pulmonary hyperlucency, 170
  subcutaneous, 200, 219
emphysematous cystitis, 311–12, *312*
enchondromatosis
  altered shape of bone, 14, 15
  metaphyses, 31
  osteolytic areas in diaphyses, 34
  osteolytic lesions, 25
  reduced radiopacity, 28
endocardial cushion defect, 167,
    183, 185
endocardial fibroelastosis, 182
endocardiosis, 181
endocarditis, bacterial, 178, 179,
    181, 184
endometritis, 322
endophthalmitis, 107
endosteum, 2
enema, 290–1
enteritis, 286
enthesiopathies
  bony masses, 20
  carpus, 65, *65*
  flexor tendon, 57
  proliferative joint disease, 44
eosinophilic bronchopneumopathy,
    153, 162, 164–5, 168
ependymoma
  spinal cord compression, 138
  spinal cord enlargement, 138
epicondylar spurs, medial, 57
epidermoid cysts, intraosseous, 24, 66
epididymitis, 326
epidural contrast leakage, 140
epidurography, 116, 132–3
epiphyseal dysplasia, 46
epiphysiolysis, femoral, 10, 70
epiphysis, 2
  lesions affecting, 29–30
  remodelling, 29
Escherichia coli, 128
ethmoturbinate polyps, 98
excretion urography, 301–2, 308
extradural spinal cord compression,
    134, 134–7, *136*
extra kidney sign, 320
extrapleural sign, 204, *204*
eye, ultrasonography, 106–9, *107*

F

fabellae, 46, 71–2, 74
facet joint osteoarthrosis, 129–30
faecal impaction, 289
faecolithiasis, 280, 282, 290
false pneumothorax, 200, *200*
fat embolism, 160
fat opacity, 202, 219, 235, 334
feline bronchial asthma, 153, 156, 168,
    207, 224
feline infectious peritonitis, 108,
    234, 300
  interstitial lung pattern, 164
  pericardial effusion, 180
feline leukaemia
  sclerotic areas in diaphyses, 34
  vertebral opacity changes, 124
feline metastatic digital carcinoma, 44
feline non-infectious erosive
    polyarthritis, 45, 46
feline non-infectious non-erosive
    polyarthritis, 46
female genital tract, 319–22
femoral head, avascular necrosis, 24,
    29, 43, 45, 69, *69*
femur, 71
fetal death, 321–2
fibrinous pleuritis, 206
fibroadenoma, 321
fibrocartilaginous embolism, 140,
    141
fibrodysplasia ossificans, 333, *333*
fibroma, 187
fibrosarcoma
  cardiac, 187
  maxilla/premaxilla, 91
  oesophageal, 218
  ribs, 221
  sternum, 222
  tracheal, 151
  vertebral opacity changes, 125
fibrous dysplasia, 24, 25
fibrous osteodystrophy
    see hyperparathyroidism
fibula, 77
filaroidiasis (*F. Hirthi, F. Milksi*), 155,
    158, 162
  geographic distribution, **349**
  interstitial lung pattern, 165
film-screen radiography faults, 341,
    345–6
fimbriation, 282
fissure fractures, 33
fissure lines, pleural, 206, *206*,
    209, *209*
fistula
  arteriovenous *see* arteriovenous
    fistula

broncho-oesophageal, 215
  contrast studies, 334
  tracheo-oesophageal, 215
  urethral, 319
fistulography, 95, 334
flail chest, 225
flail valve, 193
flat-chested conformation, 220
flexor tendon enthesiopathy, 57
fluoroscopy, 275
fluorosis, 124
foramen magnum, 88
forearm, 60–3
foreign bodies
  aspirated, 151, 154, 155, 165
  cranial radiopacity variations, 89
  gastric, 271
  intraocular, 108
  nasal, 98, 99
  nasopharyngeal, 103
  oesophageal, 149, 170, 211,
    218–19
  paravertebral soft tissues,
    130, 131
  pericardial effusion, 180
  pulmonary hyperlucency,
    168, 170
  retrobulbar, 109
  salivary gland, 110
  small intestinal, 280, *281*
  soft tissues, 336
fovea capitis, 68
fracture disease, 13
fractures, 9–14
  accessory carpal bone, 63, *64*
  antebrachium, 63
  assessment
    immediate post-operative
      radiographs, 11
    subsequent examinations, 12
    at the time of injury, 10–11, *11*
  carpus, 63–4, *64*
  causes of, 9
  classification of, 10, *10*
  elbow, 59, 59–60
  epiphyseal, 29
  fabellae, 74
  femoral, 71
  healing
    complications of, 12–13
    stages of, *11*, 11–12
    ultrasonographic assessment of,
      13–14
  hip, 70
  humerus, 55
  increased bone radiopacity, 17
  malunion, 13, *13*, 15
  mandibular, 93
  maxilla/premaxilla, 92

metacarpus/metatarsus, 67
mineralization in or near joints, 47
non-union, 12–13, *13*
patella, 74
pelvic, 68, *68*
radiographic signs, 9–10
radiography, 9
scapula, 52
sclerotic lines in diaphyses, 33–4
sesamoid, 67
shoulder, 54
stifle, 74
tarsus, *78*, 78–9
temporomandibular joint, 94
tibia/fibula, 77
tooth, 102
vertebral, 120, 121–2
vertebral opacity changes, 126
widening of physeal lines, 30
fragmentation of the medial coronoid
        process of ulna (FMCP), *56*, 56–7
Francisella tularensis, 156, 162, **349**
frontal bones, 100–1
frontal sinuses, 99–101
fused vertebrae, 118

G

gall bladder
    agenesis, 247
    duplex, 247
    obstruction, 247
    rupture, 235
gallstones *see* cholelithiasis
gas
    in the biliary tree, 242
    in the bladder, 316
    in the brain, 88
    in the colon, 290
    in joints, 41
    in the mediastinum, 105, 152, 168,
        208–9
    opacity, 235
    in paravertebral soft tissues, 130, 131
    in the pericardium, 180
    in the pleural space *see*
        pneumothorax
    in the prostate, 324
    in the small intestine, 279, *279*, 280–1
    within soft tissues, 105
    soft tissues radiopacity, 334
    in the spleen, 250
    in the stomach wall, 272
    in the uterus, 321
gastric axis, 268
gastric ulceration, 274, *274*, 277
gastrinoma, 271
gastritis, 274, *274*, 277

gastrocnemius muscle avulsion, 75–6,
    76
gastrography, 272–3, *273*
gastrointestinal tract, 260, 267–92
gastro-oesophageal intussusception,
    212, 215, 217–18
geographic distributions of diseases,
    347, **348–51**
germination, tooth, 102
giant axonal neuropathy, 140, 216
giant cell tumour *see* osteoclastoma
giant kidney worm *see Dioctophyma
    renale*
glaucoma, 107, 108
globoid cell leucodystrophy, 140
glomerulonephritis, 299
gluteal muscles, calcifying
        tendinopathy, 71
GM$_1$-gangliosidosis, 15
gonitis, juvenile, 73
granuloma
    bladder, 315, 316
    cholesterol
        ear, 96
        maxillary, 92
    diaphragmatic, 212
    eosinophilic, 158, 162, 212
    fungal, 139
    intraocular, 108
    lymphomatoid, 158
    mandibular giant cell, 93
    maxillary giant cell, 92
    mediastinal, 211, 212
    nasopharyngeal, 103
    oesophageal, 211, 214, 218, *218*
    optic, 107
    paravertebral soft tissues, 130
    peritoneal, 236
    pleural, 204
    poorly marginated pulmonary
        opacities, 158
    pulmonary, 158, 161, 170, 212
    renal, 300
    soft tissue, 105, 332
    tracheal, 151
granulomatous meningoence
        phalomyelitis, 139, 141
granulosa cell tumour, 320
gravel sign, 269, 270, *270*
greenstick fracture, 14
growth arrest lines, 17, 33, 71
growth plate closures, 3, **4**, *61*, 61–2
    delayed, 15–16
    stifle, 73, *73*
    tibia, 78
growth plates
    asymmetric bridging, 14
    closures *see* growth plate closures
    trauma, 14

H

haemangioma, 303
haemangiosarcoma, 187
    hepatomegaly, 241
    interstitial lung pattern, 164
    osteolytic lesions, 23
    pericardial effusion, 180, 181
    ribs, 221
    right ventricular enlargement, 186
    spinal cord compression, 136
    splenic, 249
    vertebral opacity changes, 125
haemarthrosis
    chronic, 43
    mixed osteolytic-proliferative joint
        disease, 45
haematoma, 336, 337
    abdominal wall, 233
    extradural, 136
    intradural, 138
    mediastinal, 211, 212
    nodular lung pattern, 163
    paravertebral soft tissues, 130, 131
    pleural and extrapleural masses, 204
    pulmonary, 161
    renal, 299, 300
    soft tissues, 105, 332
haematometra, 321, 322
haemopericardium, 180
haemoperitoneum, 234
haemophilia A
    alveolar lung pattern, 156
    interstitial lung pattern, 164
    mediastinal widening, 210
    spinal cord compression, 136
    spinal cord enlargement, 139
haemopneumothorax, 202
haemorrhage
    adrenal glands, 254
    extradural, 136
    eye, 107
    frontal sinuses, 100
    lobar, 160
    nasal, 98
    paratesticular, 326
    perirenal, 308
    pleural effusion, 204
    pulmonary, 156, 164, 168
    retroperitoneal, 236–7
    spinal cord, 139
    subretinal, 107, 108
halo artefact, 341, *344*
hamartoma
    bronchial, 170
    renal, 300
    single radiopaque lung lobe, 159
    soft tissues, 332
    tracheal, 151, 170

Hansen type I/II disc disease, 127
hard palate congenital defect, 99
head and neck, 85–111
  lymph nodes, ultrasonography, 110
  soft tissues, 105–11
heart
  enlargement *see* cardiomegaly
  malposition, 177, *177*
  neoplasia, 187–8
  normal radiographic appearance,
    175–6, *176*
  normal silhouette with cardiac
    pathology, 176–7
  reduction in size, 178, *178*
  silhouette enlargement, 178–9
  ultrasonography, 189–96
heart base tumours, 150, 187
  pericardial effusion, 180
  tracheal displacement, 149
heartworm *see Angiostrongylus*
    vasorum; Dirofilaria immitis
hemimelia, 14, 52, 60
hemithorax, 157
hemivertebrae, 117–18, *118*, 140
hepatitis
  emphysematous, 242
  hepatomegaly, 241
hepatocutaneous syndrome, 247
hepatoma, 241
hepatozoonosis
  geographic distribution, **349**
  periosteal reactions, 18
  vertebral size and shape variations,
    121
hernia
  diaphragmatic, 159, 160, 180,
    212, 224
  dynamic cervical lung, 170
  hiatal, 211, 218
  inguinal, 232, *232*
  paraoesophageal, 211
  perineal, 289
  scrotal, 326
  umbilical, 232
hiatal hernia, 211, 218
high-rise syndrome, 157
hilar masses, 171
hip, 68–71
hip dysplasia, 45, *68*, 68–9
histiocytic sarcoma, 23
histiocytosis, malignant, 210, 212,
    241, 249, 277, 307
histoplasmosis, 108
  geographic distribution, **350**
  healed, 170
  interstitial lung pattern, 164
  intrathoracic mineralized opacities,
    171
  lymphadenopathy, 212

mixed osteolytic-osteogenic
    lesions, 28
  nodular lung pattern, 162
  poorly marginated pulmonary
    opacities, 158
hock, 77–80
horseshoe kidney, 301
hound ataxia, 141
humerus, 55
hydrocephalus
  calvarium thinning, 89
  congenital, 88, *88*, 89
hydrometra, 321, 322
hydronephrosis, 299, 300, *304*, 304–5,
    306, *306*
hydroperitoneum, 234, *234*, 236
hydrophthalmos, 107
hydropneumothorax, 202
hygroma, 332
hyoid apparatus, 105
hyperadrenocorticism, 22, 253–4
  abdominal wall shape variations, 232
  hepatomegaly, 240
  increased bronchial wall visibility,
    154
  interstitial lung pattern, 165
  intrathoracic mineralized opacities,
    170
  mixed lung pattern, 168
  radiopacity of soft tissues, 332
  vascular lung pattern, 167
  vertebral opacity changes, 124
hypercalcaemia, 284
hyperdontia, 102
hyperextension, carpus, 64
hyperparathyroidism, 98
  cranial radiopacity variations, 88
  intrathoracic mineralized opacities,
    170
  mandible, 93
  maxilla/premaxilla, 91, *91*
  nutritional secondary, 21, *21*
  osteopenia, 21
  primary, 21
  radiopacity of soft tissues, 332
  renal secondary, 21, 91, *91*, 93
  teeth, 102
  vertebral opacity changes, 124
hyperplastic gastropathy, 274
hypertension
  portal, 247
  pulmonary, 166, 185
  systemic, 183, 184
hyperthyroidism
  osteopenia, 22
  vertebral opacity changes, 124
hypertrophic cardiomyopathy, 178
hypertrophic (pulmonary)
    osteopathy (HPO)

femur, 71
  periosteal reactions, 18–19, *19*
  phalanges, 66
  radius/ulna, 62
  thickening of cortices, 33
  tibia/fibula, 77
hypervitaminosis A, 46, 333
  bony masses, 20, 29
  calvarium thickening, 89
  dwarfism, 15
  elbow, 59
  intrathoracic mineralized opacities,
    170
  osteopenia, 22
  periosteal reactions, 19
  proliferative joint disease, 45
  spinal cord compression, 136
  stifle, 73
  vertebral opacity changes, 124
  vertebral size and shape variations,
    121
hypervitaminosis D
  delayed growth plates closure, 16
  dwarfism, 15
  increased bone radiopacity, 17
  osteopenia, 22
hypoadrenocorticism
  microcardia, 178
  pulmonary hyperlucency, 168
  vascular lung pattern, 167
hypoalbuminaemia
  alveolar lung pattern, 156
  pericardial effusion, 180
hypodontia, 101–2
hypoplasia, congenital, 150
hypoplastic dens, 123
hypothyroidism, acquired, 110
hypothyroidism, congenital, 119
  altered shape of long bones, 14
  delayed growth plates closure, 16
  dwarfism, 15
  epiphyses, 30
  intervertebral disc space
    abnormalities, 126
  radius/ulna, 62
  thickening of cortices, 33
  vertebral endplate irregularities, 128
  vertebral opacity changes, 124
  widening of physeal lines, 30
hypovitaminosis D
  dwarfism, 15
  widening of physeal lines, 31
hypovolaemia, 178, 200

I

idiopathic dilated cardiomyopathy, 178
idiopathic effusive arthritis, 73

idiopathic multifocal osteopathy, 24, 119
idiopathic osteodystrophy, 16
idiopathic pulmonary fibrosis, 154
  alveolar lung pattern, 157
  mixed lung pattern, 168
iliopsoas, calcifying tendinopathy, 71
immune-mediated vaccine reactions, 41, 46
indented vertebral endplates, 121
infection
  lymphadenopathy, 212
  metaphyses, 32
  mixed osteolytic-osteogenic lesions, 26–8, 34
  osteolytic areas in diaphyses, 34
  osteolytic lesions, 24
  periosteal reactions, 18
  temporomandibular joint, 94
  widening of physeal lines, 30, 31
infundibular stenosis, 186
infusion intravenous urogram, 302
inguinal hernia, 232, 232
inherited hypertrophic neuropathy, 140
insertion tendonopathies, 15
insulinoma, 253
International Elbow Working Group, elbow dysplasia, 58
interstitial lung pattern, 163–5, 164
interstitial nephritis, 299
intervertebral disc space abnormalities, 126–7
intervertebral foramen abnormalities, 128–9, 129
intraocular tumour, 107
intravenous urography (IVU), 301–2, 308, 313
intravertebral disc herniation, 124–5, 126, 127, 128
intussusception, 212, 215, 217–18, 271, 283, 283, 286, 286–7
involucrum, 13, 27, 33
iodine oesophagram, 214
iris cyst, 108
ischaemic neuromyopathy, 141

J

joint disease
  mixed osteolytic-proliferative joint disease, 45
  osteolytic (erosive), 42–4
  proliferative, 44–5
joint effusion, 41, 41
joints, 39–47
  conditions affecting multiple, 45–6

disease see joint disease
effusion see joint effusion
gas in, 41
mineralization in or near, 46–7
joint space, altered width, 41
jugular vein ultrasonography, 110
juvenile gonitis, 73
juvenile osteomalacia see rickets

K

Kartagener's syndrome, 98, 100, 154, 156
kidney(s), 298–308, 299
  acute failure, 308
  agenesis, 299
  contrast studies, 301–5
  diffuse parenchymal ultrasonographic abnormalities, 307
  ectopic, 212
  focal parenchymal ultrasonographic abnormalities, 306–7
  location variations, 301
  loss of visualization, 236, 236–7
  masses, 237, 258, 258
  measurement, 298–9, 299
  mineralization on radiographs, 261
  non visualization of, 299
  normal ultrasonographic appearance, 305–6, 306
  perirenal ultrasonographic abnormalities, 307–8, 308
  radiopacity variations, 300–1
  renal pelvis ultrasonographic abnormalities, 306, 306
  size and shape variations, 299–300
  ultrasonographic examination, 305
  see also entries beginning renal
kyphosis, 122–3

L

large intestine, 287–92
  contents variations, 289–90
  contrast studies, 290–2
  dilation, 289
  displacement, 288
  impaction, 289–90
  masses, 259, 260, 291, 291
  normal radiographic appearance, 287, 287–8
  normal ultrasonographic appearance, 292
  rupture, 290

ultrasonographic changes in disease, 292
  ultrasonographic technique, 292
  wall opacity variations, 290
larval migrans, 158, 162
larynx, 103–5
lead poisoning
  increased bone radiopacity, 17
  metaphyses, 33
  osteopenia, 22
  vertebral opacity changes, 126
left atrium
  abnormalities, 189–90, 190
  enlargement, 181–2, 182
left ventricle
  abnormalities, 191–2
  enlargement, 182–3
  hypertrophy, 182
Legg-Calvé-Perthes disease, 24, 29, 43, 45, 69, 69
leiomyoma
  bladder, 316
  gastric, 271, 277
  large intestine, 291
  oesophageal, 218
  small intestine, 283
  tracheal, 151
  uterine, 321
leiomyosarcoma
  bladder, 316
  gastric, 271
  large intestine, 291
  oesophageal, 218
  small intestine, 283
  uterine, 321
leishmaniasis, 45
  geographic distribution, **350**
  mixed osteolytic-osteogenic lesions, 28
  mixed osteolytic-proliferative joint disease, 45
  osteolytic joint disease, 44
  periosteal reactions, 18
  thickening of cortices, 33
lens, 108
leptospirosis, 162
  interstitial lung pattern, 164
  mixed lung pattern, 168
leucoencephalomyelopathy, 141
levocardia, 177
ligamentum flavum, hypertrophied/redundant, 135
linear tomography, 116
lipoma
  abdominal wall, 233
  cardiac, 187
  infiltrative, of the thigh, 71
  intradural, 138
  soft tissues, 336

lipoma (*Continued*)
  spinal cord compression, 136
  uterine, 321
liposarcoma, 23
liquid oesophagram, 214
liver, 239–48
  contrast studies, 242–4
  displacement, 239
  enlargement, 255, *256*
  lobe torsion, 246
  masses, 257
  mineralization on radiographs, 261
  normal ultrasonographic
      appearance, 245, *245*
  parenchyma, 245–7
  radiopacity variations, 242
  shape variations, 241–2
  size variations, 239–41, *240, 241*
  ultrasonographic abnormalities,
      245–7
  ultrasonographic technique, 245
  vascular system abnormalities,
      247–8
lobar vesicular gas pattern, 170
lordosis, 122
lower respiratory tract, 145–71
lumbar myelography, 131–2, *133*
lumbar sinus venography, 116
lumbosacral disc disease, 135
lumbosacral instability, 124
lumbosacral stenosis, 122
lung lobes
  consolidated, *159*, 160
  increased visibility, 205–6
  single radiopaque, *159*, 159–60
  torsion *see* lung lobe torsion
  ultrasonography of consolidated,
      160
lung lobe torsion, 153, *159*, 159–60,
      201
  alveolar lung pattern, 156, 157
  tracheal displacement, 149
lungs
  lobes *see* lung lobes
  patterns
    alveolar, 154–7, *155*
    bronchial, *153*, 153–4
    interstitial, 163–5, *164*
    mixed, 167–8
    nodular, *161*, 161–3
    vascular, 165–7, *166*
  trauma, 225
  see also entries beginning pulmonary
lungworm, feline *see* Aelurostrongylus
      abstrusus
Lyme disease, 46
  geographic distribution, **348**
  joint effusion/soft tissue swelling,
      41

lymphadenopathy
  abdominal, 234
  hilar region, 212
  mediastinal, 212
  retroperitoneal space, 237, 238
  sternal, 211, 212
  tracheobronchial, 211
lymphangiography, 334–5
lymphatic system, contrast studies,
      334–5
lymph nodes
  head and neck, ultrasonography,
      110
  mineralization on radiographs,
      261
  retroperitoneal space, 238
  ultrasonography of, 338
lymphoedema, 331, 334–5
lymphography, 334–5
lymphoma, 107
  bladder, 316
  ciliary body, 108
  gastric, 271, 277
  hepatomegaly, 240, 241
  increased bronchial wall visibility,
      154
  large intestine, 291
  lymphadenopathy, 212
  mediastinal, 210
  mixed lung pattern, 168
  nasal, 98
  osteolytic areas in diaphyses, 34
  osteolytic lesions, 23
  pericardial effusion, 180
  pulmonary, 162, 164
  reduced radiopacity, 28
  renal, 299, 300, 303, 307, 308
  retroperitoneal space, 237
  sclerotic areas in diaphyses, 34
  small intestine, 283, 285
  spinal cord compression, 136, 138
  spinal cord enlargement, 139
  splenic, 249, 251
  tracheal, 151
  vertebral opacity changes, 125
lysosomal storage diseases, 140

M

magnetic resonance imaging (MRI),
      90, 96, 116, 253, 331
male genital tract, 322–6
malignant melanoma, 66
  ciliary body, 107, 108
  maxilla/premaxilla, 91
mammary glands mineralization on
      radiographs, 262
mandible, 92–3

marble bone disease *see* osteopetrosis
Marie's disease *see* hypertrophic
      (pulmonary) osteopathy
      (HPO)
mast cell disease, 251
mast cell tumour, 151, 291
maxilla, 90–2
maxillary cholesterol granuloma, 92
maxillary giant cell granuloma, 92
medial epicondyle
  spurs, 57, *58*
  ununited, 57–8
mediastinal fluid, 148
mediastinitis, 209–10
mediastinum, 206–13
  anatomy and radiography, 206–7,
      207
  lymphadenopathy, 212
  masses, 148, 150, *210*, 210–12
  mediastinal shift, 207–8
  radiopacity variations, 208–9
  trauma, 225
  ultrasonography, 212–13
  widening, 209–10
medullary cavity, 2
medullary rim sign, 307
megacolon, hypertrophic, 291
megaoesophagus, 168, 208, *215*,
      215–16
meningioma
  calvarium thickening, 89
  cranial radiopacity variations, 89
  intervertebral foramen
      abnormalities, 129
  spinal cord compression, 136, 138
meningitis
  corticosteroid responsive, 141
  eosinophilic, 141
meningitis syndrome, 41, 46
meningocele, 119
meningoencephalomyelitis, 139, 141
meniscal calcification/ossification,
      76
meromelia, 52
mesaticephalic breeds, 87
mesenteric masses, 259
mesothelioma, 180, 181, 188, 204, 222
metacarpus, 65–7
metallosis, 13
metaphyseal osteomyelitis, 24, 29,
      32, *32*
metaphyseal osteopathy, 31–2, *32*
  femoral neck, 70
  femur, 71
  humerus, 55
  increased bone radiopacity, 17
  mixed osteolytic-osteogenic
      lesions, 28
  osteolytic lesions, 24

periosteal reactions, 18
  radius/ulna, 62
  reduced radiopacity, 28–9
  tibia, 77
metaphysis, 2
  lesions affecting, 31–3
metatarsus, 65–7
microcardia, 178, *178*
microlithiasis, bronchial, 154, 170
micromelia, 52
microphthalmos, 107
miliary nodules, 162
mirror image artefacts, 347, *347*
mitral valve
  abnormalities, *190*, 190–1
  Doppler flow abnormalities, 194–5
  dysplasia, 185
  insufficiency, 181–2
mixed lung pattern, 167–8
M-mode echocardiography, 189–94
Monteggia fracture, 60
mucocele, 247
  frontal bones variation, 101
  zygomatic, 109
mucolipidosis
  dwarfism, 15
  epiphyses, 30
  hip dysplasia, 70
mucometra, 321, 322
mucopolysaccharidosis, 46, 119
  articular facets abnormalities, 130
  delayed growth plates closure, 16
  dwarfism, 15
  epiphyses, 30
  hip dysplasia, 70
  intervertebral disc space
      abnormalities, 126
  nasal cavity variations, 97
  osteopenia, 22
  paravertebral soft tissues, 130
  periosteal reactions, 19
  proliferative joint disease, 45
  vertebral endplate irregularities, 128
  vertebral opacity changes, 124
  vertebral size and shape variations,
      121, 122
mucosal slough, *313*, 314
multifocal diseases, 28–9
multifocal idiopathic
      pyogranulomatous bone
      disease
  mixed osteolytic-osteogenic
      lesions, 28
  mixed radiopacity, 29
multilobar tumour of bone, 333
  calvarium thickening, 89, *90*
  cranial radiopacity variations,
      88–9, 89
  ribs, 221

multipartite patella, 72
multiple myeloma
  coarse trabecular pattern, 22
  osteolytic areas in diaphyses, 34
  osteolytic lesions, *23*, 23–4
  osteopenia, 22
  reduced radiopacity, 28
  ribs, 221
  sacroiliac joints, 67
  sternum, 222
  vertebral opacity changes, 124, 125
muscle(s)
  atrophy, 332
  hypertrophy, 331
  mineralization on radiographs, 261
  ultrasonography of, 337
  see also specific muscles
musculoskeletal system
      ultrasonography, 52
myasthenia gravis, congenital, 216
mycetoma, 27, 28
Mycoplasma infection, 164
Mycoplasma polyarthritis, 44, 46
myelodysplasia, 140, 289
myelography, 115–16, 131–2
  cervical, 131, 133, *133*
  complications, 132
  extradural spinal cord compression
      on, 134–7
  intradural-extramedullary spinal
      cord compression on, *137*,
      137–8
  lumbar, 131–2, *133*, 134
  miscellaneous findings, 139–40
  neurological deficits involving the
      spinal cord, 140–1
  normal appearance, 132, *132*
  spinal cord enlargement, 138–9, *139*
  technical errors, 133–4
myelolipoma, 136
myeloma, multiple *see* multiple
      myeloma
myelomalacia, 139
myelomeningocele, 119
myelopathy
  degenerative, 140, 141
  demyelinating, 141
  hereditary, 140
myocardial disease, 179
myocardial failure, 183, 186
myocarditis, 186
myositis ossificans, 47, 333
myxoma, 136, 138, 187
myxomatous atrioventricular
      valvular degeneration,
      178, 179
myxosarcoma, 109
  cardiac, 187
  spinal cord compression, 136, 138

N

nasal cavity, *97*, 97–9
nasal neoplasia, 98, *98*, 99
nasolacrimal duct
  contrast studies, 106
  cysts, 91
nasopharyngeal polyps, 103, *103*
nasopharyngeal stenosis, 103–4
near-drowning, 156
neck, 85–111
necrotizing vasculitis, 137, 141
neoplasia
  altered shape of bone, 14
  alveolar lung pattern, 156
  bladder, 313, 315, *315*
  bony masses, 19–20
  calvarium thickening, 89–90
  cardiac, 187–8
  cranial radiopacity variations, 88–9,
      89
  digits, 66
  ear, 96
  femur, 71
  frontal bones, 101
  frontal sinuses, 100
  gastric, 271, *271*
  globe, 107
  increased bone radiopacity, 16
  increased bronchial wall visibility,
      154
  interstitial lung pattern, 164
  larynx, 104
  left atrial, 190
  mandible, 92
  maxilla/premaxilla, 90–1, *91*, 92
  metaphyses, 31
  metatarsus/metacarpus, 66
  mixed osteolytic-osteogenic
      lesions, 25–6, *26*, 34
  nasal, 98, *98*, 99
  nasopharyngeal, 103
  osteolytic areas in diaphyses, 34
  osteolytic lesions, 23, *23*, 24–5
  ovarian, 320
  paravertebral soft tissues, 130
  pericardial effusion, 180, 181
  periosteal reactions, 18
  poorly marginated pulmonary
      opacities, 157
  proliferative joint disease, 44
  prostatic, 319, *319*, 323–4
  pulmonary hyperlucency, 170
  renal, 299, 300, 303, 305, *305*, 307, 308
  retroperitoneal space, 237
  right atrium, 185
  sacroiliac joints, 67
  salivary gland, 109
  sclerotic areas in diaphyses, 34

neoplasia (*Continued*)
single radiopaque lung lobe, 159
soft tissues, 105, 332, 336
solitary pulmonary nodules/
masses, 161
spinal, 120, 122
spinal cord compression, 136, 138
spinal cord enlargement, 138–9
temporomandibular joint, 94
testicular, 326
tracheal, 151
urethral, 318
uterine, 321
vertebral opacity changes, 124,
125–6
see also bone tumours; soft tissue
tumours *specific tumours*
nephroblastoma, 300, 303
spinal cord compression, 138
spinal cord enlargement, 139
nephrocalcinosis, 261, 301, 307
nephrogram, 302
abnormal timing, 303
absent, 303
uneven radiopacity, 303
nephroliths, 300, 308
nerve roots, neurological deficits, 140–1
nerves, ultrasonography of, 337
neuroaxonal dystrophy, 140
neuroblastoma, 254
neurofibroma
spinal cord compression, 136
spinal cord enlargement, 138
neurofibrosarcoma, 129
neuronopathy, progressive, 140
neutering, delayed growth plates
closure, 16
nocardiosis (*Nocardia* spp.), 128
geographic distribution, **350**
lymphadenopathy, 212
poorly marginated pulmonary
opacities, 158
nodular lung pattern, *161*, 161–3
Norberg angle, 69, *69*
notomelia, 52
nucleus pulposus mineralization,
127
nutrient foramen, 2, 33

O

obesity, 179, 209
fat opacity, 202
soft tissues of the head and neck,
105
obstipation, 290
occipital bone, thinning and caudal
bulging, 88

occipitoatlantoaxial malformations,
119
odontogenic tumours, 91, 92, *93*, 102,
103
odontoid peg, 123
odontoma, 91
oedema, 331
bronchial wall, 154
cardiogenic pulmonary, 155, 164,
168
interstitial lung pattern, 164
mediastinal widening, 210
non-cardiogenic pulmonary, 156–7,
164
pancreatic, 253
pleural, 206
pulmonary, 157
soft tissues of the head and neck,
105
spinal cord, 139
oesophagram, 214
oesophagus
cervical, 111
contrast studies, 214–15
dilation, 149, 150, 210, 215–17
foreign bodies, 149, 170, 211,
218–19
gas, 105
masses, 217–18
mediastinal masses, 211–12
normal radiographic appearance,
213–14
perforation, 105, 201, 208, 215,
218–19
radiopacity variations, 217
redundant, 216
thoracic, 213–19
oligodendroma, 138
omentum masses, 259
operative mesenteric
portovenography, 242–3
optic disc, 109
optic nerve, 109
optic neuritis, 107
orbit, ultrasonography, 106–9, *107*
orchitis, 326
Oslerus osleri, 151, 154, **350**
ossification, 3
delayed, 15–16
ossifying fibroma, 20
ossifying pachymeningitis, 126,
128–9, 140
osteitis fibrosa cystica
see hyperparathyroidism
osteoarthritis, 44
bony masses, 20
epiphyses, 29
mineralization in or near joints, 47
temporomandibular joint, 94

osteoarthrosis, 44, *44*, 45
carpus, 65
of the digits, 67
elbow, 60, *60*
facet joint, 129–30
mineralization in or near joints, 47
shoulder, *53*, 54
stifle, 76
tarsus, 79–80
osteocartilaginous exostoses, 59
osteochondritis dissecans *see*
osteochondrosis
osteochondrodysplasia
radius/ulna, 62
of the Scottish Fold cat, 45, 66
tibia, 77
osteochondrofibrosis, heterotopic,
333
osteochondroma, 46, 333
altered shape of bone, 15
bony masses, 19–20, *20*, 29
calvarium thickening, 90
cranial radiopacity variations, 89
metaphyses, 31
osteolytic lesions, 25
physeal masses, 31
proliferative joint disease, 45
ribs, 221
sacroiliac joints, 67
spinal, 120
spinal cord compression, 136
synovial *see* synovial
osteochondroma
tracheal, 151
vertebral opacity changes,
125, 126
osteochondrosarcoma, 89
osteochondrosis, 42, 45
elbow, 57, *57*
epiphyseal, 29
hip, 70
joint effusion/soft tissue swelling,
41
lumbosacral, 136
mineralization in or near
joints, 47
sacral, 119, 122, *122*, 128
shoulder, 53, *53*
stifle, 72, *72*
tarsus, 79–80
tibiotarsal joint, 77–8, *78*
osteoclastoma
epiphyseal, 29
osteolytic lesions, 24
radius/ulna, 63
osteodystrophia fibrosa, 91, *91*
osteodystrophy of the Scottish Fold
cat, 63, 78
osteogenesis, patterns of, 6–7

osteogenesis imperfecta
  altered shape of bone, 15
  osteopenia, 22
  vertebral opacity changes, 124
osteoid matrix, 1
osteoid osteoma, 18
osteolysis *see* bone loss (osteolysis)
osteolytic (erosive) joint disease,
    42–4, 45
osteolytic lesions, 21, 22–4
  expansile, 24–5, 25
  mandibular, 93
  maxilla/premaxilla, 92
  thinning of cortices, 33
osteolytic-osteogenic lesions, 25–8
osteoma
  bony masses, 20
  cranial radiopacity variations, 88–9
  frontal sinuses, 100
  proliferative joint disease, 44
  pulmonary, 162, 170
  ribs, 221
osteomalacia, 21
  definition of, 3
  juvenile *see* rickets
osteomyelitis
  altered shape of bone, 14
  cranial radiopacity variations, 89
  delayed healing, 13
  differentiating from malignant
      bone neoplasia, 28
  frontal bone variation, 101
  frontal sinuses, 100
  haematogenous, 28, 29
  increased bone radiopacity, 16
  increased radiopacity, 28
  mandible, 92
  maxilla/premaxilla, 90
  metaphyseal, 24
  mixed osteolytic-osteogenic
      lesions, 26–8, 27
  mixed radiopacity, 29
  osteolytic lesions, 24
  ribs, 221
  sclerotic areas in diaphyses, 34
  sternum, 221
  thickening of cortices, 33
  vertebral opacity changes, 125, 126
osteopathy
  craniomandibular
      see craniomandibular
      osteopathy
  hypertrophic *see* hypertrophic
      (pulmonary) osteopathy
      (HPO)
  idiopathic multifocal, 24, 119
  metaphyseal *see* metaphyseal
      osteopathy
osteopenia, 6, 21–2, 43

altered shape of bone, 15
artefactual, 21
coarse trabecular pattern, 22
definition of, 3
diffuse, 21, 29
disuse, 29
focal, 21
reduced radiopacity, 29
thinning of cortices, 33
osteopetrosis
  coarse trabecular pattern, 22
  increased radiopacity, 17–18, 28
  sclerotic areas in diaphyses, 34
  thickening of cortices, 33
  vertebral opacity changes, 124
osteoporosis, 21
  definition of, 3
  vertebral opacity changes, 124
osteosarcoma
  bony masses, 20
  cranial radiopacity variations, 89
  extraskeletal, 333
  femur, 71
  frontal sinuses, 100
  humerus, 55
  intrathoracic mineralized opacities,
      171
  juxtacortical, 20
  maxilla/premaxilla, 91
  metastases, 170
  mineralization in or near joints,
      47
  oesophageal, 218
  osteogenic, 126
  osteolytic lesions, 23, 23
  parosteal *see* parosteal
      osteosarcoma
  radius/ulna, 62
  ribs, 220
  single radiopaque lung lobe, 159
  spinal, 120
  spinal cord compression, 136
  sternum, 222
  tracheal, 151
  vertebral opacity changes, 125
osteosclerosis
  definition of, 4
  increased bone radiopacity, 18
osteosclerosis fragilis
      see osteopetrosis
otitis externa, 96
otitis media, 96, 96
otolithiasis, 96
ovaries, 319–20
  abnormalities on ultrasonography,
      320
  enlargement, 320
  masses, 259
  mineralization on radiographs, 261

normal ultrasonographic
    appearance, 320
ultrasonographic examination, 320

P

pachymeningitis, 126, 128–9, 140
palatine mass, 103
pancreas, 252–3
  masses, 257
  mineralization on radiographs, 261
  normal ultrasonographic
      appearance, 252–3
  radiology, 252
  ultrasonographic abnormalities,
      253
  ultrasonographic technique, 252
pancreatitis, 234, 252, 252, 253
panosteitis
  coarse trabecular pattern, 22
  femur, 71
  humerus, 55
  increased radiopacity, 16, 16–17, 28
  osteopenia, 22
  periosteal reactions, 18
  radius/ulna, 62
  sclerotic areas in diaphyses, 33, 34
  tibia, 77
papilloma
  renal, 303
  salivary gland, 109
Paragonimus kellicotti, 158, 163
  geographic distribution, **350**
  pulmonary hyperlucency, 169–70
paraprostatic cysts, 235, 289, 324, 324,
    325, 325
paraquat poisoning, 168
parathyroid gland
  ectopic tumour, 210
  ultrasonography, 110
paravertebral soft tissues
  lesions, 130
  ultrasonography, 130–1
paronychia, 66
parosteal osteosarcoma, 20, 44, 71,
    73–4, 74
Pasteurella multocida, 128
Pasteurella tularensis, **349**
patella, 72, 72–3
  aplasia, 72
  fractures, 74
patella alta, 72
patella baja, 72
patella cubiti, 58–9
patellar ligament rupture, 76
patent ductus arteriosus, 167, 181,
    182, 182, 185, 194
pectus carinatum, 221

pectus excavatum, 221, *221*
pelvic canal deformity, 289
pelvis, *67*, 67–8
PennHIP scheme, 69
pentalogy of Fallot, 186
periarticular fibrosis, 42
pericardial disease, 179–80, 181, *181*
pericardial effusion, 179, 180, *180*, 181, *181*, 240
pericarditis, constrictive, 178
perineal hernia, 289
periodontal disease, 91, 92, 93, 102
periosteal proliferative polyarthritis, 45, 46
periosteal reactions, *6*, 6–7, 18–19, 33
periosteum, 2
peripheral nerve sheath tumours, 138
peripheral nerve ultrasonography, 337
perirenal fluid, 299
peritoneal cavity, 233–6
  decreased radiopacity, 235
  increased radiopacity, 233–5
  mineralization on radiographs, 261
  ultrasonography, 235–6
peritoneal effusion, 232, 234
peritoneal fluid, 235–6
peritoneography, 244
peritonitis, 234
  bile, 234
  focal, 252
  sclerosing encapsulating, 279
perocormus, 119
peromelia, 52
perosomus elumbis, 116
persistent hyaloid artery, 108
persistent hyperplastic primary vitreous, 108
persistent right aortic arch, 149, 150, 184, 216
Perthes disease *see* Legg-Calvé-Perthes disease
pes varus, 77
phaeochromocytoma, 237
  adrenal glands, 254
  spinal cord compression, 136
phalanges, 65–7
pharynx, *103*, 103–5
  breed and conformational variations, 87, *87*
  perforation, 105
phocomelia, 52
phthisis bulbi, 107
physeal dysplasia
  hip, 70
  osteolytic lesions, 24
physeal line
  loss, 30
  widening, 30–1

physeal scar, 16
physis, 2
  lesions affecting, 30–1
  masses arising at, 31
  vertebral, 116
physitis, vertebral, 125
physometra, 321
plasma cell myeloma *see* multiple myeloma
plasmacytoma
  extramedullary, 151
  osteolytic lesions, 23
pleural cavity, 199–206
  anatomy and radiography, 199–200, *200*
  increased radiolucency, 200–2
  increased radiopacity, 202–4
  nodules and masses, 204
  pleural thickening, 205–6
  trauma, 225
  ultrasonography of lesions, 205
pleural effusion, *202*, 202–3, 205
pleural plaques, calcified, 162, 170
pleural thickening, 147
pleuritis, 206
pneumatocele, 169
pneumatosis coli, 290
pneumobilia, 242
pneumocephalus, 88
pneumocolon, 290
pneumoconiosis, 162, 165
Pneumocystis carinii, **350**
pneumocystogram, 312
pneumocystosis, **350**
pneumogastrography, 272
pneumohaematocele, 169
pneumomediastinum, 105, 152, 168, 208–9
pneumonia
  alveolar lung pattern, 155–6
  aspiration, 155
  bacterial, 162, 201
  haematogenous bacterial, 162
  interstitial lung pattern, 163–4
  lipid/lipoid, 165, 170
  lobar, 159, 160
  mixed lung pattern, 168
  poorly marginated pulmonary opacities, 157
  thromboembolic, 158–9
Pneumonyssus caninum, 98, **350**
Pneumonyssus carinii, 164
pneumopericardium, 180
pneumothorax, *200*, 200–1
  cardiac malposition, 177
  pulmonary hyperlucency, 168, 169
  spontaneous, 201
polioencephalomyelitis, 141

polyarteritis nodosa, 41, 46
polyarthritis, 46
  carpus, 63
  drug-induced, 41, 44, 46
  heritable, 41, 46
  joint effusion/soft tissue swelling, 41
  Mycoplasma, 44, 46
  periosteal proliferative, 45, 46
  tarsus, 78
polycystic kidney disease (PKD), 300, 303, 305
polydactyly, 52, 66
polydontia, 102
polymelia, 52
polymyositis syndrome, 41, 46
polyneuropathy, distal, 140
polypodia, 52
polyps
  bladder, 313, 314, 315, 316
  ear, 96
  gastric, 277, 283
  nasal, 98–9
  nasopharyngeal, 103, *103*
  tracheal, 151
polyradiculoneuritis, 141
popliteal muscle avulsion, 76
popliteal sesamoid, 71
portal hypertension, 247
portal vein
  obstruction, 248
  small, 248
portal venography, 242–3
portocaval shunt, 247
portosystemic shunts, 241, 242–4, *243*, *244*, 299
positive contrast canalography, 95
positive contrast gastrography, 272
positive contrast rhinography, 97
post caval syndrome, 240
pregnancy
  see also Uterus
  abdominal wall shape variations, 232
  normal uterus, 322
  uterine radiopacity, 321
premaxilla, 90–2
prepubic tendon avulsion, 68
pressure atrophy
  osteolytic lesions, 24
  thinning of cortices, 33
primary ciliary dyskinesia, 153, 154
progressive haemorrhagic myelomalacia, 139
progressive retinal atrophy, 108
proliferative joint disease, 20, 44–5
prostate, 322–5
  diffuse parenchymal changes on ultrasonography, 325
  focal parenchymal changes on ultrasonography, 325

location variations, 323
masses, 260
mineralization on radiographs, 261
neoplasia, 319, *319*
normal ultrasonographic
    appearance, 324–5
paraprostatic lesions on
    ultrasonography, 325
radiopacity variations, 324
shape variations, 324
size variations, *323*, 323–4
ultrasonographic examination, 324
prostatitis, 323, 325
pseudocysts, 300, 308
pseudogout, 47
pseudohyperparathyroidism, 21–2
radiopacity of soft tissues, 332
vertebral opacity changes, 124
pseudopolydontia, 102
pseudoulcers, small intestine, 282,
    282, 283
pulmonary alveolar proteinosis, 157,
    159
pulmonary artery
abnormalities, 194
changes in, 186
neoplasia, 186
trunk abnormalities, 186, *186*
pulmonary congestion, 166
pulmonary embolism, 159
pulmonary fibrosis, 165
pulmonary hyperlucency, 168–70, *169*
pulmonary hypoperfusion, 167
pulmonary lymphomatoid
    granulomatosis, 156
pulmonary nodules/masses
multiple, 161–3, *161*
solitary, 160–1, *161*
ultrasonography, 163
pulmonary opacities, poorly
    marginated, *157*, 157–9
pulmonary osteomata, 147–8
pulmonary thromboembolism, 160
alveolar lung pattern, 157
interstitial lung pattern, 165
vascular lung pattern, 166, 167
pulmonic valve
abnormalities, 194
Doppler flow abnormalities, 196,
    196
insufficiency, 185, 193, 194
stenosis, 184–5
pyelogram, 302, *302*
abnormalities of, 304–5
ultrasound-guided antegrade, 303
pyelonephritis, 299, 305
pyloric stenosis, 275, *275*
pylorospasm, 275
pylorus, 268

pyometra, 321, 322, *322*
pyonephrosis, 305
pyopneumothorax, 202
pythiosis (*Pythium insidiosum*), **350**

Q

quadriceps contracture, 76

R

rabbit fever, **349**
rabies vaccine, 141
radiographic faults, 341
radius, 14, 60–3
radius curvus syndrome, 61, *61*
rebound effect, 341, *344*
redundant colon, 288
redundant oesophagus, 216
Reiter's disease, 45
renal agenesis, 299
renal calculi, 305
renal cell carcinoma, 300, 303
renal dysplasia, 31
renal ectopia, 301
renal infarct, 303
renal pelvis distortion, 305, 306
resistive index (*RI*), 90
respiratory tract, lower, 145–71
restrictive cardiomyopathy, 178–9
retinal detachment, 108, *108*
retinal dysplasia, 108
retrobulbar abscess, 109
retrobulbar tissue changes, 108–9
retrograde urethrography, *317*,
    317–18
retrograde (vagino)urethrography,
    308, 317, *317*, 318–19
retroperitoneal disease, 299
retroperitoneal fluid, 131, 238, 308
retroperitoneal space, 236–9
decreased radiopacity, 238
enlargement, *236*, 236–7
increased radiopacity, 237–8
masses, 238, 259
ultrasonography, 238–9
retropharyngeal swelling, 103
rhabdomyosarcoma, 125
myocardial, 187
pericardial effusion, 180
rheumatoid arthritis, 43, *44*, 45
carpus, 63
joint effusion/soft tissue swelling,
    41
mixed osteolytic-proliferative joint
    disease, 45
tarsus, 78

rhinitis, 98, *98*
fungal, 99, *99*
lymphoplasmacytic, 99
viral, 99
rhinitis-bronchitis complex, 154, 168
rhinitis-bronchopneumonia
    syndrome, 98
rhino horn callus, 13, 19
ribs
mineralization on radiographs, 262
tumours, 210, *220*, 220–1
variations in, 220–1
rickets
altered shape of long bones, 14
delayed growth plates closure, 16
dwarfism, 15
metaphyses, 32
osteopenia, 22
radius/ulna, 62
tibia, 77
widening of physeal lines, 31, *31*
Rickettsia rickettsii, **350**
right atrium
abnormalities, 192–3
enlargement, *184*, 184–5
neoplasia, 185
right ventricle
abnormalities, 193–4
double outlet, 186
enlargement, 185–6
hypertrophy, 184–5
ring-down artefacts, 347
Rocky Mountain spotted fever, 46,
    164, **350**
rubber jaw, 91, *91*

S

sacrococcygeal dysgenesis, 119
sacroiliac joints, 67–8
salivary ducts, contrast studies, 109
salivary glands
contrast studies, 109
ultrasonography, 109–10
Salter-Harris classification of
    fractures, 10, *10*, 29
San Joaquin Valley fever, **348**
sarcoma
anaplastic, 303
histiocytic, 23, 125, 156, 157, 161, 162
injection site, 105
nasal, 98
reduced radiopacity, 28
synovial *see* synovial sarcoma
scapula, 52
Schmorl's node, 124–5, 127, 128
schwannoma, 129
scintigraphy, 274–5

scleritis, 107
sclerosing encapsulating peritonitis, 279
sclerosis
    definition of, 4
    mandible, 92, *92*
    maxilla/premaxilla, 90–1
scoliosis, 122
scrotal hernia, 326
selective renal angiography, 303
senility and osteopenia, 22
sensory neuropathy, 140
sentinel loop, 280
septic arthritis, 43, *43*
    decreased joint space width, 42
    epiphyses, 29
    joint effusion/soft tissue swelling, 41
    mixed osteolytic-proliferative joint disease, 45
sequestrum formation, 13, 27, *27*, 28
seroma, 233, 332
sesamoids, 2, 46
    elbow, 56
    metatarsus, *65*, 65–6
shock
    microcardia, 178
    pulmonary hyperlucency, 168
shock lung, 157
short urethra syndrome, 310
shoulder, *53*, 53–5, *54*
sialocele, 105
sialography, 109
sialolithiasis, 106, 109
side lobe artefacts, 347
sinography, 334
sinusitis, 100
sinus tracts, contrast studies, 334
situs inversus, 177
situs solitus, 177
skeletal dysplasia, 3, 46
skeletal system
    radiographic technique for, 1–2
    see also bone(s)
skin folds, 332
skin mineralization on radiographs, 261
skull, 85–111, 87, *87*
slice thickness artefacts, 347
slipped capital femoral epiphysis, 70, *70*
sludge, biliary tract, 247
small airway disease, 153, 168, 201
small intestine, 277–87
    abnormal arrangement on ultrasonography, 286
    contents variations, 280–2, *281*, 285
    contrast studies, 282–4
    displacement, 278

loops
    bunching of, 278–9
    increased width, *279*, 279–80
    number variations, 278
lumen dilation, 285
masses, 258–9
mucosal layer alterations, 287
normal radiographic appearance, 277–8
normal ultrasonographic appearance, 285
obstruction, 279–80
ultrasonographic technique, 285
wall
    diffuse thickening, 287
    focal thickening, 286–7
    lack of visualization, 285
soft tissues, 331–8
    callus, 41
    contrast studies, 334–6
    radiopacity variations, 332–4, *333*
    swelling, 41, *41*
    thickness variations, 331–2
    tumours *see* soft tissue tumours
    ultrasonography, *336*, 336–8, *337*
soft tissue tumours, 43, *43*
    cranial radiopacity variations, 89
    epiphyses, 29
    hindquarter, 120
    joint effusion/soft tissue swelling, 41
    mixed osteolytic-osteogenic lesions, 26, 34
    mixed osteolytic-proliferative joint disease, 45
    osteolytic areas in diaphyses, 34
    vertebral opacity changes, 125
    see also specific tumours
Spalding's sign, 322
spina bifida, 119, 139, 140
spina bifida cystica, 119
spina bifida manifesta, 119, 289
spina bifida occulta, 119
spinal arachnoid pseudocyst
    see arachnoid pseudocyst, spinal
spinal cord
    compression
        extradural, *134*, 134–7, *136*
        intradural-extramedullary, *137*, 137–8
    enlargement, 138–9, *139*
    neurological deficits, 140–1
spinal dysraphism, 122
spinal infarct, 140
spinal muscular atrophy, 140
spinal nerve tumour, 136
spinal stenosis, 118–19
spine
    conditions affecting, 115–41

radiographic technique, 115–16
spinous processes, fused dorsal, 119
spirocercosis (*Spirocerca lupi*), 120, 218, *218*, **351**
spleen, 248–52
    absence of the splenic shadow, 248
    accessory, 250
    location variations, 248–9
    masses, 257–8, *258*
    mineralization on radiographs, 261
    normal ultrasonographic appearance, 250
    radiopacity variations, 250
    size and shape variations, 249–50
    target lesions, 251
    torsion, 251
    ultrasonographic abnormalities, 250–2
    ultrasonographic technique, 250
splenoportography, 244
spondylarthrosis, 129–30
spondylitis, *120*, 120–1, 222
    paravertebral soft tissues, 130
    vertebral opacity changes, 125, 126
spondylosis, 140
    ageing, 147
    intervertebral disc space abnormalities, 127
    paravertebral soft tissues, 130
    vertebral opacity changes, 125
spondylosis deformans, *119*, 119–20
sporotrichosis (*Sporothrix schenckii*), **351**
    geographic distribution, **351**
    poorly marginated pulmonary opacities, 158
squamous cell carcinoma
    of nail bed, 66
    oesophageal, 218
    poorly marginated pulmonary opacities, 157
    premaxilla, 91, *91*
    pulmonary, 161
squamous prostatic metaplasia, 323, 324, 325
Staphylococcus aureus, 128
Staphylococcus intermedius, 128
steatitis, 180, 234
sternum
    tumour, 210
    variations in, *221*, 221–2
stiff Beagle disease, 41, 46
stifle, 71–6, *72*
stippled epiphyses, 46
stomach, 268–77
    abnormal gastric mucosal pattern, 274
    contents variations, *270*, 270–1, 276–7
    contrast studies, 272–4

dilation, 269–70, *270*
displacement, 269
gastric emptying time variations, 274–5
gastric luminal filling defects, 273–4
gastric wall
    diffuse thickening of, 277
    focal thickening of, 277
    lack of visualization of, 277
    variations, *271*, 271–2
gastrogram technical errors, 273
masses, 257
normal radiographic appearance, *268*, 268–9
normal ultrasonographic appearance, 276
polyps, 277, 283
size variations, 269–70, *270*
ultrasonographic technique, 275–6
Streptococcus spp. 128
subchondral bone, 2, 16
subchondral cysts, 44
sublumbar mass, 260, *260*
subretinal haemorrhage, 107, 108
superficial digital flexor tendon luxation, 79
supratrochlear foramen, absence of, 56
synchysis scintillans, 107
syndactyly, 52, 66
syndesmitis ossificans, 120
synostosis, radioulnar, 62
synovial cysts, 41
synovial osteochondroma, 20, 29, 45, 47, *47*, 76
synovial sarcoma, 23, 43, 59
    osteolytic lesions, 23
    stifle, 73
syringohydromyelia, 88, 122, 139, 140, 141
systemic lupus erythematosus, 45
    joint effusion/soft tissue swelling, 41
    proliferative joint disease, 45

T

tarsus, 77–80
teeth, *101*, 101–3
telangiectasia, 251, 261, 301
temporomandibular joint, 93–4, *94*, *94*
tendinopathy, calcifying
    see calcifying tendinopathy
tendon avulsions, stifle, *75*, 75–6, *76*
tendons, ultrasonography of, 337, *337*
tenosynovitis
    abductor pollicis longus, 65
    bicipital, 55

tentorium osseum, 87, *87*
teratoma, 320
testes, 325–6
    retained, 259, 260, 261
    torsion, 326
tetralogy of Fallot, 168, 185, 186, 194
thoracic wall, 219–224
    diaphragm variations, 222–3, *223*
    rib variations, *220*, 220–1
    soft tissue variations, 219–20
    sternum variations, *221*, 221–2
    ultrasonography, 222
    ultrasonography of the diaphragm, 224
    vertebral variations, 222
thorax
    border effacement in, 148, *148*
    positioning, 145–6, **147**
    radiographic technique, 145–6
    radiological changes associated with ageing, 147–8
    trauma, 225–6
    ultrasonographic technique, 146–7
    wall *see* thoracic wall
thrombocytopaenia, 136, 139
thrombus
    left atrial, 190
    pericardial effusion, 181
    right atrial, 193
thymic tumours, 171
thymoma, 210
thyroid gland
    ectopic tumour, 210
    ultrasonography, 110
tibia, 77
tibial compression radiography, 74
tibial plateau angle (TPA), 74–5, *75*
tibial tuberosity avulsion, 74, *74*
toxaemia, 180
toxoplasmosis (*Toxoplasma gondii*), 108
    geographic distribution, **351**
    increased bronchial wall visibility, 153
    interstitial lung pattern, 164
    nodular lung pattern, 162
    poorly marginated pulmonary opacities, 158
trachea, 148–52
    diameter variations, *150*, 150–1
    displacement, 148–50, *149*
    lumen opacification, 151
    perforation, 105, 201, 208
    polyps, 151
    ultrasonography, 152
tracheal collapse syndrome, *150*, 150–1
tracheal ring calcification, 147, 170
tracheal stripe sign, 151–2

tracheal wall visibility variations, 151–2
tracheobronchial lymphadenopathy, 149
traction band, 108
transitional cell carcinoma, 300, 303
    bladder, 316
    renal, 308
transitional vertebrae, 117, *117*, 140
transrectal ultrasound, 292
trauma
    alveolar lung pattern, 156
    bony masses, 19
    cranial cavity shape variations, 88
    cranial radiopacity variations, 88
    frontal sinuses, 100
    joint effusion/soft tissue swelling, 41
    mixed osteolytic-osteogenic lesions, 28, 34
    nasal cavity variations, 97
    osteolytic lesions, 24
    pericardial effusion, 180
    periosteal reactions, 18
    spinal, 123
    spinal cord compression, 136
    temporomandibular joint, 94
    thoracic, 225–6
    tooth, 103
Triadan system, 101
tricuspid valve
    abnormalities, 193
    Doppler flow abnormalities, 195–6
    insufficiency, 184, 185, 194
trilogy of Fallot, 186
tuberculosis, 46
    alveolar lung pattern, 156
    interstitial lung pattern, 164
    intrathoracic mineralized opacities, 170, 171
    lymphadenopathy, 212
    mixed osteolytic-osteogenic lesions, 28
    mixed osteolytic-proliferative joint disease, 45
    osteolytic joint disease, 44
    pericardial effusion, 180
    periosteal reactions, 18
    poorly marginated pulmonary opacities, 158
tularaemia, **349**
tumours *see* neoplasia; *specific tumours*
tympanic bulla, *96*, 96–7
typhlitis, 289

U

Überschwinger artefact, 341, *344*
ulceration, gastric, 274, *274*, 277

ulcerative gastritis, 274
ulna, 60–3
ultrasonography
    acoustic enhancement, 344, *346*
    acoustic shadowing, 343–4, *346*
    artefacts, 343–7
    comet tail and ring-down artefacts,
        347
    edge shadowing, 346, *347*
    mirror image artefacts, 347, *347*
    poor transducer contact, 343
    reverberation artefacts, 346–7
    side lobe artefacts, 347
    slice thickness artefacts, 347
    terminology, 341
ultrasound-guided antegrade
        pyelography, 303, 308
umbilical hernia, 232
ununited anconeal process, 57, *57*
ununited medial epicondyle, 57–8
urachus, persistent, 311
uraemia
    intrathoracic mineralized opacities,
        170
    pericardial effusion, 180
ureterocele, 309, 315
ureters, 308–10
    calculi, 237
    contrast studies, 302
    dilated, 309, 310
    ectopic, 305, *308*, 309
    mineralization on radiographs, 261
    normal, *308*, 309
    reflux of contrast media up, 313
    traumatic rupture, 308–9
urethra, 317–19
    calculi, 318
    contrast studies, 317–19
    displacement, 318
    mineralization on radiographs, 261
    stricture, 318
    ultrasonography, 319
urethritis, 261, 318
urethrography, retrograde, 308, *317*,
        317–19
urinary bladder *see* bladder, urinary
urinary outflow obstruction, 311

urinary retention, 311
urinary tract, 298–319
urine, retroperitoneal, 237
urinoma, 237, 308
uroabdomen, 234
urogenital tract, 297–326
uterine distension, 232
uterus, 320–2
    content variation on
        ultrasonography, 322, *322*
    dystocia and fetal death, 321–2
    enlargement, 320–1, *321*
    masses, 259–60
    mineralization on radiographs,
        261
    normal ultrasonographic
        appearance, 322
    radiopacity variations, 321
    torsion, 321
    ultrasonographic examination, 322
    wall thickening on
        ultrasonography, 322
uveitis, 108

V

vacuum phenomenon, 41
vagina, 317–19
    contrast studies, 317–19
    enlargement, 319
    ultrasonography, 319
vaginourethrography, retrograde,
        308, 317, *317*, 318–19
valgus, 52
valvular dysplasia, 178, 179
varus, 52
vascular lung pattern, 165–7, *166*
vascular malformations, 332
vascular ring anomaly, 216, *217*
veins larger than arteries, 166
venography, 335–6
ventricular septal defects, 167, 181,
        183, 185, 193, 194
ventriculomegaly, 88
vertebrae
    alignment variations, 122–4

number variations, 116
opacity changes, 124–6
size and shape variations, *117–20*,
        117–22, *122–3*
variations in thoracic, 222
vertebral canal changes, 122
vertebral endplate
    irregularities, 127–8
    sclerosis, 126
vertebral heart size measurement,
        176, *176*
vertebral physes, 116
villonodular synovitis, 43
    joint effusion/soft tissue swelling,
        41
    mixed osteolytic-proliferative joint
        disease, 45
VITAMIN D mnemonic, 7
vitamin D toxicosis, 332
vitreal syneresis, 107
vitreous detachment, 108
vitreous floaters, 107
vitreous membranes, 108
voiding urethrography, 318
volvulus
    gastric, 269, *270*
    large intestine, 289
von Willebrand disease
    alveolar lung pattern, 156
    interstitial lung pattern, 164
    spinal cord compression, 137
von Willebrand heterotopic
        osteochondrofibrosis, 47,
        68, 71

W

wobbler syndrome *see* cervical
        spondylopathy (wobbler
        syndrome)
worms, 283

Z

zygomatic sialadenitis, 108

Printed and bound by CPI Group (UK) Ltd, Croydon, CR0 4YY

08/06/2025

01896874-0008